Ischemic Heart Disease

Erling Falk
Department of Cardiology
Aarhus University Hospital (Skejby)
Aarhus, Denmark

Prediman K. Shah
Division of Cardiology
Cedars-Sinai Medical Center
Los Angeles, USA

Pim J. de Feyter
Erasmus Medical Center, Thoraxcenter
Rotterdam, The Netherlands

MANSON
PUBLISHING

ISBN-10 1–84076–052–4
ISBN-13 978-1-84076-052-1

A CIP catalogue record for this book is available from the British Library.

For full details of all Manson Publishing Ltd titles please write to:
Manson Publishing Ltd
73 Corringham Road
London NW11 7DL, UK

Tel: +44 (0)20 8905 5150
Fax: +44 (0)20 8201 9233

Email: manson@mansonpublishing.com
Website: www.mansonpublishing.com

Commissioning editor: Jill Northcott
Project manager: Paul Bennett
Text editor: Ruth C Maxwell
Layout: Initial Typesetting Services
Color reproduction: Tenon & Polert Colour Scanning Ltd, Hong Kong
Printed by: Grafos SA, Barcelona, Spain

Contents

Contributors

Ulrik Abildgaard
Department of Cardiology
Copenhagen University Hospital
(Gentofte), Denmark

Farqad Alamgir
Department of Cardiology
Castle Hill Hospital
Kingston-upon-Hull, UK

Jan Aldershvile (deceased)
Department of Medicine
Division of Cardiology
Rigshospitalet
University of Copenhagan
DK-2100 Copenhagen, Denmark

Joseph S. Alpert
Department of Medicine
University of Arizona Health Sciences Center
Tucson, Arizona, USA

Henning Rud Andersen
Department of Cardiology
Aarhus University Hospital (Skejby)
DK-8200 Aarhus N, Denmark

Joseph Aragon
Department of Cardiology
Cedars-Sinai Medical Center
Los Angeles, USA

Wilbert S. Aronow
Cardiology Clinic
Westchester Medical Center/New York
Medical College
Valhalla, USA

Juan A. Asensio
Department of Surgery
University of Southern California Keck
School of Medicine
LAC+USC Medical Center
Los Angeles, USA

Ulrik Baandrup
Department of Pathology
Aarhus University Hospital (AAKH)
DK-8000 Aarhus C, Denmark

Jeroen J. Bax
Department of Cardiology
Leiden University Medical Center
Leiden, The Netherlands

Søren Boesgaard
Department of Medicine
Division of Cardiology
Rigshospitalet
University of Copenhagen
DK-2100 Copenhagen, Denmark

Hans Erik Bøtker
Department of Cardiology
Aarhus University Hospital (Skejby)
DK-8200 Aarhus N, Denmark

Morten Bottcher
Department of Cardiology
Aarhus University Hospital (Skejby)
DK-8200 Aarhus N, Denmark

Nico Bruining
Erasmus Medical Center
Thoraxcenter and Erasmus University
Rotterdam, The Netherlands

Matthew J. Budoff
Division of Cardiology
Harbor-UCLA Medical Center Research
and Education Institute
Torrance, USA

David S. Celermajer
Department of Cardiology
Royal Prince Alfred Hospital
Sydney, Australia

Kevin S. Channer
Royal Hallamshire Hospital
University of Sheffield
Sheffield,UK

Christian Lindskov Christiansen
Department of Cardiology
Aarhus University Hospital (Skejby)
DK-8200 Aarhus N, Denmark

Andrew Clark
Department of Cardiology
Castle Hill Hospital
Kingston-upon-Hull, UK

John G.F. Cleland
Department of Cardiology
Castle Hill Hospital
Kingston-upon-Hull, UK

Filippo Crea
Institute of Cardiology
Catholic University of the Sacred Heart
Largo Agostino Gemelli
8-00168 Rome, Italy

Pim J. de Feyter
Erasmus Medical Center, Thoraxcenter
3015 GD Rotterdam, The Netherlands

R.J. de Winter
Department of Cardiology
Academic Medical Center
University of Amsterdam
The Netherlands

Dirk J.G.M. Duncker
Laboratory for Experimental Cardiology,
Cardiolog, Thoraxcenter
Cardiovascular Research Institute
COEUR
Erasmus University Medical Center
3000 DR Rotterdam, The Netherlands

Dario Echeverri
Cardiovascular Institute
University of Kentucky
Lexington, Kentucky, USA

Henrik Egeblad
Department of Cardiology
Aarhus University Hospital (Skejby)
8200 Aarhus N, Denmark

Raimund Erbel
Department of Cardiology
University Clinic Essen
D-45122 Essen, Germany

Erling Falk
Department of Cardiology
Aarhus University Hospital (Skejby)
DK-8200 Aarhus N, Denmark

John K. French
Green Lane Hospital
Auckland, New Zealand

William Ganz
Department of Cardiology
Cedars-Sinai Medical Center
Los Angeles, USA

Henry Gewirtz
Department of Medicine (Cardiac Unit)
Massachusetts General Hospital
Boston, USA

Bob Goedhart
Division of Image Processing (LKEB)
Department of Radiology
Leiden University Medical Center
Leiden, The Netherlands

Johan Herlitz
Division of Cardiology
Sahlgrenska University Hospital
SE 413 45 Göteborg, Sweden

Jonathan M. Hill
London Chest Hospital
London, UK

Sjoerd Hofma
Department of Interventional Cardiology
Erasmus Medical Center
3015 GD Rotterdam, The Netherlands

Steen E. Husted
Department of Cardiology and Medicine A
Aarhus University Hospital
DK-8000 Aarhus C, Denmark

Anne Kaltoft
Department of Cardiology
Aarhus University Hospital (Skejby)
DK-8200 Aarhus N, Denmark

Samir R. Kapadia
University of Washington
Seattle, USA

Saibal Kar
Division of Cardiology and Department of
Medicine
Cedars-Sinai Medical Center
Los Angeles, USA

Tamer Karsidag
Division of Trauma and Critical Care/
Department of Surgery
University of Southern California Keck
School of Medicine
LAC+USC Medical Center
Los Angeles, USA

Jens Kastrup
Cardiac Catheterization Laboratory
Heart Centre
Rigshospitalet
DK-2100 Copenhagen, Denmark

Steven Khan
Division of Cardiology
Cedars-Sinai Medical Center and UCLA
School of Medicine
Los Angeles, USA

Michael C. Kim
The Zena and Michael A.Wiener
Cardiovascular Institute
The Mount Sinai School of Medicine
New York, USA

Won Yong Kim
MR-Center and Department of
Cardiology
Aarhus University Hospital (Skejby)
Aarhus, Denmark

Jens H. Knudsen
Department of Cardiology
Copenhagen University Hospital
(Gentofte), Denmark

Gerhard Koning
Division of Image Processing (LKEB)
Department of Radiology
Leiden University Medical Center
Leiden, The Netherlands

R.W. Koster
Department of Cardiology
Academic Medical Center
1105 AZ Amsterdam, The Netherlands

Ingrid Bayer Kristensen
Department of Forensic Medicine
University of Aarhus
DK-8000 Aarhus C, Denmark

Kavita Kumar
Cedars-Sinai Medical Center
Los Angeles, USA

Eric J. Kuncir
Division of Trauma and Critical Care
Instructor, Department of Surgery
University of Southern California Keck
School of Medicine
LAC+USC Medical Center
Los Angeles, USA

Gaetano A. Lanza
Institute of Cardiology
Catholic University of the Sacred Heart
Largo Agostino Gemelli
8-00168 Rome, Italy

Mogens Lytken Larsen
Department of Cardiology
Aarhus University Hospital
DK-8000 Aarhus C, Denmark

Jens Flensted Lassen
Aarhus University Hospital
Aarhus, Denmark

Steve Lee
Department of Cardiology
Cedars-Sinai Medical Center
Los Angeles, USA

Howard Lewin
San Vicente Cardiac Imaging Center
Beverly Hills, USA

Peter Lukac
Arrhythmia Department
Slovak Cardiovascular Institute
SK 833 48 Bratislava, Slovakia

Rajendra Makkar
Department of Cardiology
Cedars-Sinai Medical Center
Los Angeles, USA

Bernhard Meier
Department of Cardiology
Swiss Cardiovascular Center Bern
University Hospital
Bern, Switzerland

Daphne Merkus
Laboratory for Experimental Cardiology,
Cardiolog, Thoraxcenter
Cardiovascular Research Institute
COEUR
Erasmus University Medical Center
3000 DR Rotterdam, The Netherlands

Noel Bairey Merz
Department of Cardiology
Cedars-Sinai Medical Center
Los Angeles, USA

Hans Mickley
Department of Cardiology
Odense University Hospital
5000 Odense C, Denmark

Stefan Möhlenkamp
Department of Cardiology
University Clinic Essen
D-45122 Essen, Germany

Pedro R. Moreno
Cardiovascular Institute
University of Kentucky
Lexington, USA

James E. Muller
Department of Cardiology
Massachusetts General Hospital
Boston, USA

Christian J Mussap
Department of Cardiology
Royal North Shore Hospital
Sydney, Australia

Eike Nagel
Internal Medicine Cardiology
German Heart Institute
Berlin, Germany

Morteza Naghavi
Association for Eradication of Heart
Attack
P.O. Box 20345
Houston, USA

Jens Erik Nielsen-Kudsk
Department of Cardiology
Aarhus University Hospital (Skejby)
DK-8200 Aarhus N, Denmark

Koen Nieman,
Erasmus Medical Center, Thoraxcenter
3015 GD Rotterdam, The Netherlands

Dr Nikolay Nikitin
Department of Cardiology
Castle Hill Hospital
Kingston-upon-Hull, UK

Bjarne Linde Nørgaard
Department of Cardiology
Aarhus University Hospital (Skejby)
DK-8200 Aarhus N, Denmark

William N. O'Connor
Cardiovascular Institute
University of Kentucky
Lexington, USA

Stephanie Ounpuu
Department of Medicine and Population
Health Research Institute
McMaster University, Canada

Sriram Padmanabhan
Department of Cardiology
Cedars-Sinai Medical Center
Los Angeles, USA

Anders Kirstein Pedersen
Department of Cardiology
Aarhus University Hospital (Skejby)
DK-8200 Aarhus N, Denmark

Ira Perry
1109 S. Redondo Boulevard
Los Angeles, USA

C. Thomas Peter
Clinical Electrophysiology
Cedars-Sinai Medical Center
David Geffen School of Medicine at
UCLA, Los Angeles, USA

Patrizio Petrone
Division of Trauma and Critical Care and
Department of Surgery
University of Southern California Keck
School of Medicine
LAC+USC Medical Center
Los Angeles, USA

J.J. Piek
Academic Medical Centre
University of Amsterdam
1100 DD Amsterdam, The Netherlands

Don Poldermans
Department of Cardiology
Erasmus Medical Center, Thoraxcenter
3015 GD Rotterdam, The Netherlands

Matthew J. Price
Cardiac Catheterization Laboratory
Scripps Clinic
La Jolla, California, USA

K-Raman Purushothaman
Cardiovascular Institute
University of Kentucky
Lexington, USA

Jan Ravkilde
Department of Cardiology
Aarhus University Hospital (Skejby)
DK-8200 Aarhus N, Denmark

Johan H.C. Reiber
Division of Image Processing (LKEB)
Department of Radiology
Leiden University Medical Center
Leiden, The Netherlands

Benno J. Rensing
Heart Lung Center Utrecht
St Antonius Hospital
Department of Cardiology
3435 CM Nieuwegein, The Netherlands

Mark J. Sarnak
Division of Nephrology and
Department of Medicine
Tufts New England Medical Center
Boston, USA

Johannes A. Schaar
Erasmus Medical Center, Thoraxcenter
3000 DR Rotterdam, The Netherlands

Arend F.L. Schinkel
Department of Cardiology
Thoraxcenter, Erasmus Medical Center
3015 GD Rotterdam, The Netherlands

Axel Schmermund
Department of Cardiology
University Clinic Essen
D-45122 Essen, Germany

Prediman K. Shah
Division of Cardiology and
Atherosclerosis Research Center,
Cedars Sinai Medical Center,
David Geffen School of Medicine at
UCLA, Los Angeles, California

Samin K. Sharma
The Zena and Michael A.Wiener
Cardiovascular Institute
The Mount Sinai School of Medicine
New York, USA

Erik Sloth
Aarhus University Hospital (Skejby)
Aarhus, Denmark

Allan D. Sniderman
Mike Rossenbloom Laboratory for
Cardiovascular Research
Royal Victoria Hospital
Montreal
Quebec H3A 1A1, Canada

K.E. Sørensen
Department of Cardiology
Aarhus University Hospital (Skejby)
Aarhus, Denmark

Ahmed Tawakol
Department of Medicine
(Cardiac Unit)
Massachusetts General Hospital
Boston, USA

Allen J. Taylor
Cardiology Service
Walter Reed Army Medical Center and
the Cardiovascular Division
Armed Forces Institute of Pathology
Washington, USA

Leif Thuesen
Department of Cardiology
Aarhus University Hospital (Skejby)
DK-8200 Aarhus, Denmark

Kristian Thygesen
Department of Medicine and Cardiology
Aarhus University Hospital
Aarhus, Denmark

Adam D Timmis
London Chest Hospital
London, UK

Geoffrey H. Tofler
Department of Cardiology
Royal North Shore Hospital
Sydney, Australia

Joan C. Tuinenburg
Division of Image Processing (LKEB)
Department of Radiology
Leiden University Medical Center
Leiden, The Netherlands

David Tüller
Department of Cardiology
Swiss Cardiovascular Center Bern
University Hospital
Bern, Switzerland

E.M. Tuzcu
The Cleveland Clinic Foundation
Cleveland, USA

Anne Tybjærg-Hansen
Department of Clinical Biochemistry
Rigshospitalet, Copenhagen
University Hospital
Copenhagen, Denmark

Yasumi Uchida
Jikei University School of Medicine
and Cardiovascular Center
Toho University
Tokyo, Japan

Miguel Valderrábano
Implanted Devices Clinic
UCLA Cardiac Arrhythmia Center
Division of Cardiology
Los Angeles, USA

Robert Jan M. van Geuns
Department of Cardiology and
Department of Radiology
Erasmus Medical Center
Rotterdam, The Netherlands

Renu Virmani
Cardiovascular Division
Armed Forces Institute of Pathology
Washington, USA

Frans C. Visser
Department of Cardiology
VU University Medical Center
1081HV Amsterdam, The Netherlands

M. Voskuil
Academic Medical Centre
University of Amsterdam
1100 DD Amsterdam, The Netherlands

Daniel E. Weiner
Division of Nephrology and
Department of Medicine
Tufts New England Medical Center
Boston, USA

Harvey D. White
Green Lane Hospital
Auckland, New Zealand

Salim Yusuf
Department of Medicine and
Population Health Research Institute
McMaster University, Canada

Birgitte K. Ziegler
Department of Pharmacology
University of Aarhus
DK-8000 Aarhus C, Denmark

Preface

The global burden of ischemic heart disease (IHD) is increasing. IHD is already the leading cause of death worldwide and constitutes, contrary to the general belief, a huge problem not only in the affluent and developed countries but also in many developing countries with enormous and rapidly changing populations. IHD will remain the leading cause of death for years, with cerebrovascular disease ranking second, and is expected to become the leading cause of disability/morbidity worldwide within the next few decades because of an aging population and increasing urbanization, sedentary life style, obesity, and smoking. The purpose of this book is to provide a solid foundation of knowledge to cope with this alarming pandemic of IHD.

The format of this color-illustrated handbook of IHD is unique. More than 100 world authorities from four continents have provided clinically-oriented concise and highly illustrated overviews, covering all aspects of IHD, including pathogenesis, clinical presentation, diagnosis, treatment, and prevention. Special problems are dealt with in separate chapters. The clinical pictures are of high quality, and figures and tables have been redrawn in a consistent style to ensure a comprehensible and useful layout.

High quality illustrations are, of course, especially important in the field of IHD where diagnosis and treatment are based on an accurate understanding and interpretation of a variety of graphic waveforms, images, decision trees, and pathologic specimens. Thus, this color handbook has been designed to provide a brief but comprehensive text highlighted by a detailed visual exposition of all aspects of IHD.

This color handbook is aimed at the practicing clinician and at trainees and students of cardiology and internal medicine, who want a concise, straightforward guide to the recognition and management of IHD. The unique format of the book should make it easy to find and comprehend the information that is useful for everyday patient care. All of us who have been engaged in this exciting project hope that this book will be valued by those who are responsible for the care of patients with IHD.

Erling Falk
Prediman K. Shah
Pim J. de Feyter

Abbreviations

3D 3-dimensional
AII angiotensin II
ABI ankle brachial index
AC alternating current
ACC American College of Cardiology
ACE angiotensin-converting enzyme
acetyl-CoA acetyl coenzyme A
ACS acute coronary syndromes
ADP adenosine diphosphate
AED automatic external defibrillator
AF atrial fibrillation
AHA American Heart Association
ALS advanced life support
AMI acute myocardial infarction
APD action potential duration
apoB apoB100 protein
aPTT activated partial thromboplastin time
ARA aldosterone receptor antagonist
ARB angiotensin receptor blocker
ATP adenosine triphosphate
AV atrioventricular
AVN atrioventricular node
BARI Bypass Angioplasty Revascularization Investigation
BBB bundle branch block
BLS basic life support
BMIPPA betamethyl-iodo-phenylpentadecanoic acid
BNP brain natriuretic peptide
BP blood pressure
CABG coronary artery bypass grafting
CAC coronary artery calcification
CAD coronary artery disease
CAG coronary angiography
CBF coronary blood flow
CCS(C) Canadian Cardiovascular Society (class)
CCU Coronary Care Unit
CETP cholesterol ester transfer protein
CFR coronary flow reserve
CHB complete heart block
CHD coronary heart disease
CHF chronic heart failure/congestive heart failure
CI confidence interval
CK creatine kinase
CKD chronic kidney disease
CKMB creatine kinase MB fraction
CMC cardiomyocyte
CMRI cardiovascular magnetic resonance imaging
CPB cardiopulmonary bypass
CPU Chest Pain Unit
CPR cardiopulmonary resuscitation
CREB cyclic AMP response element-binding protein
CRP C-reactive protein

CT computed tomography
cTn cardiac troponin
CVC central venous catheter
CVD cardiovascular disease
CVP central venous pressure
Cx circumflex artery
DGGE dideoxy gradient gel electrophoresis
dHPLC denaturing high performance liquid chromatography
DNA deoxyribonucleic acid
DS diameter stenosis
DVT deep vein thrombosis
E(max) (maximum)elastance
EBA electron-beam angiography
EB(C)T electron-beam (computed) tomography
ECG electrocardiogram
ECM extracellular matrix
ED Emergency Department
EDHF endothelium-derived hyperpolarizing factor
EDT Emergency Department thoracotomy
EDTA ethylene diamine tetra acetic acid
EECP enhanced external counterpulsation
EF ejection fraction
EMD electromechanical dissociation
EMS Emergency Medical System
EP electrophysiologic
ESC European Society of Cardiology
ET endothelin
FABP fatty acid binding protein
FDA Food and Drug Administration
FDG fluorodeoxyglucose
FGF fibroblast growth factor
FH familial hypercholesterolemia
FLDB familial ligand-defective apolipoprotein B
GCV great cardiac vein
GE gradient echo
GFR glomerular filtration rate
GP glycoprotein
G-CSF granulocyte colony-stimulating factor
HbA1c glycated hemoglobin
HCM hypertrophic cardiomyopathy
HDL (C) high-density lipoprotein (cholesterol)
HLA human leukocyte antigen
HRT hormone replacement therapy
5-HT serotonin
HU Hounsfield units
IABP intra-aortic balloon pump
IAP intra-arterial blood pressure
ICD implantable cardioverter-defibrillator
ICUS intracoronary ultrasound
IFCC International Federation of Clinical Chemistry
IHD ischemic heart disease

INR international normalized ratio
IV intravenous
IVS interventricular septum
IVUS intravascular ultrasound
JAK janus kinase
JL Judkins left (catheter)
JNC 7 Seventh Joint National Committee
JNK (SAPK) cJUN NH2-terminal kinase
LA left atrium
LAD left anterior descending artery
LAFB left anterior fascicular block
LAO left anterior oblique
LAP left atrial pressure
LBBB left bundle branch block
LC1 light chain isotype 1
LCA left coronary artery
LCx left circumflex artery
LD1 lactate dehydrogenase isoenzyme 1
LDL (C) low-density lipoprotein
  (cholesterol)
LDLR low-density lipoprotein receptor
LIMA left internal mammary artery
LMT left main trunk
Lp(a) apolipoprotein (a)
LPFB left posterior fascicular block
LV left ventricle
LVEDP left ventricular end-diastolic pressure
LVFW left ventricular free wall
LVH left ventricular hypertrophy
LVOT left ventricular outflow tract
LVSD left ventricular systolic dysfunction
MACE major adverse cardiac events
MAPK(K) mitogen activated protein kinase (kinase)
m-ASAT mitochondrial aspartate aminotransferase
MCA minimal cost analysis
MCP-1 monocyte chemotactic protein-1
METS metabolic equivalents
MI myocardial infarction
MMP matrix metalloproteinase
MP multi-purpose
MPR multi-planar reconstruction
MRA magnetic resonance angiography
MRCA magnetic resonance coronary angiography
MRI magnetic resonance imaging
mRNA messenger ribonucleic acid
MSCT multi-slice computed tomography
MV mitral valve
MVO_2 myocardial oxygen consumption
NACB National Academy of Clinical Biochemistry
$NADH_2$ nicotinamide adenine dinucleotide
NHANES National Health and Nutrition
  Examination Survey
NKF National Kidney Foundation
NIRS near-infrared spectroscopy
NO nitric oxide
NSTEMI non-ST segment elevation myocardial infarction
OCT optical coherence tomography
OP-CAB off-pump coronary artery bypass
PA pulmonary artery
PAC pulmonary artery catheter
PAI-1 plasminogen activator inhibitor 1
PAOP pulmonary artery occlusion pressure
PAPP-A pregnancy-associated plasma protein A
PCI percutaneous coronary intervention
PCR polymerase chain reaction

PDA posterior descending artery
PE pericardial effusion
PEA pulseless electrical activity
PET positron emission tomography
PICAB percutaneous *in situ* coronary artery bypass
PICVA percutaneous *in situ* coronary venous arterialization
PKC protein kinase C
PLC phospholipase C
PN Purkinje network
PSA pseudoaneurysm
PTCA percutaneous transluminal coronary angioplasty
PVC premature ventricular complex
PVD peripheral vascular disease
QCA quantitative coronary arteriography
QRS-VD QRS vector difference
RA right atrium
RAO right anterior oblique
RBBB right bundle branch block
RBC red blood cell
RCA right coronary artery
RCT randomized controlled trial
REM rapid eye movement
RV right ventricle
RVH right ventricular hypertrophy
RVOT right ventricular outflow tract
SAC stretch activated channel
SAN sinoatrial node
SCD sudden cardiac death
sCD40L soluble CD40 ligand
SCS spinal cord stimulation
SD sudden death
SDF stromal-derived factor
SFR stenotic flow reserve
SMI silent myocardial ischemia
SNR signal-to-noise ratio
SPECT single photon emission computerized tomography
SPIO superparamagnetic iron oxide
SSCP single strand conformation polymorphism
STAT signal transducers and activators of transcription
STEMI ST segment elevation myocardial infarction
ST-VM ST vector magnitude
SVG saphenous vein graft
SvO_2 central venous oxygen saturation
SVR systemic vascular resistance
T3 tri-iodothyronine
T4 thyroxine
TEE transesophageal echocardiography
TENS transcutaneous electrical nerve stimulation
TG triglyceride
TIMI Thrombolysis In Myocardial Infarction (Trial)
TIMP tissue inhibitor of matrix metalloproteinase
TLC therapeutic lifestyle change
tPA recombinant tissue plasminogen activator
TXA_2 thromboxane A_2
UAP unstable angina pectoris
US ultrasound
VCATS volume coronary angiography using
  targeted scans
VEGF vascular endothelial growth factor
VF ventricular fibrillation
VLDL very low-density lipoprotein
VSD ventricular septal defect
VT ventricular tachycardia
WHO World Health Organization

Chapter One

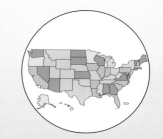

Burden of Ischemic Heart Disease

BURDEN OF ISCHEMIC HEART DISEASE

ERLING FALK, MD, PREDIMAN K. SHAH, MD AND PIM J. DE FEYTER, MD

INTRODUCTION

Ischemic heart disease (IHD) is a condition characterized by inadequate myocardial perfusion caused by reduced blood supply or increased myocardial oxygen demand, or both. Coronary artery disease (CAD), by compromising the blood supply, is by far the most frequent cause of myocardial ischemia, which is why IHD is also called coronary heart disease (CHD). CAD is often present without limiting the flow of blood (subclinical CAD), but when it does, preclinical CAD has usually existed and progressed over decades before CHD/IHD ultimately develops. CAD, CHD, and IHD share a nearly uniform underlying cause, coronary atherosclerosis, with or without superimposed thrombosis.

Cardiovascular disease (CVD), of which IHD and stroke are the two most important components, contributed to nearly one-third of all deaths in 2001 worldwide[1]. Death rates for CVD and the contributions of IHD and stroke differ markedly among populations and nations (1). Regarding IHD, the highest (Russia and other eastern European countries) and lowest (Japan, South Korea, and France) death rates differ by more than 10-fold (1, 2).

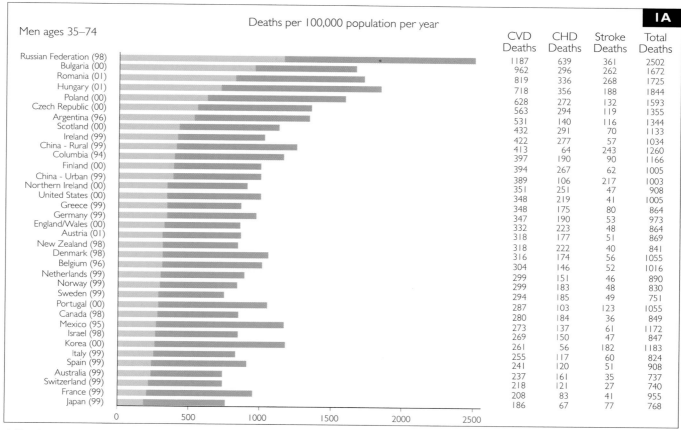

	CVD Deaths	CHD Deaths	Stroke Deaths	Total Deaths
Russian Federation (98)	1187	639	361	2502
Bulgaria (00)	962	296	262	1672
Romania (01)	819	336	268	1725
Hungary (01)	718	356	188	1844
Poland (00)	628	272	132	1593
Czech Republic (00)	563	294	119	1355
Argentina (96)	531	140	116	1344
Scotland (00)	432	291	70	1133
Ireland (99)	422	277	57	1034
China - Rural (99)	413	64	243	1260
Columbia (94)	397	190	90	1166
Finland (00)	394	267	62	1005
China - Urban (99)	389	106	217	1003
Northern Ireland (00)	351	251	47	908
United States (00)	348	219	41	1005
Greece (99)	348	175	80	864
Germany (99)	347	190	53	973
England/Wales (00)	332	223	48	864
Austria (01)	318	177	51	869
New Zealand (98)	318	222	40	841
Denmark (98)	316	174	56	1055
Belgium (96)	304	146	52	1016
Netherlands (99)	299	151	46	890
Norway (99)	299	183	48	830
Sweden (99)	294	185	49	751
Portugal (00)	287	103	123	1055
Canada (98)	280	184	36	849
Mexico (95)	273	137	61	1172
Israel (98)	269	150	47	847
Korea (00)	261	56	182	1183
Italy (99)	255	117	60	824
Spain (99)	241	120	51	908
Australia (99)	237	161	35	737
Switzerland (99)	218	121	27	740
France (99)	208	83	41	955
Japan (99)	186	67	77	768

I Death rates in selected countries, ages 35–74 years (most recent year available). Age-adjusted (European standard population) death rates for cardiovascular disease (CVD), coronary heart disease (CHD), stroke, and total deaths **A**: men; **B**: women.

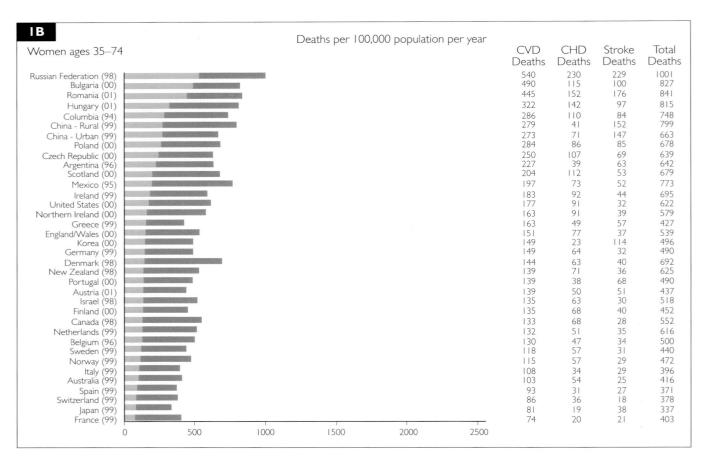

IB	Deaths per 100,000 population per year	CVD Deaths	CHD Deaths	Stroke Deaths	Total Deaths
Women ages 35–74					
Russian Federation (98)		540	230	229	1001
Bulgaria (00)		490	115	100	827
Romania (01)		445	152	176	841
Hungary (01)		322	142	97	815
Columbia (94)		286	110	84	748
China - Rural (99)		279	41	152	799
China - Urban (99)		273	71	147	663
Poland (00)		284	86	85	678
Czech Republic (00)		250	107	69	639
Argentina (96)		227	39	63	642
Scotland (00)		204	112	53	679
Mexico (95)		197	73	52	773
Ireland (99)		183	92	44	695
United States (00)		177	91	32	622
Northern Ireland (00)		163	91	39	579
Greece (99)		163	49	57	427
England/Wales (00)		151	77	37	539
Korea (00)		149	23	114	496
Germany (99)		149	64	32	490
Denmark (98)		144	63	40	692
New Zealand (98)		139	71	36	625
Portugal (00)		139	38	68	490
Austria (01)		139	50	51	437
Israel (98)		135	63	30	518
Finland (00)		135	68	40	452
Canada (98)		133	68	28	552
Netherlands (99)		132	51	35	616
Belgium (96)		130	47	34	500
Sweden (99)		118	57	31	440
Norway (99)		115	57	29	472
Italy (99)		108	34	29	396
Australia (99)		103	54	25	416
Spain (99)		93	31	27	371
Switzerland (99)		86	36	18	378
Japan (99)		81	19	38	337
France (99)		74	20	21	403

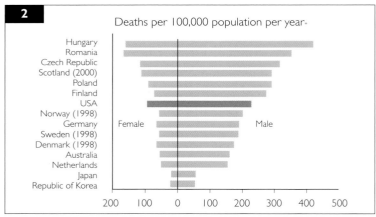

2 Death rates for coronary heart disease, ages 35–74 years, 1999. Age-adjusted (European standard population) death rates for CHD in 15 industrialized countries, CHD-prone ages (35–74 years), year 1999 unless otherwise noted in parentheses.
(Source: Chart 3-31 at: http://www.nhlbi.nih.gov/resources/docs/02_chtbk.pdf)

ISCHEMIC HEART DISEASE IN DEVELOPED COUNTRIES

In the USA, IHD caused more than 1 of every 5 deaths in 2001, totalling 502,189 deaths of which 50.6% involved males[2]. The overall IHD death rate was 177.8 per 100,000 population but, as shown in **3**, death rates by state varied markedly. The five highest-ranking states were New York, Oklahoma, Tennessee, West Virginia, and Mississippi. The five lowest-ranking were Utah, Hawaii, Minnesota, Puerto Rico, and Alaska[3].

The average age of a person having a first heart attack is 65.8 years for men and 70.4 years for women. The incidence of total IHD in women lags behind men by 10 years and by as much as 20 years for more serious events such as myocardial infarction (MI) and sudden death[2]. Because the risk of IHD increases markedly with aging and life expectancy for women is greater than for men, almost as many women ultimately die of IHD as do men (248,184 versus 254,005 in 2001)[2]. IHD is the leading cause of

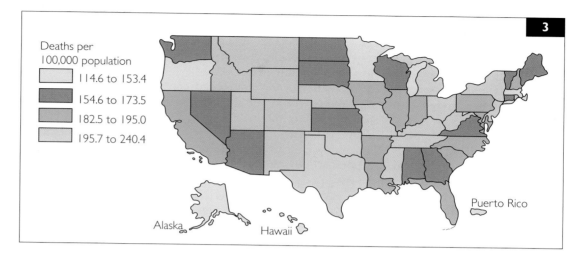

3 Death rates for coronary heart disease in the USA, 2000. Age-adjusted (USA standard population 2000) death rates for CHD by state in the United States. In 2001, the overall CHD death rate was 177.8 per 100,000 population/year[3].

Deaths per 100,000 population
- 114.6 to 153.4
- 154.6 to 173.5
- 182.5 to 195.0
- 195.7 to 240.4

Alaska
Hawaii
Puerto Rico

premature, permanent disability in the USA labor force, accounting for 19% of disability allowances by the Social Security Administration[2].

Regarding race and ethnicity, there are much greater differences in the distribution of risk factor levels within a specific race and ethnic group than between USA populations[4]. There are also very large differences in levels of risk factors for IHD between specific ethnic migrant populations such as black people in Africa versus those in the USA, or Japanese people in Japan versus those in Hawaii and California. Differences in distribution of risk factors and IHD between racial and ethnic groups are a function of the frequency of specific genotypes and interaction with environmental factors. Several of the most important differences between racial groups are higher blood pressure, lower triglycerides and higher high-density lipoprotein cholesterol among black people, higher prevalence of diabetes and insulin resistance among Mexican Americans and American Indians, and higher triglyceride levels among the Japanese. Many of the reported ethnic differences in risk factors and IHD in USA populations are primarily a function of differences in education, socioeconomic variations, and utilization of preventive and clinical treatments[4].

In Europe, IHD alone is the most common cause of death, accounting for nearly 2 million deaths each year[1]. More than 1 in 5 deaths of women (22%) and men (21%) are from IHD[1]. Death rates vary tremendously with alarmingly high values in many eastern European countries and Scotland and low values in France, Portugal, Italy, and Spain (**1**, **2**). IHD death rates in the Russian Federation are among the highest in the world and are even higher than those of Finland and the USA at their peak in the late 1960s.

The IHD death rates of other developed countries, including Japan, Australia, and New Zealand, are also shown in **1** and **2**. In all countries, age-adjusted IHD death rate is lower in women than in men.

ISCHEMIC HEART DISEASE IN DEVELOPING COUNTRIES

Death rates for total CVD are high in China (many strokes) but those for IHD are relatively low (**1**) as in most low- and middle-income developing countries. Among MONICA Project populations, the coronary event rate (per 100,000) in men was lowest in China (Beijing, 81) and highest in Finland (North Karelia, 835)[5]. For women, the event rates were also the lowest in China (Beijing, 35), and Spain (Catalonia, 35), whereas they were the highest in the United Kingdom (Glasgow, Scotland, 265).

TRENDS OVER TIME

Since the 1960s, the age-adjusted death rate for IHD has declined by 50% in the USA, followed by a similar decline in many other developed countries. From the mid 1980s to mid 1990s, the WHO MONICA Project monitored IHD events (nonfatal MI and coronary death) and classic IHD risk factors among men and women aged 35–64 years in 37 populations from 21 countries[6]. The MONICA Project was designed to answer the key question: are reported declines in IHD mortality genuine, and if they are, how much is attributable to improved survival (reflecting better acute management and secondary prevention) rather than to declining coronary event rates (reflecting mainly primary prevention)? Overall, the MONICA data showed that, in populations with declining IHD death rates, about two-thirds of the decline was attributable to a decrease in incidence rates and one-third to declining case fatality. In populations with increasing IHD death rates, these were attributed to a combination of increases in incidence and case fatality. The change in case fatality appears to be closely related to the changes in intensity in acute coronary care, the populations with the fastest change in treatment intensity having the fastest decline in case fatality. In most of eastern Europe, acute coronary care improved little during the MONICA monitoring period and case fatality remained high. High case fatality explains why IHD death rates are high in eastern European countries, despite incidence rates not being exceedingly high.

CAUSE-OF-DEATH STATISTICS

Coding rules and practices are not universal, limiting the usefulness of cause-of-death statistics[7]. Comparisons of mortality data among countries are affected by differences in diagnostic practices and physician training, interpretation of internationally recommended rules for coding a cause of death, availability of diagnostic aids, and the use of autopsies. The Global Burden of Disease Study highlighted that the official coding of death certificates is notoriously variable for CVD[8]. For example, deaths from heart failure, ventricular arrhythmias, general atherosclerosis, and ill-defined descriptions and complications of heart disease of likely ischemic origin are not always coded as deaths caused by IHD. The IHD death rates before and after correction of miscoding, shown in **4**, indicate that Japan and France rank low. However, the differences between these and highest rank nations with good vital registration are probably not as great as indicated by the officially certified cause of death. After correction for this undercoding of IHD, the death rate for IHD in Japan increased by a factor of 2.8 and also increased in southern Europe, mitigating the so-called French paradox (**4**).

GLOBAL BURDEN OF ISCHEMIC HEART DISEASE

IHD is the leading cause of death worldwide and constitutes, contrary to the general belief, a huge problem not only in the affluent and developed countries but also in many developing countries because of their enormous and rapidly changing populations[9]. For example, more than one-third of the world's population live in China (1.3 billion) and India (1 billion), and their total numbers of deaths from IHD are already disturbingly high despite relatively low, but increasing, IHD death rates.

The Global Burden of Disease Study revealed that IHD will remain the leading cause of death for the next several decades, with cerebrovascular disease ranking second, and it will also be the leading cause of disability/morbidity worldwide in the year 2020 (*Table 1*)[9]. The main reasons for this grim outlook are the increasing longevity of the world's population, declining mortality from malnutrition and infection in childhood and infancy, urbanization leading to physical inactivity, obesity and metabolic syndromes, and increasing use of tobacco worldwide [9,10]. Tobacco-attributable mortality is projected to increase from 3.0 million deaths in 1990 to 8.4 million deaths in 2020[9]. The largest increases in this alarming epidemic of tobacco-related mortality will be in India, China, and other Asian countries.

Table 1 Most important causes of death worldwide

Disorder	Ranking 1990	2020	Change in ranking
Within top 15			
Ischemic heart disease	1	1	0
Cerebrovascular disease	2	2	0
Lower respiratory infections	3	4	↓1
Diarrhoeal diseases	4	11	↓7
Perinatal disorders	5	16	↓11
Chronic obstructive pulmonary disease	6	3	↑3
Tuberculosis	7	7	0
Measles	8	27	↓19
Road-traffic accidents	9	6	↑3
Trachea, bronchus, and lung cancers	10	5	↑5
Malaria	11	29	↓18
Self-inflicted injuries	12	10	↑2
Cirrhosis of the liver	13	12	↑1
Stomach cancer	14	8	↑6
Diabetes mellitus	15	19	↓4
Outside top 15			
Violence	16	14	↑2
War injuries	20	15	↑5
Liver cancer	21	13	↑8
HIV	30	9	↑21

A RACE AGAINST TIME

The last decade of the twentieth century greatly enhanced our awareness of the hitherto unrecognized global dimensions of the CVD epidemic[9]. Of the 50 million deaths a year worldwide, 40 million occur in developing countries and a substantial proportion of these deaths are already due to CVD. Hypertension and stroke play a major role in addition to IHD. The report 'A race against time: The challenge of cardiovascular disease in developing economies' was released April 2004[11]. It documented that the global CVD epidemic in the near future will kill or disable an extraordinarily high number of working age people, predominantly affecting developing countries. In China, for example, it is projected that by 2030 over one-half of all CVD deaths will be among those in the prime working ages of 35–64 years. The low-income (about 2.5 billion people in 61 countries) and middle-income (about 2.7 billion people in 65 countries) countries currently contribute about 80% of global CVD-related deaths and 87% of CVD-related disabilities, and the escalating CVD epidemic in many of these countries poses a serious threat to their development[11]. Projections suggest that for IHD, an important subset of CVD, the mortality for all developing countries between 1990 and 2020 will increase by 120% for women and 137% for men[11]. Never before in the course of the cardiovascular epidemic have so many people been at risk of premature death (5), but also never before has such a vast body of knowledge been available which empowers societies to reduce that risk. Despite these sobering statistics, it is heartening that the majority of CVD, including IHD, is preventable.

4 Undercoding of deaths caused by ischemic heart disease. Age-standardized death rates by country for IHD before and after adjustment for miscoding, men and women aged >30 years, about 1990[8].

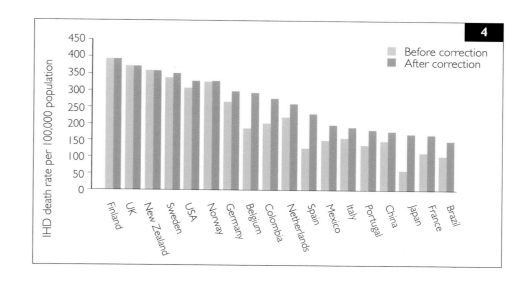

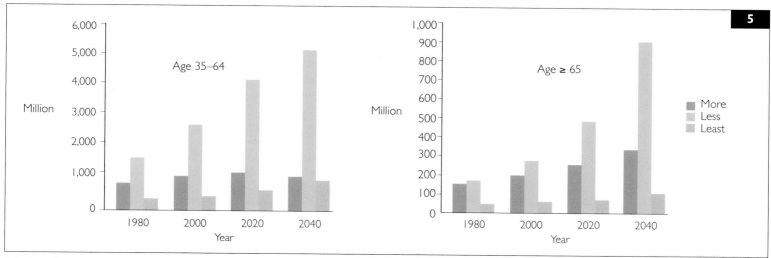

5 Projected increases in world population. Projected increase in the population aged 35–64 years (left), the peak productive years, and >65 years (right) from 1980 to 2040 in more-, less-, and least-developed countries[11].

Chapter Two

Anatomy of the Heart

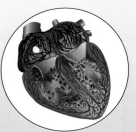

CORONARY ARTERIES

SAIBAL KAR, MD

INTRODUCTION
The heart, like all other tissues of the body, requires oxygen-rich blood to maintain its function. The oxygenated blood is supplied to the heart by two arteries, namely the left and right coronary arteries. These two vessels, which are the first branches of the aorta, encircle or 'coronate' the heart and through their branches supply blood to the myocardium (6–9)[1,2].

LEFT CORONARY ARTERY
The left coronary artery (LCA) arises from the left sinus of Valsalva of the ascending aorta (6–8). The left main coronary artery passes behind the pulmonary trunk and then divides into two major branches, the left anterior descending (LAD) and left circumflex (LCx) arteries. The LAD travels along the anterior interventricular groove towards the apex of the heart and, in most cases, courses

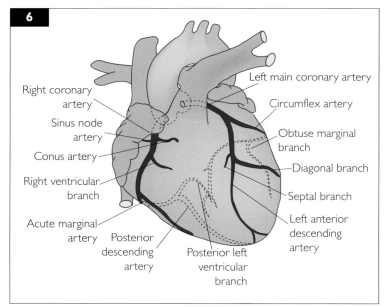

6 Schematic diagram of the coronary arteries.

around the apex and ends on the diaphragmatic surface of the heart, where it meets the posterior descending artery (PDA). The PDA usually arises from the right coronary artery (RCA). The major branches of the LAD are the septal and diagonal branches. The septal branches are variable in number and pass through the interventricular septum where they can form anastomoses with similar branches from the PDA. The first septal branch is often the largest and constitutes the most important communication between the RCA and LCA. The diagonal branches of the LAD, usually two to six in number, run across the anterolateral surface of the heart, to supply the anterolateral wall.

The LCx originates at bifurcation of the left main coronary artery. It passes down the left atrioventricular groove and turns to end posteriorly where it meets the RCA. Two to three obtuse marginal branches arise from the LCx and supply the lateral and posterior walls of the left ventricle (LV). The other important branches of the LCx include the left atrial circumflex branch and, in 40–50% of subjects, the sinus node artery. In 20% of subjects the LCx is a dominant vessel and gives rise to the PDA, which supplies the inferior portion of the left ventricle.

As expected, the LCA is larger then the RCA and supplies most of the LV, except for a small portion of the inferior surface. In 20% of cases where the LCA is the dominant vessel, the entire LV is supplied by this artery.

RIGHT CORONARY ARTERY
The RCA arises from the right aortic sinus of Valsalva at a level lower than the origin of the LCA (6, 7, 9). The RCA traverses down the right atrioventricular groove towards the crux, a point on the diaphragmatic surface of the heart where the right and left atrioventricular grooves and the posterior interventricular groove come together. This artery supplies the right atrium (RA), right ventricle (RV) and some of the inferior portion of the LV.

The first branch of the RCA is the conus artery, which runs anteriorly to supply the right ventricular outflow tract. In 40% of subjects, the conus branch can arise separately from the right aortic sinus. This branch often runs across the anterior surface of the RV and meets with a branch from the LAD. Thus, the conus branch can be an important source of collateral blood supply in patients with a proximal occlusion of the LAD.

The second branch of the RCA is usually the sinus node artery, which arises from the RCA in 60% of subjects and from the LCx in 40%. This branch courses posteriorly and supplies the RA and

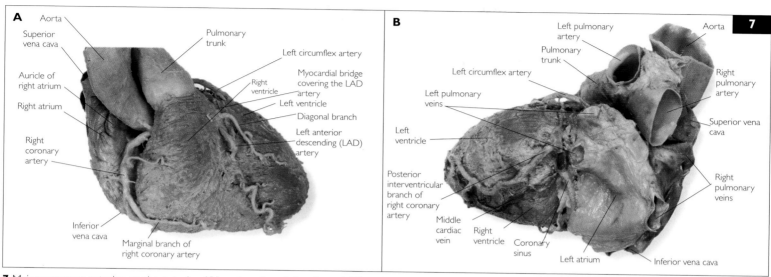

7 Major coronary arteries on the anterior (**A**) and postero-infero-lateral (**B**) surface of the heart. LAD: left anterior descending artery. (From McMinn *et al.* [1998]. *The Concise Handbook of Human Anatomy.* Manson Publishing, London).

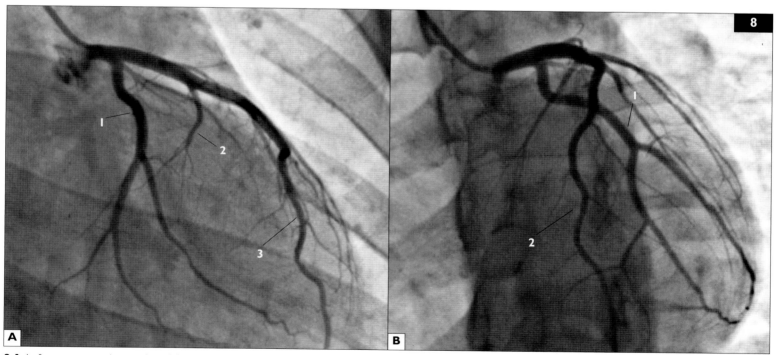

8 A: Left coronary angiogram in a right anterior oblique projection. **B**: Left coronary angiogram in a left anterior oblique projection.
A 1: Left circumflex artery; 2: septal artery; 3: left anterior descending artery. **B** 1: left circumflex artery; 2: left anterior descending artery

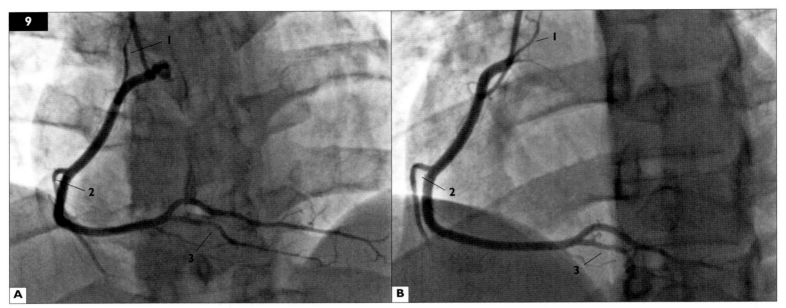

9 A: Right coronary angiogram in a right anterior oblique projection. **B**: Right coronary angiogram in a left anterior oblique projection. **A** 1: sinus node artery; 2: right ventricular artery; 3: posterior descending artery. **B** 1: sinus node artery; 2: right ventricular artery; 3: posterior descending artery

sinus node. The mid portion of the RCA gives rise to one or more medium-sized acute marginal branches which supply the anterior wall of the RV.

The next important branch of the RCA is the PDA. This branch arises from the RCA at the crux and runs forward along the posterior interventricular groove to meet the LAD. It gives off short septal branches that supply the inferior/posterior portion of the interventricular septum, and important anastomoses can be established here between the RCA and LCA. After giving rise to the PDA, the RCA continues to the left and terminates in posterior left ventricular branches which supply the infero-posterior wall of the LV. At or near the crux, the atrioventricular nodal artery, which supplies the atrioventricular node (AVN) and His bundle, arises.

DOMINANCE OF CIRCULATION

Dominance of circulation is a term used to describe which artery gives rise to the PDA. In 80% of subjects, the RCA gives rise to the PDA and the circulation is known as right dominant. In 20% of subjects, the PDA arises from the LCx artery and the coronary circulation is termed left dominant. In a small proportion of cases, both the RCA and LCx arteries give rise to two parallel PDAs, and the circulation is then termed codominant.

HISTOLOGY OF A NORMAL CORONARY ARTERY

The coronary artery, similar to other arteries, contains three distinguishable concentric layers (**10**): the inner intima, the media, and the outer adventitia. The intima consists of a single layer of endothelial cells and thin layer of subendothelial connective tissue. The endothelium forms a smooth inner semipermeable lining of the vessel that separates blood from the structures of the vessel wall. The endothelium secretes several important hormones and vasoactive substances which modulate coagulation, smooth muscle cell growth, platelet function, and vasomotor tone of the vessel.

The intima is separated from the media by a fenestrated sheet of elastic tissue termed the internal elastic lamina. The media consists of multiple layers of helically arranged smooth muscles interspersed with connective tissue. The media is separated from the adventitia by the external elastic lamina. This thin fenestrated layer of elastic tissue allows neurotransmitters to diffuse from the adventitia into the media, thus modulating the vasomotor tone of the vessel. The adventitia consists of fibrous tissue (collagen and elastic fibers) surrounded by vasa vasorum, nerves, and lymphatics. The loose consistency of this layer allows continual changes in diameter of the coronary artery.

ANOMALIES OF THE CORONARY ARTERIES

In 1–2% of subjects, there is a significant variation of coronary anatomy sufficient to qualify as coronary anomalies (see Chapter 4, Coronary Artery Anomalies). One of these is shown in (**11**). Even though most of these rare anomalies are benign and merely form a challenge to the angiographer, there are a few anomalies which are associated with early myocardial infarction (MI) or sudden cardiac death (SCD). The two most common anomalies are separate ostia for the LAD and LCx, and an abnormal origin of the LCx from the RCA or the right aortic sinus. A rare but important cause of sudden death in young people is an abnormal origin of the LCA from the right coronary ostium and the LCA traverses between the aorta and pulmonary trunk. This can lead to compromise of flow in the LCA during exercise and can trigger sudden death.

CLINICAL IMPLICATIONS

Proper communication among clinicians and researchers regarding the localization of lesions in the coronary arterial tree requires an unambiguous terminology. The system developed by the BARI (Bypass Angioplasty Revascularization Investigation) investigators (**12**)[3] was endorsed in recent guidelines[4].

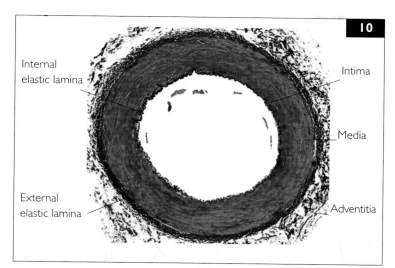

10 Histological section of a normal epicardial coronary artery.

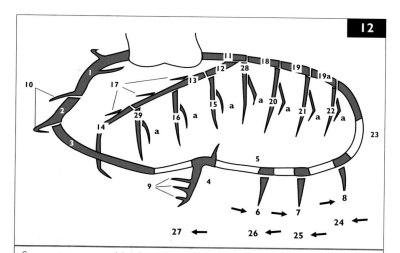

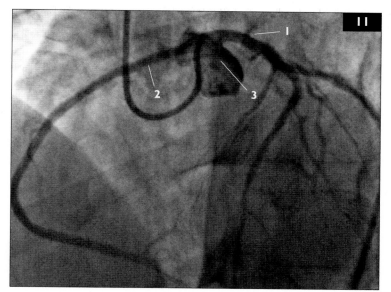

11 Coronary angiogram in a left anterior oblique projection showing an anomalous origin of the right coronary artery (RCA) from the left aortic sinus just adjacent to the origin of the left main coronary artery. 1: left main; 2: right coronary artery (RCA); 3: left aortic sinus.

12 The coronary artery map used by the Bypass Angioplasty Revascularization Investigation[3], and the names of the coronary artery segments numbered on the map.

Segment	Map Location
1	Proximal right coronary artery conduit segment
2	Mid-right coronary artery conduit segment
3	Distal right coronary artery conduit segment
4	Right posterior descending artery segment
5	Right posterior atrioventricular segment
6	First right posterolateral segment
7	Second right posterolateral segment
8	Third right posterolateral segment
9	Posterior descending septal perforator segments
10	Acute marginal segment(s)
11	Left main coronary artery segment
12	Proximal LAD artery segment
13	Mid-LAD artery segment
14	Distal LAD artery segment
15	First diagonal branch segment
15a	Lateral first diagonal branch segment
16	Second diagonal branch segment
16a	Lateral second diagonal branch segment
17	Left anterior descending septal perforator segments
18	Proximal circumflex artery segment
19	Mid-circumflex artery segment
19a	Distal circumflex artery segment
20	First obtuse marginal branch segment
20a	Lateral first obtuse marginal branch segment
21	Second obtuse marginal branch segment
21a	Lateral second obtuse marginal branch segment
22	Third obtuse marginal branch segment
22a	Lateral third obtuse marginal branch segment
23	Circumflex artery AV groove continuation segment
24	First left posterolateral branch segment
25	Second left posterolateral branch segment
26	Third left posterolateral branch segment
27	Left posterior descending artery segment
28	Ramus intermedius segment
28a	Lateral ramus intermedius segment
29	Third diagonal branch segment
29a	Lateral third diagonal branch segment

AV—atrioventricular; LAD—Left anterior descending.

MYOCARDIUM

SAIBAL KAR, MD AND PREDIMAN K. SHAH, MD, FACC

INTRODUCTION

The human heart is a remarkably efficient and durable pump that propels several hundreds of liters of blood daily during an individual's lifetime, supplying the necessary nutrients to all the tissues of the body. The basis of the heart's function is the near-inexhaustible cardiac muscle, the myocardium, which is composed of a collection of branching and anastomosing striated muscle cells tethered together in a collagen network and with other supporting cells (**13**, **14**). The atrial myocardium is thinner than the ventricular myocardium. The ventricular myocardium is much thicker in the LV (**15**). These muscle fibers are arranged in a spiral form such that during contraction of the cells, an effective pump is created that helps in propelling blood into the systemic or pulmonary circulation.

STRUCTURE OF CARDIAC MYOCYTE

Each cardiac myocyte is a branching striated muscle cell that comes in contact with other adjacent cells through an intercalated disk (**13**). Each cell contains five major components: (1) cell membrane (sarcolemma) and T tubules of impulse transmission; (2) sarcoplasmic reticulum, a calcium reservoir needed for contraction; (3) contractile elements; (4) mitochondria; and (5) the nucleus. Cardiac myocytes have many more mitochondria than skeletal muscles, reflecting the extreme dependence on aerobic metabolism.

The functional intracellular contractile unit of a cardiac muscle is the sarcomere (**16**). It consists of an orderly arrangement of thick filaments composed primarily of *myosin*, thin filaments containing *actin*, and certain regulatory proteins, namely *troponins* and *tropomyosin*. The myosin molecule resembles a golf club with two large bulbous heads protruding from one end of a straight shaft. The heads contain an actin-binding site and a site for adenosine triphospate- (ATP-) ase activity. The Z line to which the actin filaments are anchored marks the ends of a sarcomere. A sarcomere is the area from one dark Z line to an adjacent Z line, with a length that varies between 1.6 and 2.2 μm. A thin dark M line lies across the center of the sarcomere. The tropomyosin molecule lies alongside the actin molecules and prevents the active site of the actin molecule from coming in contact with a myosin molecule. Troponins are relaxing proteins associated with tropomyosin, forming the troponin–tropomyosin complex. Troponin T aids in the binding of the troponin complex to actin and tropomyosin; troponin I inhibits the ATPase of actomyosin; and troponin C contains binding sites for the calcium ions involved in contraction. On depolarization of the sarcolemma, calcium is mobilized into the areas of the myofibrils. Calcium binding to troponin inhibits troponin C (which enhances troponin I–actin binding). These in turn cause tropomyosin to move away, thus uncovering the myosin-binding site on actin. ATP can be dephosphorylated to adenosine diphosphate (ADP), releasing the energy required for contraction. Sliding of the thick and thin filaments can now occur, and the muscle contracts. During relaxation, calcium is actively pumped out of the myofibrils. Troponin releases calcium, and the tropomyosin complex blocks the active sites of actin to interact with myosin, and thus relaxation occurs. As expected, the greater the separation of the actin and myosin fibers at rest, the greater is the force and length of contraction, a phenomenon described as the Frank–Starling phenomenon. Thus moderate dilatation of the ventricle is often associated with an increase in stroke volume. This compensatory

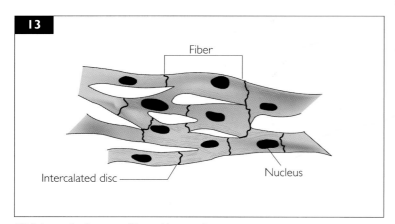

13 Schematic diagram of branching cardiac myocytes.

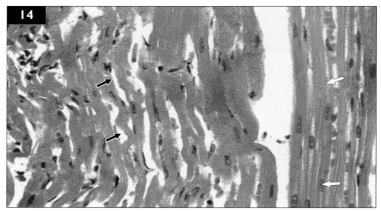

14 Histology of the myocardium. Note the wavy appearance of the cells and spaces between cells in the left half (black arrows), suggesting acute ischemia. On the right side (white arrows), the myocardium is normal. (Courtesy of Prof. Michael Fishbein, Department of Pathology, UCLA School of Medicine.)

mechanism plays an important role during various diseased states of the myocardium and valves. The process of relaxation is a calcium-dependent active process requiring ATP.

Functional integration of cardiac myocytes is brought about by unique structures, the intercalated disks, which connect one cell to the other (**13**). Intercalated disks are thickened portions of the sarcolemma that enable electrical impulses to spread quickly in a continuous cell-to-cell (syncytial) fashion. The intercalated disks contain two junctions: desmosomes, which attach one cell to another; and gap junctions, which allow the electrical impulse to spread from cell to cell. They allow electrical coupling and free ion exchange between myocardial cells, allowing synchronous contraction of myocardium. Functional disturbances of gap junctions and their respective proteins are responsible for the electromechanical dysfunction in patients with ischemic heart disease and cardiomyopathy.

EXTRACELLULAR MATRIX AND THE CYTOSKELETON

Although cardiac myocytes make up the bulk of the cardiac mass by volume, they are tethered in an extensive extracellular network of collagen and other structural proteins, including fibronectins and proteoglycans. Collagen production, synthesized principally by fibroblasts, can occur in response to a variety of pathologic stimuli, including oxidative and mechanical stress, ischemia, and inflammation. The increased fibrosis can produce increased myocardial stiffness and arrhythmogenesis in ischemic heart disease, cardiac hypertrophy, and congestive heart failure. Collagen synthesis can be continuously offset by extracellular matrix resorption, mediated by matrix metalloproteinases (MMPs). The activity of these enzymes is increased in dilated cardiomyopathy. Conversely, the activity of a class of enzymes known as tissue inhibitors of matrix metalloproteinases (TIMPs) is reduced in this setting. The resultant excessive collagen lysis may induce myofibrillar slippage and contributes to the dilated thin walled chamber geometry that characterizes acute and chronic heart failure. This process is termed chamber remodeling.

Cardiac myocytes are tethered to the extracellular matrix by membrane-spanning proteins called integrins. Various pathologic states of the myocardium are associated with changes in the relative abundance of these various intra- and extracellular structural proteins.

CARDIAC HYPERTROPHY

From birth to adulthood, there is an increase in chamber size primarily due to an increase in numbers of cardiac myocytes. Cardiac hypertrophy, however, is a process involving an increase in chamber mass produced largely by an increase in size of terminally differentiated cardiac myocytes. Cardiac hypertrophy can be categorized as either physiologic or pathologic. Pathologic hypertrophy is an important adaptive response to abnormal global or regional increases in cardiac work (**15**). Initially, the increase in cardiac mass helps to normalize wall stress and permit normal cardiovascular function. If the stimuli are intense and prolonged, decompensated hypertrophy and heart failure may ensue. Current information suggests that mechano-transduction and a number of interrelated autocrine, paracrine, and endocrine effects of growth factors and hormones mediate hypertrophy.

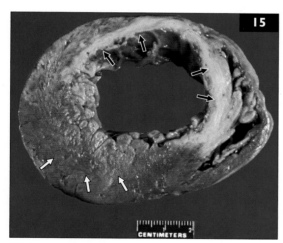

15 Cross section of the heart at mid ventricular level. Note the acute anteroseptal myocardial infarction which extends from the anterolateral wall and involves most of the interventricular septum (black arrows). There is thinning of the expanded infarcted segment. Also note the compensatory hypertrophy of the posterolateral wall (white arrows). (Courtesy of Prof. Michael Fishbein, Department of Pathology, UCLA School of Medicine.)

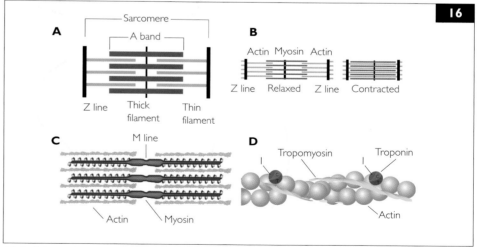

16 A: Schematic diagram of a sarcomere of a cardiomyocyte showing arrangements of thick (myosin) and thin (actin) fibers. **B**: Sliding of actin on myosin during muscle contraction. **C**: Detail of the relation between actin and myosin. Note myosin molecules reverse their polarity at the M line. **D**: Schematic diagram of actin fibers showing the regulatory proteins tropomyosin and troponins C, T, and I.

MYOCARDIAL METABOLISM

The myocardium has an abundant blood supply, numerous mitochondria, and a high content of myoglobin. In normal circumstances <1% energy liberated is provided by anaerobic metabolism. Therefore, under totally anaerobic conditions, the energy liberated is inadequate to sustain ventricular contractions. At rest and under basal conditions, most of the energy is derived from oxidative metabolism of fats. However, in stressful situations and in severe myocardial ischemia, energy is also derived from carbohydrates and ketones (see Chapter 4, Anaerobic Myocardial Metabolism). The myocardium extracts a large portion of oxygen from the circulation; therefore, the only way that an actively beating heart can increase its energy production is by increasing coronary blood flow. This explains the importance of the coronary circulation in the preservation of the functional integrity of the myocardium, at health and in diseased states.

CONDUCTION SYSTEM

**MIGUEL VALDERRÁBANO, MD AND
C. THOMAS PETER, MD**

INTRODUCTION

The conduction system is comprised of the sinoatrial node (SAN), the interatrial conduction pathways, atrioventricular node (AVN), the His bundle, the bundle branches, and the distal Purkinje network (PN) (**17**). The SAN, which contains the leading pacemaker, generates the impulse. The impulse is subsequently conducted, via the atrial myocardium, which in this sense is part of the conduction pathway as well, toward the AVN. With a delay, the impulse is then rapidly transmitted from the AVN via the bundle branches and PN to ensure a coordinated activation of the ventricular myocardium from apex to base.

SINOATRIAL NODE

The SAN is a spindle-shaped structure found at the junction of the superior vena cava and the RA (**18**). It is composed of nodal or 'P' cells and transitional 'T' cells: 'P' cells are small, ovoid, and located in clusters in the center of the SAN, and are thought to be the source of impulse formation; T cells are located in the periphery connecting with the neighboring atrial myocytes. There is a relative paucity of gap junctions between cells in the SAN, which underlies slow conduction within it. Of the gap junction

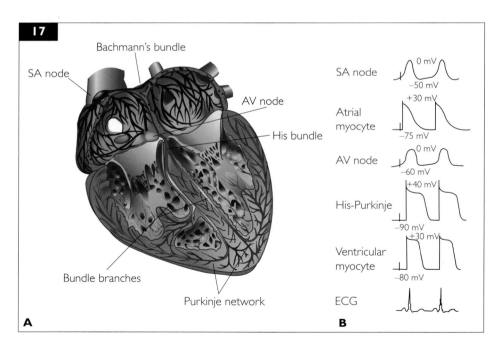

17 A: Macroscopic delineation of the conduction system.
B: Action potential morphology in the different components of the conduction system. AV: atrioventricular; ECG: electrocardiogram; SA: sinoatrial

components, connexin 40 and 45 are the predominant isoforms (as opposed to connexin 43, the predominant isoform in gap junctions of working myocytes). The blood supply to the SAN is provided by the RCA in 55% of subjects, from the LCx in 35%, and has a dual supply from both arteries in 10% (**19**). The SAN is richly innervated by both sympathetic and parasympathetic systems.

INTERNODAL AND INTRAATRIAL CONDUCTION PATHWAYS

The presence of preferential pathways connecting the SAN with the AVN is still controversial. Such pathways are not distinct anatomically, but a functional preferential conduction is indeed present which may be due to myocyte fiber orientation, size, and geometry. Three pathways have been described:

1. The anterior internodal tract goes from the anterior margin of the SAN around the superior vena cava towards the interatrial septum. There it connects with the Bachmann bundle which spreads through the LA. The anterior internodal pathway connects with the superior margin of the AVN.
2. The middle internodal tract begins at the superior and posterior margins of the sinus node and travels behind the superior vena cava to the interatrial septum. It descends in the septum and connects with the superior aspect of the AVN.
3. The posterior internodal tract starts at the posterior margin of the SAN and descends along the crista terminalis to the Eustachian ridge and then into the interatrial septum above the coronary sinus, where it joins the posterior portion of the AVN. Interatrial conduction has been demonstrated through the roof of the coronary sinus.

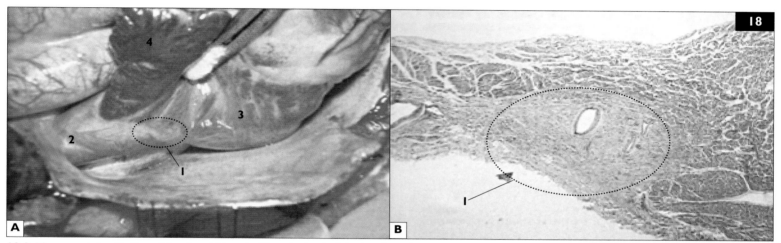

18 A: Macroscopic localization of the sinoatrial node (1) at the level of the junction of the superior vena cava (2) and the right atrium (3). 4: Right atrial appendage. **B**: Microscopic view of the sinoatrial node (1) traversed by the sinus node artery.

19 Blood supply of the conduction system.

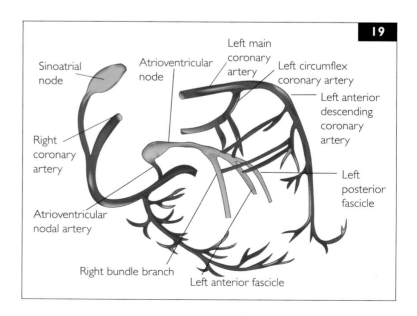

ATRIOVENTRICULAR NODE

The AVN is located in the posteroseptal aspect of the RA, anterior to the coronary sinus os at the apex of the triangle of Koch. The triangle of Koch is formed by the tendon of Todaro superiorly, the septal leaflet of the tricuspid valve inferiorly, and the coronary sinus os posteriorly. The tendon of Todaro is an extension of the Eustachian valve that connects with the heart's central fibrous body. The AVN has been divided into two zones: the transitional zone, composed of the insertions of internodal tracts, and the compact AVN whose fibers penetrate the central fibrous body to become the His bundle (20). Gap juctions are scarce, consistent with slow conduction, and connexin 40 and 45 predominate. The AVN receives blood supply from the AV nodal artery, which is a branch of the RCA in 80% of subjects, originates from the LCx in 15%, and has a dual supply in 5% (19). The AVN is richly innervated by both the sympathetic and the parasympathetic systems.

HIS BUNDLE AND BUNDLE BRANCHES

The His bundle connects with the distal part of the compact AVN, perforates the central fibrous body, and continues through the annulus fibrosus, where it is called the nonbranching portion as it penetrates the membranous septum. It passes adjacent to the noncoronary cusp of the aortic valve. It receives blood supply from the AV nodal artery and septal perforators from the LAD (19). The His bundle separates into the right and left bundle branches (R/LBBs). The RBB runs within the interventricular septum close to the right ventricular subendocardium and exits at the level of the anterior papillary muscle, forming the echocardiographically distinct moderator band. The LBB spreads in a fan-like fashion along the left side of the interventricular septum and divides into the anterior and superior fascicles. The anterior fascicle travels along the left ventricular outflow tract towards the anterolateral papillary muscle. The posterior fascicle takes a posteroinferior direction towards the posteriomedial papillary muscle. The RBB and left anterior fascicle receive blood supply predominantly from septal perforator branches of the LAD, whereas the supply for the left posterior fascicle derives from septal branches of the LAD and the PDA (19).

The BBs give rise to a subendocardial network of Purkinje fibers that form a discontinuous coat under the endocardium (21A). At discrete locations (between endocardial trabeculae and the base of the papillary muscles, for example) this network gives rise to penetrating Purkinje fibers that form Purkinje–muscle junctions (21B). The distal Purkinje system selectively expresses connexin 40 in its gap junctions, enabling microscopic identification (21).

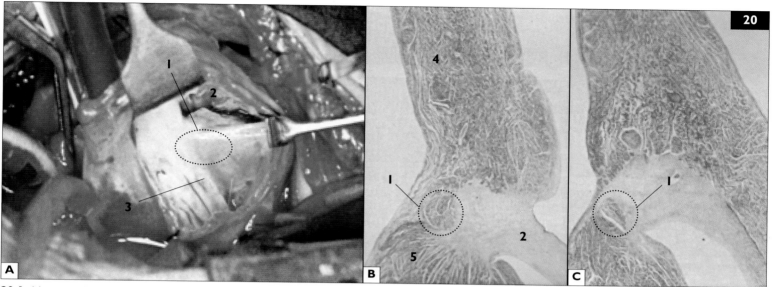

20 A: Macroscopic localization of the atrioventricular node (1) at the vertex of the triangle of Koch, which is formed by the septal leaflet of the tricuspid valve (2) inferiorly, the tendon of Todaro (3) superiorly, and the coronary sinus os posteriorly. **B, C:** Microscopic view of the atrioventricular node (1) as it traverses through the fibrous skeleton of the heart. 4: right atrium; 5: right ventricle.

21 Immunohistochemical staining of connexin 40.
A: Subendocardial Purkinje cells. **B**: Purkinje–muscle junctions at the level of the papillary muscle root.

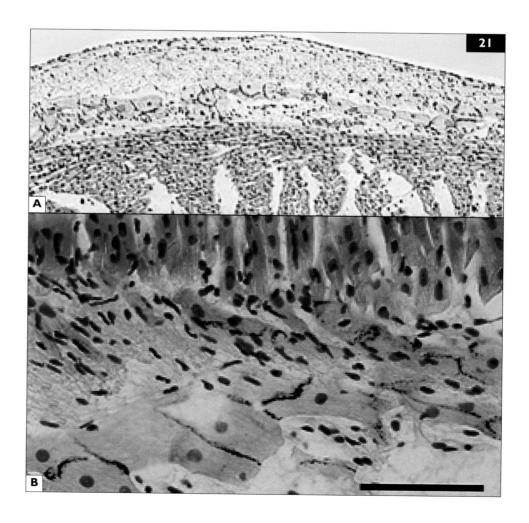

Chapter Three

Physiology of the Heart

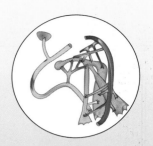

CORONARY CIRCULATION

DIRK J.G.M. DUNCKER, MD, PhD AND
DAPHNE MERKUS, PhD

INTRODUCTION

The heart depends principally on aerobic metabolism as it can obtain a maximum of 7% of its adenosine triphospate (ATP) requirement through anaerobic glycolysis. In contrast to skeletal muscle, the cardiac muscle never stops working and pumps blood with approximately 60–70 beats per minute under resting conditions. Consequently, oxygen consumption normalized per gram of myocardium is 20-fold higher than that of skeletal muscle. One way the heart has adapted to the high oxygen demand is by achieving a high level of oxygen extraction, reaching as much as 70–80% of the arterially delivered oxygen, as compared to 30–40% in skeletal muscle. This high level of oxygen extraction is facilitated by a high capillary density: 3000 per mm^2 compared to 400 per mm^2 in skeletal muscle. Since the heart extracts already 70–80% of the delivered oxygen, it follows that a 4–5-fold increase in oxygen demand, as occurs during maximum exercise, can only be met by an increase in oxygen delivery, i.e. an increase in coronary blood flow (CBF). Indeed, despite the high resting flows in the heart (0.7–0.8 ml/min/g of myocardium, compared to 0.05–0.10 ml/min/g of skeletal muscle), coronary blood flow can still increase 4–5-fold during exercise.

CORONARY BLOOD FLOW

CBF is determined by the pressure drop across the coronary bed (perfusion pressure) and total coronary vascular resistance ($R_{coronary}$):

$$CBF = Perfusion\ pressure\ /\ R_{coronary}$$

Perfusion pressure and extravascular compressive forces

Since the coronary vasculature is embedded in the myocardium, it is continuously exposed to intramyocardial pressure and the effective perfusion pressure is not equal to the difference between the arterial and venous pressures. During systole, the contracting myocardium of the left ventricle (LV) generates a high level of intramyocardial pressure that compresses the coronary circulation.

Consequently, blood is squeezed out of the LV intramyocardial vessels during systole, and arterial inflow into the large epicardial conductance arteries such as the left anterior descending coronary artery (LAD) is markedly impeded (**22**). Thus, only 15–20% of coronary flow to the LV occurs during systole (time period encompassed by each pair of green lines in **22**) and 80–85% during diastole. Blood is also squeezed out of the LV intramural venules into the epicardial veins, resulting in venous blood flow through the great cardiac vein (GCV) that is largest in systole. In contrast, pressure generation by the right ventricle (RV) is lower than in the LV. Consequently, right coronary artery (RCA) arterial inflow follows the pattern of aortic pressure.

Since the intramyocardial pressure during systole is greatest in the subendocardium (equalling systolic pressure in the ventricular lumen), blood from vessels within these innermost layers is squeezed back into the more superficial subepicardial arterial vessels during each systole and the subendocardial vessels have to be refilled in diastole (analogous to the emptying and filling of a capacitor). Consequently, (1) systolic arterial inflow is directed towards the subepicardium, while subendocardial blood flow occurs exclusively during diastole, and (2) with a shortening of diastole (as occurs when heart rate increases) a significant part of diastole is used for refilling the subendocardial vessels, thereby delaying net forward flow in the subendocardial microcirculation and potentially compromising subendocardial blood flow.

Diastolic flow is determined by the diastolic pressure gradient across the vascular bed and the coronary vascular resistance. The pressure at the entrance of the coronary bed is the diastolic arterial pressure, whereas the effective back pressure is not the venous pressure in the coronary sinus, but the diastolic intramyocardial pressure. The diastolic intramyocardial pressure in the endocardium equals the diastolic pressure in the intraventricular lumen, while in the epicardium it equals intrapericardial pressure. Under normal circumstances, the average diastolic pressures in the ventricles are negligible but in situations of elevated intraventricular pressures (e.g. aortic regurgitation or heart failure) perfusion of particularly the subendocardium can become compromised.

Resistance

Total coronary resistance is the sum of both passive (structural) and active (smooth muscle tone) components. In the completely vasodilated bed, flow to the different regions of the heart is determined by the length of the vasculature, the diameter of the vessels, and the number of parallel vessels that supply a certain perfusion territory. Measurements of intravascular pressure have shown that 90% of resistance resides in the small arteries (100–400 μm in diameter) and arterioles (<100 μm), hence the term resistance vessels (23). The main part of coronary resistance is located in the coronary arterioles, as is evidenced by the large pressure-drop that occurs across these vessels. However, during maximal coronary vasodilation (dotted line), the large and small coronary arteries also contribute significantly to total resistance. Since the smallest arterioles are in closest proximity to the tissue, they are most sensitive to metabolic dilators. An increase in

metabolism therefore results in vasodilation of the smallest arterioles, which decreases coronary resistance and results in an increase in flow. This increase in flow then recruits the large arterioles and small arteries, which are more sensitive to flow-dependent dilation, to further decrease coronary resistance. The myogenic response, an increase in diameter in response to a decrease in pressure that contributes to autoregulation, is strongest in the arterioles of intermediate size.

The total length of the vessels supplying the subendocardium is longer than that of those supplying the epicardium. Also, because the vasculature is compressed during each contraction the diameter of the vessels changes, resulting in an increase in resistance and a decrease in flow to especially the subendocardium. To compensate for this, the subendocardium has a 10% higher arteriolar and capillary density. Thus, during complete vasodilation, flow to the subendocardium is similar to flow to the subepicardium.

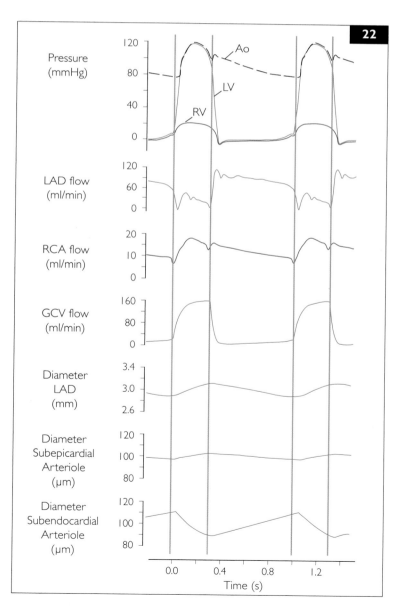

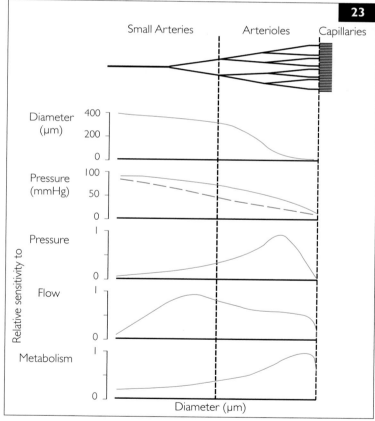

23 Sensitivity of the coronary resistance vessels to various physiological stimuli. (Modified from Jones *et al.* [1995]. Regulation of coronary blood flow: coordination of heterogeneous control mechanisms in vascular microdomains. *Cardiovasc. Res.* **29**:585–596.)

22 Phasic patterns of coronary blood flow and diameters in relation to aortic and ventricular pressures. Ao: aorta; GCV: great cardiac vein; LAD: left anterior descending artery; LV: left ventricle; RCA: right coronary artery; RV: right ventricle.

REGULATION OF CORONARY RESISTANCE

Under basal resting conditions and intact vascular smooth muscle tone, 70–80% of coronary resistance resides in the coronary arterioles (**23**). Regulation of coronary vascular resistance is the result of a balance between a myriad of vasodilator and vasoconstrictor influences, which are exerted by the myocardium, endothelium, and neurohumoral system. This way, the myocardium can match its blood supply to its requirement of oxygen and nutrients.

Myocardial metabolism

The high level of basal oxygen extraction requires an increase in coronary blood flow to accommodate any major increase in myocardial oxygen demand. Since mean aortic pressure increases only by 10–20% and average extravascular compressive forces increase during exercise, it is clear that any increase in coronary blood flow must be accommodated by a decrease in coronary vascular resistance. However, the traditional view of a homogeneous array of resistance vessels that act principally in response to local myocardial needs, but which can also respond weakly to systemic vasomotor influences, is incorrect. Metabolic regulation of coronary vascular resistance occurs principally in coronary arterioles (<100 μm) to tightly couple oxygen demand and supply, whereas the small arteries respond much less to local metabolic influences (**23**). Proposed mediators of metabolic vasodilation are adenosine (resulting from ATP breakdown), carbon dioxide, pH, and potassium. Several of these mediators have been shown to cause opening of K^+_{ATP} channels, K^+_{Ca} channels, or K^+_V channels in the vascular smooth muscle membrane, leading to hyperpolarization and vasodilation (**24**). Unraveling of the exact mechanism of metabolic vasodilation has been difficult, probably because blockade of a single pathway results in compensatory increments in the contribution of other pathways (redundancy evolution).

Endothelium

The endothelium produces vasoactive factors that influence platelet aggregation, vascular remodeling and growth, and vascular tone. Among these factors are prostaglandins (prostacyclin, PGI_2), endothelium-derived hyperpolarizing factor (EDHF), nitric oxide (NO), and endothelin-1 (ET) (**24**). The production of NO is related to shear stress, and thus to the velocity of blood in the vasculature. When the distal arterioles dilate in response to a metabolic stimulus the downstream resistance decreases, resulting in an increase in blood flow in the more proximal vessels (**23**). This causes an increase in shear stress which increases NO production, thereby recruiting the vasodilator response of the more proximal small arteries and further decreasing resistance.

Neurohormones

The coronary bed is richly innervated by sympathetic and parasympathetic nerve fibers. The role of the parasympathetic system (which can exert vasodilator influences via production of NO) is not clear since its activity wanes during increasing levels of exercise. Conversely, under resting conditions the sympathetic influence is negligible but during exercise sympathetic activation results in stimulation of α- and β-adrenoceptors (**24**). The net result of sympathetic activation is metabolic vasodilation due to β-adrenoceptor-mediated increases in heart rate and contractility. However, α-adrenergic vasoconstriction limits the increase in coronary blood flow during exercise, necessitating a small increase in myocardial oxygen extraction, which is in part counteracted by direct β-adrenergic vasodilation. In addition to these autonomic influences, coronary resistance vessel tone is also modulated by endo- and paracrine factors such as angiotensin II, bradykinin, histamine, thromboxane A_2 (TXA_2), serotonin (5-HT) (**24**).

CORONARY ARTERY STENOSIS

Autoregulation is defined as the capacity to maintain blood flow constant in the face of a changing perfusion pressure (with constant metabolic needs). The vasomotor mechanisms that underlie autoregulation are probably the same as for metabolic regulation but also probably involve the myogenic response. Normally, the large epicardial 'conductance' coronary arteries do not contribute to total coronary resistance. However, autoregulation becomes clinically important when atherosclerosis causes narrowing of a large coronary artery and obliterates >75% of the lumen cross sectional area (50% diameter reduction). Such a stenosis results in a significant increase in resistance and creates a decrease in distal coronary perfusion pressure. Although autoregulation preserves basal CBF, the maximum CBF (as measured with intracoronary administration of adenosine) is reduced (**25**). Consequently, coronary flow reserve (the ratio of maximum over basal CBF) is attenuated. When poststenotic pressure decreases to <40 mmHg (5.3 kPa), vasodilator reserve is exhausted and basal flow decreases, resulting in myocardial hypoperfusion. Autoregulatory reserve is not homogeneously distributed across the LV wall. Due to the higher extravascular compressive forces in the subendocardium, the autoregulation curve is shifted to the right (with the break-point at 40 mmHg [5.3 kPa]) compared to that in the subepicardial layers (break-point at 25 mmHg [3.3 kPa]).

The influence of various degrees of coronary artery stenosis, exercise, and exogenously administered coronary vasodilators on pressure–flow relationships in the left coronary vasculature is shown in **25**. Maximal flow (for example through administration of exogenous vasodilators) to the heart depends on coronary perfusion pressure and is higher in the subepicardium (Epi_{max}) than in the subendocardium ($Endo_{max}$) due to differences in extravascular compressive forces. Also note that, due to these compressive forces, a back-pressure is generated that causes flow to stop at a pressure (zero-flow pressure) that is higher than central venous pressure. Under normal circumstances, flow is determined by the metabolic demands of the myocardium, and flow to the subendocardium ($Endo_{auto}$) is slightly higher than flow to the subepicardium (Epi_{auto}). Coronary flow reserve is determined by the ratio of maximal and basal flow (a′/a), and is therefore larger in the subepicardium than in the subendocardium. The presence of a stenosis (left panel) results in a decrease in coronary artery pressure (distal to the stenosis), which, in the case of a mild

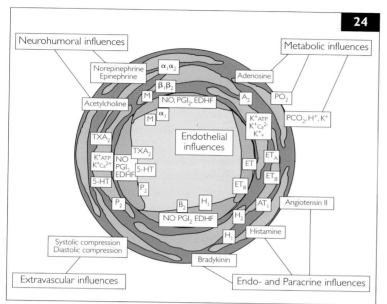

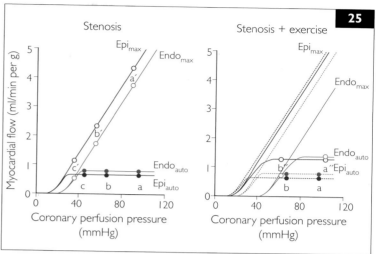

25 Influence of various degrees of coronary artery stenosis, exercise, and exogenously administered coronary vasodilators on pressure–flow relationships in the left coronary vasculature (see text).

24 Diameter of the coronary arteries and arterioles is influenced by mechanical forces (compression) and determinants of vascular smooth muscle tone. α_1, α_2, β_1, β_2: adrenergic receptors; A_2: adenosine A_2 receptor; AT: angiotensin; ATP: adenosine triphosphate; B_2: bradykinin B_2 receptor; EDHF: endothelium-derived hyperpolarizing factor; $ET_{A,B}$: endothelin A,B receptors; $H_{1,2}$: histamine $H_{1,2}$ receptors; 5-HT: serotonin; M: muscarinic receptor; NO: nitric oxide; P_2: purinergic P_2 receptor; PGI_2: prostacyclin; TXA_2: thromboxane A_2.

stenosis (b), does not compromise normal myocardial perfusion but does decrease flow reserve (b′/b). With a critical stenosis, administration of an exogenous vasodilator (e.g. adenosine) to recruit vasodilator reserve may cause adverse effects through coronary steal (c). Thus, the increase in flow to the subepicardium will increase the pressure gradient across the stenosis (δP= flow × resistance), and thereby decrease poststenotic perfusion pressure and hence subendocardial blood flow. Since subendocardial vasodilator reserve is exhausted, flow to the subendocardium will decrease in parallel to the decrease in perfusion pressure (c′), whereas flow to the subepicardium will increase (c′), hence the term 'steal'.

When myocardial oxygen consumption increases (e.g. during exercise), the autoregulatory plateau will be shifted upward, as is shown by the higher level of $Endo_{auto}$ and Epi_{auto} (a″). In addition, the increase in heart rate, which results in an increase in average myocardial tissue pressure (by spending relatively more time in systole), shifts the pressure–flow relation to the right, particularly in the subendocardial layers. This explains why a subcritical coronary artery stenosis (that has no effect on basal CBF) can result in selective subendocardial hypoperfusion (b″) during exercise. Resting pressure–flow relations have been depicted as dotted lines.

Ischemia has generally been assumed to render the coronary resistance vessels maximally vasodilated and unresponsive to vasoconstrictor stimuli. However, recent observations have demonstrated that during ischemia the coronary microvessels retain some degree of vasodilator reserve and remain responsive to vasoconstrictor stimuli. Thus, vasoconstrictor influences resulting from α-adrenergic receptor activation, thromboxane A_2 (TXA_2), and serotonin can compete with endogenous vasodilator mechanisms such as ATP-sensitive K^+ channels, adenosine, and NO which are recruited during ischemia. Indeed, recent studies have demonstrated that in the coronary arterioles which are responsive to the metabolic state of the myocardium, vasoconstrictor influences can compete with metabolic vasodilator activity. Moreover, because small arteries (which contribute significantly to coronary resistance) respond only weakly to metabolic dilator influences, these vessels are even more susceptible to these vasoconstrictor influences.

The finding that vasoconstrictor tone can persist in microvessels within ischemic myocardium raises the question whether pharmacologic vasodilators acting at the microvascular level might be therapeutically useful. In clinical situations in which myocardial ischemia results from a flow-limiting coronary stenosis, pharmacologic vasodilation of the arterioles causes several effects that can even worsen ischemia. Thus, as explained above, vasodilation of the resistance vessels can cause redistribution of the limited blood flow toward the subepicardium, thereby worsening subendocardial ischemia. Furthermore, resistance vessel dilation can cause a decrease of intravascular pressure that allows recoil of a compliant stenosis, thereby worsening stenosis severity. A pharmacologic agent that causes selective vasodilation of the coronary arteries (including the small arteries), but which does not interfere with metabolic vasoregulation by the arterioles, would be predicted to have anti-ischemic effects. Selective dilation of the small arteries in an adequately perfused region would be countered by compensatory vasoconstriction of the arterioles to maintain blood flow appropriate for local myocardial requirements, thereby preventing overperfusion that can result in coronary steal. In contrast, in ischemic regions where the arterioles have already undergone metabolic vasodilation, removing residual vasoconstrictor tone in the small arteries would have the potential for increasing blood flow. The critical property of an effective agent would thus be lack of interference with metabolic vasoregulation at the level of the arterioles.

MYOCARDIUM AND DETERMINANTS OF OXYGEN DEMAND

HENRY GEWIRTZ, MD AND AHMED TAWAKOL, MD

INTRODUCTION
The vast majority of oxygen consumed by the heart is required for contraction. Only a small amount (~20%) is needed for basal requirements[1]. Further, under basal conditions, pressure work done by the heart (i.e. generation of tension) consumes roughly four times the oxygen that volume work (shortening against load) needs and so is far more costly in terms of oxygen consumption (**26**)[1]. Moreover, oxygen (and substrate) delivery is dependent on myocardial blood flow with only modest room to increase oxygen supply by enhanced extraction. Accordingly, increased myocardial oxygen demand must be met by increased myocardial blood flow. More generally, the level of myocardial blood flow is regulated to meet the prevailing level of myocardial oxygen demand.

SUBSTRATE UTILIZATION BY THE MYOCARDIUM
The ATP required to fuel myocardial contraction and basal requirements is derived primarily from the oxidative metabolism of long chain fatty acids and glucose. While the amount of ATP needed to perform a given amount of work is fixed, oxygen consumption may vary depending on the mixture of fuels (fatty acids versus glucose) employed. Thus, for a given ATP requirement exclusive metabolism of a fatty acid such as palmitate would consume ~13% more oxygen than glucose[2], since one glucose molecule yields 38 ATP with consumption of six oxygen molecules ($0.16 \ O_2/ATP$) in comparison with 129 ATP from 23 oxygen molecules ($0.18 \ O_2/ATP$) for one palmitate molecule (**27**)[2].

While fatty acids, nonetheless, are the preferred metabolic substrate of the heart, glucose is also used under normal conditions, especially after meals when glucose and insulin levels are elevated and during catecholamine stimulation with exercise[3]. Indeed, the interplay between glucose and fatty acid metabolism is complex and, depending on conditions, each has the potential to inhibit metabolism of the other. Thus, under low flow ischemic conditions fatty acid metabolism is inhibited and glucose uptake and utilization are stimulated[3]. Enhanced production of malonyl-CoA from lactate inhibits transport of fatty acyl moieties into the mitochondria where β-oxidation occurs, while at the same time ATP stores decline which facilitates glycolysis by reversal of the Pasteur effect (ATP inhibition of glycolysis)[3].

MAJOR DETERMINANTS OF MYOCARDIAL OXYGEN CONSUMPTION (MVO$_2$)

Contractile state
While a number of indices of myocardial contractility have been proposed, the majority suffer from the limitation of being load dependent and thus do not provide a good measure of contraction

velocity, perhaps the best indicator of contractile state. In intact animals and humans the left ventricular end-systolic pressure-volume relationship has been employed as a load-independent measure of myocardial contractility[4]. The ratio of left ventricular pressure to volume (elastance, E) varies throughout the cardiac cycle and is near maximum at end-systole (E_{max}). A given contractile state is defined by a series of end-systolic pressure–volume points (**28**) which form a straight line, whose slope (E_{es}) is an index of contractility[4]. The line becomes steeper when contractility increases and flatter with myocardial depression. Changes in contractility generally produce directly proportional changes in MVO_2[1].

Heart rate

The frequency of cardiac contraction has a direct influence on MVO_2. Increasing heart rate results in a proportionate increase in MVO_2 and *vice versa*[1]. In the intact animal or human, the manner in which heart rate is increased, however, may have a substantial effect on MVO_2. Thus, atrial pacing, which artificially elevates heart rate without change in contractility will augment MVO_2

much less than if heart rate is increased by an intervention which also augments contractility (e.g. catecholamine stimulation).

Systolic wall tension

Tension (T) generated by the myocardial wall during systole may be approximated, assuming spherical geometry, by the LaPlace equation:

$$T = P \times r/2h; \text{ where } P = \text{intracavitary pressure,}$$
$$r = \text{chamber radius, and } h = \text{wall thickness.}$$

Though left ventricular afterload is commonly equated with systolic arterial pressure, systolic wall tension is a more accurate measure since it incorporates wall thickness. In the case of left ventricular hypertrophy, wall tension may be returned toward baseline despite elevation of LV systolic pressure due to increase in wall thickness.

Preload is approximated by LV end-diastolic or mean pulmonary capillary wedge pressure, and is determined in part by LV

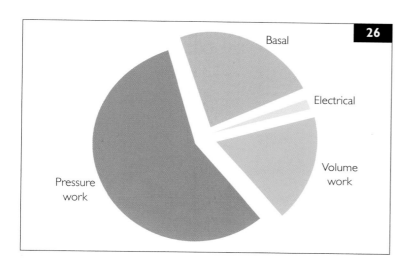

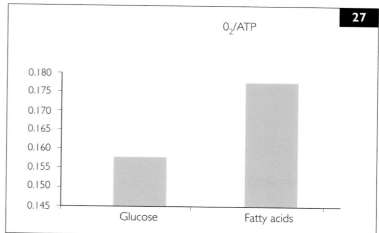

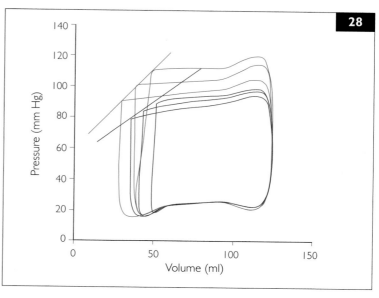

26 Pie chart illustrating the relative contribution, under basal conditions, of essential cardiac functions to global myocardial oxygen consumption. Note that pressure work is by far the most costly activity.

27 Bar chart illustrating the oxygen cost of generating adenosine triphosphate (ATP) from glucose in comparison with fatty acid. To generate an equivalent number of moles of ATP, approximately 13% more oxygen is required using fatty acid in comparison with glucose.

28 A series of hypothetical pressure–volume loops for two different contractile states are shown here. Note that the end-systolic pressure volume points lie on a straight line, the slope of which (E_{es}) is a measure of myocardial contractility. The family of red loops has steeper slope (and is left shifted) in comparison with those in blue and defines a state of greater contractility.

volume. Accordingly, an increase in LV volume will increase chamber radius and hence systolic wall tension. Thus, LV preload is an important determinant of systolic wall tension.

The manner in which systolic wall tension is altered has an important influence on MVO_2. Augmentation of intracavitary pressure (pressure load) by 50% will generally result in a proportionate increase in MVO_2. In contrast, increase in chamber volume alone by 50% (volume load) results in only a small increase (~5%) in MVO_2. Thus, imposition of a pressure load is much more costly in terms of oxygen consumption than volume load[1].

PHYSIOLOGIC HETEROGENEITY OF MYOCARDIAL OXYGEN DEMAND

While myocardial oxygen demand is defined for the entire LV in terms of global parameters such as contractility, heart rate, and systolic wall tension, it is important to note that the problem is more complex. First, since wall tension is greater at the endocardial compared with epicardial surface of the LV, myocardial oxygen demand generally is thought to be greater in the endocardium[1, 5]. Greater wall tension and hence oxygen demand may in part account for greater endocardial versus epicardial blood flow in the heart. In addition to heterogeneity across layers of the LV wall, heterogeneity of myocardial blood flow on a scale of <1% of LV mass has also been described and has been shown to correlate with evidence of proportionate microvariation in myocardial oxygen demand[6, 7]. The range of variability is rather large, from <50% to more than 250% of the mean[7]. Relatively constant ATP levels in such small tissue samples indicate that myocardial oxygen supply and demand are in balance and that low flow zones (i.e. <50% of mean flow) are not ischemic[7]. The physiologic basis for such heterogeneity in the normal heart remains uncertain and is an active area of investigation.

CLINICAL IMPLICATIONS

Many of the recent advances in the treatment of both acute and chronic coronary syndromes involve improvements in supply-side therapy. Examples include stents (both passive and drug-eluting) for percutaneous coronary intervention (PCI), new thrombolytics and antiplatelet drugs, statins for improvement of endothelial function[8] and even angiogenesis[9]. However, therapies which reduce myocardial oxygen demand continue to play an essential role in the management of both acute and chronic coronary disease. Beta blockers effectively lower arterial pressure and heart rate, reduce myocardial contractility, and antagonize adverse metabolic effects of catecholamine stimulation. Angiotensin-converting enzyme (ACE) inhibitors and angiotensin receptor blockers (ARB) control arterial pressure and also have important biologic properties, notably anti-oxidant effects, which help to preserve endothelial function and vascular integrity. Metabolic therapy of acute myocardial infarction(MI) with glucose–insulin–potassium solution has also shown some promise and is under consideration again[10]. Finally, in the acute setting, demand-side interventions such as IV beta blockers and nitrates have immediate onset and thus protect the myocardium while PCI, the preferred supply-side therapy, is being mobilized or thrombolysis takes effect.

CONDUCTION SYSTEM

PETER LUKAC, MD, PhD AND ANDERS KIRSTEIN PEDERSEN, MD, DMSC

INTRODUCTION

The electrical impulse initiating the cardiac contraction begins in the sinoatrial node (SAN). The activation wavefront is then conducted through the atrial myocardium to the atrioventricular node (AVN), possibly by preferential internodal tracts. Conduction from the AVN to the ventricles proceeds through the His bundle and the specialized conducting tissue in the ventricles, termed the His–Purkinje system, which begins as the left and right bundle branches. The left bundle branch (LBB) divides into a larger posterior and smaller anterior fascicle and the His–Purkinje system ends in contact with ventricular muscle fibers[1]. The arterial blood supply of the conduction system is depicted in **29**.

SINOATRIAL NODE

Pacemaker activity of SAN cells is the result of a spontaneous process called phase 4 diastolic depolarization caused by a net sum of different ionic currents[2]. When the membrane potential reaches threshold, initiation of a slow Ca^{++}-dependent action potential

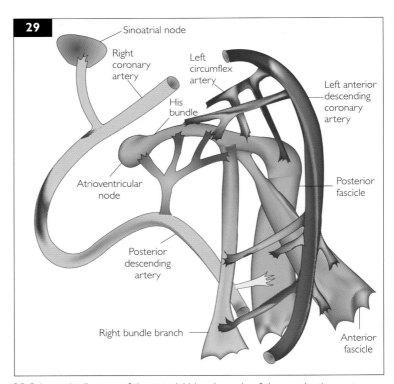

29 Schematic diagram of the arterial blood supply of the conduction system. Interindividual variations exist.

results (**30**). The action potential conducts via gap junction channels built from hexameric connexin arrangements to adjacent cells. Phase 4 diastolic depolarization is not limited to SAN cells. However, the SAN maintains dominance over latent pacemaker sites in the AVN and His–Purkinje system because it depolarizes more rapidly.

The rate of SAN depolarization is influenced by various factors. Electrotonic interactions between the cells of the SAN modulate the rate of spontaneous activity, so that faster discharging cells are slowed by cells that discharge more slowly and *vice versa*[3]. Another factor is the level of sympathetic and parasympathetic tone. Adrenergic stimulation speeds the sinus discharge rate. The vagus modulates cardiac sympathetic activity and leads to slowing of the SAN depolarization rate and prolongation of intranodal and sinoatrial conduction time up to the point of exit block. A third mechanism which is not completely understood is the so-called mechanical-electrical feedback, leading to an increase in heart rate in response to increased atrial pressure.

ATRIOVENTRICULAR NODE

In the absence of an accessory pathway, the AVN is the only normal electrical connection between the atria and the ventricles. Atrial connections to the AVN, the AVN itself, and the His bundle represent an intricate structure with complex electrophysiologic properties[4]. The atrial connections determine the particular pattern of atrial–AVN engagement and may be part of the anatomical substrate for dual pathway AVN physiology. At least two populations of isolated AVN cells (rod-shaped and ovoid) with distinct action potentials, ionic current profiles, and morphology significantly different from either atrial or ventricular myocytes, have been characterized[5]. Conduction through the AVN is much less rapid than conduction through the working muscle or the His–Purkinje system owing to slow Ca^{++}-dependent action potential conduction through at least a portion of the AVN tissue (**30**).

The electrical conduction properties of the AVN and other cardiac tissues are commonly studied during clinical electrophysiologic studies. The time between the onsets of the atrial and His spike (i.e. the AH interval) in the His bundle recording represents AVN conduction (**31**). The AVN exhibits decremental conduction properties, i.e. with rapid atrial pacing or premature atrial stimuli the AH interval increases and the delay is inversely related to the prematurity of the impulse. This phenomenon is related to slow recovery of excitability of AVN cells. The cellular response to a premature stimulus applied before full recovery exhibits decreased action potential amplitude and reduced rate of depolarization. Dual pathway AVN physiology manifests as sudden prolongation of the AH interval in response to a slightly more premature atrial stimulus, corresponding to change from fast pathway conduction to slow

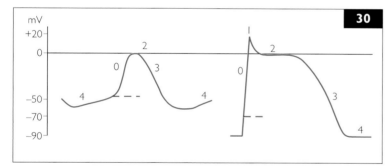

30 Two types of action potentials in cardiac cells and their phases. Slow Ca^{++}-dependent action potential of sinoatrial and atrioventricular nodal cells (left), in comparison to fast Na^+-dependent action potential of working myocardium and His–Purkinje system (right) shows spontaneous phase 4 depolarization, slow upstroke (phase 0), absence of phase 1, and virtual absence of plateau (phase 2). Resting potential is less negative.

31 Schematic diagram of the cardiac conduction system in relation to intracardiac recordings. The heart is shown in the right anterior oblique view. A, H, and V – atrial, His bundle, and ventricular activation in the His bundle electrogram; AH: AH interval; AVN: atrioventricular node; HB: His bundle electrogram (recording catheter position is depicted); HIS: His bundle; HRA: electrogram recorded from the high right atrium near the SAN; HV: HV interval; RA: right atrium; RBB: right bundle branch; RV: right ventricle; SAN: sinoatrial node.

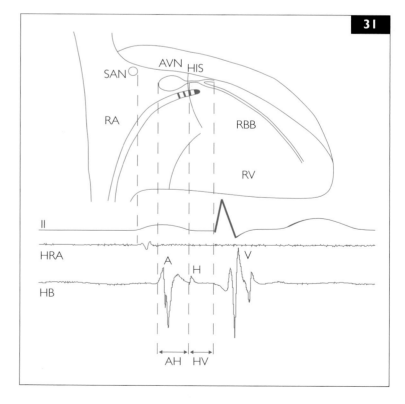

pathway conduction (**32**)[6]. This phenomenon is the physiologic basis for the establishment of slow–fast conduction reentry in AVN tachycardia.

As with the SAN, the AVN is rich in sympathetic and parasympathetic innervation and its conduction properties are exquisitely sensitive to changes in autonomic tone. Enhanced sympathetic and reduced parasympathetic activation shorten the AVN conduction time and refractory periods.

HIS–PURKINJE SYSTEM
Conduction through the His–Purkinje system is particularly rapid because the fibers here utilize fast Na^+-dependent action potentials and have the largest diameter and lowest longitudinal resistance which, according to cable theory, allows the fastest conduction (**30**). This leads, in the absence of conduction disturbances, to rapid almost simultaneous activation of the working ventricular muscle. Action potential duration and refractory periods gradually increase from proximal to the distal sites in the His–Purkinje system[7]. The His bundle is not affected by the level of autonomic tone and does not exhibit decremental conduction. The His–Purkinje system, however, may exhibit decremental conduction properties under certain conditions, such as ischemia and long QT syndrome[8]. Class I antiarrhythmic drugs are Na^+-channel blockers and slow phase 0 in the action potential, leading to slowed conduction speed. Excessive or toxic effects are seen in the surface electrocardiogram (ECG) as widening of the QRS complex. K^+-channel blockers (class III drugs) prolong the repolarization phase and thereby the refractory period; this effect is observed in the surface ECG as QT prolongation.

The time between the onset of the His spike in the His bundle recording and the earliest activation of the ventricles (onset of the QRS complex) is termed the HV interval (**31**). It represents the time required for the electrical impulse to conduct through the His–Purkinje system and has prognostic implications[9].

CLINICAL IMPLICATIONS
Myocardial ischemia may cause dysfunction of the conduction system either directly by ischemia of its components or by reflex mechanisms. Abnormal myocytes perfused by a normal (e.g. healed MI) or abnormal (e.g. acute myocardial ischemia and infarction) milieu display reduced resting membrane potentials. Reduced action potential amplitude and rate of depolarization follow and in turn lead to slowing of the propagated impulse up to the point of block. Any part of the conduction system may be affected and both acute and chronic ischemic syndromes may be the cause.

Coronary artery disease (CAD) has been implicated in the genesis of the sick sinus syndrome, although the causal relationship remains controversial[10–12]. Extrinsic SAN dysfunction may be caused by vagotonia with inferior MI, which is a manifestation of the Bezold–Jarisch reflex[13]. AVN conduction disturbances early in the course of inferior MI may also be caused by increase in vagal tone and usually respond to atropine. Later, AV block may be secondary to ischemia induced by occlusion of the AV nodal artery and is less sensitive to atropine[14]. In patients with anterior MI, conduction disturbances are usually distal to the AVN, are caused by ischemia of parts of the His–Purkinje system, and are an especially ominous sign (**33**)[15].

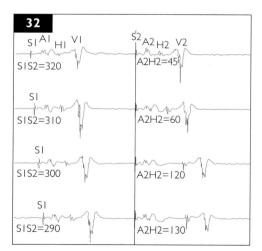

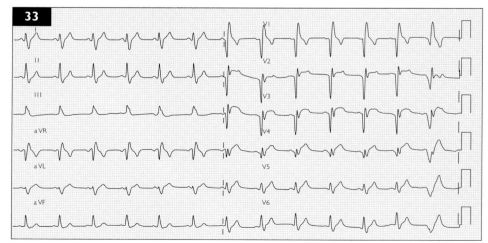

32 Decremental conduction properties of the atrioventricular node and dual pathway atrioventricular node physiology. After a fixed pacing drive (S1, only the last beat shown), a progressively premature impulse (S2) is introduced. His bundle recordings of four consecutive sequences, aligned for S2, are shown. Note gradual prolongation of the AH interval for the first two sequences and sudden 'jump' during the third, when the effective refractory period of the fast pathway is reached and conduction shifts to the slow pathway. A1, H1, V1, A2, H2, V2: atrial, His bundle, and ventricular activation of a basic cycle beat and premature beat, respectively (in milliseconds).

33 Electrocardiogram depicting acute anterior myocardial infarction due to occlusion of the left anterior descending coronary artery before the first septal perforating branch. Right bundle branch block (prolongation of the QRS complex to 120 ms with rSR′ pattern in lead V1) and left posterior fascicular block (right axis deviation) are present.

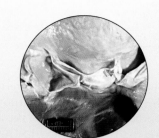

Chapter Four

Pathophysiology of Myocardial Ischemia

CORONARY ARTERY ANOMALIES

ALLEN J. TAYLOR, MD AND RENU VIRMANI, MD

INTRODUCTION

Coronary artery anomalies are rare. Since estimates of the prevalence of coronary artery anomalies are derived from autopsy or angiographic series, their true incidence is unknown. Coronary artery anomalies are found in approximately 1% of patients undergoing coronary angiography[1–3] and in approximately 0.3% of autopsies[4].

Although the majority of coronary anomalies are benign, some are a potential cause of cardiovascular morbidity and mortality. The described spectrum of symptoms arising from coronary anomalies includes angina, syncope, congestive heart failure, myocardial infarction, and sudden death[5]. Sudden cardiac death (SCD) is the most dramatic presentation for a Coronary anomaly. Coronary artery anomalies are particularly prevalent among young patients with sports-related SCD (*Table 2*).

CLINICAL PRESENTATION

In general, coronary artery anomalies may present with symptoms that include angina, shortness of breath, and syncope. More severe presentations include clinical syndromes of either myocardial infarction (MI), congestive heart failure, or SCD, generally occurring during or shortly after strenuous physical exertion. Overall, symptoms are present in approximately one-third of patients. In the Armed Forces Institute Pathology (AFIP) pathology series[5] the majority of cases with sudden death (62%) were asymptomatic. Symptoms were most commonly reported in cases of ectopic origin of the left main from the right aortic sinus (50%). In comparison, no patients with ectopic origin of the right coronary artery (RCA) were symptomatic. This suggests that a greater extent of myocardium at risk, such as in cases of anomalous left main origin or when the anomalous vessel is dominant in the coronary circulation[6], can determine symptoms and outcomes.

ANOMALOUS ORIGIN OF ONE OR MORE CORONARY ARTERIES FROM THE AORTA

Left main and right coronary artery from the right aortic sinus
Anomalous origin of the left main from the right aortic sinus (**34, 35**) is classified further based on the course of the anomalous artery: (a) between the aorta and pulmonary trunk; (b) anterior to the

Table 2 Coronary artery anomalies

Definition
- Abnormalities in the origin, course, or distribution of the coronary arterial circulation.

Key features
- Rare form of congenital heart disease affecting approximately 1% of the population.
- Second most common cause of sports-related sudden cardiac death in the young.
- Many are benign, but some, particularly origin of the left or right coronary artery from the contralateral coronary cusp, are potentially serious.
- Clinical presentations of coronary anomalies range from asymptomatic to angina, myocardial infarction, congestive heart failure, and sudden cardiac death.

Therapy
- Surgical correction generally indicated for serious anomalies when causing symptoms or when identified in youth.

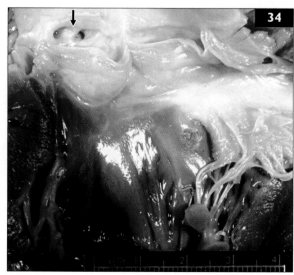

34 View of the left ventricular outflow tract and aorta of a 14-year-old boy who died suddenly while playing soccer, showing left and right coronary ostia arising from the right coronary sinus (arrow).

pulmonary trunk; (c) posterior to the aorta; and (d) posterior to the right ventricular outflow tract within the interventricular septum. In 60% of cases, the anomalous left main most commonly courses between the aorta and pulmonary trunk[5]. This anomaly accounts for 2.8% of serious coronary anomalies, and occurs with an incidence of 1 in 12,500[3]. Although this anomaly is relatively uncommon in angiographic series, it is significantly overrepresented in pathology series because of its clear association with SCD. SCD is most common (82%) when the anomalous artery courses between the aorta and pulmonary trunk[5].

Left main and right coronary artery from the left aortic sinus

Anomalous origin of the RCA from the left aortic sinus (**36**, **37**) is the most common and potentially serious coronary artery anomaly, accounting for 8.1% of serious coronary anomalies[3]. Such an anomaly is more than twice as common as anomalous origin of the left main or left anterior descending (LAD) arteries. Sudden death is observed in approximately 25% of cases, with roughly half of these in association with exercise[5].

DIAGNOSIS AND PATHOPHYSIOLOGY

Increasingly, noninvasive imaging modalities are used to diagnose coronary anomalies. Modalities include transesophageal echocardiography, magnetic resonance imaging (MRI), and electron beam computed tomography (CT). There are a number of candidate pathologic variables of significance in cases of an anomalous coronary artery arising from the contralateral coronary sinus and coursing between the great vessels[7]. These include the size of the slit-like coronary orifice (transverse ostial dimension), the angle at which the anomalous coronary artery arises from the aorta, the distance that the coronary artery is contained within the aortic wall, fibrous ridges at the coronary ostium, and degree of displacement of the anomalous artery from the appropriate coronary sinus. Theoretically, some of the variables, if more severe, could predispose patients to SCD, and therefore provide insight into prognosis. However, a recent study found no differences in the severity of these variables in patients with and without anomaly-related SCD[8]. Furthermore, these pathologic features showed a high degree of variability between patients (**38**). Thus, the accurate identification of patients at increased risk of SCD will be difficult at best.

ORIGIN OF THE LEFT MAIN CORONARY ARTERY FROM THE PULMONARY TRUNK

This rare anomaly is the most common anomaly involving a coronary artery arising from the pulmonary trunk. It is very commonly fatal[9], including a predominance of death during early childhood from myocardial ischemia and systolic dysfunc-tion, resulting in congestive heart failure and sudden death. Electrocardiographic findings, including broad, deep Q waves can aid in the differentiation of this anomaly from myocarditis or dilated cardiomyopathy[10]. In a minority of cases (approximately 20%), sufficient myocardial collaterals develop from the normally-arising RCA, and survival into adulthood may occur. In these cases, a continuous murmur may be present and symptoms (angina pectoris, MI, dyspnea, syncope, and sudden death) are generally present[11–14]. Angiography accurately diagnoses this anomaly, with the demonstration of collateral channels from the RCA to the left coronary system with drainage to the pulmonary trunk. Ischemia arises from either shunting of blood into the pulmonary trunk or insufficient myocardial blood flow from some other mechanism[14].

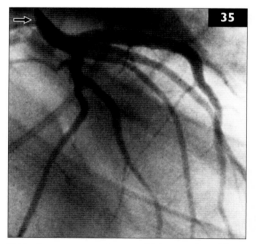
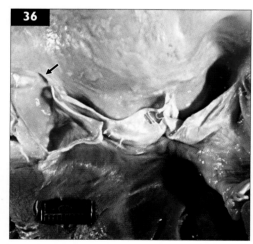
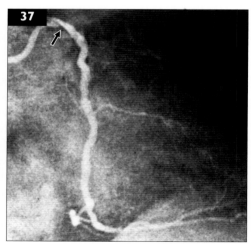

35 Left coronary angiogram (right anterior oblique projection) of an anomalous left main coronary artery from the right coronary sinus. The presence of a crescent-shaped orifice (arrow) suggests the presence of an ostial ridge. (From Taylor *et al.* [1997]. Myocardial infarction associated with physical exertion in a young man [clinical conference]. *Circulation* **96**:3201–3204.)

36 View of the left ventricular outflow tract and aorta showing left and right coronary arteries arising from the left coronary sinus. A slit-like coronary orifice and ostial ridge are present at the right coronary ostium (arrow).

37 Left coronary angiogram (right anterior oblique projection) showing an anomalous right coronary artery arising from the left coronary sinus. The proximal right coronary artery is visibly narrowed (arrow) from the slit-like coronary orifice and aortic intramural course.

Echocardiography can also diagnose this anomaly, through demonstration of an enlarged RCA relative to the aortic size[15], and by abnormal flow on Doppler echocardiography[16,17]. Treatment for this anomaly involves surgical closure of the left main artery with or without a concomitant bypass graft to the LAD. An alternative procedure is primary reanastomosis of the anomalous artery from the pulmonary trunk to the aorta or subclavian artery[11]. Since there is a persistent risk for late cardiac death after left main artery ligation alone, the definitive approach for long-term survival involves establishment of a two-coronary artery system with reimplantation techniques. Long-term results from these procedures appear favorable[18].

SINGLE CORONARY ARTERY

The coronary circulation may be entirely supplied by a single coronary artery arising from either the right, left, or posterior aortic sinus. The course of the coronary arteries can be highly variable. Single coronary artery is uncommon as an isolated, congenital coronary anomaly, occurring in 1 in 2250 patients undergoing angiography[3]. In a compilation of 142 cases, there was an approximately equal distribution between origin from the right and left coronary sinus[19]. Single coronary artery can be associated with sudden death (6 of 44 cases [14%] in the AFIP series)[5], with a greater incidence of sudden death when the single coronary artery arises from the right aortic sinus. Since there is no currently available option for surgical correction of this anomaly, the use of medications to treat ischemic heart disease should be considered.

MANAGEMENT

In the past, the diagnosis of a coronary artery anomaly was most frequently made in symptomatic patients or as an autopsy finding in cases of sudden death. In the future, it is reasonable to anticipate that an increasing number of patients will be prospectively and coincidentally identified with these anomalies by cardiovascular imaging procedures such as echocardiography and electron beam CT. The management of these cases will be difficult in the absence of controlled data to guide treatment decisions, for example whether patients undergo surgical correction of coronary anomalies. Surgically-correctable anomalies include anomalous origin of one or more coronary artery from the pulmonary trunk, and ectopic origin of a coronary artery from the aorta. All patients with origin of a coronary artery from the pulmonary trunk should be strongly considered for surgical correction. In contrast, management decisions in cases of ectopic coronary artery origin can be difficult. Case series clearly document heterogeneity in the clinical course of patients with anomalous RCA or LCA. Thus, while some patients die suddenly, others can live a normal lifespan with an unrepaired anomalous coronary artery[20,21].

The precise risk for SCD in an individual patient is difficult to determine, and thus management decisions should be highly individualized. In the asymptomatic patient, considerations in the decision on 'prophylactic' correction include the known risk for SCD, the inability to risk-stratify the patient by morphologic criteria, and patient age. While the need for prophylactic surgical correction is most compelling in a young patient, there is little question that anomaly-related SCD can occur regardless of patient age. However, this risk does appear to decrease with advancing age. Overall, it is

likely that the risk for SCD attributable to the coronary anomaly in an older patient is low, although the precise magnitude of risk is unknown due to the influence of selection bias and unknown denominator size in an autopsy series. How to relate this risk to the risk of surgical correction with coronary bypass surgery is unknown and should be a highly individualized decision in an older, asymptomatic patient[22,23]. The impact of symptoms on risk for SCD is unknown. When symptoms are present, the argument supporting surgical correction is aided by the goal of symptom relief. Lastly, for the patient with an uncorrected coronary artery anomaly arising from the contralateral coronary sinus and coursing between the aorta and pulmonary trunk, avoidance of strenuous activity may be prudent given the known propensity for SCD to occur in relation to exercise.

SUMMARY

Coronary artery anomalies are a rare form of congenital heart disease affecting approximately 1% of the population (*Table 2*). They encompass a wide range of abnormalities in the origin, course, or distribution of the coronary arterial circulation. Most coronary anomalies are benign, but some, including origin of a coronary artery from the pulmonary trunk, ectopic origin of a coronary artery, and single coronary artery can result in cardiovascular symptoms and even SCD. The pathophysiology of symptoms lies in abnormalities in coronary flow including shunting (in cases with the origin of a coronary artery from the pulmonary trunk), and limited coronary flow reserve (in cases with ectopic coronary artery origin). Surgical correction is generally indicated for patients with symptoms or when these anomalies are identified in youth.

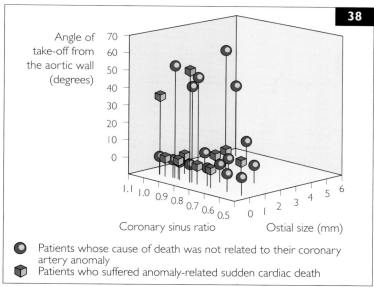

38 Three-dimensional plot of anatomic variables: ostial size (mm), coronary sinus ratio (calculated as the distance from the nearest commissure of the noncoronary cusp to the center of the anomalous coronary ostium divided by the size of the coronary sinus of origin), and angle of take-off from the aortic wall (degrees) for all cases of anomalous right or left coronary artery from the contralateral coronary sinus. (From Taylor *et al.* [1997]. Anomalous right or left coronary artery from the contralateral coronary sinus: 'high-risk' abnormalities in the initial coronary artery course and heterogeneous clinical outcomes. *Am. Heart J.* **133**:428–435[24].)

ANEROBIC MYOCARDIAL METABOLISM

FRANS C. VISSER, MD, PhD

INTRODUCTION

In contrast to skeletal muscle, which derives its energy almost exclusively from oxidation of glucose, the heart is able to use a large variety of substrates[1]. Glucose, pyruvate, fatty acids, lactate, ketone bodies, and even amino acids can all be used for oxidative metabolism. In general, the substrate with the highest concentration is preferentially used. For example, after a carbohydrate-rich meal glucose is the main source of energy. In contrast, during fasting when fatty acid levels are high, fatty acids are mainly oxidized. During exercise, when lactate is released by skeletal muscles, this substrate is mainly used. Overall, however, the main energy sources under normal conditions are glucose and fatty acids. The energy metabolism of the heart is more dependent on fatty acid metabolism than on glucose metabolism because glucose oxidation is inhibited by metabolites of fatty acid metabolism. Both fatty acids and glucose not only are oxidized but a variable amount can be stored, as triglycerides and glycogen respectively.

After a series of metabolic steps each substrate is converted into acetyl-coenzyme A (acetyl-CoA), and enters the final common pathway, the citric acid cycle (Krebs cycle). In the citric acid cycle the energy of acetyl-CoA is transformed to energy-rich phosphate bonds (ATP) using oxygen (**39**). This process takes place in the mitochondria; oxidation of one molecule of glucose yields 38 ATP molecules, one molecule of lactate yields 18 ATP molecules, and the fatty acid molecule palmitate yields 129 ATP molecules. Although fatty acids are the major source for energy production, metabolism of fatty acids requires more oxygen than glucose and as such are less efficient substrates than glucose.

CARDIAC ENERGY METABOLISM DURING ISCHEMIA

Ischemia is a condition in which the flow and supply of oxygen is inadequate for the demand of the tissue. Ischemia causes profound alterations in metabolism. Fatty acid oxidation is reduced or stops and free fatty acids and metabolites such as fatty acids bound to acetyl-CoA accumulate in the myocardium. Triglyceride content in the myocardium is also increased. The accumulation of these metabolites is detrimental as they may cause arrhythmias and cause breakdown of phospholipids, a major component of the cellular membranes. Oxidation of glucose is reduced and anaerobic glycolysis is increased (**40**). Glycolysis indicates the process of metabolic steps leading to the formation of lactate during ischemia. The glycolytic pathways use two ATP molecules and produce four ATP, thus the net production is two ATP. When glycogen is the source of glucose (glycogenolysis), three ATP molecules are produced. However, the side-effect of this anaerobic glycolysis is the formation of lactate and protons (H^+), which lower the intracellular pH and inhibit enzyme activity. For anaerobic glycolysis to produce as much ATP as is produced during aerobic oxidation of glucose, an increase in the ATP production rate of almost 20 times is needed, which is unrealistic.

Nevertheless, ischemia has a biphasic effect on glycolysis. During mild ischemia glucose uptake and glycolysis are enhanced, leading to an increase in anaerobic ATP production. The end products, lactate and protons, are washed out of the cell. The

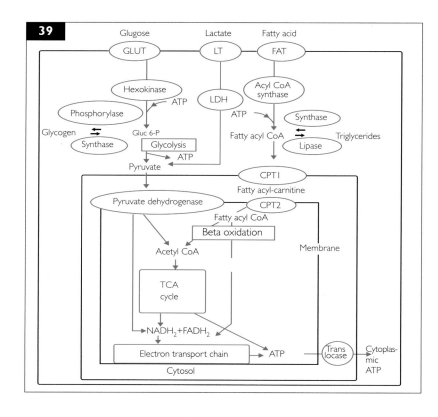

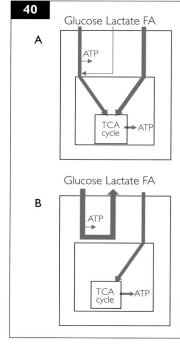

39 Schematic representation of energy metabolism pathways under normal oxygen conditions. CPT 1,2: carnitine palmitoyl transferase 1,2; FAT: fatty acid transporter; Gluc 6-P: glucose-6-phosphate; GLUT: glucose transporter; LDH: lactate dehydrogenase; LT: lactate transporter; $NADH_2$: nicotinamide adenine dinucleotide; TCA: tricarboxylic acid.

40 Changes in metabolism during mild/moderate ischemia (**B**) compared with normal conditions (**A**). The same format as in **39** is used. Arrows indicate the contributions of the different nutrients to adenosine triphosphate (ATP) production.

benefit of this anaerobic glycolysis is increased ATP production, yet the amount is insufficient to maintain the energy needs of the normally contracting myocardium. Therefore, contractile dysfunction occurs. It must be remembered that the formation of ATP by glycolysis does not occur in the mitochondria. It is postulated that formation of ATP occurs near the cell membrane (sarcolemma) and may help to maintain crucial membrane functions such as the maintenance of Na^+ and K^+ gradients (ATP-sensitive Na^+/K^+ pumps).

Under normal conditions, fatty acid oxidation inhibits glucose oxidation. The same mechanism is present during ischemia. If there is residual oxidation, fatty acids effectively compete with glucose for the residual oxygen. Since fatty acid oxidation is less efficient, relatively more glycolysis is needed for the same (i.e. diminished) ATP production. Moreover, the acidosis itself results in sodium and calcium accumulation. This requires more energy (ATP) for homeostasis, aggravating the cardiac inefficiency.

During an episode of severe ischemia, flow is inadequate for washout of metabolites. Thus protons, CO_2, lactate, and $NADH_2$ accumulate inside the cell with resulting severe acidosis inside the cell. Moreover, the metabolites themselves inhibit glycosis. If severe ischemia persists or no reperfusion is attained, metabolism enters a negative spiral and ultimately the cell is irreversibly damaged, resulting in necrosis.

CLINICAL IMPLICATIONS

The understanding of cardiac metabolism is used both for diagnostic purposes and for therapeutic interventions.

Diagnostic purposes

As mentioned above lactate is produced by anaerobic glycolysis during ischemia and is washed out of the cell. This lactate release can be sampled during catheterization, when arterial and coronary venous blood samples are simultaneously taken during provocation of ischemia by pacing. However, this technique is not frequently used because the procedure is invasive, difficult, and expensive, the sensitivity of the test is limited, and because there are other established techniques such as flow-velocity reserve and fractional flow reserve.

Another approach is to label glucose and fatty acids with radioactive isotopes which can then be visualized using a conventional gamma camera or positron emission tomograph (PET)[2]. Indeed, radiolabeled glucose and fatty acids have given important information about the pathophysiology of myocardial ischemia, infarction, hypertrophy, and cardiomyopathies in humans. Also, radiolabeled acetate imagin (a precursor of acetyl-CoA) reflects the turnover rate of the citric acid cycle and therefore regional myocardial oxygen consumption. Moreover, glucose imaging with ^{18}F-fluorodeoxyglucose (FDG) is an established technique to assess myocardial viability, with a sensitivity of 88% and a specificity of 73% to detect improvement of left ventricular function after revascularization. Also fatty acid uptake may be used to detect myocardial viability, but this approach is less validated than FDG[3]. Examples of glucose and fatty acid uptake in the myocardium are given (**41**, **42**).

Therapeutic purposes

There are now metabolic agents (trimetazidine and ranolazine) which interact with cardiac metabolism without any hemodynamic effect. Experimental studies with trimetazidine have shown that it partially inhibits fatty acid oxidation and increases glucose oxidation[4]. Both agents decrease objective and subjective signs of ischemia in patients with exercise-induced ischemia.

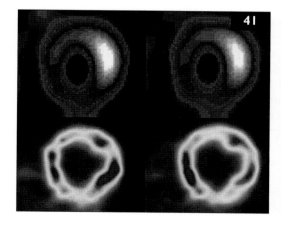

41 Short-axis slice imaging of glucose uptake (FDG) in the myocardium. **Upper**: Perfusion abnormalities in the anterior wall, septum, and inferior wall in a patient with previous anterior and inferior infarction. **Lower**: FDG positron emission tomography shows relatively increased uptake of FDG in areas with perfusion abnormalities, indicating the presence of viable tissue. FDG: fluorodeoxyglucose.

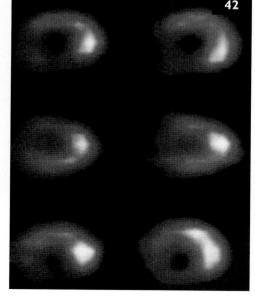

42 Short-axis slice imaging of glucose uptake (FDG) and fatty acid uptake of a modified fatty acid (betamethyl-iodo-phenylpentadecanoic acid:BMIPPA) in the myocardium. **Upper**: Perfusion abnormalities in the septum and inferior wall in a patient with previous inferior infarction. **Middle**: Increased uptake of FDG in the inferior wall, indicating presence of viable tissue using SPECT. **Lower**: BMIPPA uptake in the same area; inferior wall and septum uptake is lower compared to perfusion and FDG uptake, a sign of viable tissue. FDG: fluorodeoxyglucose; SPECT: single photon emission computerized tomography.

COLLATERAL DEVELOPMENT

STEVE LEE, MD, RAJENDRA MAKKAR, MD AND WILLIAM GANZ, MD

INTRODUCTION

Coronary collaterals are vascular pathways that help supply blood to the myocardium in the setting of severe ischemia. They are a common finding at angiography in patients with coronary stenoses, and can help limit the severity of myocardial ischemia and infarction by providing an alternative supply of blood to the jeopardized myocardium. Collaterals exist in many different animal species, and have been known for quite some time to exist in humans. More recently, details regarding their physiology and development have been elucidated.

Collaterals are now known to be preexisting conduits that are closed under normal conditions, but in the setting of ischemia open and develop rapidly to provide a channel for blood flow from a coronary artery to the ischemic coronary artery. Prior to the maturation of these collaterals, the preexisting structures are not angiographically visible, although they have been demonstrated on autopsy. At least a 90% stenosis of a coronary artery is required before a coronary collateral will open and develop.

MECHANISM OF COLLATERAL FORMATION

Once a significant stenosis develops, a series of changes occur within the collateral that ultimately leads to the development of a mature coronary vessel. Under normal circumstances when coronary blood flow is not significantly limited, there is no pressure gradient between coronary arteries; therefore the preexisting collateral channels between them remain closed. However, when a coronary occlusion occurs, the pressure distal to the occlusion drops and therefore a pressure gradient between arteries develops, causing the collaterals to open almost immediately. These collaterals progressively dilate and soon are visible angiographically.

The process of collateral maturation from a closed pre-existing structure to a fully developed vascular conduit occurs in three stages. The first stage occurs in the first 24 hours and involves passive widening of the collateral vessel with concomitant increased blood flow. This increased blood flow leads to activation of the endothelium and the secretion of proteolytic enzymes, which then dissolve local tissue and create space for the developing vessels. The second stage occurs in the next 3 weeks and is marked by an inflammatory response during which monocytes secrete cytokines and growth factors, leading to cellular proliferation. The third stage occurs in the next 6 months and involves further cellular proliferation and vessel thickening, ultimately leading to a vessel with a normal three-layer structure and vasoactive properties similar to a normal coronary artery. Mature coronary collaterals can reach up to 1 mm in luminal diameter.

CLINICAL SIGNIFICANCE

The clinical benefits of coronary collaterals are numerous and are predicated on the provision of an alternative supply of blood to myocardium that would otherwise be compromised (**43, 44**). It is not uncommon for patients to be found at angiography to have a high-grade stenosis in a major coronary artery but yet have relatively minor clinical symptoms because of the existence of a well-developed collateral supply of blood. In studies such as the Thrombolysis in Myocardial Infarction (TIMI) phase I trial, the existence of coronary collaterals has been shown to decrease the size of MI following a coronary occlusion and to improve left ventricular (LV) function after infarction. Collaterals also decrease the chance of LV aneurysm formation, improve long-term survival, decrease the likelihood of subsequent infarction, and improve the likelihood of successful coronary bypass surgery. Studies have also shown that in chronic total occlusion of coronary arteries, collaterals can provide complete preservation of myocardium.

The significance of coronary collateral vessels can further be inferred from animal studies in which species such as pigs, which have essentially no collaterals, develop significant myocardial infarction following coronary artery occlusion. However, guinea pigs, which have a very well developed system of collaterals, develop essentially no infarction following coronary artery occlusion. In humans, patients with diabetes mellitus have a reduced ability to develop coronary collaterals in the setting of myocardial ischemia. It is not clear why some patients are able to develop effective coronary collaterals to ischemic vessels whereas other patients cannot.

Once developed, coronary collaterals have been demonstrated to regress once blood flow is restored through the ischemic lesion. Studies have shown that the same collaterals may then reappear if myocardial ischemia redevelops. However, patients have been reported to suffer MI without the redevelopment of previously established collateral bridging as early as 1 month following percutaneous transluminal angioplasty.

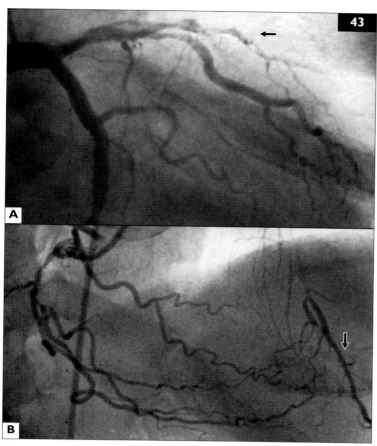

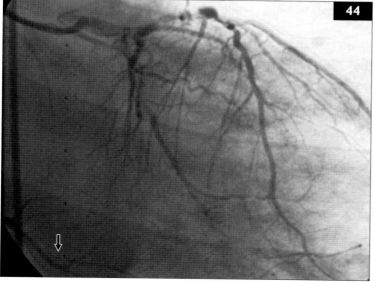

43 A: Severely diseased left anterior descending coronary artery (arrow).
B: Collateral bridging from the right coronary artery to the distal left anterior descending artery (arrow).

44 Collateral bridging to the right coronary artery (arrow) from the left anterior descending coronary artery, which is itself diseased.

PRECONDITIONING, STUNNING, AND HIBERNATION

SRIRAM PADMANABHAN, MD, MS, HOWARD LEWIN, MD AND PREDIMAN K. SHAH, MD, FACC

ISCHEMIC PRECONDITIONING

A large number of recent experimental studies have shown that short periods of coronary occlusion before a more sustained coronary artery occlusion (lasting 1.5–3 hours followed by reperfusion) result in a substantive reduction in myocardial infarct size, independent of collateral flow. These observations have led to the concept that brief episodes of myocardial ischemia protect the myocardium against subsequent prolonged myocardial ischemia, a phenomenon labeled 'ischemic preconditioning'.

Two types of preconditioning have been described, classic (early) and delayed. In classic preconditioning, myocardial protection occurs if the longer occlusion occurs within 5–60 minutes after brief occlusive episodes. However, this effect wanes and then disappears if the duration between brief and long occlusions is extended to a few hours. In delayed preconditioning, protection returns if the long occlusion is made 24–96 hours after the brief occlusions. This is also referred to as the second window of protection, and may involve different mechanisms compared with classic preconditioning. The precise biochemical mediators of this interesting phenomenon are not fully understood; potential mediators include activation of an energy-sparing ATP-activated potassium channel, slowing of glycolysis with attenuation of intracellular acidosis, and molecular adaptation with induction of heat shock protein (*Table 3*).

The evidence for the existence of the phenomenon of ischemic preconditioning in humans is mostly indirect. For example, the reduced infarct size, better preserved ventricular function, and lower mortality of Q wave acute MI patients in whom the infarction was preceded by preinfarction angina (the clinical surrogate for brief periods of ischemia) compared with those without antecedent preinfarction angina, represent a potential example of ischemic preconditioning. Similarly, angina early during exercise necessitating a brief rest followed by resumption of activity without further angina (so-called 'warm-up phenomenon') may represent yet another clinical manifestation of ischemic pre-

Table 3 Potential molecular mechanisms of ischemic preconditioning

- Second-messenger pathways involving adenosine receptors, G proteins, PKC isoforms, and ATP-dependent potassium channels.
- Heat shock proteins.
- Nitric oxide.

conditioning (*Table 4*). Another example of clinical ischemic preconditioning may be the observation that during repeated balloon inflation during coronary angioplasty, ST elevation, chest pain, and lactate production are reduced on subsequent inflations.

STUNNED MYOCARDIUM

Numerous studies have demonstrated that brief episodes of severe myocardial ischemia can lead to prolonged systolic and diastolic dysfunction that outlasts the duration of ischemia, a state referred to as myocardial stunning (**45**). This phenomenon results in prolonged myocardial dysfunction with gradual but eventual recovery over hours, days, or weeks. The intensity and duration of ischemia appear to be the major determinants of the degree of postischemic reversible dysfunction. Despite lack of contractile function at rest after termination of myocardial ischemia, the myocardium remains responsive to inotropic stimulation. Stunned myocardium is typified by normal or near normal regional blood flow. Thus, there is a mismatch between flow and function such that despite restoration of flow, function remains depressed. Clinically, myocardial stunning is often seen during unstable angina as a result of intermittent episodes of ischemia at rest, after an acute MI accompanied by spontaneous or therapeutic reperfusion with delayed recovery of function, after ischemic cardiac arrest during cardiopulmonary bypass and cardiac surgery, and in some cases after cardiac arrest. Stunning can also be demonstrated in patients undergoing stress testing, where ischemia-induced wall-motion abnormalities may last 30 minutes or more after test completion (**46**). In the patient in **46**, although wall motion was normal prior to stress testing, it became abnormal during stress testing and remained abnormal for several minutes after the stress test was over. Wall-motion analysis after stress testing showed moderate–severe hypokinesis of the same areas, which is representative of poststress stunning. Coronary angiography showed a subtotal occlusion in the LAD.

Ischemia during coronary angioplasty is usually too short to induce stunning characterized by systolic dysfunction, but brief balloon inflations may induce prolonged diastolic dysfunction. An experimental clinical study demonstrated that angioplasty consisting of prolonged (5 minutes) balloon inflation resulted in systolic stunning, requiring up to 36 hours for recovery. The precise mechanism responsible for prolonged dysfunction after relief of ischemia is not known, although increased cytosolic calcium and free-radical formation upon reperfusion has been postulated to be one potential mechanism.

CHRONIC MYOCARDIAL ISCHEMIA AND HIBERNATING MYOCARDIUM

Chronic or repetitive reduction of myocardial perfusion because of severe coronary stenoses or collateralized total occlusion may lead to depressed contractile function and adaptive changes in myocardial metabolism, resulting in a state of myocardial 'hibernation' with noncontractile but viable myocardium (**47**). Proof of viability is provided if these nonfunctional myocardial

---

Table 4 Potential clinical correlates of ischemic preconditioning

- ANGINA: Angina patients often exhibit the 'warm up' phenomenon where exertional angina, followed by rest for a few minutes, permits them to continue the activity without further angina. This 'warm up' phenomenon may represent ischemic preconditioning.
- ANGIOPLASTY: Repeated angioplasty balloon inflations in the coronaries reduce the degree of chest pain, ST segment elevation, and lactate production. This phenomenon is independent of coronary collateral flow recruitment.
- THROMBOLYIS: In several thrombolytic trials, preinfarct angina was associated with smaller infarcts, less in-hospital mortality, fewer arrhythmias and improved LV function. Preinfarct angina may represent episodes of brief ischemic preconditioning or may have enhanced thrombolysis.
- CABG and MI: Adenosine, a preconditioning mimetic agent, administered prior to CABG, reduced the need for high-dose inotropic agents intra- and post-operatively. In the AMISTAD I trial, adenosine administered to AMI patients reduced infarct size in patients with anterior infarctions.

---

segments recover their contractile function when blood flow is restored through revascularization. From a clinical standpoint, patients with coronary artery disease with severely depressed ventricular function and chronic congestive heart failure may benefit both symptomatically and with an improved prognosis with revascularization, when noninvasive imaging studies provide evidence of viability in noncontractile myocardial segments. A number of noninvasive techniques are used to assess myocardial viability in poorly functioning myocardial segments. These include: (i) rest and redistribution or reinjection myocardial perfusion imaging with various radioactive perfusion tracers such as thallium 201 or technetium sestamibi, showing tracer uptake in areas of reduced function as a marker of viability; (ii) positron emission tomography (PET) using radiolabeled ammonia (NH_3) to assess myocardial blood flow and radiolabeled FDG to assess myocardial metabolism, with viable areas showing reduced flow and function with intact metabolism (**48**). A perfusion–metabolism mismatch is suggestive of viable but ischemic myocardium (hibernating myocardium); (iii) low-dose dobutamine and contrast echocardiography to demonstrate contractile reserve upon inotropic stimulation; myocardium that does not contract at rest, but contracts with low-dose dobutamine, suggests viability. However, high-dose dobutamine can worsen ischemia. This biphasic response to dobutamine is highly suggestive of tissue viability and hibernating myocardium, and may indicate the need for revascularization.

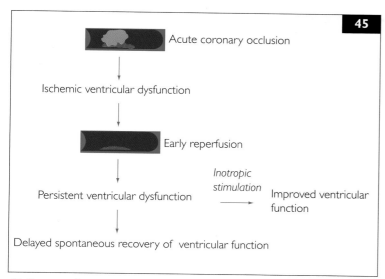

45 Conceptual model of myocardial stunning.

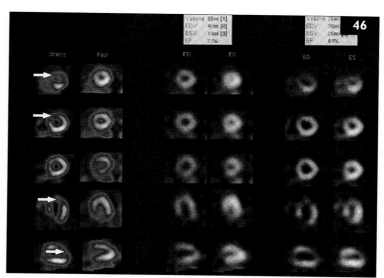

46 Perfusion images during stress sestamibi myocardial imaging show severe perfusion defects in the anterior, septal, and apical regions (white arrows), representative of left anterior descending artery ischemia.

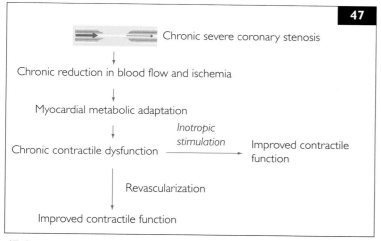

47 Conceptual model of hibernating myocardium and its detection by noninvasive imaging.

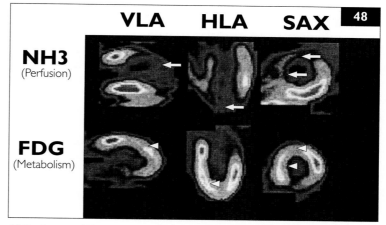

48 Positron emission tomography imaging for myocardial viability in a 58-year-old male with a history of myocardial infarction and coronary artery bypass graft, who presented with chronic heart failure. Perfusion imaging using ^{13}N ammonia (NH$_3$; top row) showed an extensive and severe perfusion defect involving the apex, anterior, and septal walls (white arrows). Metabolic images using 18-fluorodeoxyglucose (FDG; bottom row) demonstrated disproportionately enhanced uptake when compared to the perfusion study (white arrows). HLA: horizontal long axis; VLA: vertical long-axis; SAX: short-axis.

Other noninvasive methods available to identify hibernating myocardium include cardiac MRI (**49**) and rest-redistribution thallium imaging (**50**).

CLINICAL IMPLICATIONS

Preconditioning-mimetic pharmacologic agents are being studied for their potential to limit ischemic damage. Recent trials with adenosine administered prior to coronary artery bypass graft (CABG), reduced the need for high-dose inotropic agents. In the AMISTAD-1 study, adenosine administered to acute MI patients reduced infarct size in patients with anterior infarctions. An ongoing trial, AMISTAD-2, is investigating the effects of adenosine on outcomes after acute MI.

There are several areas where administration of such agents would be potentially beneficial: administering these agents prior to a known episode of ischemia or low flow (e.g. prior to cardiopulmonary bypass); prior to a heart being removed for transplantation; during unstable angina; and in patients with threatened MI may result in clinical benefit. In chronic stable angina, an adequate warm-up phase prior to vigorous exertion may help by stimulating preconditioning.

In the past, LV regional wall-motion abnormality was thought to represent infarcted/scarred myocardium or acute ischemia. It is now understood that other conditions involving viable myocardium can be associated with regional wall-motion abnormalities. In both stunning and hibernation, the myocardium can be stimulated to contract with appropriate inotropic interventions such as dopamine, dobutamine, and postextrasystolic potentiation. In several clinical situations, stunning may need to be treated temporarily with inotropic agents if it is contributing to acute hemodynamic compromise. This may occur after cardiopulmonary bypass, after cardiac arrest, or following reperfusion therapy for acute MI.

In severe chronic heart failure associated with ischemic heart disease, it becomes imperative to diagnose nonfunctional but viable myocardium using noninvasive techniques, since revascularization may provide significant improvement. Patients who have evidence of chronic wall-motion abnormalities and reduced blood flow and tissue viability have a high likelihood of recovering function following revascularization. Areas that lack tissue viability in general do not recover function following revascularization. **51** represents a meta-analysis of PET (see Chapter 8, Positron Emission Tomography), single photon emission computerized tomography (SPECT; see Chapter 8, Myocardial Scintigraphy) using thallium 201, and dobutamine echocardiography for detection of viable (hibernating) myocardium and prediction of improved regional LV function after revascularization.

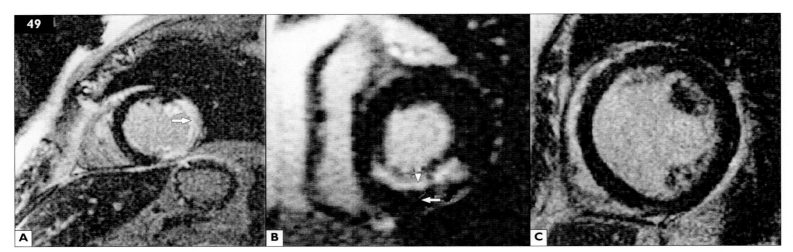

49 Assessment of viability by contrast MRI. **A**: a transmural infarct, involving the left circumflex territory, which has taken up gadolinium-diethylenetriamine penta acetic acid (Gd-DTPA) in its entire thickness (arrow), leaving no viable tissue in the infarcted region. **B**: a subendocardial infarction (arrow head) in the inferior-posterior wall. Only one-third of the wall has taken up contrast, suggesting necrotic tissue. The rest is viable tissue (arrow). **C**: no enhancement of myocardial tissue in a patient with dilated cardiomyopathy, suggesting a nonischemic pathology.

50 Rest-redistribution Tl-201 imaging for viability. A resting Tl-201 scan showed perfusion defects (arrow heads) in the apical and distal anterior segments. A 24-hour redistribution scan was performed which showed filling in of the defects seen in the resting scan (white arrows). This is suggestive of viable myocardium (hibernating myocardium).

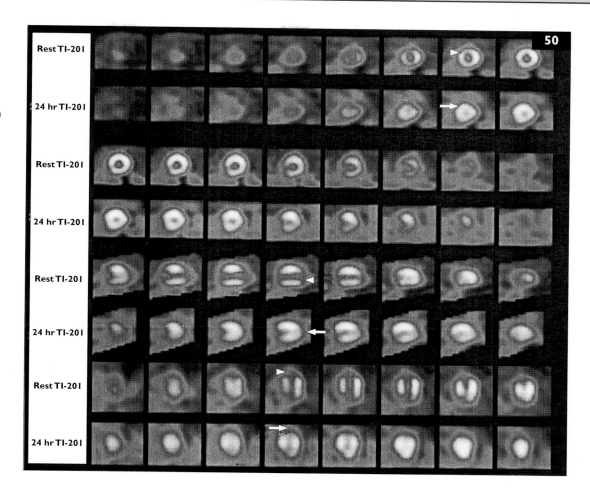

51 Comparison of noninvasive methods for detection of nonfunctional but viable myocardium that improves with revascularization. PET: positron emission tomography; SPECT: thallium single photon emission computerized tomography. (Modified from Bonow [1996]. Identification of viable myocardium. *Circulation* **94**:2674–2680.)

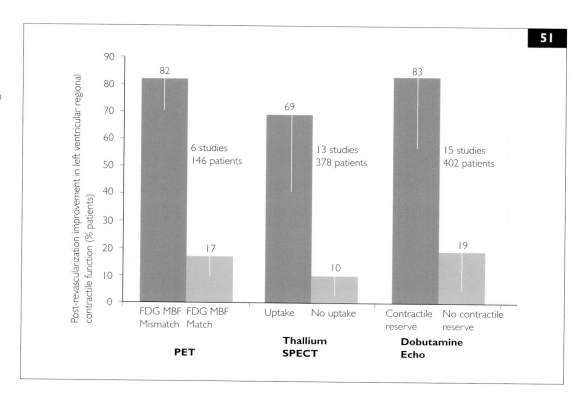

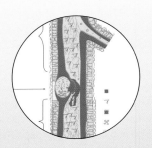

Chapter Five

Myocardial Ischemia: Compromised Supply

ATHEROTHROMBOSIS

JENS FLENSTED LASSEN, MD, PhD AND ERLING FALK, MD, PhD

DEFINITION

Atherosclerosis is a chronic and multi-focal immuno-inflammatory disease fueled by lipids[1–3]. It affects primarily the intima of medium-sized and large arteries, resulting in intimal thickening that may lead to luminal narrowing and inadequate blood supply. As the name implies, mature atherosclerotic plaques consist typically of two main components: one is lipid-rich and soft (*athére* is Greek for gruel or porridge) and the other is collagen-rich and hard (*skleros* is Greek for hard) (**52**).

Thrombosis is defined as the formation of a solid mass within the bloodstream during life from components of the blood.

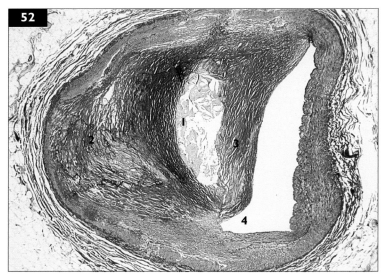

52 In coronary atherosclerosis, atherosclerotic plaques consist typically of two main components: one is lipid-rich and soft (*athére*: 1) and the other is collagen-rich and hard (*skleros*: 2). The soft lipid-rich core is separated from the lumen by a cap of fibrous tissue: (3). (Trichrome stain, rendering collagen blue and lipid colorless.) 4: lumen.

Atherosclerosis begets thrombosis, but when and to what extent are difficult to know in the individual patient. Thus atherothrombosis is indeed an appropriate term for clinically significant vessel wall disease.

EPIDEMIOLOGY

Coronary atherosclerosis is the underlying cause of nearly all cases of ischemic heart disease (IHD), and superimposed thrombosis is the proximate cause of the great majority of the life-threatening acute coronary syndromes (ACS: unstable angina, myocardial infarction [MI], and sudden cardiac death [SCD])[4–6]. The pathogenesis of peripheral arterial disease and, to a great extent, that of ischemic stroke are similar. Thus, atherosclerosis with superimposed thrombosis (atherothrombosis) is the leading cause of death and severe disability in affluent countries, and will soon be so worldwide, due to the pandemic growth of obesity, insulin resistance, and type 2 diabetes mellitus.

The burdens of atherosclerosis and IHD increase markedly with age, regardless of sex and ethnic background. Although the major cardiovascular risk factors are similar for both sexes, men develop IHD 10–15 years earlier than women. By age 60 years, in the United States only 1 in 17 women has had a coronary event, as compared with 1 in 5 men. After age 60 years, however, IHD becomes the leading cause of death among women as well as among men, and as many women as men eventually die of the disease. Diabetes mellitus is a particularly strong risk factor among women, nearly eliminating the normal protection offered by female sex.

CARDIOVASCULAR RISK FACTORS

Besides age, sex, and family history of premature IHD, several major and independent risk factors for the clinical manifestations of atherosclerosis have been identified, including elevated serum low-density lipoprotein (LDL) cholesterol, low serum high-density lipoprotein (HDL) cholesterol, cigarette smoking, elevated blood pressure, and type 2 diabetes mellitus. If left untreated, any of these major risk factors has the potential to produce clinical disease. Nevertheless, in principle, only a single absolutely necessary and truly independent etiologic agent for atherosclerosis exists, namely a high level of serum LDL cholesterol (or its surrogate, serum total cholesterol). Both human and experimental studies strongly indicate that a certain serum cholesterol level (~4 mmol/l; 150 mg/dl) needs to be present to initiate and drive atherogenesis. Below that level IHD is rare, regardless of other risk factors. Although the individual susceptibility varies greatly, atherosclerosis increases with age, and the speed of progression is accelerated by hypertension, type 2 diabetes, and low HDL levels. High HDL levels may inhibit many essential steps in atherogenesis and promote reverse cholesterol transport from the vessel wall to the liver[7]. Cigarette smoking is probably not atherogenic as such but markedly increases the risk of superimposed thrombosis causing ACS[8].

ATHEROGENESIS

Atherosclerosis is a complex multi-factorial disease driven by atherogenic lipoproteins in the blood, particularly high levels of LDL cholesterol (*Table 5*)[1–3]. The concentration and size of LDL particles in the blood determine the amount within intima, where LDL is retained and modified (e.g. oxidized), making it cytotoxic, chemotactic, proinflammatory, and prothrombotic. The dyslipidemia seen with obesity, metabolic syndrome, and type 2 diabetes appears to be extraordinarily atherogenic (small dense LDL, high triglycerides, low HDL).

Fatty streaks

The endothelium is intact, but activated and dysfunctioning during the early stage of atherosclerosis[9]. Monocyte-derived macrophages (inflammation) and T-cells (immune response) are recruited via local expression of adhesion molecules on the endothelium. Within intima, activated macrophages engulf the modified LDL by scavenger receptors and become stuffed with lipid (foam cells) giving rise to the earliest lesions of atherosclerosis, fatty streaks.

The expression of scavenger receptors is not down-regulated by intracellular lipid accumulation, and the macrophages engulf lipid until they die, giving rise to a soft pool of foam cell debris, the lipid-rich core of the advanced lesion (**52**).

Advanced plaques

Inflammation is followed by healing and repair, mediated by the vascular smooth muscle cells that function as fibroblasts in the vessel wall (*Table 5*). When lipids begin to accumulate extracellularly, then atherogenesis has passed beyond the fatty-streak stage. Besides lipids, connective tissue produced by the vascular smooth muscle cells also accumulates, giving rise to very heterogeneous atherosclerotic lesions. Some plaques are lipid rich, whereas others are lipid poor, and morphologically dissimilar plaques may evolve next to each other. The endothelium is intact during early atherogenesis, but denuded areas, often related to superficial foam cell infiltration (inflammation), with adherent platelets are later seen over mature plaques[10]. Growth factors released from these adherent platelets and microthrombi may stimulate the smooth muscle cells within the plaques to produce more connective tissue matrix. The advanced lesions may cause luminal narrowing, inadequate blood supply, and ischemic symptoms.

Table 5 Atherothrombosis

- Inflammation:
  Endothelial activation; monocyte and T-cell adhesion and recruitment.
  Generation of cytokines, growth factors, and tissue factor.

- Growth:
  Smooth muscle cell activation, proliferation, migration, matrix synthesis (fibrosis).

- Degeneration:
  Lipid accummulation.
  Calcification.
  Cell death (apoptosis and necrosis).

- Complications:
  Plaque rupture, hemorrhage, and thrombosis.
  Plaque erosion and thrombosis.

Vulnerable plaques

A subset of the advanced lesions is particularly dangerous, 'vulnerable plaques', because they are at high risk of becoming complicated by luminal thrombosis (**53–56**). Rupture of vulnerable plaques with superimposed thrombosis is the most frequent cause of ACS[4–6].

Plaque rupture

The risk of plaque rupture depends more on plaque vulnerability (plaque type) than on degree of stenosis (plaque size); lipid-rich, soft plaques are more vulnerable and prone to rupture than collagen-rich, hard plaques. Furthermore, they are highly thrombogenic after rupture. There seem to be three major determinants of a plaque's vulnerability to rupture (**55**):
- Size and consistency of the lipid-rich core.
- Thickness of the fibrous cap covering the core.
- Ongoing inflammation and repair processes within the fibrous cap.

Lipid accumulation, cap thinning, loss of smooth muscle cells, and macrophage-related inflammation destabilize plaques, making them vulnerable to rupture. In contrast, smooth muscle cell-mediated healing and repair processes stabilize plaques, protecting them against rupture. Although vulnerable plaques are relatively large, they are often invisible angiographically due to compensatory vascular enlargement (positive remodeling), which partly explains why most ACS originate from plaques that were nonstenotic before the acute event (**57**). Most myocardial infarctions (68 + 18 = 86%, see **57**) are caused by thrombosis superimposed on atherosclerotic lesions that, prior to the acute events, were only mildly to moderately stenotic (and probably asymptomatic). Although stenotic lesions are at higher individual risk of occlusion, nonstenotic lesions by far outnumber the stenotic ones and, furthermore, nonstenotic lesions are often thrombosis-prone because vulnerable plaques tend to remodel outward, mitigating luminal narrowing[11]. When severely stenotic lesions occlude, they often do so silently because of preexisting collateral vessels.

Remodeling and stenosis

Rupture-prone plaques (large lipid-rich core, thin cap, ongoing inflammation) and those responsible for ACS are usually relatively large and are associated with compensatory enlargement of the artery (positive remodeling), which tends to preserve the lumen despite the presence of significant and potentially dangerous vessel wall disease. In contrast, plaques responsible for stable angina are usually smaller but, nevertheless, often cause more severe luminal narrowing because of concomitant local shrinkage of the artery (negative remodeling). The reason for these different modes of remodeling is unknown, but processes in the adventitia could play a critical role.

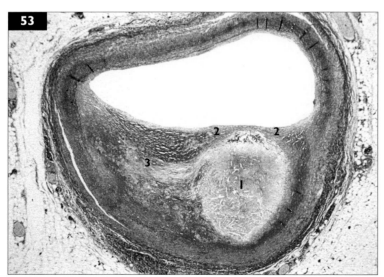

53 Cross section of a coronary artery containing a rupture-prone plaque, consisting of a relatively large lipid-rich core (1) covered by a thin and fragile fibrous cap (2). (Trichrome stain, rendering collagen blue and lipid colorless.) 3: fibrosis.

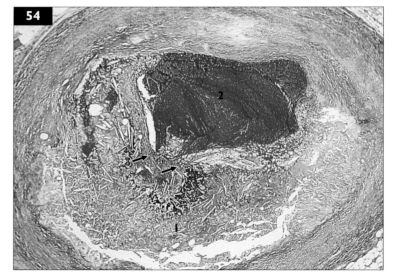

54 Cross section of a coronary artery containing a lipid-rich plaque (1) with ruptured surface (between arrows) and an occlusive thrombosis superimposed (2), the most frequent cause of an acute coronary syndrome. (Trichrome stain, rendering thrombus red, collagen blue, and lipid colorless.)

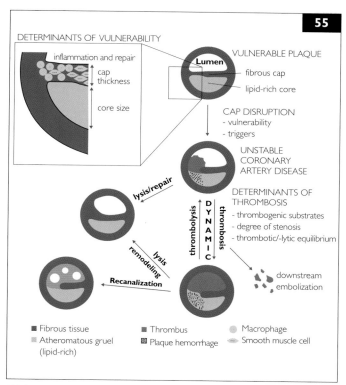

DETERMINANTS OF VULNERABILITY

inflammation and repair

cap thickness

core size

Lumen

VULNERABLE PLAQUE
- fibrous cap
- lipid-rich core

CAP DISRUPTION
- vulnerability
- triggers

UNSTABLE CORONARY ARTERY DISEASE

DETERMINANTS OF THROMBOSIS
- thrombogenic substrates
- degree of stenosis
- thrombotic/-lytic equilibrium

lysis/repair

DYNAMIC
thrombolysis
thrombosis

lysis

remodeling

Recanalization

downstream embolization

- Fibrous tissue
- Atheromatous gruel (lipid-rich)
- Thrombus
- Plaque hemorrhage
- Macrophage
- Smooth muscle cell

55 Schematic diagram to show the relationship between plaque vulnerability, rupture, and thrombosis.

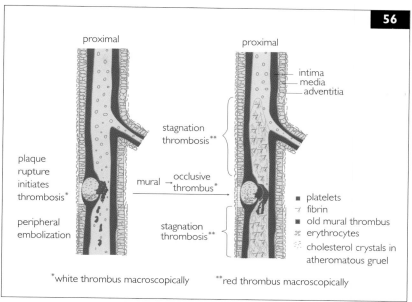

proximal   proximal

intima
media
adventitia

stagnation thrombosis**

plaque rupture initiates thrombosis*

mural → occlusive thrombus*

peripheral embolization

stagnation thrombosis**

- platelets
- fibrin
- old mural thrombus
- erythrocytes
- cholesterol crystals in atheromatous gruel

*white thrombus macroscopically   **red thrombus macroscopically

56 Schematic diagram to show the pathogenesis of coronary thrombosis. Plaque rupture precipitates ~75% of thrombi responsible for acute coronary syndromes. The primary flow obstruction is caused by aggregated platelets which later become stabilized by fibrin (white thrombus). Secondarily, the blood may stagnate and coagulate, giving rise to a red venous-type thrombus.

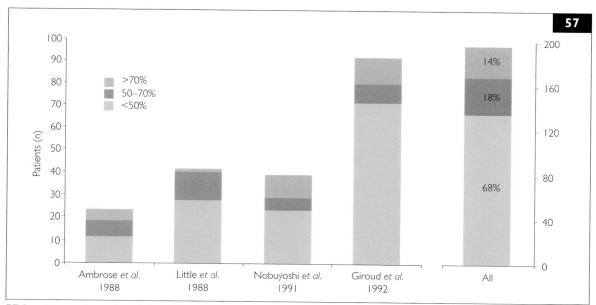

57 Bar chart to show the relationship between preexisting coronary stenosis and myocardial infarction.

THROMBOGENESIS

Plaque rupture is the major cause of coronary thrombosis, being responsible for approximately 75% of all fatal thrombotic events (**54**). Plaque rupture is a more frequent cause of coronary thrombosis in males (~80%) than in females (~60%). The term plaque erosion has gained popularity for the minority of thrombi not precipitated by plaque rupture (~20% in males and ~40% in females) (**58**). There are three major determinants of the thrombotic response to plaque rupture or the amount of thrombosis formed on top of an eroded plaque (**55, 56**):
- Local thrombogenic substrate.
- Local flow disturbances.
- Systemic thrombotic propensity.

Local thrombogenic substrate

Ongoing inflammation, in particular macrophage infiltration and activation, and lipid accumulation not only destabilize plaques making them vulnerable to rupture, but these plaque components also appear to be highly thrombogenic when exposed to the flowing blood after plaque rupture. Activated macrophages express tissue factor, and the lipid-rich atheromatous core contains a lot of active tissue factor, probably originating from dead macrophages[12]. Culprit lesions responsible for ACS contain more tissue factor than plaques responsible for stable angina. Tissue factor is a very potent generator of thrombin via the extrinsic coagulation pathway, and thrombin is a key mediator in arterial thrombosis due to its powerful effects on both platelets (aggregation) and fibrinogen (fibrin formation).

Local flow disturbances

In contrast to venous thrombosis, rapid flow and high shear forces promote arterial thrombosis, probably via shear-induced platelet activation (**59**). A platelet-rich thrombus may indeed form and grow within a severe stenosis, where the blood velocity and shear forces are highest. Irregularities of the exposed surface also increase platelet-mediated thrombus formation.

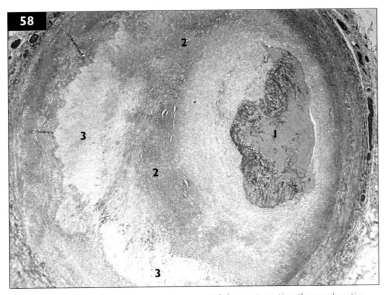

58 Cross section of a coronary artery containing a stenotic atherosclerotic plaque with an occlusive thrombosis (1) superimposed. The endothelium is missing at the plaque–thrombus interface but the plaque surface is otherwise intact (so-called plaque erosion). Thus, there is no obvious local cause such as plaque rupture beneath the thrombus. (Trichrome stain, rendering thrombus red, collagen blue, and lipid colorless.) 2: fibrosis; 3: lipid.

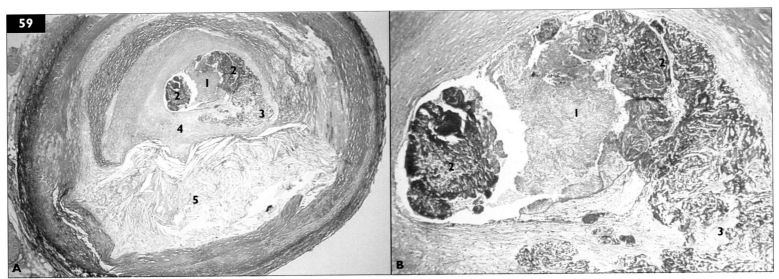

59 Cross section of a coronary artery occluded by a layered thrombus (**A**), indicating episodic growth of the thrombus over a period of time. At least three episodes (1–3) can readily by identified with the most recent part of the thrombus located centrally and consisting of aggregated platelets (**B**). The older parts of the thrombus near the vessel wall and partly incorporated into the plaque (organizing) are homogeneous, indicating that fibrin has stabilized the platelet-rich thrombus. (Trichrome stain, rendering thrombus red, collagen blue, and lipid colorless.) 1: platelets; 2: platelets/fibrin; 3: organizing thrombus; 4: fibrous cap; 5: lipid-rich core.

Although platelet aggregation plays a critical role initially during the evolution of a coronary thrombus, blood stagnation and coagulation contribute significantly to the overall thrombotic burden once the platelet-rich thrombus totally occludes the lumen (**60**). Lack of side branches favors blood stagnation and an enormous amount of thrombus may develop in occluded large-caliber saphenous vein grafts.

Systemic thrombotic propensity

The state (activation) of platelets, coagulation, and fibrinolysis is critical for the outcome of plaque rupture, documented by the protective effect of antiplatelet agents and anticoagulants in patients at risk of coronary thrombosis. Tissue factor and thrombin generation probably play an important prothrombotic role both locally (expressed by macrophages in the culprit lesion) and systemically (expressed by activated leukocytes in the peripheral blood)[12].

Dynamic thrombosis and microembolization

The thrombotic response to plaque rupture is dynamic, giving rise to changing chest pain and dynamic ischemic electrocardiogram (ECG) changes during the course of an ACS. Thrombosis and thrombolysis, often associated with vasospasm, tend to occur simultaneously, causing intermittent flow obstruction and distal embolization (**61**). The latter leads to microvascular obstruction, which may prevent myocardial reperfusion despite a 'successfully' recanalized infarct-related artery[13].

In coronary thrombosis, the initial flow obstruction is usually caused by platelet aggregation, but fibrin is important for the subsequent stabilization of the early and fragile platelet thrombus (**59**). Thus, both platelets and fibrin are involved in the evolution of a stable and persisting coronary thrombus.

VASOSPASM IN ACUTE CORONARY SYNDROMES

Dynamic flow reductions in ACS encompass elements of thrombosis and vasoconstriction superimposed on atherosclerotic lesions. Thrombosis may in fact induce vasospasm. Local platelet activation and thrombus formation generate serotonin, thromboxane A_2, and thrombin which can cause vasoconstriction not only at the site of thrombosis but also downstream. In this manner, a thrombus upstream in a coronary artery might propagate spasm to the distal smaller vessels. Vasodilator drugs, when given systemically, seldom overcome the effect of locally produced vasoconstrictor substances[14].

Multiple active lesions in acute coronary syndromes

The risk of recurrent ischemic events is particularly high during the first month after ACS. It has generally been assumed that the

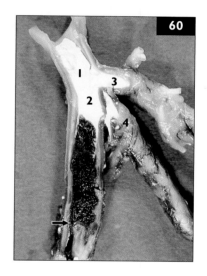

60 Thrombosed coronary artery cut open longitudinally, illustrating a voluminous erythrocyte-rich stagnation thrombosis (dark red) that has developed secondarily to blood stagnation caused by an occlusive platelet-rich thrombus (white) formed on top of a severely stenotic and ruptured plaque (arrow). The white material in the lumen is contrast medium injected postmortem. 1: left main stem; 2: left anterior descending coronary artery; 3: circumflex branch; 4: first diagonal branch.

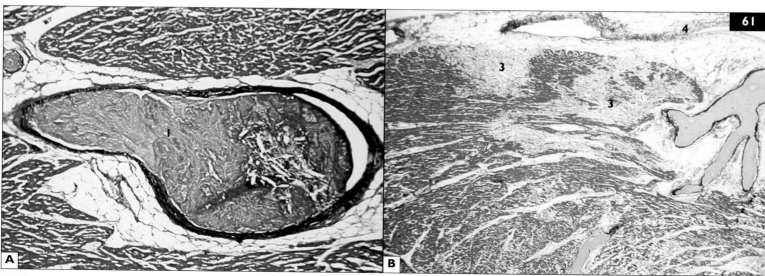

61 Coronary thrombosis is a dynamic process. Thrombosis and thrombolysis, often associated with vasospasm, tend to occur simultaneously, causing intermittent flow obstruction and distal embolization. The latter leads to microvascular obstruction (**A**) which may cause microinfarction (**B**) and troponin elevations in acute coronary syndromes without ST segment elevation (usually associated with a patent culprit artery). 1: platelets; 2: atheromatous gruel embolized from a ruptured plaque upstream in the supplying artery; 3: micro-infarct; 4: epicardium.

same atherothrombotic plaque, the culprit lesion, is responsible not only for the initial heart attack but also for early recurrent events if they occur. Recent observations indicate, however, that not just one but multiple 'active', complex, and rapidly progressing coronary lesions are often present in patients with ACS[15–18].

TRIGGERING

The onset of an ACS does not occur at random. Onset of ACS is more likely in the morning (soon after awakening), in the winter, on Mondays, and during heavy physical exertion (especially in those unaccustomed to regular physical activity) and emotional stress (anger, earthquakes, missile attacks), in acute infections, and sexual activity[19]. To explain these observations the 'triggering-concept' has been introduced, drawing attention to acute risk factors that may trigger disease onset if a vulnerable plaque is present. Triggering of disease onset could be mediated via activation of the sympathetic nervous system and catecholamines causing sudden rupture of a vulnerable plaque, acute thrombosis, and/or coronary spasm, so leading to sudden coronary occlusion.

CLINICAL IMPLICATIONS

Coronary atherosclerosis is the underlying cause of nearly all cases of ischemic heart disease, and superimposed thrombosis is the usual proximate cause of the ACS[4–6]. Coronary thrombosis is precipitated by plaque rupture in ~75% of cases.

Atherothrombosis is a multi-focal immunoinflammatory disease fueled by lipid, and inflammation is particularly frequent and intense in ruptured plaques beneath coronary thrombi. In contrast, the role of inflammation in thrombosis not caused by plaque rupture (plaque erosion) is controversial. Many patients with ACS have signs of pancoronary inflammation with multiple 'active', complex, and rapidly progressing coronary plaques rather than just a single culprit lesion[15–18].

The culprit lesion responsible for an ACS is frequently 'dynamic', leading to intermittent flow obstruction and peripheral microembolization, and the clinical presentation and the outcome depend on the location of the obstruction and the severity and duration of myocardial ischemia. A nonocclusive or transiently occlusive thrombus most frequently underlies ACS without ST segment elevation, whereas a more stable and occlusive thrombus prevails in ST segment elevation myocardial infarction (STEMI), overall modified by vascular tone and collateral flow. A critical thrombotic component is also frequent in culprit lesions responsible for out-of-hospital cardiac arrest and SCD.

Manifest atherothrombosis is a widespread disease that always needs systemic treatment. An invasive approach may be needed to obtain rapid, complete, and sustained reperfusion of infarct-related arteries (primary angioplasty) or to 'pacify' one or a few complex lesions that pose a particularly high short-term risk in unstable coronary syndromes. However, a target lesion-based approach alone will not eliminate the threat posed by all the other existing coronary plaques, and their overall risk determines the prognosis long term (**57**). Therefore, a global (systemic) approach is always of paramount importance for both prevention and treatment of this disease.

CORONARY VASOCONSTRICTION AND SPASM

FILIPPO CREA, MD AND GAETANO A. LANZA, MD

DEFINITION

The term coronary artery spasm indicates a sudden, intense, occlusive or subocclusive vasoconstriction of a segment of an epicardial coronary artery, resulting in a dramatic reduction of coronary blood flow which causes transmural myocardial ischemia, typically manifested by ST segment elevation on the ECG (**62**)[1].

Spasm may occur at the level of coronary stenoses of variable severity or in totally normal coronary vessels. In some patients, the spasm may involve more segments of the same or different epicardial coronary arteries (multi-focal spasm) (**63**), or may involve one or more coronary artery branches diffusely, a condition more frequently reported in Japanese than in Caucasian people[2].

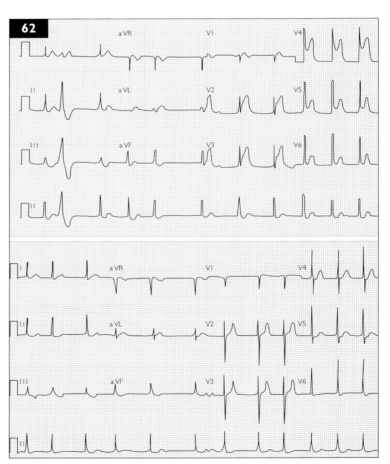

62 Electrocardiogram tracing of anterolateral ST segment elevation documented during an anginal attack in a patient with vasospastic angina (**upper tracing**). Both angina and ST changes disappeared spontaneously within 1 minute (**lower tracing**).

Coronary spasm must be distinguished from coronary vasoconstriction, which is characterized by a mild to moderate reduction of the lumen of the vessel[3]. Coronary vasoconstriction at the level of a stenosis often modulates the threshold and severity of effort-induced myocardial ischemia but, when severe enough, it may also cause subendocardial ischemia at rest, typically manifested by ST depression on the ECG.

EPIDEMIOLOGY

There are scarce data on the incidence of vasospastic angina. In a review of clinical records from 1991–1996 a yearly incidence of about 1.0% of the hospital admissions to the authors' institute was observed[4]. The incidence, however, might be higher in Japanese than in Caucasian people.

Vasospastic angina usually occurs at age 50–60 years, but it can also be observed in both younger or older people, with a 5:1 prevalence of male gender in the authors' experience[4]. Smoking is the only accepted risk factor for vasospastic angina, but use of some substances (e.g., alcohol, cocaine, 5-fluorouracil, sumatriptan) may favor or unmask coronary spasm, and therefore their use should be sought for in these patients. In rare cases, variant angina has been reported to be associated with systemic vasomotor disorders such as migraine and Raynaud's phenomenon, suggesting the presence of a general vascular disorder.

Coronary vasoconstriction modulates the critical reduction of coronary blood flow at the level of coronary stenoses in about 75% of patients with stable coronary syndromes. Furthermore, it may contribute significantly to the reduction of coronary blood flow at the site of the culprit coronary lesion responsible for an ACS, although the exact prevalence of this phenomenon is unknown.

PATHOGENESIS

Coronary spasm results from the interaction of two components: (1) a local abnormality which makes smooth muscle cells of a coronary segment hyperreactive to vasoconstrictor stimuli, and (2) transient vasoconstrictor stimuli which trigger the spasm in the hyperreactive segment[5].

The vascular smooth muscle hyperreactivity is likely due to an alteration of the intracellular pathways involved in the regulation of myofibril contraction. Indeed, coronary spasm can be induced by a variety of stimuli acting through different mechanisms and different cellular receptors, and vasodilators which act by blocking specific cellular receptors (e.g. α-blockers, 5-HT antagonists) have limited effect in preventing symptoms in patients with variant angina. Recently, the intracoronary infusion of fasudil, an inhibitor of the intracellular enzyme rho-kinase, has been shown to prevent acetylcholine-induced coronary spasm in patients with vasospastic angina, suggesting that an increased activity of this enzyme, which reduces myosin-phosphatase activity 'sensitizing' smooth muscle cell myofibrils to calcium, may contribute to the hyperreactivity of spastic segments[6].

Several vasoconstrictor stimuli may induce coronary spasm when acting at the site of hyperreactive coronary segments. Adrenergic and vagal autonomic nervous activation are both believed to be important triggers of spasm. Adrenergic activity acts through α-stimulation and is responsible for coronary spasm during exercise, stress conditions, and cold pressor test; furthermore, spontaneous ischemic episodes have been shown to be preceded by changes in the sympato-vagal balance towards a prevalence of the adrenergic activity[7]. Vagal activation may also trigger the spasm by direct stimulation of muscarinic receptors on smooth muscle cells, as suggested by the possibility of inducing spasm by cholinergic drugs and the prevalence of anginal attacks during sleep found in several patients (**64**)[8]. Other possible triggering stimuli *in vivo* include local vasoconstrictors released by activated endothelial cells (e.g. endothelin-1 [ET]) or platelets (e.g. thromboxane A_2 [TXA_2], 5-HT).

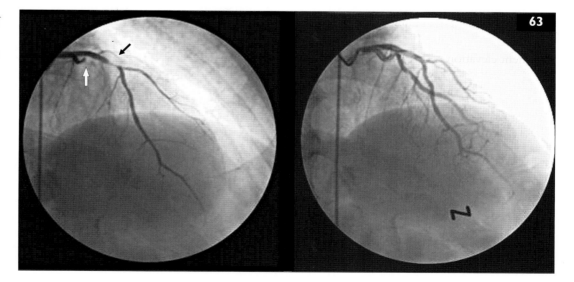

63 Left: spontaneous subocclusive spasm of the left anterior descending coronary artery (black arrow) and occlusive spasm of the left circumflex coronary artery (white arrow) occurring during coronary angiography in a patient with variant angina. **Right**: both coronary spasms were relieved by intravenous nitroglycerin administration.

Coronary vasoconstriction in atherosclerotic coronary vessels of patients with stable coronary syndromes is believed to be mainly caused by endothelial dysfunction, whereas at the site of the culprit lesion of patients with ACS it is probably caused by a complex interaction of endothelial dysfunction, platelet activation, and activated inflammatory cells.

CLINICAL PRESENTATION

Vasospastic angina should be suspected in patients with anginal episodes occurring exclusively or predominantly at rest, without any apparent triggering cause. Anginal attacks are usually short in duration (2–5 minutes, but sometimes only 30 seconds) and may recur in clusters of 2–4 or more within 20–30 minutes. They usually respond promptly to sublingual nitrates and show a circadian pattern with a typical prevalence in the early morning hours or at night (**64**). Effort tolerance is often well preserved in patients with vasospastic angina, particularly in those with normal coronary arteries. However, exercise may induce spasm in about 25% of patients.

The clinical diagnosis can be confirmed by the documentation of transient ST segment elevation (1–2 mm up to 20–30 mm) on the ECG during an anginal attack (**62**). When it is difficult to record standard ECG during angina, the diagnosis can usually be obtained by 24–48-hour ambulatory ECG recording, which also allows assessment of the total ischemic burden and daily distribution of the ischemic episodes, 75–80% of which are silent (**64**).

When typical transient ST elevation cannot be demonstrated even by ambulatory ECG monitoring, vasospastic angina can be diagnosed by a pharmacologic provocative test. Intracoronary or IV administration of ergonovine or intracoronary infusion of acetylcholine can be used to induce and demonstrate coronary spasm during coronary angiography. The IV ergonovine test can also be performed noninvasively, under careful clinical and ECG monitoring, with spasm induction indicated by the appearance of angina and ST segment elevation.

In some patients, severe ventricular tachyarrhythmias may develop during myocardial ischemia caused by coronary spasm (**65**)[9]. These patients may present with syncope or presyncope associated with angina, and are at risk of sudden death. Severe bradyarrhythmias (sinus arrest, atrioventricular [AV] block) may also occur during transmural myocardial ischemia, in particular in patients with inferior ischemia.

Coronary artery spasm is usually highly sensitive to calcium antagonists (**66**). Nevertheless, in rare cases spasm can be refractory to maximally tolerated vasodilator treatment. Coronary angioplasty with stent implantation may be helpful in favoring the prevention of segmental spasm by drug therapy in these patients[10].

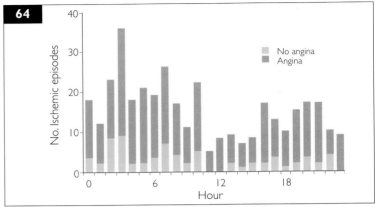

64 Circadian distribution of 301 episodes of ST segment elevation detected during 24 hour electrocardiogram Holter recording in 26 patients with Prinzmetal's variant angina. Note the high prevalence of nocturnal and early morning ischemic attacks and the prevalence of silent episodes, compared to symptomatic episodes.

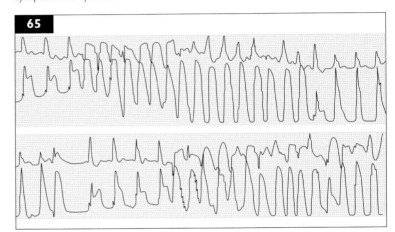

65 Electrocardiogram documentation of nonsustained ventricular tachycardia during transient transmural ischemia caused by coronary artery spasm in a patient with a history of frequent anginal attacks at rest, which were often associated with syncope or presyncope.

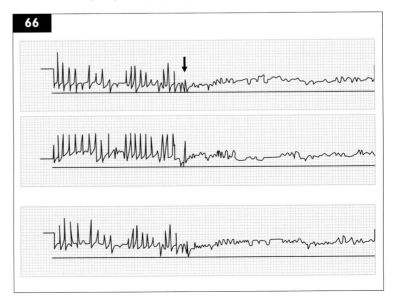

66 ST segment trend of a 24-hour ambulatory electrocardiogram (ECG) recording in a patient with *de novo* diagnosis of vasospastic angina. Frequent episodes of ST segment elevation can be observed in the first 10 hours of the ECG recording, often involving all three monitored ECG chest leads. After starting a standard dose of diltiazem (120 mg q8h, arrow), there was complete abolition of ischemic episodes.

NONATHEROTHROMBOTIC CORONARY ARTERY DISEASE

ULRIK BAANDRUP, MD, PhD AND INGRID BAYER KRISTENSEN, MD

INTRODUCTION

Nonatheromatous coronary artery disease is markedly less common than atherothrombotic coronary disease. However, there are many causes of nonatheromatous coronary disease and these diseases can be just as life-threatening (*Table 6*). Identification and correct diagnosis are therefore essential for reasons of optimal therapy and understanding.

Coronary vasculitis spans the entire spectrum of infectious and inflammatory/immunologic vasculitides. Some of these disorders are still of unknown cause. Most of them only rarely affect the coronary arteries but all can. Kawasaki's disease has a special predilection for the coronary arteries of children (**67**).

The many diagnostic, invasive and operative techniques of the coronary arteries and the heart pose a risk of their own, which rarely may give rise to iatrogenic coronary obstruction and myocardial

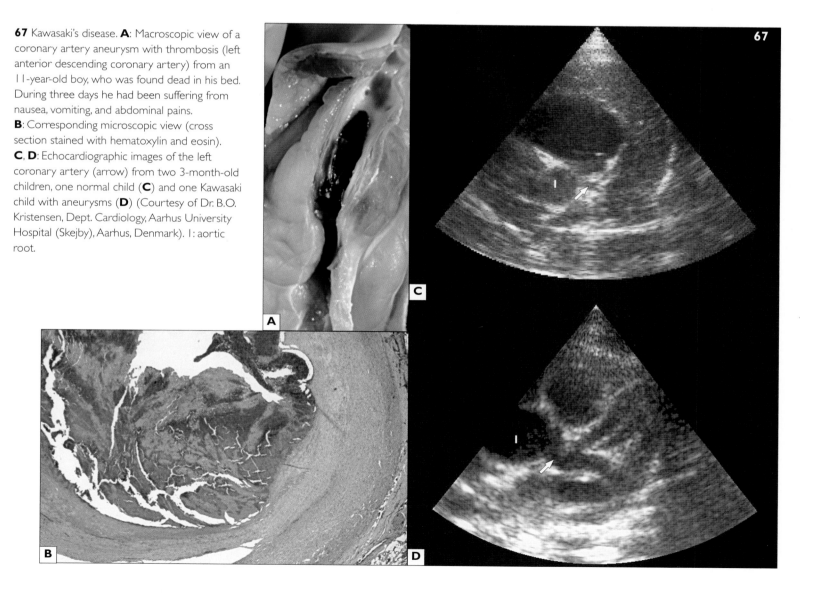

67 Kawasaki's disease. **A**: Macroscopic view of a coronary artery aneurysm with thrombosis (left anterior descending coronary artery) from an 11-year-old boy, who was found dead in his bed. During three days he had been suffering from nausea, vomiting, and abdominal pains.
B: Corresponding microscopic view (cross section stained with hematoxylin and eosin).
C, **D**: Echocardiographic images of the left coronary artery (arrow) from two 3-month-old children, one normal child (**C**) and one Kawasaki child with aneurysms (**D**) (Courtesy of Dr. B.O. Kristensen, Dept. Cardiology, Aarhus University Hospital (Skejby), Aarhus, Denmark). I: aortic root.

Table 6 Causes of nonatherothrombotic coronary artery disease

Arteritis
- Infection:
  Bacterial.
  Fungal.
  Viral.
  Rickettsial.
  Spirochetal.
- Immunological
  Immune complex-mediated: lupus vasculitis, hepatitis B
    microscopic polyarteritis.
  Direct antibody attack-mediated: Kawasaki
    (antiendothelial antibodies).
  ANCA associated (mediated): Wegener's granulomatosis.
  Cell-mediated: best known is allograft organ rejection.
  Hypersensitivity reaction: drugs.
- Unknown:
  Polyarteritis nodosa (classic).
  Giant cell arteritis.
  Takayasu's arteritis.

Embolism
- Infectious endocarditis.
- Nonbacterial thrombotic endocarditis (NBTE).
- Parasitic disorders.
- Vegetations on catheters or fragments of catheters:
  iatrogenic material.
- Tumors:
  Myxoma.
  Paradoxical embolus.
  Foreign bodies, including gas.

Occlusion of the coronary arterial orifice
- Thrombus from stalky endocarditic excrescence.
- Papillary fibroelastoma: papillary tumor of the leaflet.
- Surgical material:
  Felt pads, which can also be embolic.
  Suture material gripping the coronary artery in
    relation to arterioplastic operations or bypass.

Dissection
- Spontaneous.
- Marfan.
- Hypertension.

Miscellaneous
- Congenital coronary anomalies:
  Arteriovenous malformation.
  Anomalous origin of coronary arteries.
- Fibromuscular dysplasia/hyperplasia.
- Perivascular/vascular fibrosis in hypertrophic cardiomyopathy.
- Endocrine and metabolic disorders:
  Diabetes, hypothyroidism.
  Homocysteinemia, mucopolysaccharidoses.

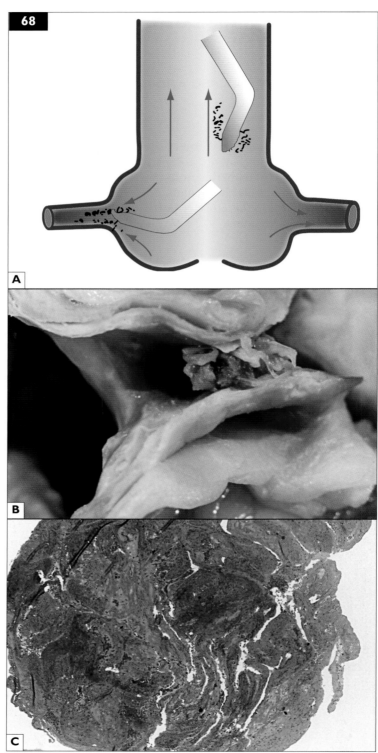

68 A: Schematic diagram of iatrogenic thromboembolism. **B**: Macroscopic view of a thromboembolus impacted in the left main coronary artery causing sudden death during coronary intervention. **C**: Microscopic cross section of the thromboembolus.

ischemia (**68, 69**). During coronary interventions, thrombotic material may form around a catheter tip. Usually the material will be carried into the aorta, but it may enter a coronary ostium. Many other disorders can alter coronary flow due to narrowing of the arteries. Trauma and transplantation are specifically dealt with elsewhere in this book (see Transplant Vasculopathy, and Traumatic Coronary Artery Disease; Allograft Coronary Artery Disease, Chapter 19. The list of nonatherothrombotic coronary artery diseases (CADs) described in *Table 6* is not complete, and only a few cases are illustrated (**67–71**).

In general, most of these diseases rarely affect the coronary arteries but if they do, myocardial ischemia, infarction, and/or sudden death may occur. The reader is directed toward major textbooks for information on the incidence, pathogenesis, diagnosis, treatment, and prognosis of the individual diseases. Sometimes nothing or very little is known, or knowledge is based on case reports only. Many of these disorders may reveal hereditary or mutational defects as more is understood of the molecular pathology.

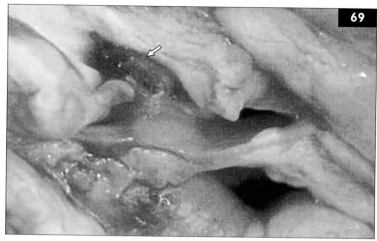

69 Iatrogenic coronary occlusion in a patient who had aortic valve replacement. After the operation he developed signs of acute myocardial infarction and died. At autopsy an intracoronary felt pad intended for anchoring the new valve was found at the bifurcation of the left main coronary artery. (arrow).

70 A: Obstruction from stalky endocarditic excrescence in a previously healthy 38-year-old male who complained of sudden severe chest pain and died. There was no history of cardiovascular symptoms or rheumatic disease. On the left aortic valve, a friable stalky excrescence (18 mm × 3 mm) was located. The mobile part of this nonbacterial thrombotic excrescence had occluded the left main coronary artery. **B**: Close-up view.

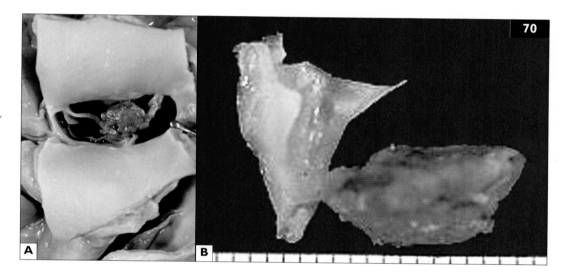

71 Spontaneous coronary dissection in a 48-year-old male with fatal dissection of the left anterior descending coronary artery and the circumflex branch, causing massive myocardial infarction. The nonstenotic atherosclerotic plaque in intima is unrelated to the dissecting hemorrhage between tunica media and adventitia. The cause of the dissection is unknown. (Hematoxylin and eosin stain.)

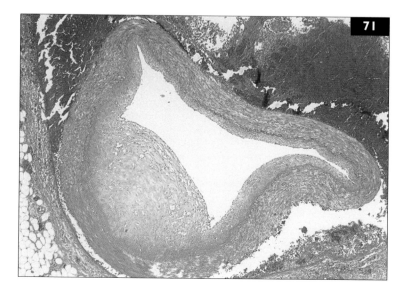

MICROVASCULAR DISEASE

HANS ERIK BØTKER, MD, PhD

DEFINITION
Microvascular disease is defined as reduced coronary perfusion caused by coronary microvascular dysfunction in patients with nonstenotic epicardial arteries on the coronary angiogram.

EPIDEMIOLOGY
Between 10 and 30% of patients who undergo coronary angiography because of angina pectoris have normal-appearing epicardial coronary arteries on angiogram. Disturbances of the microcirculation are frequently secondary to specific cardiac or generalized vascular or nonvascular diseases that affect the heart, but may also be manifest without concomitant diseases as in some patients with cardiac syndrome X (see Chapter 9, Cardiac Syndrome X).

PATHOGENESIS
The microvascular bed includes prearterioles, arterioles, and capillaries. Coronary blood flow is regulated in proportion to the need of the myocardium for oxygen, which is closely related to cardiac work. The mechanisms ensure that coronary auto-regulation maintains coronary flow over a wide range of perfusion pressures. The microvasculature allows an increment of myocardial blood flow between three and six times its basal level. The amount by which coronary blood flow increases in response to maximal arteriolar dilatation reflects the vasodilator capacity of the heart and is defined as the coronary flow reserve (CFR). CFR >2.5 is most frequently used to characterize a normal microvascular function even though this definition contains conceptual limitations because the CFR does not result from a simple monodimensional comparison of two flow values, but rather from the area limited by the pressure–flow relations obtained in the presence and absence of arteriolar tone (72).

A reduction in the cardiac vasodilator capacity may cause inadequate coronary blood flow in relation to the metabolic demand of the heart. At least four factors may disturb this relationship: (1) the vascular component, (2) the myocardial component, (3) the metabolic component, and (4) the rheological component (*Table 7*). The impairment of the CFR is frequently not caused by a single mechanism, but involves both vascular and myocardial components, which may explain that microvascular pathology by histology is scarce in many cases of microvascular dysfunction. However, media hypertrophy is considered the main mechanism for microvascular dysfunction in arterial hypertension (73), because angina pectoris and the impairment of the CFR can be present in the absence of myocardial hypertrophy. The microangiopathy of diabetes mellitus may produce a thickening of the arteriolar wall in the myocardium and involves both the tunica media and the perivascular connective tissue (74A,B). Ventricular enlargement and dilatation, as in aortic stenosis, result in increased wall tension such that the myocardial component reduces CFR, while hypertrophic and dilated cardiomyopathies may also involve inadequate growth of microvessels in relation to hypertrophied myocytes ('capillary rarefaction').

In inflammatory vascular disease, disturbance of the coronary microcirculation can be caused by a primary vascular inflammation

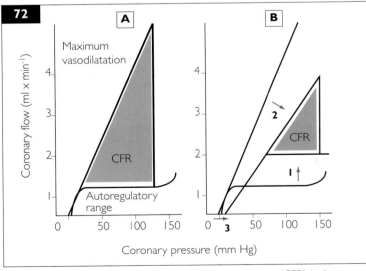

72 Pressure–flow relationships. The coronary flow reserve (CFR) is the amount by which coronary flow increases in response to maximal arteriolar dilatation. Mechanisms for reduction of the CFR: 1. upward shift of autoregulation curve, as in conditions with an increase in metabolic demand; 2. decreased slope in the absence of arteriolar tone; and 3. increase in the pressure value at zero flow (i.e. the critical closing pressure), with vascular abnormalities.

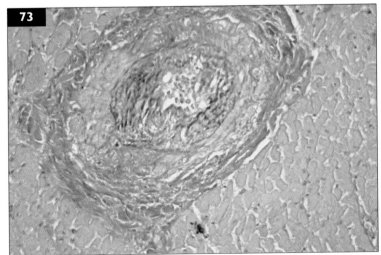

73 Histological section (elastic Van Gieson stain) showing thickening of the coronary arteriolar tunica media in a patient with severe arterial hypertension. Intimal thickening is also present. (Courtesy of Associate Prof. Ulrik Baandrup, MD, PhD, Department of Pathology, Aarhus University Hospital, Aarhus, Denmark.)

or by a secondary vascular reaction in diseases not primarily vascular in nature. Such diseases are mainly viral, toxic, and drug-induced forms of immune complex vasculitis and the vascular lesions in systemic immunologic disease. The coronary reserve is usually severely reduced or completely absent in such disorders.

Myocardial hypertrophy, dilatation and an abnormal myocardial composition caused by deposit disorders, infiltration, and inflammation can lead to limitation of the minimal attainable coronary resistance and consequently a reduction of the CFR. Diastolic compression of the coronary vasculature is considered to be the main mechanism but, as illustrated by cardiac amyloidosis, compression of the arterioles by amyloid infiltration may not be the sole mechanism since CFR is also impaired by reduced compliance of the vessel wall due to amyloid deposits (75).

The third group of disturbances of the coronary micro-circulation is metabolic in nature. The classic example is

Table 7 Sources of disturbed coronary microcirculation

Vascular abnormalities
- Microangiopathy:
    Arterial hypertension.
    Diabetes mellitus.
- Capillary rarefaction:
    Hypertrophic and dilated cardiomyopathy.
- Inflammation:
    Vasculitis.
    Immunocomplex diseases.

Myocardial abnormalities
- Hypertrophy of myocytes:
    Arterial hypertension.
    Aortic stenosis.
    Hypertrophic cardiomyopathy.
- Abnormal composition of the myocardium:
    Deposit disorders.
- Infiltrating interstitial processes:
    Collagen.
    Amyloidosis.
    Parasitosis.
- Inflammatory processes:
    Myocarditis.

Metabolic abnormalities
- Increased oxygen consumption:
    Increased ventricular wall stress.
    Hyperthyroidism.

Rheological abnormalities
- Increased blood viscosity:
    Paraproteinemia.
    Polyglobulia and polycythemia.
    Hyperlipidemia.

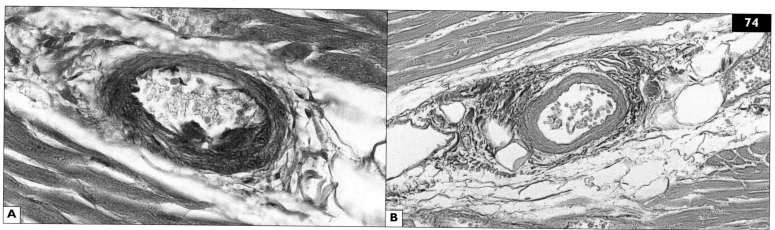

74 Histological sections showing characteristics of diabetic microangiopathy in the heart. **A**: PAS-positive thickening of the coronary arteriolar tunica media. **B**: Gieson-Sirius Red staining demonstrating accumulation of perivascular connective tissue. (Courtesy of Prof. Thomas Ledet, MD, PhD.)

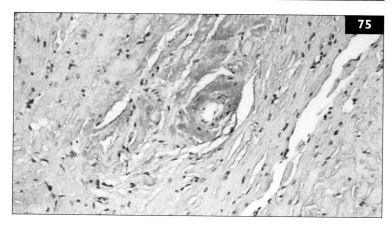

75 Biopsy specimen (Congo red stain) with cardiac amyloidosis characterized by amyloid deposit in the coronary arterioles and amyloid infiltration in the myocardium. (Courtesy of Associate Prof. Ulrik Baandrup, MD, PhD, Department of Pathology, Aarhus University Hospital, Aarhus, Denmark.)

thyrotoxicosis, characterized by elevated heart rate, high filling pressure, and high end-diastolic and end-systolic wall tensions. Myocardial oxygen consumption is augmented in these cases and reduction of the CFR results from an increased blood flow at rest. There is usually no genuine reduction of the coronary conductance, because the minimal attainable coronary resistance is within normal range.

Finally, impairment of coronary microcirculation can be rheological in origin and results from abnormal flow characteristics of the blood. Clinically relevant and diagnostically identifiable disorders are paraproteinemia, polycythemia, and hyperlipidemia.

PRESENTATION

Angina pectoris due to microvascular dysfunction manifests as chronic stable angina pectoris comparable to that caused by epicardial coronary stenoses. Even though ischemic manifestations such as congestive heart failure and arrhythmia are not always clinically overt, many patients may have slightly augmented heart rate, elevated filling pressure, and increased end-diastolic and end-systolic ventricular wall tensions, which explains the fact that the precordial complaints are frequently accompanied by dyspnea and fatigue.

The crucial question when angiography reveals normal coronary arteries in a patient referred due to angina pectoris is whether additional diagnostic procedures are necessary. The purposes of further procedures are: (1) to establish the diagnosis, (2) to clarify whether the symptoms are part of a cardiac or generalized disorder of which identification has therapeutic consequences, and (3) to clarify whether the patient has microvascular dysfunction. Persistent symptoms may rationalize additional diagnostic procedures able to demonstrate disturbances of the microcirculation, in particular if an exercise stress test reveals ST segment depression suggestive of ischemia, because some of the abnormalities are accessible for specific treatment.

A thorough medical history and clinical examination often uncover the presence of a generalized disorder, which may affect the coronary microcirculation. If appropriate, serologic markers must be measured. Echocardiography can clarify whether specific cardiac diseases such as valvular disease, cardiomyopathies, deposit diseases, and pericardial diseases are present. An endomyocardial biopsy may be necessary in selected patients. Epicardial spasms are excluded by provocative spasm test.

The demonstration of microvascular dysfunction relies on measurement of the CFR using flow measurements at rest and after maximum vasodilatation following administration of one of the vasodilatory compounds papaverine, dipyridamole, or adenosine. Invasive techniques for measurement of flow velocities comprise the thermodilution method in the coronary sinus and intracoronary Doppler measurements. The most convenient method is noninvasive measurement of perfusion with positron emission tomography (PET) using perfusing markers such as ^{13}N-ammonia and ^{15}O-water.

A normal coronary angiogram is usually associated with a benign prognosis *quo ad vitam*, but the prognosis in microvascular angina depends on the underlying disease.

SYSTEMIC CAUSES OF COMPROMISED SUPPLY

KAVITA KUMAR, MD

INTRODUCTION

Anemia and hypotension are among the most frequent systemic conditions that may lead to inadequate myocardial oxygen supply in the absence of CAD.

ANEMIA

Anemia is defined as a decrease in the hemoglobin content in an erythrocyte or in the volume of circulating erythrocytes (hematocrit). Anemia occurs when there is decreased erythrocyte production or increased erythrocyte destruction. The effects on the cardiovascular system vary depending upon the degree of anemia and the severity of underlying CAD.

Pathogenesis

Myocardial ischemia results from an imbalance in the myocardial oxygen supply versus myocardial oxygen demand. Myocardial oxygen supply is governed by the coronary blood flow, arterial oxygen content, and the myocardial oxygen extraction. Coronary blood flow is directly related to the perfusion or driving pressure and is inversely related to coronary vascular resistance. The vascular resistance depends on the vascular tone, autoregulation, epicardial coronary stenosis, and the myocardial compressive force. Arterial oxygen content is determined by the hemoglobin concentration and the oxygen saturation. Changes in any of the above parameters could alter myocardial oxygen supply. Oxygen demand, on the other hand, is determined by the heart rate, contractility, and wall stress (directly related to ventricular developed pressure and volume and inversely related to wall thickness). An increase in any of these parameters could increase the myocardial oxygen demand (**76**).

Cardiovascular effects

In a normal cardiovascular system, mild or moderate degrees of anemia have little effect. As the anemia becomes more severe, with the hemoglobin level decreasing below 9 g/dl (90 g/l), the cardiac output begins to increase. The cardiac output continues to increase as the hemoglobin concentration decreases. The lower blood viscosity and the lower systemic vascular resistance cause a decrease in the afterload. The increased venous return causes an increase in the stroke volume. Consequently, the cardiac output rises. This high-output state may eventually lead to congestive heart failure.

In response to the anemia there are structural and functional changes. A compensatory increase in the microvascular density and collateral circulation occurs. Additionally, there is a shift in the oxygen dissociation curve to maintain tissue oxygen delivery. Patients without underlying coronary disease tolerate anemia without developing ischemia, with the possible exception of patients with sickle cell anemia.

In patients with underlying CAD, however, ischemia may be precipitated by anemia. The combination of decreased oxygen-carrying capacity and flow-limiting stenosis creates a milieu for reduced myocardial oxygen delivery, thereby resulting in myocardial ischemia. Acute and chronic anemia have different impacts on the cardiovascular system. Acute anemia, from acute blood loss, results in hypovolemia and hypotension, thereby decreasing the coronary perfusion pressure and coronary blood flow. In response to the hypotension, catecholamine levels increase causing a reflex tachycardia, which increases myocardial oxygen demand. Anemia leads to a lower oxygen content and thereby lower tissue oxygen delivery. The decreased coronary blood flow, decreased oxygen content, and increased oxygen demand lead to myocardial ischemia (77).

In chronic anemia, on the other hand, hypotension does not play a significant role. Chronic anemia reduces oxygen content of the blood but its adverse impact on tissue oxygen delivery is partially offset by an increase in cardiac output and blood flow due

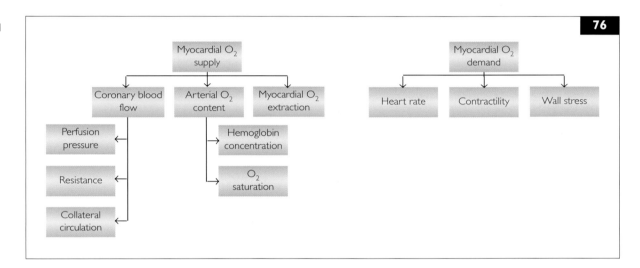

76 Determinants of myocardial oxygen supply and demand.

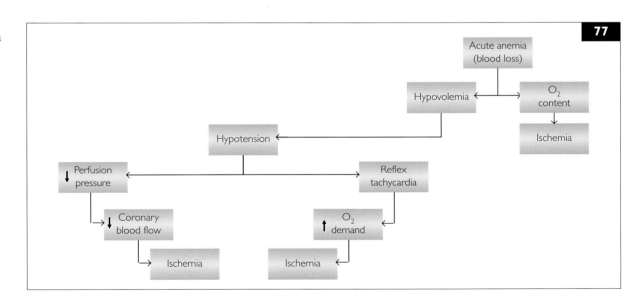

77 The effects of acute anemia on myocardial oxygen supply and demand.

to reduced viscosity; however, if the anemia is severe and/or CFR is exhausted due to a severe underlying epicardial coronary stenosis, myocardial ischemia may be precipitated (**78**).

Sickle cell anemia
In patients with sickle cell anemia resulting from hemo-globinopathy, hypoxia leads to sickling of the abnormal red cells. This phenomenon, in combination with platelet aggregation and fibrin deposition, leads to coronary microvascular occlusion. Epicardial coronary artery thrombosis, however, is rare. Additionally, endothelial proliferation and fibromuscular dysplasia have been documented in coronary arteries of patients with sickle cell anemia. The combination of reduced oxygen delivery and vaso-occlusion creates an ischemic milieu. These vaso-occlusive events also occur in the pulmonary vasculature, leading to pulmonary infarctions and eventually pulmonary hypertension and cor pulmonale (**79**).

HYPOTENSION
Hypotension can be defined as low blood pressure associated with clinical manifestations of reduced organ perfusion. The symptoms can range from mild, such as lightheadedness, to severe, i.e. shock, a state that produces widespread organ dysfunction as a result of inadequate tissue perfusion.

Pathogenesis
The various etiologies of shock include cardiogenic, obstructive, hypovolemic, and distributive (*Table 8*). Cardiogenic shock can be the result of a massive MI or mechanical complications of an MI. It can also occur when there is cardiac inflow or outflow obstruction. Extracardiac obstruction, as seen in massive pulmonary embolism (**80**) and cardiac tamponade, can also result in shock. Hypovolemic shock occurs when there is a >20% decrease in blood volume, as a result of trauma or vascular catastrophe. In the case of distributive shock, there is inappropriate peripheral vasodilatation and inadequate tissue oxygen delivery. This state can result from anaphylaxis, sepsis, massive neurologic insults, or endocrine failure such as adrenal crisis.

Etiology of shock
In this chapter, cardiogenic shock will be excluded since it is the ischemia or infarction that usually causes cardiogenic shock. Regardless of the etiology of shock, the problem lies in the mismatch between inadequate tissue oxygen delivery and increased metabolic demands (**81**). High levels of circulating catecholamines increase the heart rate and contractility, thereby increasing the cardiac workload and myocardial oxygen demand. Flow-limiting stenoses create an impediment to increasing blood supply in the

---

Table 8 Etiologies of shock.

Cardiogenic (*low cardiac output, high wedge pressure*)
- Acute myocardial infarction.
- Mechanical complications of acute MI (acute mitral regurgitation, acute VSD).
- LV outflow obstruction (Aortic stenosis, HCM).

Obstructive (*low cardiac output, high or normal wedge pressure*)
- Pericardial tamponade.
- Massive pulmonary embolism.

Hypovolemic (*low cardiac output, low wedge pressure*)
- Hemorrhage.
- Volume depletion.

Distributive (*high or normal cardiac output, low wedge pressure*)
- Sepsis.
- Anaphylaxis.
- Neurogenic.
- Endocrinologic.

HCM: hypertrophic cardiomyopathy; LV: left ventricle; VSD: ventriculoseptal defect.

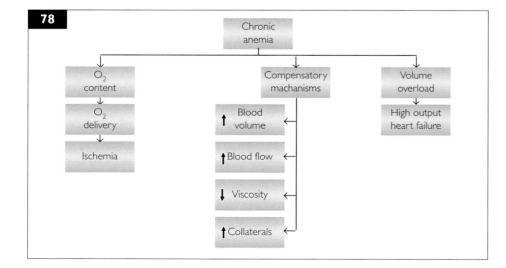

78 The effects of chronic anemia on myocardial oxygen supply and demand.

face of increasing oxygen demand. Hypotension decreases the coronary perfusion pressure, mainly involving the subendocardium, thus further contributing to an ischemic environment. In addition to the above mechanisms for ischemia, the inflammatory milieu during septic shock propagates thrombosis and microvascular obstruction which further contribute to an ischemic environment.

Clinical presentation

Shock is defined clinically as hypotension with a systolic blood pressure <90 mmHg (12 kPa) and tachycardia with a heart rate >100 beats per minute. Additionally, patients are usually tachypneic and may have an altered level of consciousness. End-organ damage may also be manifest in the form of oliguria. Other signs and symptoms will be manifest depending on the underlying etiology of shock. Correcting the underlying etiology is necessary to relieve the ischemia.

79 Relationship between sickle cell anemia and myocardial ischemia.

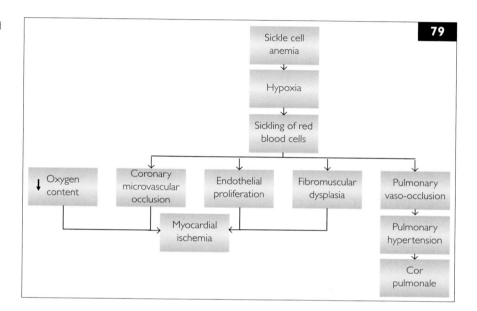

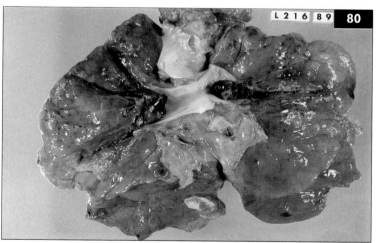

80 Autopsy specimen from a patient who died of thromboemboli that blocked the pulmonary arteries to both lungs. The emboli originated from a thrombosed femoral vein.

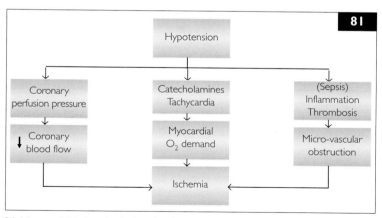

81 Myocardial ischemia during shock.

TRANSPLANT VASCULOPATHY

SAMIR R. KAPADIA, MD AND E. MURAT TUZCU, MD

DEFINITION

Allograft vasculopathy refers to accelerated intimal hyperplasia of the coronary arteries seen after cardiac transplantation (See Chapter 19, Allograft Coronary Artery Disease). Transplant coronary disease includes lesions of allograft vasculopathy and lesions of conventional atherosclerosis pre-existent in donor coronary arteries at the time of transplantation (**82A–C**)[1].

Histologically, end-stage allograft vasculopathy lesions are characterized by concentric intimal proliferation and diffuse narrowing involving the entire length of the vessel. This is quite different from the focal, eccentric lesions usually seen in native CAD. Other histologic features of allograft vasculopathy that distinguish it from conventional atherosclerosis include intact internal elastic lamina, rarity of calcification, and severe involvement of small intramyocardial vessels (**83**)[2]. However, it is important to note that the early lesions of transplant vasculopathy, although more diffuse and concentric, cannot always be differentiated from atherosclerosis lesions by morphology alone (**84**)[3].

EPIDEMIOLOGY

Atherosclerotic lesions are frequently present in the donor heart despite adequate screening and even normal angiogram[4]. These lesions are angiographically undetectable because these early atherosclerotic lesions typically do not encroach upon the lumen of coronary arteries, a process described as arterial remodeling[5]. Intravascular ultrasound (IVUS) examination of coronary vessels, which allows *in vivo* visualization of vessel walls, has demonstrated that atherosclerotic lesions are frequently transmitted to recipients despite normal coronary angiogram of the donor hearts[6]. Donor age and presence of CAD risk factors have been associated with more frequent transmission of donor atherosclerotic lesions.

Angiographic evidence of allograft vasculopathy is present in 50% of transplanted hearts in 5 years[7,8]. However, angiography is even more limited in defining allograft vasculopathy lesions compared to conventional atherosclerotic lesions because the vasculopathy lesions tend to involve the entire vessel diffusely. The prevalence of vasculopathy lesions is almost 50% at 1 year and 80% at 5 years when investigated with intravascular ultrasound[9].

Numerous risk factors have been associated with the development of allograft vasculopathy. These factors cause endothelial injury and can be classified as those unique to transplantation and those implicated in conventional atherosclerosis (*Table 9*). Most transplant-related injuries are immunologically mediated whereas most conventional atherosclerosis risk factors may have nonimmunologic mechanism of injury, but this distinction is probably an oversimplification.

PATHOGENESIS

The process of allograft vasculopathy is thought to begin with endothelial injury[9–12]. This injury probably begins in the donor with brain death. Ischemia during organ preservation and reperfusion injury with transplantation of the organ exacerbates the injury. After transplantation, acute cellular and humoral rejection, viral infections, and even immunosuppressive agents can lead to ongoing endothelial cell injury with resulting intimal hyperplasia. Other well-known endothelial insults such as hyperglycemia, hypertension, smoking, and hyperlipidemia accentuate the injury and its consequences.

The mechanism of intimal proliferation after endothelial injury in allograft vasculopathy has many similarities to the mechanism of lesion generation in conventional atherosclerosis or after balloon angioplasty. Endothelial cell injury causes a cascade of responses involving coagulation proteins, activation of complement, platelet activation, expression of selectins and adhesion molecules, recruitment and activation of proinflammatory cells, and subsequent increase in inflammatory mediators and cytokines. The multiple growth factors and cytokines lead to cell migration and proliferation, causing a typical lesion of allograft vasculopathy. As the initial events are generalized, the lesions involve the entire coronary vasculature in a diffuse pattern. Platelet activation and clotting play a role in total obliteration of the lumen with MI (**85**). Due to denervation of the heart, these events can be clinically

---

Table 9 Risk factors for allograft vasculopathy

Risk factors unique to transplantation
- Ischemic time.
- Activated cellular immunity:
    Increased cellular rejections.
    Increased IL-2 levels.
- Activated humoral immunity:
    Increased cytotoxic B-cell antibodies.
    Increased anti HLA antibodies.
- Infection:
    CMV infection.
- Gender mismatch.

Risk factors for conventional atherosclerosis that affect allograft vasculopathy
- Recipient age and gender.
- Diabetes.
- Hypertension.
- Hyperlipidemia (LDL, triglyceride).
- Smoking.
- Obesity.

HLA: human leukocyte antigen; LDL: low density lipoprotein.

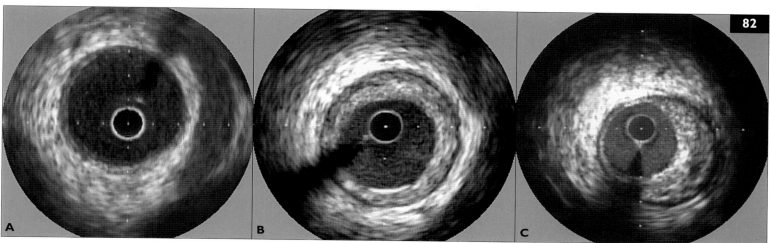

82: Intravascular ultrasound image of the proximal left anterior descending artery (LAD) 15 days (**A**) and 1 year (**B**) after transplantation to show allograft vasculopathy lesion. The same site is identified one year later by the intravascular ultrasound landmarks such as side branches and relation to pericardium. At 1-year follow-up there was a new plaque formed at a previously normal site. Intravascular ultrasound image of the proximal LAD 15 days after transplantation (**C**). This eccentric lesion is an example of a pre-existing atherosclerotic lesion in the donor heart.

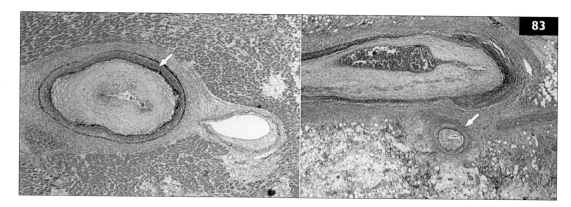

83 Cross section of an intramyocardial artery with severe intimal hyperplasia and obliteration of lumen (Verhoeff von Gieson stain). Note that the internal elastic lamina is intact (arrow). There is no calcification at the lesion site. (Courtesy of Dr. Corinne L. Fligner, Associate Prof. Department of Pathology, University of Washington Medical Center, Seattle, Washington.)

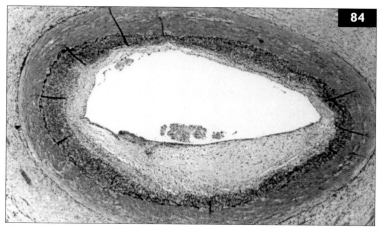

84 Cross section of a major epicardial artery with an eccentric plaque of transplant vasculopathy (Verhoeff von Gieson stain). (Courtesy of Dr. Corinne L. Fligner, Associate Prof. Department of Pathology, University of Washington Medical Center, Seattle, Washington.)

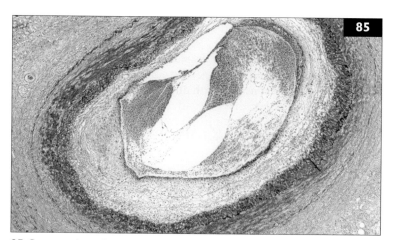

85 Cross section of a coronary artery with intense intimal hyperplasia and thrombus formation with obliteration of lumen (Verhoeff von Gieson stain). Platelet activation and thrombus formation are not uncommon events in the late stages of allograft vasculopathy. (Courtesy of Dr. Corinne L. Fligner, Associate Prof. Department of Pathology, University of Washington Medical Center, Seattle, Washington.)

silent and may only present as heart failure at a late stage. The role of donor atherosclerotic lesions in the generation of allograft vasculopathy is not entirely clear but it appears that early atherosclerotic lesions do not predispose to allograft vasculopathy. This is substantiated by the fact that the incidence of detectable transplant coronary disease on angiography at 5 years follow-up is similar in recipients of older hearts compared to those from younger donors[13].

CLINICAL PRESENTATION

Most typically, allograft vasculopathy is silent and is brought to attention by posttransplant surveillance testing. In the event that it is not clinically silent, it commonly presents with symptoms of heart failure including dyspnea on exertion, orthopnea, decreased exercise tolerance, and fatigue. About 10–30% of the heart recipients develop reinnervation of the transplanted heart and some of these patients can present with anginal symptoms, although this is rare[14]. Unfortunately, in a subset of patients the initial presentation could be SCD.

Most commonly, the allograft vasculopathy is suspected from new wall motion abnormalities, positive stress test, or surveillance angiography. The definitive noninvasive diagnosis of transplant vasculopathy is difficult because none of the tests are very sensitive or specific[15,16]. Even angiography is not always reliable because it is not able to detect early changes of allograft vasculopathy. IVUS is the most sensitive and specific method to identify and quantify lesions of transplant vasculopathy.

IVUS studies have significantly enhanced the understanding of the disease process[17,18]; allograft vasculopathy lesion morphology, long-term natural history of lesions, and role of remodeling have been studied extensively. IVUS continues to play a major role in investigating the effectiveness of various therapies to influence vasculopathy. Importantly, IVUS findings are shown to predict long-term clinical outcomes in heart transplant recipients[19,20]. Overall, IVUS provides an important clinical and research imaging tool to study allograft vasculopathy.

The optimal treatment regimen to prevent allograft vasculopathy has not been established. Various immunosuppressive regimens are under investigation. The conventional atherosclerosis risk factor modification is probably effective in retarding the progression of vasculopathy. The early use of diltiazem, pravastatin, or simvastatin has been demonstrated to be effective in reducing the development of vasculopathy[21,22]. The modification of potential risk factors that may help, but has not yet been proven, in allograft vasculopathy includes aggressive treatment of hypertension, obesity, diabetes, regular exercise, and abstinence from smoking. Percutaneous or surgical revascularization has been attempted to treat advanced allograft vasculopathy but with very limited success[23,24]. Retransplantation remains a viable treatment option but with obvious logistic limitations.

TRAUMATIC CORONARY ARTERY DISEASE

JUAN A. ASENSIO, MD, FACS, ERIC J. KUNCIR, MD, FACS, TAMER KARSIDAG, MD, AND PATRIZIO PETRONE, MD

INTRODUCTION

Penetrating cardiac injuries remain a difficult challenge to both trauma surgeons and trauma centers. They are one of the leading causes of death in the arena of urban violence. Improvements in emergency medical services systems over the past few years along with the applied principle of rapid transport have been responsible for an increasing number of cardiac injury patients arriving in impending or full cardiopulmonary arrest at busy urban trauma centers. Overall, cardiac injuries remain uncommon except in areas where penetrating trauma predominates.

Great difficulties exist in evaluating the results of many series. Over the past two decades, more than 30 series describing patients with penetrating cardiac injuries have been reported in the English language literature. Upon close scrutiny of these series, flaws become apparent; most series are retrospective reviews originating from institutions treating <15 cases of cardiac injuries annually. Furthermore, many serial and overlapping studies from few institutions account for a significant proportion of these reports.

High survival rates in selected reports tend to convey the erroneous impression that the lethal nature of cardiac injuries has significantly diminished. Invariably, all of these series omit data on the physiologic status upon initial presentation of these patients and are biased towards the reporting of patients with lesser degrees of anatomic severity and physiologic compromise.

There are three prospective studies in the literature dealing with cardiac injuries. The first study was reported by Buckman *et al.* in 1993 and consisted of 66 consecutive patients sustaining cardiac injuries, of whom 70% were admitted with gunshot wounds[1]. They reported an overall survival rate of 38%. When stratified to mechanism of injury, 80% of the patients sustaining stab wounds survived versus 20% of those that sustained gunshot wounds. In the second prospective cardiac injury study in the literature, 60 patients were included, 58% of whom had sustained gunshot wounds of the heart[2]. For the total number of patients, there was a reported overall survival rate of 37%. When stratified according to mechanism of injury, 68% of patients with stab wounds and 14% of patients with gunshot wounds survived. In this study, 62% of the patients underwent emergency department thoracotomy (EDT) with a 16% survival rate. Also in this study, five patients were studied with associated coronary artery injuries with an 80% mortality.

In the third prospective cardiac injury study in the literature 105 penetrating cardiac injuries were studied in a 2-year period[3]. Of these 105 patients, 65% had received gunshot wounds and 35% had received stab wounds. Seventy-one of the 105 patients (68%)

underwent EDT with a 14% survival rate. The overall survival was 33%, with a 16% survival rate for gunshot wounds and a 65% survival rate for stab wounds to the heart. In this study the authors reported nine penetrating coronary artery injuries with only one survivor, i.e. a 90% mortality rate.

INCIDENCE

Traumatic injury to the coronary arteries is extremely uncommon and is usually associated with a very poor prognosis. Rea *et al.*[4] reported 22 coronary artery injuries from penetrating trauma in a series of 500 patients, i.e. an incidence of 4.4%. Another study reported that of 76 patients treated over a 4-year period, nine had associated coronary artery injuries, an incidence of 12%. This is the highest incidence reported in the literature[5]. Wall *et al.*[6] reported 711 cardiac injuries in a period of over 20 years. In this series, 39 patients sustained associated penetrating coronary artery injuries, giving an incidence of 5%. This compares with nine patients out of 105 sustaining penetrating coronary artery injuries in a 2-year prospective study, an incidence of 9%[3].

In the military arena, no coronary artery injuries have been reported from the American experiences in World War II[7], the Korean war[8], or from the Vietnam war[9], this describing 96 cardiac injuries.

MECHANISM OF INJURY

Coronary artery injuries are extremely rare. Penetrating injuries (**86–89**) are by far more common than blunt injuries

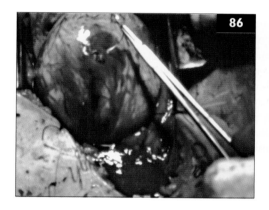

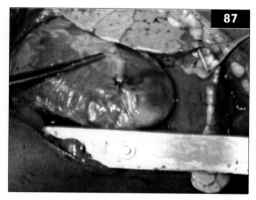

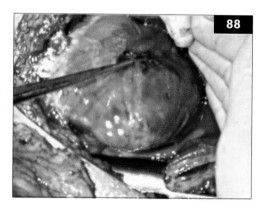

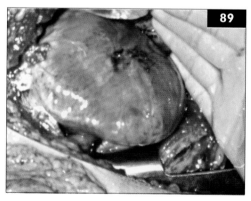

86 Laceration to the left ventricle and the distal third of the left anterior descending coronary artery (LAD) with a clot in a young male presenting with hypotension after sustaining a single stab wound to the precordium. After an immediate median sternotomy the patient underwent successful left ventricular cardiorraphy with ligation of the distal third of the LAD which he tolerated well. He was discharged home.

87 A 49-year-old male was admitted in full cardiopulmonary arrest after sustaining a stab wound to the left chest. Was intubated in the field and required closed cardiopulmonary resuscitation. Upon arrival in the Emergency Department (ED) the patient underwent ED thoracotomy, aortic crossclamping, open cardiopulmonary resuscitation and left ventricular cardiorraphy and ligation of the distal third of the left anterior descending coronary artery (LAD). A blood pressure was recovered and the patient was rushed to the operating room for further revision of his left ventricular cardiorraphy. The forceps points to the LAD as well as an area of scar secondary to an old and silent myocardial infarction. Associated injuries included a laceration to the left lower lobe of the lung which was repaired primarily. After ligation of the distal LAD, the patient experienced left ventricular dysfunction and required intraoperative pressors to allow him to reach the Intensive Care Unit. He required pressors for the first two days postoperatively and had diminished cardiac output /cardiac index which eventually corrected. Pressors were weaned succesfully. Patient survived with no neurological sequelae.

88 Young male who had received multiple stab wounds to the left chest and sustained a cardiopulmonary arrest. He required Emergency Departement (ED) intubation and ED thoracotomy, aortic crossclamping, and open cardiopulmonary resuscitation. He had sustained a biventricular laceration adjacent to the middle third of the left anterior descending coronary artery involving two septal branches. These lacerations were stapled temporarily and a blood pressure was recovered. The patient was rushed to the operating room.

89 The same patient as in **88**. Most staples were removed. The septal branches from the left anterior descending artery (LAD) were ligated and a biventricular cardiorraphy was performed with 2-0 polypropylene monofilament sutures, passing the sutures below the bed of the LAD to prevent inadvertent occlusion or narrowing. The patient required intraoperative pressors which were progressively discontinued. He recuperated fully.

(**90**). Penetrating coronary artery injuries are only reported from a few of the major urban trauma centers that have sufficiently large experience with the management of penetrating cardiac injuries. The incidence ranges from 5 to 12% of all associated penetrating cardiac injuries.

Penetrating coronary artery injuries usually consist of either a partial laceration, total transection or, rarely, coronary artery injury fistulas to the pulmonary artery and/or ventricles. Similarly, retained missiles in the heart encroaching upon the coronary vessels have been reported to initiate local arteriosclerosis at a time remote from the original injury[10]. Blunt coronary artery injuries are even more infrequent, with approximately 30 cases reported in the literature[11]. Blunt trauma to the coronary arteries can result in complete occlusion, transection with thrombosis, dissection, and pseudoaneurysm formation[12].

SURGICAL MANAGEMENT

The vast majority of patients with coronary artery injuries will also have an associated cardiac injury. Patients with penetrating coronary artery injuries will arrive at busy urban trauma centers 'in extremis' or in full cardiopulmonary arrest. Patients presenting with pericardial tamponade or hypotension should be immediately transported to the operating room for immediate median sternotomy.

The techniques for EDT and those required for the management of penetrating cardiac injuries have been described (**86–89**)[3]. For the purposes of injury description and surgical management, the coronary artery is divided into the upper third, middle, and lower third. These injuries should also be conceptualized as either injuries to the right or left coronary arteries (RCA or LCA), or to their main branches.

Techniques

Repairing the periventricular wounds adjacent to coronary artery injuries can be quite challenging. Isolated coronary artery injuries in the absence of a myocardial injury have not been reported. Injudicious placement of sutures may narrow or occlude a coronary artery or one of its branches. Therefore, it is recommended that sutures be placed underneath the bed of the coronary. The authors recommend the utilization of 2-0 polypropylene monofilament sutures to repair the associated cardiac injury.

Primary repair of a lacerated coronary artery that is actively bleeding is extremely difficult, if not impossible, without the use of cardiopulmonary bypass. Consequently, lacerations in the upper third of a coronary artery that are actively bleeding will require ligation and demand the use of cardiopulmonary bypass for repair, but few patients survive to be placed on pump. Lacerations of the middle third of the coronary artery that are actively bleeding will also require ligation. This often results in an immediate MI at the operating table, often requiring vasopressors. To maintain tissue perfusion, these patients may benefit from the immediate institution of intraaortic balloon counterpulsation, and/or aortocoronary bypass. Injuries to the distal one-third of the coronary arteries will usually tolerate ligation and may or may not require the institution of vasopressors.

The majority of blunt injuries to the coronary artery resulting in lacerations, thrombosis, aneurysms, or fistulas will require utilization of cardiopulmonary bypass and aortocoronary bypass grafting. Adjunct utilization of intra-aortic balloon counterpulsation may be required in selected cases.

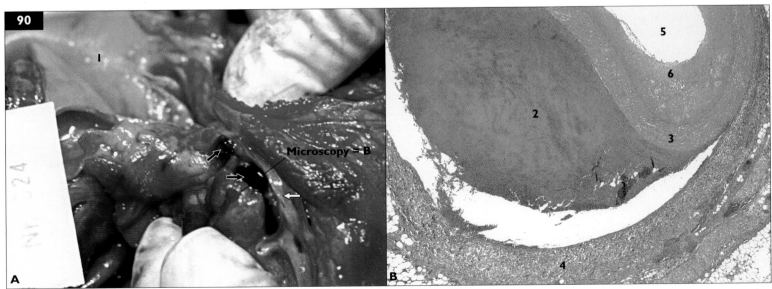

90 A 35-year-old pedestrian was hit frontally by a moped (blunt chest injury). At hospital admission, the electrocardiogram showed extensive ST segment elevation (transmural ischemia of the anterior wall) followed by a rapid rise in blood markers of myocardial necrosis. He died suddenly 8 days later. Autopsy revealed transmural infarction with myocardial rupture and hemopericardium. **A**: The left anterior descending coronary artery (white arrow) was patent without thrombosis but surrounded (compressed) proximally by a hematoma (black arrows). **B**: Microscopic examination revealed that the hematoma seen macroscopically was a hemorrhagic dissection (2) between tunica media (3) and adventitia (4) (traumatic coronary artery dissection). There was no significant preexisting arterial disease. 1: aorta; 5: left anterior descending artery lumen; 6: intima. (Courtesy of Dr. Ingrid Bayer Kristensen, MD, Institute of Forensic Medicine, University of Aarhus.)

MANAGEMENT

Review of the literature shows that outcome depends on the vessel injured and on the location of the injury in relation to the origin of the vessel. Rea et al.[4] in 1969 reported the first series of 22 penetrating coronary artery injuries in the era of early cardiac surgery. Overall mortality was 55% and the majority of injuries were to the LCA system, as would be expected from its more anterior location. Ligation of injured coronary arteries was employed predominantly with only one person placed on emergency cardiopulmonary bypass. The ten survivors uniformly were found to have distal coronary artery injury, which tolerated vessel ligation and produced nonfatal MI. The patient who was placed on bypass died of intractable fibrillation.

Espada et al.[5] reported on a series of nine patients. Six patients had injury to the left anterior descending coronary artery (LAD) and two had injury to the RCA with only one injury to the left circumflex artery (LCx). All patients presented with signs of life, four were in severe shock, and all had ECG abnormalities consisting of bundle branch block or ST- and T-wave changes. Eight patients underwent vessel ligation and one was successfully placed on bypass, with only one death occurring to a patient who had RCA ligation. The authors determined that, despite rapid improvement in the technique of cardiac bypass, its utilization in this setting was still limited. The patient who was placed on bypass had a proximal LAD injury with shock, which prompted placement on bypass utilizing standby portable equipment. They concluded that suture ligation of the cut ends is the treatment of choice for small distal coronary vessels. More proximal injuries may also be ligated; however, if signs of cardiac failure occur then bypass is advocated.

In a series of 39 cases[6], an overall mortality of 69% was reported, and 58% of patients required EDT. Mortality clearly depended on the vessel injured, with LAD injury resulting in 76% mortality, LCx/obtuse marginal artery injury with 71% mortality, and right/posterior descending coronary artery with 62% mortality. All but two patients underwent vessel ligation, and only one of the bypassed patients survived. Bypassed patients again presented with high proximal LAD lesions with obvious ventricular dysfunction and with sufficient signs of life to warrant emergent coronary bypass grafting. The authors concluded that despite large numbers of cardiac injuries, injury to the coronary arteries remains rare. Many patients self-triage, with those with more complex injuries often found dead at the scene or presenting in extremis. Consequently, the utilization of bypass should still be limited because survivors tend to tolerate distal vessel ligation without significant cardiac dysfunction. Marginal cardiac dysfunction can be successfully temporized using intra-aortic balloon pump in an attempt to avoid bypass surgery. Bypass for proximal vessels is still sometimes necessary and survival is not always guaranteed due to complications of bypass, such as heparinization[13].

Blunt chest trauma resulting in coronary artery injury is rare. The most frequently injured vessel is the LAD (76%), followed by the RCA (12%), and LCx (6%)[14]. Mechanism of injury is due to direct deceleration forces and occlusion is most likely due to response to intimal tears, subintimal hemorrhage, thrombosis, and disruption of a pre-existing atherosclerotic plaque[11].

Resultant MI from blunt trauma can represent coronary artery injury and should be considered by the trauma surgeon. The injury can be recognized early, presenting with an abnormal admission ECG with ST–T changes or, more frequently, acute MI pattern[11]. Secondary survey may or may not reveal signs of blunt chest injury. The patient may not have a history of prior chest pain or coronary disease, prompting the surgeon to investigate further the new ECG changes. Workup with transthoracic and transesophageal echocardiography (TEE) has been reported, although TEE enables the differentiation of simple myocardial contusion, coronary artery dissection, or aortic dissection involving the coronary artery[15]. Cardiac catheterization is used when TEE is not available or in order to plan surgical intervention[14].

Alternative treatments have been reported in the literature. The use of thrombolytic treatment would not be advocated by most surgeons because of the risk of hemorrhage from other injuries[14]. Reperfusion by percutaneous transluminal coronary angioplasty (PTCA) has also been assessed but it must be performed within the standard time window of 6 hours after onset of symptoms[11]. Case reports of stenting of occluded dissections after blunt trauma also exist, although anticoagulation is also necessary and is frequently restricted secondary to concomitant injuries[14]. Reports of coronary bypass also exist but the majority are for treatment of mechanical defects resulting from the injured coronary vessel, such as aneurysms, septal defects, or fistulas, rather than for acute treatment of posttraumatic angina[12, 14–16].

Alternatively, medical therapy can be used in the absence of ongoing ischemia[12], with some intimal injuries demonstrated to have completed healing in 6 months on serial cardiac catheterization[14]. This conservative approach is not uniformly advised, however, as 30% of patients develop aneurysmal disease with case reports of dissection evolving into permanent poor ventricular function[14].

Chapter Six

Myocardial Ischemia: Morbid Demand

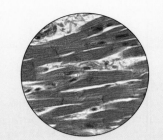

CARDIAC HYPERTROPHY

**K-RAMAN PURUSHOTHAMAN, MD,
WILLIAM N. O'CONNOR, MD, DARIO ECHEVERRI, MD
AND PEDRO R. MORENO, MD**

DEFINITION

Myocardial hypertrophy is defined as excessive cardiomyocyte growth with protein synthesis and organization of sarcomeres, accompanied by interstitial collagen deposition and growth of the vascular compartment[1]. This is a self-limited response triggered by elevated extrinsic or intrinsic biomechanical stress within the myocardium. In the human ventricle, parallel and reproducible increases in cell diameter, volume, and nuclear area characterize 'hypertrophic' growth but are accompanied by extracellular matrix (ECM) and interstitial changes that ultimately 'stiffen' the hypertrophied myocardium, which affects diastole, resulting in clinical symptoms. Macroscopically, hypertrophy is characterized by wall thickening and near obliteration of the ventricular cavity (**91**). Classification of cardiac hypertrophy is divided into physiologic and pathologic conditions (*Table 10*).

EPIDEMIOLOGY

The prevalence of left ventricular hypertrophy is 14.9% for men and 9.1% for women[2]. The epidemiology of cardiac hypertrophy is related to specific etiology. The most common major cause of hypertrophy is systemic hypertension. Valvular heart disease and primary hypertrophic cardiomyopathy are second and third causes and affect a lower percentage of the population.

PATHOGENESIS

Two major concepts define hemodynamic parameters related to wall stress, preload, and afterload. Preload, defined as the wall stress at the end of diastole and therefore at the maximum resting length of the sarcomere, is dependent on left ventricular-end diastolic volume[3]. Because volumes are difficult to measure, a common surrogate of preload is the end-diastolic pressure, prior to isovolumetric contraction. Afterload is defined as the wall stress in systole induced by the load of the ventricle during contraction. Wall stress is directly proportional to the radius of the ventricle and intra-cavitary pressure and is inversely proportional to wall thickness. Hence, physiologic hypertrophy compensates for increased wall stress. Compensatory hypertrophy presents as concentric and eccentric patterns. Concentric hypertrophy is defined as an increase in myocardial mass by the addition of parallel arrayed cardiomyocytes in width, without an increase in end-diastolic volume (pressure overload). Eccentric hypertrophy is defined as an increase in myocardial mass by the addition of longitudinal and serial arrayed cardiomyocytes, accompanied by increased end-diastolic volume (volume overload)[4].

Myocardial oxygen supply versus demand

Ischemia-driven cardiac hypertrophy is either due to decreased supply of oxygen (coronary artery disease [CAD], atherothrombosis, and coronary arteriovenous fistulas) or due to increased demand for oxygen (aortic stenosis, hypertrophic obstructive cardiomyopathy, systemic hypertension, aortic incompetence).

When oxygen demand outstrips oxygen supply to the myocardium, there is a state of ischemia that alters relaxation,

---

Table 10 Classification of cardiac hypertrophy

Physiologic:
- Exercise-induced (athletics).
- Growth, age, gender, hormone related.

Pathologic:
- Increased preload: aortic and mitral incompetence.
- Increased afterload:
  - Systemic hypertension.
  - Left ventricular outflow obstruction (aortic stenosis).
  - Coarctation of aorta.
- Cardiac muscle disease:
  - Hypertrophic cardiomyopathy (contractile protein defects).
- Systemic extracardiac factors:
  - Thyrotoxicosis.
  - Increases in catecholamines, corticotrophins, and growth hormone.

stiffens the myocardium, and increases wall stress, perpetuating hypertrophy. The major components of myocardial oxygen demand are determined by: (1) preload; (2) afterload; (3) contractility; and (4) heart rate. Coronary flow is mostly autoregulated but may be influenced by humoral factors and metabolic and neural control. Myocardial oxygen supply, provided by 4000 capillaries/mm^2 of myocardium, is progressively reduced in hypertrophy, contributing to the supply/demand mismatch characteristic of this entity. **92** summarizes the relationship between oxygen supply and demand[5].

CELLULAR BASIS OF HYPERTROPHY

Linzbach[6] previously assessed the critical left ventricular (LV) weight leading to pathologic hypertrophy, and found a cut-off point of 400 g. Addition of new myofibril contributes half the bulk up to a 300% increase in the contractile proteins. Sarcomerogenesis can increase by up to 40% in addition to augmentation/ proliferation of mitochondria and the capillary bed[7].

Ultrastructurally, progressive hypertrophy shows a gradual and ultimately self-limiting increase in the proportion of mitochondria to myofilaments within each cardiomyocyte (**93**). Under normal physiologic conditions, mitochondria occupy 30% and myofilaments 70% of the total cytoplasmic volume. Thus the early, or evolving phase of hypertrophy exhibits structural and biochemical remodeling of the myocyte and the ECM.

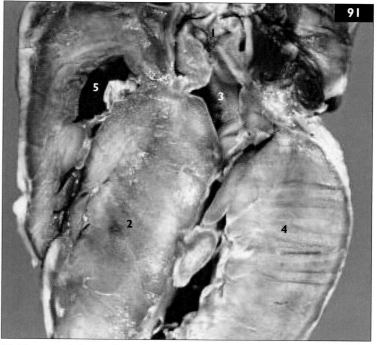

91 Macroscopic long axis view of hemi-sectioned, autopsy heart displaying primary hypertrophic cardiomyopathy with small left ventricular (LV) cavity and markedly thickened LV free wall. 1: aortic valve; 2: interventricular septum; 3: left ventricular outflow tract; 4: left ventricular free wall; 5: right ventricular outflow tract.

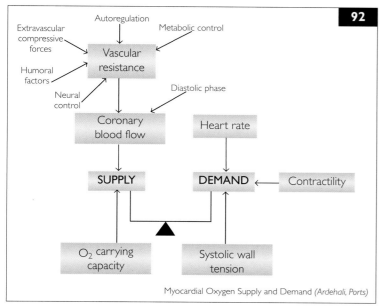

Myocardial Oxygen Supply and Demand (Ardehali, Ports)

92 Diagram to show the factors that influence myocardial oxygen supply and the demand elicited by the systolic wall tension, contractility, and heart rate. (From Ardehali and Ports [1990][5]. Myocardial oxygen supply and demand. *Chest* **98**:703. With permission.)

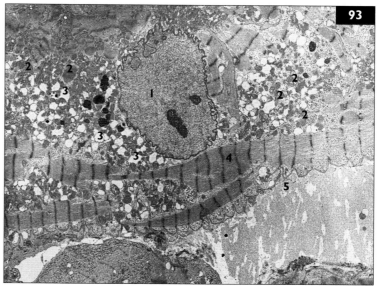

93 Electron micrograph of advanced hypertrophy, with a cardiomyocyte showing mitochondriosis with increased cell volume occupied by proliferated mitochondria, splitting and disorganization of myofibrils (X6000). 1: nucleus; 2: mitochondria; 3: sarcotubules (holes with fluid); 4: myofilaments; 5: cell membrane.

Ventricular pump function and oxygen delivery remain normal[8]. Ultrastructurally, the early, compensated hypertrophied cardiomyocyte consists of 50% mitochondria and 50% myofilaments. Remodeled myocardium may revert to normal if the trigger loading condition is removed, resulting in a stage of coordinated balance (**94A**). Myocardial contractility may be abnormal if the cellular mechanisms reach the maximum physiologic compensatory hypertrophy[8]. If the loading conditions persist, an end-stage or pathologic phase develops, characterized by imbalanced structural and biochemical remodeling of the myocyte and ECM (**94B**), and resulting in depressed myocardial contractility. Ultrastructurally, the late, uncompensated hypertrophied cardiomyocyte shows a ratio of 70% mitochondria to 30% myofilaments. By then, abnormal systolic function affects oxygen delivery[8], leading to peripheral muscle wasting and clinical signs of advanced heart failure.

MOLECULAR BASIS OF HYPERTROPHY

Activation of mechanoreceptors induces cytoplasmic signals through the cell membrane. Growth factors initiate the phosphorylation of tyrosine kinases, in addition to the activation of protein kinase C by angiotensin II, endothelin-1 (ET), α_1-adrenergic receptors, and stretch receptors resulting in the activity of mitogens and oncoproteins, causing signal transduction of hypertrophy through the nucleus to produce early response genes[9]. Transcriptional activity by messenger ribonucleic acid (mRNA) and protein synthesis leads to fetal gene phenotype formation, angiotensin II, and growth factors leading to cardiac remodeling and hypertrophy (**95**)[10].

CLINICAL PRESENTATION AND SIGNIFICANCE OF CARDIAC HYPERTROPHY

The early or evolutionary phase, where workload exceeds the work output, leads to a stable, compensatory state where myocyte growth counteracts increased workload/cardiac mass ratio[11]. This is characterized by delayed relaxation and diminished coronary vascular reserve. Clinical manifestations of this compensated phase may be absent (silent hypertrophy) or may be manifested by dyspnea associated with physical activity and decreased exercise capacity. The end-stage, heart failure/decompensated phase, where the workload cannot compensate for the work output, leads to a progressive decreased ability of the heart to fill normally and to generate force. Clinical manifestations of this decompensated phase include dyspnea at rest, orthopnea, paroxysmal nocturnal dyspnea, and peripheral edema. Cardiac arrhythmia and sudden death may be the terminal events.

Major advances in diagnosis and treatment of heart failure are rapidly evolving. However, prevention is the most effective approach against this lethal disease, and stabilization/reversal of hypertrophy with early diagnosis and treatment of causative agents are crucial to achieving this goal.

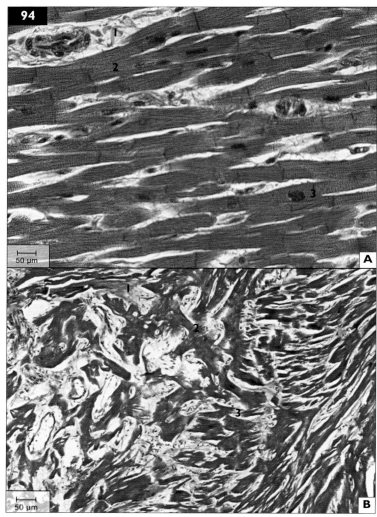

94 A: Compensated hypertrophy: an elastic trichrome-stained section of left ventricular cardiac hypertrophy (hypertension-related) shows parallel array of cardiomyocytes 30–40 μm diameter, box-shaped nuclei, and increased interstitial matrix (×40). **B**: Decompensated hypertrophy: an elastic trichrome-stained section from b-myosin heavy chain disease in hypertrophic obstructive cardiomyopathy shows nonparallel myofiber disarray (up to 90° intersection of enlarged cardiomyocytes) with irregular deposition of extracellular collagen matrix (×40). 1: collagen; 2: cardiomyocyte; 3: nucleus .

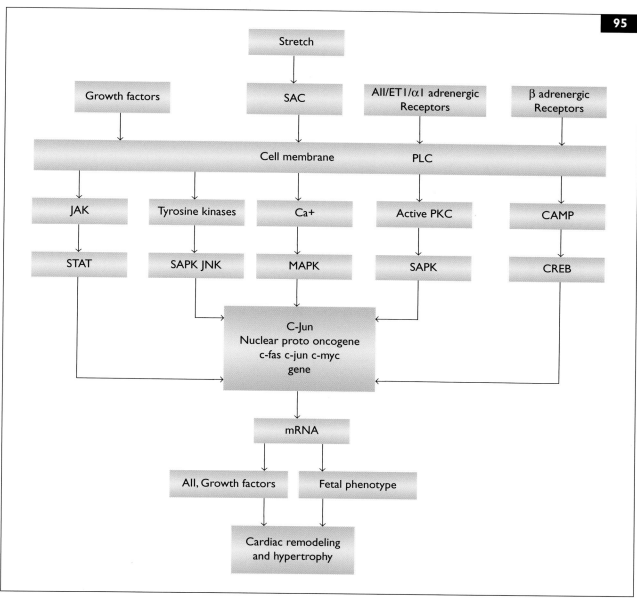

95 Cell signals in response to hypertrophic stimuli induce transcription of protooncogene through the nucleus and initiation of mRNA for the fetal phenotype gene and angiotensin II and growth factors, resulting in cardiac hypertrophy and remodeling. AII: angiotensin II; ET: endothelin-1; JAK: janus kinase; STAT: signal transducers and activators of transcription; JNK (SAPK): cJUN NH2-terminal kinase; α_1: α_1-adrenergic activity; SAC: stretch activated channel; PLC: phospholipase C; CREB: cyclic AMP response element-binding protein; MAPK: mitogen activated protein kinase; PKC: protein kinase C. (Adapted and modified from Opie [1997]. Overload hypertrophy and its molecular biology. In: *The Heart: Physiology, from Cell to Circulation*, 3rd edn. LH Opie (ed). Lippincott-Raven, Philadelphia, pp. 391–418.)

SYSTEMIC CAUSES OF INCREASED DEMAND

KAVITA KUMAR, MD

INTRODUCTION
Hypertension and hyperthyroidism are among the most frequent systemic conditions that may lead to an abnormal, high myocardial oxygen demand.

HYPERTENSION
The definition of hypertension is based on the level of blood pressure that carries a doubling of long-term cardiovascular risk. A patient is diagnosed with hypertension when at least two blood pressure measurements obtained over a 3-month period are at a level that increases long-term risk. Based on the Seventh Joint National Committee (JNC 7) guidelines, normal blood pressure is a systolic pressure <120 mmHg (16 kPa) and a diastolic pressure <80 mmHg (10.7 kPa) (*Table 11*). A new category has been introduced in JNC 7 in the classification of blood pressure, prehypertension, in order to increase awareness that these patients are at higher risk of progressing to overt hypertension and should implement lifestyle modifications at an earlier phase.

Additionally, stages 2 and 3 in JNC 6 have been combined into one stage in JNC 7, as outlined in *Table 11*. When systolic and diastolic pressures fall into different stages, the higher stage is used to classify the patient's hypertension. According to JNC 7, the risk of cardiovascular diseases doubles in an incremental fashion for each increase of 20/10 mmHg (2.7/1.3 kPa). As the blood pressure increases, so does the risk of developing progressive cardiovascular and renal dysfunction.

Epidemiology
The Third National Health and Nutrition Examination Survey (NHANES) studied the prevalence of hypertension in the adult population in the United States from 1988 to 1991. This study indicated that the age-adjusted prevalence was highest amongst non-Hispanic blacks (32.4%), followed by non-Hispanic whites (23.3%) and Mexican Americans (22.6%). Overall, the prevalence of hypertension was slightly higher in men than in women. An increase in age correlated with an increase in prevalence and severity of hypertension, regardless of gender or race. Diastolic pressure, however, increased into the fifth decade, but then decreased, consequently increasing the pulse pressure.

Observational studies have shown a direct association between elevated diastolic pressure and coronary artery disease. Prolonged elevation of diastolic pressure of 5–10 mmHg (0.7–1.3 kPa) was associated with at least 21–37% increase in coronary heart disease risk and 34–56% increase in stroke risk.

Pathogenesis
Hypertension in the long run causes end-organ damage as manifest by LV hypertrophy (LVH), coronary artery disease, carotid wall thickness, nephropathy, and retinopathy. Hypertension increases the left ventricular wall tension, which results in myocardial hypertrophy (**96**). It also increases the wall tension and shear stress on the vascular smooth muscle. As a result, there is an increase in vascular smooth muscle cell proliferation, hypertrophy, and hyperplasia. Consequently, atherosclerosis is accelerated and ischemia results from endothelial dysfunction and impaired coronary vasodilation. This process affects not only the epicardial vessels, but also the microvasculature. Additionally, in the presence of LVH there is increased myocyte hypertrophy and decreased microvascular density, which can result in extrinsic compression of the microvasculature. All these processes create a mismatch between increased demand and inadequate supply, resulting in myocardial ischemia (**96**).

Clinical presentation
The clinical presentation of hypertension can range from asymptomatic to sudden death. Studies have shown that hypertensive patients develop silent infarcts more frequently than nonhypertensive patients. They can also present with either stable or unstable angina. Myocardial ischemia also places these patients at higher risk of ventricular arrhythmias. Long-standing hypertension leads to LVH (**97A,B**), diastolic dysfunction, and eventually systolic dysfunction and congestive heart failure. Other manifestations of hypertension include stroke and renal disease. Thus, the goals for treatment of hypertension should focus on the prevention of end-organ damage.

Table 11 Blood pressure classification

Category	Systolic BP (mmHg)		Diastolic BP (mmHg)
Normal	<120	AND	<80
Pre-hypertension	120–139	OR	80–89
Hypertension			
Stage I	140–159	OR	90–99
Stage II	≥160	OR	≥100

(From Chobanian *et al.* [2003]. National Heart, Lung, and Blood Institute Joint National Committee on Prevention, Detection, Evaluation, and Treatment of High Blood Pressure; National High Blood Pressure Education Program Coordinating Committee (2003). The seventh report of the Joint National Committee on prevention, detection, evaluation, and treatment of high blood pressure: the JNC 7 report. *JAMA* **289**:2560–2572.)

HYPERTHYROIDISM

The thyroid gland secretes thyroxine (T4) and tri-iodothyronine (T3). T4, which is a prohormone, is deiodinated to form T3, the final mediator of biologic effects of thryroid hormones. T3 and T4 help regulate oxidative and metabolic processes in the body. Hyperthyroidism results from excessive T3 production as well as increased deiodination of T4 to T3. The excess T3 has both direct and indirect effects on the heart, which result in a hyperdynamic circulation.

Epidemiology

Hyperthyroidism has a prevalence of approximately 1%. Younger women (aged 30–50 years) are more frequently affected. Some causes include Graves' disease and multi-nodular goiter. Cardiac

96 Pathogenesis of myocardial ischemia secondary to hypertension. LV: left ventricle; LVH: left ventricular hypertrophy.

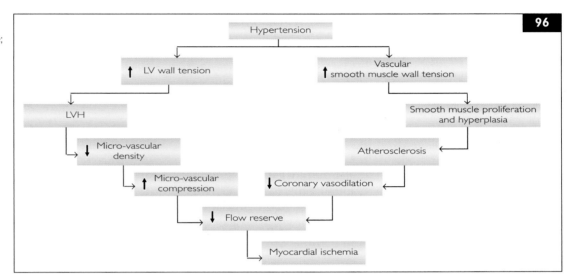

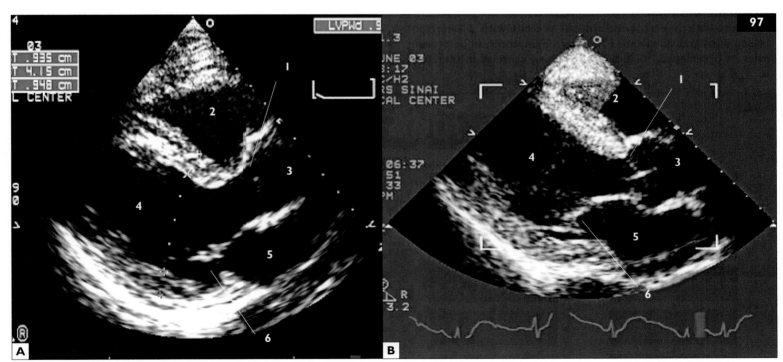

97 A: Parasternal long axis echocardiographic view of a normal heart showing left ventricular wall thickness ~ 1 cm (normal <1.1 cm). **B**: The same parasternal long axis echocardiographic view of a heart with left ventricular hypertrophy (LVH) secondary to hypertension. The left ventricular wall thickness measures ~ 1.5 cm. 1: aortic valve; 2: right ventricle; 3: aorta; 4: left ventricle; 5: left atrium; 6: mitral valve.

involvement is frequent, with arrhythmias being the most common manifestation. Myocardial ischemia and heart failure are less common.

Pathogenesis

Thyroid hormone affects both the heart and the systemic vasculature (**98**). T3 binds to nuclear receptor proteins of cardiac myocytes. These proteins then bind to the thyroid hormone response elements, which are specific deoxyribonucleic acid (DNA) sequences on target genes. These genes are responsible for encoding myosin heavy chain, sarcoplasmic reticulum calcium-activated ATPase, phospholamban, and Na/K ATPase. These proteins are involved in the structure and regulation of cardiac contractile function. In addition to these direct effects on the heart, T3 also causes relaxation of the vascular smooth muscle cells, thereby resulting in a decrease in the systemic vascular resistance (SVR) by as much as 50–70%. T3 causes vasodilation by direct stimulation of the smooth muscle and by endothelial release of vasodilators such as nitric oxide. This decrease in systemic vascular resistance consequently results in an increased cardiac output. The hyperthyroid state is similar to other states resulting from increased catecholamine stimulation. However, in hyperthyroidism there is no significant increase in the circulating catecholamines; instead, there is believed to be an increase in the number of β-catecholamine receptors. Ischemia results from inadequate blood supply and tissue oxygenation in the setting of a hyperdynamic circulation (**98**).

Clinical presentation

A patient with hyperthyroidism can present with a variety of cardiac signs and symptoms (*Table 12*). Symptoms, in decreasing order of prevalence, include palpitations, exercise intolerance, dyspnea on exertion, angina, and orthopnea. Patients commonly experience palpitations and an increase in their resting heart rate. Atrial tachyarrhythmias can also occur.

Chest pain also occurs in hyperthyroid patients (*Table 12*), and may be secondary to myocardial ischemia. Ischemia likely to be the result of a mismatch in supply and demand. Hyperthyroidism causes an increase in the cardiac workload and myocardial oxygen demand; however, this increase in demand is not met by an equal increase in supply. Coronary spasm may be another reason for myocardial ischemia. The electrocardiogram (ECG) may reveal characteristic changes of myocardial ischemia. Younger patients may not have significant coronary disease, but older patients may have underlying CAD that is unmasked by hyperthyroidism. In addition to ischemia, hyperthyroidism creates a high-output state and, if left uncorrected, can lead to dilated cardiomyopathy and heart failure.

Table 12 Hyperthyroidism: cardiac manifestations and prevalence

Symptoms		Signs	
• Palpitations	~85%	• Tachycardia	~95%
• Exercise intolerance	~65%	• Hyperdynamic precordium	~75%
• Dyspnea on exertion	~45%	• Wide pulse pressure	~75%
• Angina	~3–5%	• Murmurs	~50%
• Orthopnea		• Atrial fibrillation	~5–15%
		• Pedal edema	~5%
		• S_3	~3%

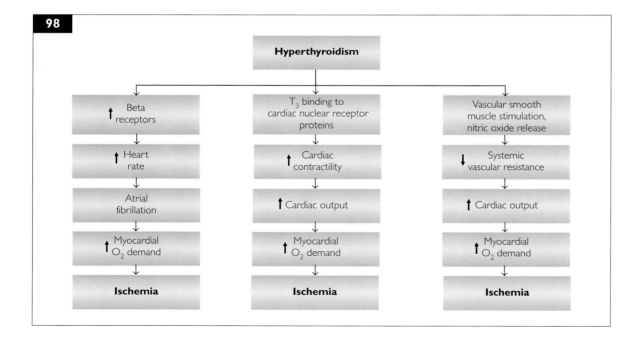

98 Pathogenesis of ischemia in hyperthyroidism.

Chapter Seven

Detection of Coronary Artery Disease

DIAGNOSTIC CORONARY ANGIOGRAPHY

JENS KNUDSEN, MD, PhD AND ULRIK ABILDGAARD, MD, DMSC

TECHNIQUE

The percutaneous approach to left heart catheterization achieves access by needle puncture of the femoral artery or radial/brachial (*ad modum* Sones) artery, or even the lumbar aorta. An introducing sheath is placed in the vessel over a guide wire. The femoral approach (*ad modum* Seldinger) with sheath has become the dominant approach to coronary angiography (CAG). In Europe, nearly 80% of the CAG procedures are performed in outpatient clinics and the patient is discharged the same day.

It is very important to perform the puncture at the correct level (i.e. 1–2 cm inferior to the inguinal ligament) to avoid vascular complications. If the puncture site is too inferior there is a chance that the needle will puncture the superficial or profunda branches which may cause vascular complications afterwards. If the puncture site is too cranial, a retroperitoneal hematoma may develop after removal of the sheath. The procedure is terminated with removal of the sheath during compression of the puncture site of the artery. Insignificant compression predisposes to complications (hematoma and pseudoaneurysm).

From the peripheral artery specially curved catheters (Judkins, Amplatz, Castillo, Sones, multi-purpose [MP], hockey-stick shape, internal mammary) can be advanced into the ascending aorta and into the ostium of the left and right coronary artery respectively. The 'Judkins left' (JL) is the standard catheter for the left coronary ostium. A JL with a 4-cm curve (JL4) will engage the left coronary main stem without further manipulation when it is advanced down into the aortic root. 'Judkins right' is the standard catheter for the right coronary ostium.

Ionic or nonionic contrast medium (iodine concentration of 320 mg/ml) is injected into the coronary artery. A new X-ray installation provides both 'live' fluoroscopy and cineangiography by digital encoding.

It is important that all segments of the coronary artery are visualized without shortening (axial X-rays) or with other artery branches overlaying the artery in question. Therefore, to obtain a complete visualization of epicardial coronary arteries without foreshortening or overlap, the image intensifier of the X-ray equipment is sequentially positioned in combinations of cranially, caudally, left, and right sided views.

A standard CAG often comprises 11 standardized angiograms: one ventriculography and seven different views of the left coronary artery (LCA) and three views of the right coronary artery (RCA). The different views of the coronary arteries visualize different segments of the vessels. Furthermore, viewing of the coronary artery from different angles is important because most atherosclerotic lesions are eccentric, resulting in an elliptic lumen rather than a circular lumen. The eccentric nature of stenoses makes them prone to erroneous evaluations, e.g. the stenosis may look severe as the angle shows the small stenotic lumen of the stenosis, or the stenosis can hardly be seen as the angle shows the largest diameter of the artery lumen (**99–102**).

INDICATIONS

In general both symptomatic as well as asymptomatic patients with suspected coronary artery disease should undergo CAG (*Table 13*)[1].

Table 13 Indications for coronary angiography

Symptomatic patients
- Patients with angina pectoris.
- Patients with NSTEMI.
- Patients with postinfarct angina pectoris during rest or during exercise-ECG or with silent ischemia during exercise-ECG.
- Patients with STEMI or patients with chest pains with presumed new LBBB who can undergo PTCA within 12 hours of onset as an alternative to thrombolytic therapy.

Asymptomatic patients
- Diabetic patients with silent ischemia or reversible defects by myocardial scintigraphy.
- Patients with postinfarct exercise test with silent ischemia.

ECG: electrocardiogram; LBBB: left bundle branch block; NSTEMI: non-ST elevation myocardial infarction; PTCA: percutaneous transluminal coronary angioplasty; STEMI: ST elevation myocardial infarction.

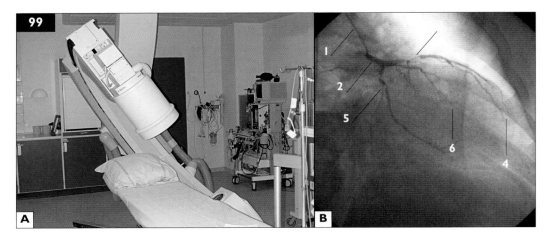

99 A: Image intensifier to the right of the patient viewing the heart in the 35/0 right anterior oblique (RAO) view, designating rotation 35° to the right without cranial or caudal rotation. The X-ray tube is to the left and beneath the table. **B**: The left coronary artery from the RAO 35/0 view.
1: Judkins catheter; 2: left main stem; 3: severe stenosis of the proximal left anterior descending artery; 4: distal left anterior descending artery; 5: circumflex artery with two stenoses; 6: intermedius artery with an offspring from the left main stem between the left anterior descending artery and the circumflex artery (see **100B**).

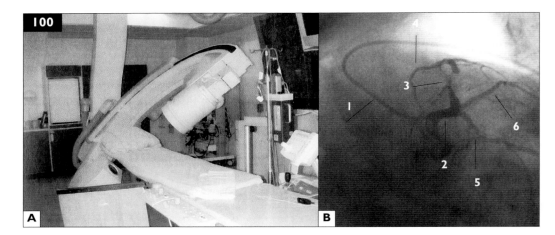

100 A: Image intensifier to the left and caudally of the patient viewing the heart in the left anterior oblique (LAO 45/30) view, i.e. 45° to the left and 30° caudally. **B**: Left coronary artery from the LAO 45/30 view (arrows: see legend to **99B**).

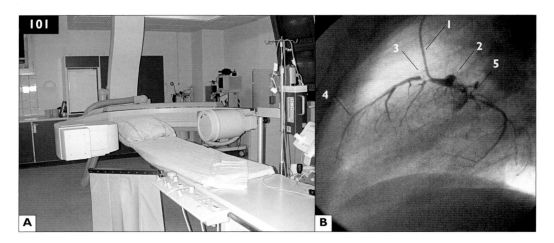

101 A: Image intensifier to the left of the patients viewing the heart in the left anterior oblique (LAO 90/0) view, i.e. 90° to the left and 0° caudally. **B**: Left coronary artery from the LAO 90/0 view (arrows: see legend to **99B**).

102 Right coronary artery in the RAO 35/0 view.
1: right Judkins catheter;
2: right coronary artery;
3: posterior descending artery with septal branches.

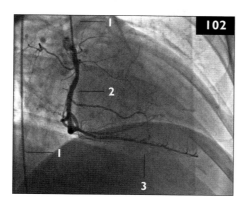

Table 14 presents specific indications for the use of CAG. These include acute coronary syndromes (ACS), patients with suspected ischemic heart disease, patients with dyspnea or angina pectoris who have previously been treated with coronary artery bypass graft (CABG) or percutaneous transluminal coronary angioplasty (PTCA), patients with heart failure or other heart diseases, and various miscellaneous conditions.

Table 14 Specific indications for coronary angiography

Patients with ACS:
- Patients with STEMI who can undergo primary PTCA as an alternative to thrombolytic therapy.
- Patients with STEMI who are unstable despite PTCA or thrombolytic treatment (persistent pain, hemodynamic instability, recurrent ischemia refractory to medical treatment).
- Angina pectoris during rest >36 hours after debut of symptoms with STEMI.
- Heart failure development days/weeks after STEMI: CAG within few weeks.
- Patients with NSTEMI and unstable angina refractory to medical therapy: acute/subacute CAG.
- Patients with NSTEMI stabilized on treatment: CAG within 72 hours.
- Patients with unstable angina pectoris with typical chest pains and ST-segment depression >1mm in >2 leads: CAG within 72 hours.
- Patients with typical chest pain without elevated markers or significant ST/T segment changes, stabilized on medical treatment: CAG depending on the result from noninvasive test(s).
- Patients with presumed unstable angina pectoris, refractory to medical treatment: CAG acute/subacute.
- Patients with chest pain during several admissions without elevated markers or significant ECG changes: CAG before discharge.
- Patients (<75 years) with acute MI within 36 hours who develop cardiogenic shock within 12 hours: CAG acutely if the plan is invasive treatment.
- Patients with suspected acute stent thrombosis or acute graft thrombosis: acute CAG.

Patients with suspected ischemic heart disease:
- Patients with typical chest pain refractory to medical treatment.
- Asymptomatic patients in antiangina medical treatment with abnormal exercise testing (<4 METS or decreasing blood pressure >30 mmHg [4 kPa], or development of ST segment depression >1 mm in >2 leads or insufficient increase in pulse frequency).

Patients with dyspnea or angina pectoris who have previously been treated with CABG or PTCA:
- Patients who have recently undergone complicated CABG or PTCA: CAG can be performed before discharge.

Patients with heart failure:
- Patients with decreased EF of the LV (<40%) for unknown reasons.

Other heart diseases:
- Patients (>40 years old) with heart valve disease before aVR or MVR or if ischemic heart disease is suspected: CAG electively before valve replacement.
- Hypertrophic obstructive cardiomyopathy in preparation for possible alcohol ablation of septal branch(es): CAG electively.
- Before heart- or lung-transplantation: CAG subacute/electively.

Miscellaneous:
- Patients resuscitated after sudden death with acute MI: CAG subacutely.
- Patients with nonsustained polymorph VT or sustained monomorph VT.

ACS: acute coronary syndromes; aVR: aortic valve replacement; CABG: coronary artery bypass graft; CAG: coronary angiography; ECG: electrocardiogram; EF: ejection fraction; LV: left ventricle; METS: metabolic equivalents; MI: myocardial infarction; MVR: mitral valve replacement; NSTEMI: non-ST elevation myocardial infarction; PTCA: percutaneous transluminal coronary angioplasty; STEMI: ST elevation myocardial infarction; VT: ventricular tachycardia.

CONTRAINDICATIONS

Absolute contraindications include refusal of the patient or absence of a qualified operator. Contraindications to coronary angiography are relative and include:

- Uncontrolled systemic hypertension.
- Fever or untreated infection.
- Decompensated congestive heart failure.
- Active bleeding and/or anemia with hemoglobin <6 mmol/l (8 g/dl).
- Severe coagulopathy.
- Electrolyte imbalance.
- Digitalis toxicity.
- Contrast allergy (not with pretreatment with corticosteroids and antihistamines).
- Ongoing stroke.
- Acute renal failure.
- Chronic renal failure (secreatinine >250 μmol/l [2.8 mg/dl]).
- Active endocarditis.
- Advanced age as well as severe medical conditions (e.g. advanced cancer).

These patients should be monitored closely for 18–24 hours after CAG. CAG performed under emergency conditions is associated with a higher risk of complications. Risks and indications should be discussed carefully with the patient before the investigation.

LIMITATIONS

CAG provides two-dimensional information on the luminal characteristics of the coronary vessels. Information is restricted to describing the lumen but not the vessel wall. Therefore, often the CAG cannot differentiate a normal artery from an artery with an unstable plaque (**103A**). Furthermore, it may be similarly difficult to differentiate the vessel with a stable plaque from a vessel with an unstable plaque (**103B**). Thus, a 'normal' CAG may hide even severe atherosclerotic vessel wall disease. The 'complex' plaque can only be disclosed by other techniques (e.g. angioscopy or intravascular ultrasound [IVUS]).

COMPLICATIONS

Major complications of CAG are rare and occur with an incidence of <1% (*Table 15*). Two registers have reported that in CAG patients death occurs with a frequency of 0.1–0.14%, myocardial infarction (MI) with a frequency of 0.06–0.07%, neurological complications with a frequency of 0.07–0.14%, adverse reactions to contrast with a frequency of 0.23%, and local vascular complications in 0.24–0.46%[2,3].

Certain factors increase the risk associated with CAG. Death occurred most frequently in patients who had: (1) stenosis of the left main stem (0.55%), (2) decreased systolic function of the left ventricle (LV) with a LV ejection fraction (EF) <30% (0.3%), and (3) congestive heart failure NYHA class IV (0.29%).

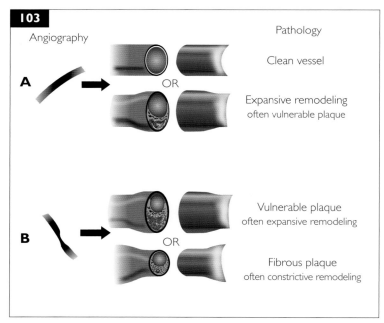

103 Diagram to show the interpretations of angiography. Although the dangerous vulnerable plaques in general are larger than the stable fibrous plaques, the former are often invisible angiographically because of expansive (positive) remodeling which tends to preserve the lumen (**A**). Angiography depicts only the lumen and cannot distinguish between stenoses caused by stable plaques and those caused by vulnerable plaques (**B**). (Original artwork by Dr. J.F. Bentzon.)

Table 15 Complications of coronary angiography

Complications	Incidence
Local vascular problems: pseudoaneurysm, hematoma (with need for blood transfusion)	0.43%
Serious arrhythmias	0.38%
Allergic reactions: local anesthetic, contrast agents, protamine sulfate	0.23%
Neurological events: transient, persistent	0.10%
Myocardial infarction	0.06%
Death	0.12%

QUANTITATIVE CORONARY ARTERIOGRAPHY

JOHAN H.C. REIBER, PhD, JOAN C. TUINENBURG, MSC, GERHARD KONING, MSC AND BOB GOEDHART, PhD

INTRODUCTION

Quantitative coronary arteriography (QCA) has been developed and used over the years as a tool for routine diagnosis, for clinical decision-making in the catheterization laboratory (vessel sizing), for the assessment of the efficacy of an interventional procedure, for teaching interventional cardiology, and for clinical research in interventional trials carried out mostly in Core-laboratories. Optional tools have been created for applications in brachytherapy and, most recently, for drug-eluting stenting.

TECHNIQUE

In the modern era of digital catheterization laboratories, the images are made available at a resolution of 512×512 pixels $\times 8$ bits on most X-ray systems, or up to 1024×1024 pixels $\times 12$ bits on some other X-ray systems at an acquisition rate of typically 12 or 15 frames/second, and stored on the high-speed disks of the digital imaging system for subsequent review and possibly quantitative analysis. An entire patient study can be stored in DICOM format on CD-R after the procedure for off-line review and analysis.

For QCA it is important that the vessel segments of interest are depicted with minimal foreshortening, and that the vessel segment is well filled with the contrast agent. A typical QCA procedure consists of calibration and vessel analysis phases, each of which will be described in more detail below.

Calibration procedure

Calibration of the image data is performed on a nontapering portion of a contrast-filled catheter, using an edge-detection procedure similar to that applied to the arterial segment. In this case, however, additional information is used in the edge-detection process because this part of the catheter is known to be characterized by parallel boundaries. It should also be recognized that the catheter calibration procedure is the weakest link in the analysis chain, because of the variable image quality of the displayed catheters. Another potential problem with calibration is the out-of-plane magnification, which occurs when the catheter and the coronary segment of analysis are positioned at different distances from the image intensifier. Biplane calibration could overcome this problem but is rarely applied in routine QCA. From observation and validation studies, the authors have concluded that it is recommended that contrast-filled catheters of the exact same type (size [minimally 6F], material, and manufacturer) should be used for both baseline and follow-up measurements[1].

Basic principles of automated contour detection and vessel analysis

The general principles and characteristics of a modern QCA software package can best be illustrated by the QCA-CMS® (Cardiovascular Measurement System, Medis medical imaging systems bv, Leiden,

the Netherlands) algorithms developed in the authors' laboratory. The QCA operator selects the coronary segment to be analyzed in the image (**104A**) by using the computer mouse to define the start and end points of that segment. Next, an arterial pathline through the segment of interest is computed automatically by using the wavefront propagation algorithm[2]. The contour-detection procedure is carried out in two iterations relative to a model. In the first iteration, the detected pathline is the model. To detect the contours, scanlines are defined perpendicular to the model (**104B**). For each point or pixel along such a scanline, the corresponding edge-strength value (local change in brightness level) is computed as the weighted sum of the corresponding values of the first- and second-derivative functions applied to the brightness values along these scanlines (**105**). The resulting edge-strength values are input to the so-called Minimum Cost Analysis (MCA) contour-detection algorithm, which searches for an optimal contour path along the entire segment (**104C**). The individual left and right vessel contours detected in the first iteration now serve as models in the second iteration, in which the MCA contour-detection procedure is repeated relative to the new models. If the QCA operator does not agree with one or more parts of the detected contours, they can be edited in various ways (**104D**).

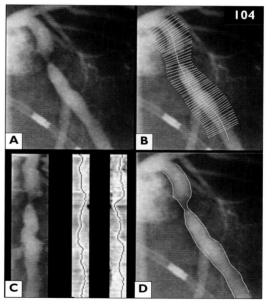

104 Basic principles of the Minimum Cost Analysis (MCA) contour-detection algorithm as demonstrated in digitized cinefilm images. **A**: Image shows the segment to be analyzed. **B**: After the pathline has been detected, scanlines are defined perpendicular to this first model (i.e. the pathline). **C**: The image is resampled along the scanlines and corresponding gray-level values stored in a rectangular matrix (see straightened vessel segment, left). Next, the changes in gray-level values (edge-strength values) along the horizontal lines are calculated in this rectangular matrix and stored in separate 'cost' matrices for the left- and the right-hand contours (right). The MCA algorithm searches for optimal contour paths in these cost matrices (curves). A similar procedure is followed in the second iteration, using these contours as models. **D**: Finally, the detected contours are transformed back to the original image and the diameter measurements can be performed.

For complex vessel morphology, the so-called Gradient Field Transform (GFT®) has been developed as an additional option. Whereas the standard MCA contour-detection allows only one left and one right contour point to be detected per scanline, the GFT has more degrees of freedom in the sense that multiple contour points are allowed per scanline and that even the search direction can be reversed[3]. This approach enables the GFT to follow more irregular arterial boundaries and by reversal of the contour direction, for example, to follow flaps. An illustrative example of the GFT is given in **106**.

From the left- and right-hand contours of an arterial segment, a diameter function is determined (**107**). The minima in the diameter function represent positions of local obstructions. The most widely used parameter to describe the severity of a coronary obstruction is the percentage diameter narrowing. Calculation of this parameter requires that a reference diameter value is computed, for which two options are available: (1) a user-defined reference diameter as positioned by the user at a so-called 'normal' portion of the vessel, and (2) the automated or interpolated reference diameter value. In practice, this last approach is preferred because it requires no user interaction and takes care of any tapering of the vessel. For that purpose, a reference diameter function is calculated by an iterative regression technique and displayed in the diameter function as a straight line (red line in diameter function). The iterative approach has been used to exclude the influence of any obstruction or ectatic area as much as possible, so that it

represents a best approximation of the vessel size before the occurrence of the focal narrowing. Now that the reference diameter function is known, reference contours can be reconstructed around the actual vessel segment, representing the original size and shape of the vessel before the focal disease occurred (**108**). Finally, the difference in area between the detected lumen contours and the reference contours is a measure of the atherosclerotic plaque area in this particular angiographic view, shaded in **107**. The actual reference diameter value corresponding with a selected obstruction is now taken as the value of the reference diameter function at the site of the obstruction, so that neither overestimation nor underestimation occurs. From the reference diameter value and the obstruction diameter, the percentage diameter narrowing is calculated.

Additional derived indices include the length of the obstruction, the stenotic flow reserve (SFR), and others. The SFR describes, on the basis of a mathematical/physiologic model, how much the flow can possibly increase under maximal hyperemic conditions in that particular coronary segment due to that single obstruction; it can also be described as a wind tunnel test of that stenosis under standardized conditions (**109**). In a disease-free segment, the SFR equals 4–5, a value that decreases as the severity of the obstruction increases. Finally, **110** shows a typical example of a QCA analysis pre- and postintervention.

The analysis of a coronary segment treated with brachytherapy or with a drug-eluting stent follows the same principles. However, in these cases the user is allowed to define multiple boundaries along the segment of interest, so that the various geographic miss, geographic hit, geographic extensions, and various edge effects can be studied in great detail[4].

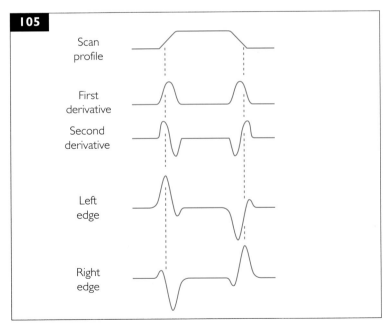

105 Schematic presentation of the brightness profile of an arterial vessel, assessed along a scanline perpendicular to the local pathline direction, and the computed 1st-derivative, 2nd-derivative and the combinations of these 1st- and 2nd-derivative functions. The maximal values of the last functions determine the edge positions.

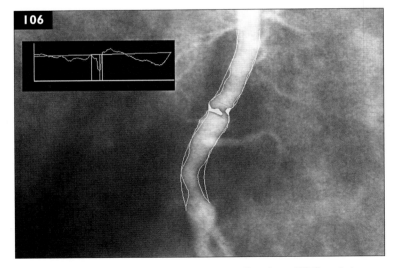

106 Example of the outcome of a Gradient Field Transform (GFT) analysis on a vessel segment with very severe complex stenosis. Conventional approaches with the MCA algorithm are not able to follow automatically the abrupt changes in morphology.

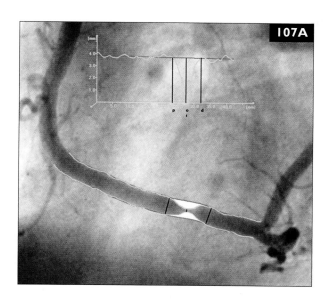

107A

107A: Results of a QCA analysis, including the reconstructed original vessel contours, plaque area (shaded), and the diameter function, are presented for QCA-CMS V5.3. **B**: All the derived absolute and relative parameters are presented in the Segments-tab of the QCA report. QCA: quantitative coronary arteriography.

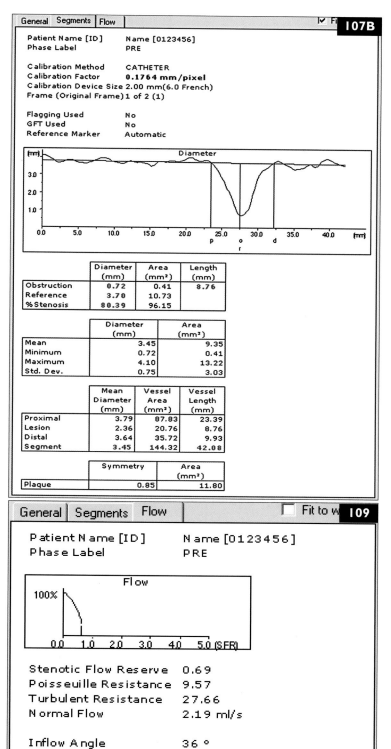

107B

General | Segments | Flow

| Patient Name [ID] | Name [0123456] |
| Phase Label | PRE |

Calibration Method	CATHETER
Calibration Factor	0.1764 mm/pixel
Calibration Device Size	2.00 mm(6.0 French)
Frame (Original Frame)	1 of 2 (1)

Flagging Used	No
GFT Used	No
Reference Marker	Automatic

	Diameter (mm)	Area (mm²)	Length (mm)
Obstruction	0.72	0.41	8.76
Reference	3.70	10.73	
% Stenosis	80.39	96.15	

	Diameter (mm)	Area (mm²)
Mean	3.45	9.35
Minimum	0.72	0.41
Maximum	4.10	13.22
Std. Dev.	0.75	3.03

	Mean Diameter (mm)	Vessel Area (mm²)	Vessel Length (mm)
Proximal	3.79	87.83	23.39
Lesion	2.36	20.76	8.76
Distal	3.64	35.72	9.93
Segment	3.45	144.32	42.08

	Symmetry	Area (mm²)
Plaque	0.85	11.80

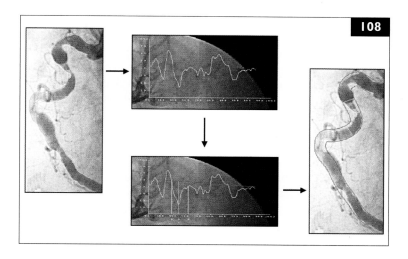

108

108 Diameter function calculation. Given the detected left and right vessel contours (**left image**) the diameter function is determined (**upper center image**). In an iterative way, a reference diameter function (the straight red line in the **lower center image**) is calculated automatically, excluding the influence of obstructions and ectatic areas, and representing the original size of the vessel as best as possible. From the reference diameter function, two reference contours are reconstructed around the vessel segment, representing the original shape of the vessel (red curved lines in **right hand image**).

General | Segments | **Flow** — Fit to w **109**

| Patient Name [ID] | Name [0123456] |
| Phase Label | PRE |

Flow

Stenotic Flow Reserve	0.69
Poisseuille Resistance	9.57
Turbulent Resistance	27.66
Normal Flow	2.19 ml/s
Inflow Angle	36 °
Outflow Angle	33 °

109 Functional data of a QCA analysis, including the stenotic flow reserve (SFR), are presented in the Flow-tab of the QCA report. The results presented are part of the QCA analysis of **107**. QCA: quantitative coronary arteriography.

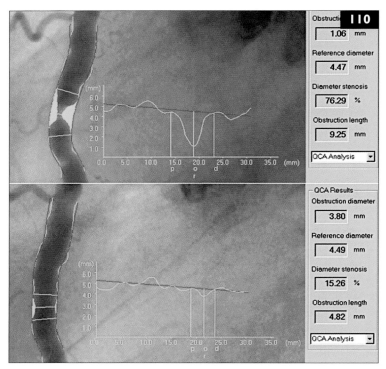

110 Typical example of pre- and postintervention QCA analyses. Preintervention, the obstruction diameter is 1.06 mm, the interpolated reference diameter 4.47 mm, and the percentage diameter stenosis 76.3%. Postintervention, the obstruction diameter has increased to 3.80 mm, with an almost unchanged interpolated reference diameter of 4.49 mm, resulting in a percentage diameter stenosis that has decreased to 15.3%.

Guidelines for QCA acquisition procedures

The primary objective of QCA measurements in clinical trials is to allow more precise and reliable analyses of the real changes after interventions, namely, acute lumen gain and late lumen loss expressed in millimeters. This is best achieved when exactly the same setting is applied during the procedure and at the follow-up studies, that is, replication of the same X-ray views, same doses of intracoronary nitroglycerin, same contrast medium, same catheter type or material, and, if feasible, same catheterization room[5].

ADDITIONAL REMARKS

- Semi-automated segmentation techniques are able to trace the luminal boundaries of coronary arteries from two-dimensional cine film or digital X-ray arteriograms after minimal user interaction.
- QCA allows the derivation of such luminal dimensions and derived indices with small systematic and random errors as demonstrated by a range of validation studies.
- QCA can be used in an off-line mode for clinical research studies and in an on-line mode during the interventional procedure to support the clinical decision-making process and for teaching purposes.

MAGNETIC RESONANCE CORONARY ANGIOGRAPHY

ROBERT JAN M. VAN GEUNS, MD, PhD

INTRODUCTION

Invasive selective CAG is the gold standard for the assessment of the coronary artery. However, it is associated with significant radiation exposure and a small risk (1.7%) of serious complications. Therefore, noninvasive CAG is highly desirable. In the development of noninvasive CAG techniques, the specifications of conventional selective CAG have to be kept in mind. CAG is a projectional technique that covers the complex tortuous epicardial course of the coronary arteries with a high spatial resolution (up to 5 line pairs/mm, approximately 0.1 mm) and a high temporal resolution (up to 50 frames/second). These specifications are almost unbeatable.

Magnetic resonance imaging (MRI) is a truly noninvasive technique that may serve as an alternative. It has a natural high contrast between different types of soft tissue and can be acquired in any desired imaging plane through the heart. The major disadvantage of MRI is the relatively low temporal resolution, which makes it sensitive to cardiac and respiratory motion. To obtain images without motion artifacts several acquisition strategies have been developed, each with a different trade-off between resolution, coverage, and image quality.

TECHNIQUE

2D Imaging during breath holding

MRI of the abdominal aorta and renal arteries using breath-hold contrast-enhanced magnetic resonance angiography without cardiac gating has been widely accepted for the diagnosis of atherosclerotic arterial disease. For magnetic resonance coronary angiography (MRCA), cardiac motion related to respiration and cardiac contraction have both to be minimized and therefore determine the major settings of all techniques. During cardiac contraction an acquisition window of <50 ms is highly desirable but a window of approximately 100 ms during mid to late diastole, which does induce minimal image blur, must be accepted for current noninvasive techniques.

Respiration related motion can be reduced with breath-hold or complicated respiratory gating techniques. Initially MRCA was performed with a technique that allowed the acquisition of a single 2D slice in approximately 20 seconds, allowing imaging during suspension of breathing. During diastases of each cardiac cycle, eight image lines of a gradient echo technique (2D-GE) image can be acquired with a repetition time of 14 ms that resulted in an acquisition window of 112 ms. These settings resulted in a resolution of $1.9 \times 0.9 \times 3$ mm that is sufficient to visualize the proximal coronary arteries (**111**). To cover a single branch of the coronary artery tree, multiple parallel images had to be obtained. This resulted in a long imaging protocol with possible malalignment of the individual slices due to different levels of expiration for each slice. Although initial results were promising, later studies where not able to reproduce these results. With the development of faster MRI scanners, this technique has been abandoned.

In conclusion, it appears that with the 2D imaging technique, images can be obtained with adequate quality and minimal or no cardiac or respiratory motion artifacts in the majority of cases. However, the overall robustness and reliability of the visualization of the complex 3D anatomy of the coronary arteries is not sufficient, mainly because of the collection of data during several breath holds. This has restricted its clinical utility and alternatives have been developed.

3D Imaging with respiratory gating

The 3D MRI technique should resolve the difficulties of 2D imaging. It requires the acquisition of more signals to complete the data for the desired volume. This considerably lengthens the acquisition time beyond breath-holding possibilities using conventional MR systems. To minimize respiratory blurring, Li *et al.*[1] used averaging of multiple acquisitions, but images still remained too blurred for clinical use.

To improve the image quality of 3D imaging, respiratory gating can be used. Initial attempts with a belt around the abdomen did not give reliable results. Respiratory gating by measuring the diaphragm movement with an MRI technique (MR-navigator) is much more reliable. A diamond-shaped region of tissue through the dome of the right hemidiaphragm is selectively imaged. All the data are frequently resampled to ensure that expiration data are acquired; in general, depending on the respiration frequency, 5–6 times. Retrospectively, a special algorithm selects only the data from expiration to generate the image. A volume of 32 mm thickness with a resolution of 1.9 × 1.25 mm requires 10–12 minutes' acquisition time. However, to image the whole heart three or four volumes are needed so that the total imaging time is 40–50 minutes. Postprocessing of these 3D datasets allows reconstruction of images along the coronary arteries (multi-planar reconstruction, MPR) with resulting images being comparable with 2D imaging (**112A**), and 3D impressions using dedicated software (volume rendering techniques) to produce images comparable to anatomical atlases (**112B**). With this technique sometimes excellent images of severe coronary artery stenoses were obtained (**113**). The results from several clinical studies will be discussed later.

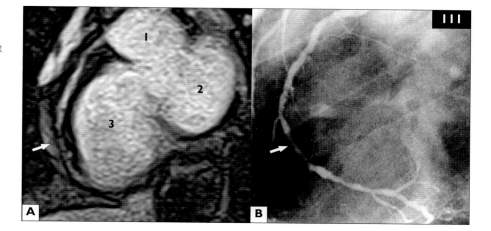

111 A: Example of a 2D segmented GE image with signal loss (arrow) occurring just beyond a stenosis in the right coronary artery (RCA). Note that the distal segment of the RCA runs out of the imaging plane and is not visualized in this 2D image. **B**: Corresponding conventional coronary angiogram. 1: aorta; 2: left ventricle; 3: right ventricle.

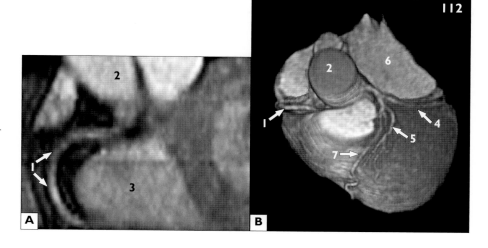

112 A: Reconstruction of an image from a 3D-navigator technique along the right coronary artery (1). **B**: Three-dimensional representation with a volume-rendering technique of a 3D-navigator dataset. 2: aorta; 3: right ventricle; 4: circumflex coronary artery; 5: great cardiac vein; 6: left atrium; 7: left anterior descending artery. The auricle of the LA is manually removed from the data set. (Reprinted from van Geuns *et al.* [1999]. Magnetic resonance imaging of the Coronary arteries: techniques and results. *Progr. Cardiovasc. Dis.* **42**. 156–166, with permission from Elsevier.)

A recent modification of the navigator technique allows correcting for the occurrence of shift of the heart and coronary arteries caused by respiratory motion. Wang *et al.*[2] have studied the extent of the shift of coronary arteries with respiration. The shift of the proximal coronary arteries in craniocaudal direction was 60% of the diaphragm movement and the shift of the apex was 90% of the diaphragm displacement. Slice position correction technique combined with the faster gradient system were thus introduced in clinical imaging and as a result imaging time for navigator techniques was dramatically reduced. However, image quality is still dependent on regular breathing patterns not always present in nonselected patients.

3D Imaging within a breath-hold

With the introduction of faster MRI systems the possibilities of breath-hold MRCA increased, which resulted in better image quality. For breath-hold MRCA a new 3D sequence was developed that uses small, targeted volumes of 24 mm thickness to cover the major coronary artery branches in a few breath-holds. This sequence is known as VCATS (volume coronary angiography using targeted scans). Presently it is possible to scan up to 21 image lines within a time window of 110 ms during every heartbeat with conventional GE techniques.

Imaging a segment of a coronary artery in one breath-hold eliminates the problems of inconsistent breath holding, introducing artifacts in breath-hold 2D-GE imaging. With this technique it is possible to image a coronary artery segment with a resolution of $1.9 \times 1.25 \times 1.5$ mm within 21 heartbeats. **114** is an example from a transversal data set positioned at the left main and proximal anterior descending coronary artery. **115** is an illustration of an angulated volume along the RCA. Postprocessing with dedicated programs allows the integration of the separate images into a single image for easy evaluation (**116**).

In general, seven targeted volumes are sufficient to visualize the important coronary artery segments. In an initial study using VCATS, the authors showed that visualization of >90% of the proximal coronary artery segments and proximal coronary artery stenosis was possible[3]. This technique follows the course of the coronary arteries better, and may reduce false-positive diagnosis of a severe stenosis due to running out of the imaging plane of a coronary artery.

CLINICAL RESULTS

Coronary artery bypass grafts

Saphenous vein and internal mammary artery bypass grafts are easier to image than coronary arteries using conventional MRI techniques due to their larger size (5–10 mm in diameter) and lesser mobility associated with cardiac and respiration motion. The first study was published by White *et al.* in 1987[4]. They used a conventional spin-echo sequence to assess bypass graft patency and achieved a sensitivity of 86% and a specificity of 59%. With increasing experience and faster sequences, such as GE, results improved (*Table 16*). However, these examinations only provide information on bypass patency and no information about graft patency distal to the first coronary anastomosis or nonoccluding stenoses within the graft, limiting the application in clinical practice. Major obstacles to bypass graft imaging are the local image artifacts associated with metallic hemostatic clips, sternal wires, and graft markers. Although internal mammary artery grafts can also be visualized, so far this has only been studied in limited numbers of patients due to the abundant image artifacts related to the presence of hemostatic clips. With the VCATS technique it is possible to image a sequential venous bypass graft with a few targeted 3D volumes and confirm its patency (**117**).

Table 16 Sensitivity, specificity, and accuracy of techniques in the assessment of coronary artery bypass graft patency using magnetic resonance imaging

First author	Year	Technique	Grafts	Patency (%)	Sensitivity (%)	Specificity (%)	Accuracy (%)
White[4]	1987	Spin-echo	72	69	86	59	78
Rubinstein[11]	1987	Spin-echo	47	62	90	72	83
Jenkins[12]	1988	Spin-echo	41	63	89	73	83
Frija[13]	1989	Spin-echo	52	83	98	78	94
Galjee[14]	1996	Spin-echo	98	74	98	85	96
White[15]	1988	GE	28	50	93	86	89
Aurigemma[16]	1989	GE	45	73	88	100	91
Galjee[14]	1996	GE	98	74	98	88	96
Kalden[17]	1999	Fast spin-echo	59	44	95	93	95
Vrachliotis[18]	1997	3D-GE	44	29	93	97	95
Wintersperg[19]	1998	3D-GE	76	60	95	81	92
Kalden[17]	1999	3D-GE	59	44	93	93	93
Langerak[20]	2002	3D-GE-Nav	50	89	98	83	96
Bunce[37]	2003	3D-GE	79	86	85	74	84

Grafts: number of grafts evaluated; Patency: percentage of patent grafts; GE: gradient-echo; 3D-GE- Nav: three-dimensional gradient-echo imaging with respiratory gating.

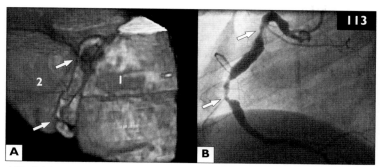

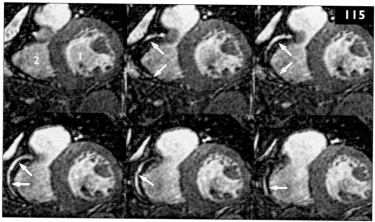

113 A: Magnetic resonance coronary angiography with a 3D-navigator technique. Detailed view of the right coronary artery in the atrioventricular groove between the right ventricle (1) and atrium (2). The arrows indicate stenoses in the proximal and mid segment. B: Corresponding conventional coronary angiogram. (Reproduced with permission, BMJ Publishing Group, from van Geuns et al. [1999]. Magnetic resonance imaging of the Coronary arteries: clinical results from three dimensional evaluation of a respiratory gated technique. *Heart* **82**:515–519.)

115 Six slices obtained from a targeted volume along the right coronary artery (arrows). It is clearly shown that, due to the complex course of the coronary artery, the different segments of the artery are only visualized in particular slices and 'disappear' in other slices. 1: left ventricle; 2: right ventricle. (From van Geuns et al. [1999]. Magnetic resonance imaging of the Coronary arteries: techniques and results. *Progr. Cardiovasc. Dis.* **42**(2):156–166.)

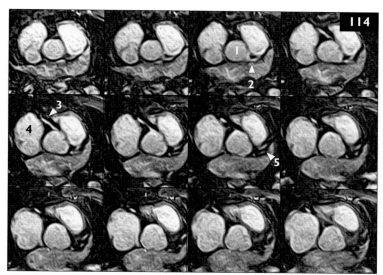

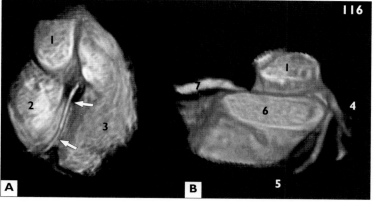

114 Example of 12 slices from a volume of 16 slices obtained in a single breathhold targeted for the aortic root from cranial to caudal. 1: aorta; 2: left main artery; 3: right coronary artery; 4: right artrium; 5: left anterior descending artery. (Reproduced with permission, Kluwer Academic Plenum Publishers from van Geuns et al. [2001]. VCATS: volume coronary angiography using targeted scans: a new strategy in MR coronary angiography. *Int. J. Cardiol. Imag.* **17**(5):405–410.)

116 A: Volume-rendered reconstruction of an image from a breath-hold, targeted volume image of a nondiseased right coronary artery (arrows) in a 43 year-old male. Right anterior view. B: Anterior cranial volume-rendered image of a targeted volume of the aortic root in the same patient. 1: aorta; 2: right atrium; 3: right ventricle; 4: left circumflex coronary artery; 5: left anterior descending coronary artery; 6: right ventricular outflow tract; 7: right coronary artery. (Reprinted with permission, RSNA from van Geuns et al. [2000]. MR coronary angiography with breath-hold targeted volumes: preliminary clinical results. *Radiology* **217**:270–277.)

117 A: Magnetic resonance image (MRI) of a partially occluded venous graft using a targeted volume technique acquired during a breath-hold of 20 seconds. The proximal segment to the first anastomosis is patent (arrows) while the second segment is patent but with diminished image quality. B: Second MRI volume targeted for the third anastomosis demonstrating the occlusion of the graft distal to the anastomosis. C: Corresponding conventional coronary angiography confirming the patency of the proximal graft segments, the diseased third segment, and occluded distal segments. 1: aorta; 2: pulmonary artery.

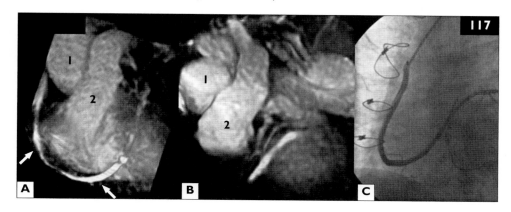

Coronary artery anomalies

Among adults referred for contrast X-ray CAG, anomalous origins of the coronary arteries are found in 0.6–1.2% of the patients. Fortunately, the majority of these anomalies are clinically benign. However, origin of the LCA from the contralateral side, with subsequent course posterior to the pulmonary artery and anterior to the ascending aorta is associated with sudden death. MRI is an ideal technique to evaluate such patients. In a double-blinded study with 2D-GE sequences involving 35 patients with anomalous aortic origins of the coronary arteries, MRCA identified the anomalous coronary artery course in 97% of the cases[5]. It may be concluded that MRCA may be used as a screening tool in young patients with unexplained arrhythmias or syncope during exercise (**118**).

Coronary artery stenosis

Manning *et al.* published in 1993 the first study on 39 patients referred for elective coronary angiography[6]. In this study they used the segmented 2D-GE technique with fat suppression. In a blinded analysis, sensitivity and specificity of the 2D-MRI technique for the detection of significant stenosis (>50% diameter reduction) on conventional contrast X-ray angiography were 90% and 92%, respectively, and positive and negative predictive values were 0.85 and 0.95, respectively. Using similar techniques Pennell[7], Duerinckx[8], and Post[9] were not able to confirm these surprisingly good results. These studies demonstrated a sensitivity varying from 63% to 85% (*Table 17*).

The differences of the results can be partially explained by bias due to different patient selection criteria, but they also reflect the present lack of robustness of the 2D-GE imaging technique. In its present state, 2D-GE MRI cannot yet be considered a reliable alternative to conventional angiography for imaging of coronary artery stenoses.

3D retrospective respiratory gated techniques have also been used for patient studies. The specificity is high (94–95%) for most studies, but sensitivity varies from 38% to 83% (*Table 17*). Image quality is negatively affected by residual respiratory blur and irregular respiration patterns or by involuntary patient motion during the relatively long acquisition time. An additional problem with MRI results from the imaging of veins, which can easily be mistaken for arteries, and imaging of the pericardial sac causing misjudgement.

Only a few centers have experience with breath-hold 3D technique (**119**) and their results have been included in *Table 17*. The publication of the first multi-center study on MRCA field by Kim *et al.* (2001)[10] is important as it included the largest number of patients. Unfortunately, the results of this study are not convincing in advocating the use of this technique as a first-line investigation in expected CAD.

FUTURE DEVELOPMENTS

MRCA needs to be improved before it will be accepted as a useful imaging tool. Most importantly the resolution has to improve. The signal-to-noise ratio (SNR) is the limiting factor to reducing the pixel size. MRI contrast agents may be used for this purpose. These agents boosted the implementation of MRI angiography of the aorta and the peripheral vessels but have not yet provided the definite answer for MRCA. Gadolinium based agents used for contrast enhanced

magnetic resonance angiography of the aorta and peripheral vessels are distributed initially within the intravascular compartment but diffuse rapidly throughout the extracellular (vascular plus interstitial) space. This limits their possible use in the long acquisition times frequently used in coronary imaging. Therefore, intravascular MRI contrast agents have been developed and do improve image quality as expected. However, Food and Drug Administration (FDA) approval has not yet been acquired.

The most exciting new possibility of MRI is the ability to study noninvasively the components of the arterial wall. The composition of the atherosclerotic plaque, rather than the degree of vessel stenosis, is known to modulate the risk of rupture and subsequent intravascular thrombus. Superficial vessels, such as the carotid and femoral arteries, have been studied using externally placed coils, and to overcome the SNR barrier for deeper arteries intravascular catheter MRI probes were used. By changing imaging parameters image contrast can be modified to highlight the different components on the basis of biochemical structure. It appeared that it was possible to characterize accurately and quantify atherosclerotic lesions using T1-, proton density-, and T2-weighted imaging

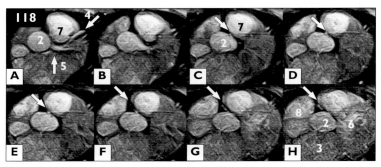

118 MRCA at several different axial levels (**A–H** caudal to cranial) of a coronary anomaly where the right coronary artery (arrows) originates from the left coronary cusp. In total 16 images were obtained during a breath-hold of 21 seconds. The RCA has a course between the aorta and pulmonary artery (**C–H**) and may be compressed during exercise. This type of anomaly is known to be associated with sudden death. 2: aorta; 3: left atrium; 4: left anterior descending coronary artery; 5: left main artery; 6: left ventricle; 7: pulmonary artery; 8: right atrium.

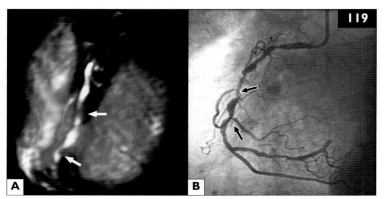

119 A: MRCA with a targeted volume technique identifying two consecutive stenoses in the middle part of the right coronary artery (arrows). **B**: Corresponding conventional coronary angiogram.

sequences. For the coronary arteries it has not yet been possible to identify the different components in the arterial wall but the presence of plaques and nonobstructing wall remodeling has been demonstrated *in vivo* (**120**). This technique may yet become a major tool with which to study atherosclerosis more closely.

SUMMARY

MRI is a generally accepted imaging technique used to evaluate a wide range of diseases of the central and peripheral vasculature, and is presently replacing conventional contrast angiography. Noninvasive CAG is much more complex due to cardiac motion during respiration and the cardiac contraction cycles. MRI is presently insufficiently reliable to replace conventional selective CAG. Multi-slice CT has a higher resolution and SNR and may replace invasive CAG sooner. MRI has some additional features such as flow imaging and vessel wall imaging and may be combined in a full cardiovascular evaluation of patients in a single examination. This will include not

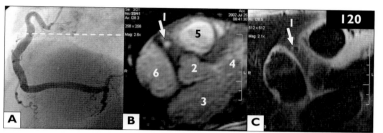

120 Noninvasive vessel wall imaging with MRI. **A**: Conventional coronary angiography of a nondiseased right coronary artery (1). The dashed line indicates the location of the MRI images. **B**: 2D-gradient echo image perpendicular to the middle segment of the RCA. **C**: High-resolution (0.5 × 0.5 mm in-plane) black blood MRI with suppression technique for the epicardial fat surrounding the vessel at the same location. Even in this nondiseased vessel the very thin wall of the artery is visualized. 2: aorta; 3: left atrium; 4: left ventricle; 5: pulmonary artery; 6: right atrium.

Table 17 Sensitivity, specificity, and accuracy of techniques in the assessment of stenosis in native coronary arteries using magnetic resonance imaging

First author	Year	Technique	Subjects	Lesions	Sensitivity (%)	Specificity (%)
Manning[6]	1993	2D-BH	39	52	90	92
Duerinckx and Urman[8]	1994	2D-BH	20	27	63	71
Pennell[7]	1996	2D-BH	39	55	85	95
Post[9]	1997	2D-BH	35	35	63	89
Yoshino[21]	1997	2D-BH	36	31	88	98
Post[22]	1996	3D-Nav retro	20	21	38	95
Müller[23]	1997	3D-Nav retro	30	54	83	94
Kessler[24]	1997	3D-Nav retro	73	43	65	n.a.
Sandstede[25]	1999	3D-Nav retro	30	37	81	89
Huber[26]	1999	3D-Nav retro	20	53	73	50
van Geuns[27]	1999	3D-Nav retro	29	26	50	91
Sardanelli[28]	2000	3D-Nav retro	42	67	82	89
Nikolaou[29]	2002	3D-Nav retro	20	39	79	70
Regenfus[30]	2002	3D-Nav retro	32	25	60	89
Wittlinger[31]	2002	3D-Nav retro	20	24	75	100
Lethimonnier[32]	1999	3D-Nav pros	20	17	65	93
Kim[10]	2001	3D-Nav pros	109	94	83	70
Weber[33]	2002	3D-Nav pros	15	16	88	94
Plein[34]	2003	3D-Nav pros	50	35	74	88
van Geuns[35]	2000	3D-BH	34	31	68	97
Regenfus[36]	2000	3D-BH	30	31	77	94
Bogaert[38]	2003	3D-Nav pros	19	29	56	84
Jahnke[39]	2004	3D-Nav pros	40	36	72	92
Gerber[40]	2005	3D-Nav pros	26	58	62	84
Sakuma[41]	2005	3D-Nav pros	20	17	82	91
Jahnke[42]	2005	3D-Nav pros	32	55	78	91
Jahnke[43]	2004	3D-BH	40	36	63	82
Herborn[44]	2004	3D-BH	20		80	93
Yang[45]	2003	Multi 2D-BH	40	41	76	91

2D-BH: two-dimensional gradient echo during breath holding; 3D-Nav: three-dimensional gradient echo imaging with respiratory gating; retro: retrospective gating; pros: prospective gating; 3D-BH: three-dimensional gradient echo during breath holding.

only MRCA but also functional parameters such as (regional) left ventricular function, myocardial perfusion and viability, and angiography of the aorta, carotid, and peripheral arteries.

NONINVASIVE MULTI-SLICE SPIRAL COMPUTED TOMOGRAPHY

KOEN NIEMAN, MD AND PIM J. DE FEYTER, MD, PhD

INTRODUCTION
Current multi-slice spiral computed tomography (MSCT) scanners are able to visualize the coronary artery lumen and detect obstructions. Atherosclerotic material can be visualized and the potential of MSCT plaque characterization is currently being explored. Using retrospective electrocardiogram (ECG) gating multiple cardiac phases can be reconstructed, providing the opportunity to evaluate ventricular function characteristics.

MULTI-SLICE SPIRAL COMPUTED TOMOGRAPHY IMAGING
Technique
The MSCT scanner is a spiral computed tomography (CT) scanner that acquires multiple parallel slices while the patient moves continuously through the scanner gantry. The ECG, which is recorded during the scan, is used for retrospective ECG-gated image reconstruction. Most currently used MSCT scanners acquire up to four slices of 1.0 mm at a rotation time of 500 ms. The data acquisition is performed during a single, but long, breath-hold of up to 40 seconds. The coronary lumen is enhanced by intravenous injection of an iodine-containing contrast medium.

The recently introduced generation of 16-slice MSCT scanners are equipped with an extended number of submillimeter slices and a further increased rotation speed. Besides an improvement in the image quality, these scanners also decrease the total scan time down to approximately 20 seconds and consequently require a lower dose of contrast medium. After the acquisition of data, ECG-synchronized image reconstruction is performed to create a stack of isocardiophasic slices[1]. To obtain nearly motion-free images, the image reconstruction interval is positioned within the mid- to end-diastolic phase, when coronary displacement is minimal. Because MSCT is a mechanical scanner, the temporal resolution is modest (200–250 ms) compared to electron beam CT (100 ms) or MRI (100–150 ms). Therefore, MSCT is more vulnerable to residual cardiac motion artifacts, which can be reduced by administration of beta-receptor blocking medication prior to the scan, in order to extend the diastolic period.

Advanced postprocessing applications
The high-resolution, high-contrast 3D data set consists of near-isotropic voxels, or 3D pixels with near-equal dimensions, which lend themselves well to advanced image processing applications. A number of postprocessing applications, such as multi-planar reconstruction (MPR), maximum intensity projection and volume rendering are illustrated (**121–123**).

MULTI-SLICE SPIRAL COMPUTED TOMOGRAPHY CORONARY IMAGING
Coronary artery obstructions
Contrast-enhanced CT angiography is reported to be a robust method to visualize the coronary artery and to depict narrowing of the vessel lumen (**121**)[2–5]. Semiquantitative assessments are possible in the proximal and middle main branches. The small diameters of the end-segments and side branches prevent evaluation beyond the assessment of patency with the current four-slice scanners. The diagnostic accuracy to detect significant lumen narrowing is good in scans of acceptable image quality. However, in studies published up till now a substantial number of coronary arteries were regarded as nonassessable. One cause of image degradation is motion artifact, particularly in patients with fast heart rates, and most pronounced in the RCA. Therefore, MSCT is most reliable in patients with low heart rates. Also the assessment of coronary arteries with advanced atherosclerotic disease and extensive presence of calcified deposits is not always satisfactory.

Angiographic evaluation after coronary revascularization
Patients who previously underwent percutaneous coronary intervention can be assessed by MSCT. However, the metal alloys in coronary stents create high-density artifacts, which limit the assessability of the in-stent lumen. While obstructions can generally be detected, particularly in stents with a larger diameter, smaller stents and discrete neo-intimal hyperplasia cannot be reliably assessed (**122**).

Venous bypass grafts are more easily visualized compared to coronary arteries, because of their larger diameter and lesser displacement (**123**). Using single-slice CT, including conventional, spiral, and electron beam, it has been shown that occlusion of venous and arterial bypass grafts can accurately be detected[6–12]. Because of the thin slices and extended scan range, MSCT allows a complete 3D angiographic evaluation of coronary bypass grafts (CABG)[13]. In addition to graft patency, noncomplete graft obstruction can also be assessed. Compared to the venous grafts, the arterial conduits with a small diameter are more difficult to assess, which is partly due to the metal vascular clips in the proximity of the artery. Additionally, the native coronary arteries in postbypass surgery patients tend to be small, diffusely diseased, severely calcified, and therefore often not reliably assessable.

Visualization of coronary plaque
Besides the contrast-enhanced lumen, MSCT allows visualization of the coronary artery wall. Calcified deposits in the vessel wall are easily recognized and provide unmistakable evidence for the presence of coronary atherosclerosis. The detection and semiquantification of coronary calcium have been used for exclusion of CAD in symptomatic patients and for coronary risk stratification in nonsymptomatic individuals[14–17]. The noncalcified components have a CT density that is lower than calcium or contrast, but higher

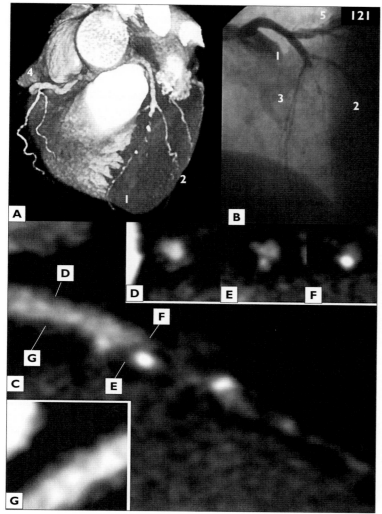

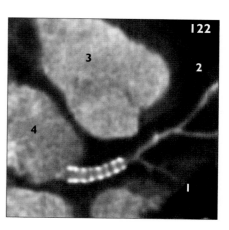

122 Coronary stent placed in the left main coronary artery. Although high-grade obstruction can be excluded in this particular case, subtle restenosis would not be detected due to the high-density artifacts in the proximity of the stent struts. 1: circumflex artery; 2: left anterior descending coronary artery; 3: right ventricular outflow tract; 4: aorta.

121 MSCT coronary angiography and plaque visualization. MSCT (**A**) and conventional (**B**) angiography show the left anterior descending coronary artery (LAD, 1), which is occluded just distal from the diagonal (2) and septal (3) branches. **C**: Longitudinal view of the diffusely diseased and occluded LAD. The cross sectional views **D**, **E**, and **F**, the locations of which are indicated (**C**), show the various plaque morphology. In the proximal LAD the plaque only consists of noncalcified tissues (**D**, **G**), while near the occlusion the plaque is predominantly calcified (**E**, **F**). The right coronary artery (4), including ventricular branches, can be observed in the three-dimensional MSCT angiogram (**A**). 5: circumflex artery; MSCT: multi-slice spiral computed tomography.

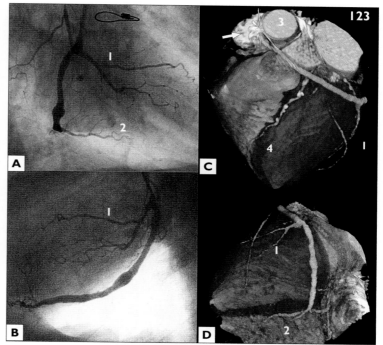

123 Coronary artery bypass grafts. Both multi-slice spiral computed tomography (MSCT) (**C**, **D**) and conventional angiography (**A**, **B**) show a venous bypass graft that is connected to a marginal branch (1) from the left circumflex artery and the posterior descending coronary artery (2). The metal indicator at the anastomosis with the aortic root (3) causes metal artifacts (**C**). A diffusely diseased left anterior descending coronary artery (4) can be observed in the MSCT angiogram (**C**).

than the fat tissue that surrounds the coronary artery (**121**). Within a narrow range the exact CT density of so-called 'soft plaques' correlates with the echogenicity as evaluated by intracoronary ultrasound[18]. Preliminary reports have shown that the *ex vivo* CT and histopathologic studies correlate well[19].

LEFT VENTRICULAR PERFORMANCE

During the spiral CT scan, data are acquired throughout the cardiac cycle, and images can be reconstructed at any point within the R- to R-wave interval. By reconstructing an end-systolic and end-diastolic volume, a 3D assessment of the ventricular cavity dimensions, stroke volume, and ejection fraction (EF) can be performed. Because of the relatively low temporal resolution of MSCT (250 ms), it is not possible to completely freeze the end-systolic phase and dynamic evaluations require substantial temporal overlap. However, MSCT does allow high spatial resolution and high contrast-to-noise images that can be assessed in a 3D fashion without geometric assumptions that restrict reliability in irregularly-shaped ventricles (**124**).

CARDIAC ANATOMY

The diastolic images also allow for morphologic assessment of the heart and great vessels. With the exception of the tricuspid valves, which are subject to incompletely dissolved contrast medium,

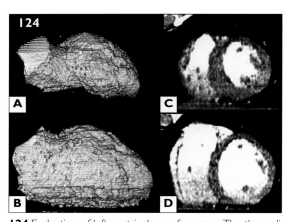

124 Evaluation of left ventricular performance. The three-dimensional view of the left ventricular cavity during the end-systolic (**A**) and end-diastolic phases (**B**) show an aneurysmatic left ventricle with absent contraction of the anterior apical wall. The short axis images confirm the absent ventricular wall thickening of the anterior wall during systole (**C**, **D**).

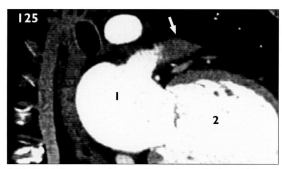

125 Atrial thrombus. A nonenhanced area in the atrial appendix suggests the presence of thrombotic material (arrow). 1: left atrium; 2: left ventricle.

thickening and calcification of the cardiac valves can be assessed. Relevant applications of cardiac CT could be the detection of thrombotic material in the cardiac cavities, particularly in the left atrium, and inflammatory disease of the pericardium (**125**).

INTRACORONARY ULTRASOUND

NICO BRUINING, PhD

INTRODUCTION

While contrast angiography is still considered to be the gold standard imaging technology to guide therapy for interventional coronary procedures, intracoronary ultrasound (ICUS) has evolved to become a valuable additional imaging tool in the catheterization laboratory. While angiography alone only shows a 2D silhouette image of the coronary lumen (**126A**), ICUS allows transmural, highly detailed imaging of the coronary vessel wall (**126B,C**). This provides insights into the pathology of vessel wall disease by defining its geometry and showing major components of atherosclerotic plaques. It is also very useful to show pathologies sometimes difficult, or even impossible, to visualize with angiography alone, such as left main stem disease, plaque rupture, and vessel remodeling. The advantages of ICUS have been described in many publications[1–3]. The ability of ICUS to detect and show small amounts of intima hyperplasia and the availability of quantitative ICUS software[4–6] have made this technique an important tool to visualize and quantify results of new interventional techniques and pharmaceutical therapies (**126D,E**).

TECHNIQUE
Intracoronary ultrasound basics

Ultrasound (US) images are created by sending electrical current through a piezoelectric (pressure-electric) element, causing expansion and contraction of this element, resulting in emission of high frequency sound waves. After being excited to send a sound wave, the element also receives the reflected sound wave (i.e. sound energy) back. If an US wave encounters a boundary between tissues, the beam will be partially transmitted and partially reflected (every tissue has its own so-called acoustic impedance) (**127**). The amount of the wave reflected depends on the mechanical characteristics of the tissue; soft tissue reflects low levels of the beam back while calcification reflects (or even blocks) the complete beam, causing so-called acoustic shadowing. These differences in received sound reflections are translated into gray value images with low levels appearing dark and high levels appearing white. The wave will be attenuated while passing through the different layers of tissue and, finally, in the far field the beam will be absorbed. The higher the operating frequency, the better the axial resolution but the penetration depth will be lower.

The electronics within the US console translates the received sound pressure into gray value images after heavily processing the signal. There are basically two different types of ICUS console (**128**) and catheter: (1) mechanical systems, where a relatively large piezoelectric element is mounted on the tip of a catheter and the

126 A: Angiogram of an implanted stent made during a 6-months follow-up procedure. Narrowing of the lumen can be observed both proximal and distal from the stented segment. Luminal diameters, at the sites indicated by the arrows, seem to be almost similar. **B**: Cross sectional ultrasound image of the proximal narrowing. **C**: Cross sectional ultrasound image of the distal narrowing. It can be observed that the luminal area is indeed almost similar at both sites; however, the ultrasound images show clearly that the plaque burden proximal is much larger than distal, which is missed by using angiography alone. **D, E**: Quantitative area measurements that can be made on-line as well as off-line. EEM: external elastic membrane. Top green circle: EEM area 19.8mm^2; top red circle: Lumen 3.3mm^2; bottom green circle: EEM area 11.5mm^2; bottom red circle: lumen 2.9mm^2

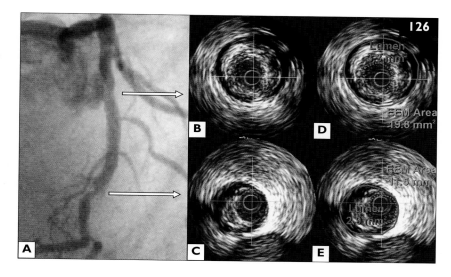

127 A: Reflection and refraction of ultrasound (US) waves. The US waves will pass tissues with different acoustical impedances, indicated by Z1–3. The differences in these impedances cause the wave to break and the beam is partially reflected, partially refracted, and partially scattered. This shows on the US images as identifiable boundaries with different gray value intensities (**B**). Roughness of tissue surface will cause diffuse reflection. 1: blood; 2: external elastic membrane; 3: fibrotic tissue; 4: soft tissue.

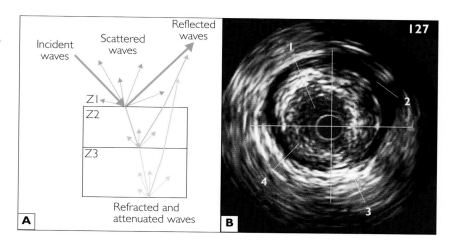

128 A: Boston Scientific Corporation Galaxy ultrasound (US) console, which drives the catheter mechanically. **B**: In-Vision Gold system of Volcano. This system operates the catheters electronically. **C**: Close-up of the mechanical ultrasound transducer that cooperates with the US console in **A**. **D**: Transducers used with the system in **B**. Both systems are so-called fully digital, thus the centre of the system is a computer, and both have on-line basic measurement capabilities on-board. Besides storing the image data on SVHS videotape both can store the data digitally on CD-ROM in the medical DICOM image format.

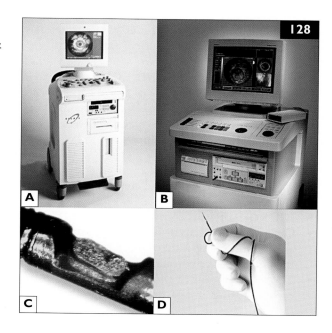

US beam is projected to the vessel wall by means of a mechanically rotated mirror with 1,800 rpm, and (2) electronic systems, where multiple (64) elements are mounted on the tip of a catheter and the elements are excited one by one or pair-wise, resulting in an electronically rotating beam. The ICUS catheters operate on frequencies between 20 (phased array catheters) and 40 MHz (mechanical catheters), resulting in a resolution of approximately 80 μm axially and 200–250 μm laterally. Higher frequency operating catheters will show more vessel wall details in the US images[7].

Intracoronary ultrasound in the laboratory

The mechanical catheter design has a sonolucent distal sheath preventing contact of the US transducer with the vessel wall. Since US requires an air-free medium to transmit and receive the US waves, this sheath must be flushed with saline and cleared of air before inserting the catheter over a guide wire into the patient. When the catheter is positioned under angiographic guidance distal from the segment to be analyzed, the guide wire must be retracted to make way for the US element. The phased array catheter can be inserted directly over the guide wire into the patient.

The ICUS catheter can then be pulled back manually to interrogate the coronary vessel. Images can be stored on videotape and modern ICUS consoles also store the images digitally (**128**). To get a more comprehensive view of the analyzed segment and to perform more accurate quantitative measurements, the catheter should be pulled back with a motorized device pulling the catheter with a uniform speed of 0.5 mm/second or ECG-gated and triggered[8] in small discrete steps (0.2 mm) (**129**). This allows building of computer reconstructed longitudinal views (L-views) for a more comprehensive visual assessment and for quantitative analysis[9] (**130, 131**). Modern ICUS consoles provide this measurement functionality built-in for on-line use in the catheterization laboratory, helping to guide the procedure.

INDICATIONS

Possible indications for the use of ICUS catheters can be divided into diagnostic and interventional applications (*Table 18*).

CONTRAINDICATIONS AND COMPLICATIONS

Contraindications for the use of ICUS catheters are presented in *Table 19*. While the use of ICUS catheters has been described as safe[10,11], according to the manufacturers the complications described in *Table 20* can occur.

LIMITATIONS

Although an important tool in coronary imaging, ICUS has some limitations:
- ICUS cannot cross coronary stenoses with diameters <1 mm.
- Quantitative analysis of ICUS images requires more skills, thus also training, and it takes more time to perform the analyses than quantitative coronary arteriography (QCA).
- The axial motion of the ICUS catheters during the cardiac cycle, causing image artifacts when applying longitudinal

reconstructed images for quantitative analysis, can make these analyses difficult and time-consuming. Applying an ECG-gated and triggered pullback, at the cost of some extended pullback time, can solve this problem[8].
- Since CAG and QCA are still regarded as the gold standards to study CAD and the effects of new therapeutic strategies, only a very limited number of manufacturers are investing in the development of ICUS equipment and additional analysis software.

Table 18 Indications for the use of intracoronary ultrasound catheters

Diagnostic applications
- Assessment of apparently angiographically normal coronary vessels (e.g. transplanted heart).
- Assessment of angiographically nonsignificant stenoses.
- Interrogation of unstable lesions.

Interventional applications
- Preinterventional imaging (e.g. determination of exact lesion length).
- Guidance during angioplasty.
- Progression/regression studies.

Table 19 Contraindications for the use of intracoronary ultrasound catheters

- Bacteria or sepsis.
- Abnormalities in the coagulation system.
- Unsuitability for coronary artery bypass surgery.
- Total occlusion.
- Hemodynamic instability or shock.
- Coronary artery spasm.
- Myocardial infarction.
- Unsuitability for balloon angioplasty.

Table 20 Complications in the use of intracoronary ultrasound catheters

- Vessel dissection or perforation.
- Total occlusion.
- Ventricular fibrillation.
- Unstable angina.
- Abrupt closure.
- Death.

129 Ultrasound catheter pullback device setup for the pullback of a mechanical ultrasound (US) catheter. 1: The outer sheath of the catheter must be clamped. 2: The connector which connects the driving cable (rotating the US element) to the motor device, 3: The US motor device transports the radio frequency ultrasound waves to the US element. 4: The flush channel used to clear the sonolucent distal catheter lumen of air by filling it with saline. 5: The motor unit carriage device which can be moved backwards and forwards by rotating a driving shaft, indicated by 6: This shaft is driven by use of an electro- (0.5mm/second pullback) or a stepping-motor (ECG-gated pullback) in 7.

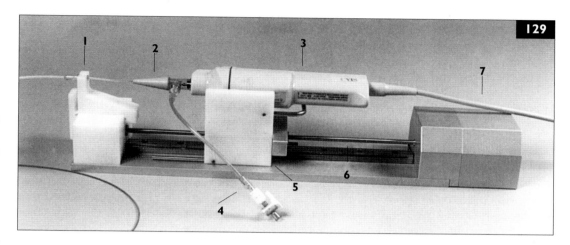

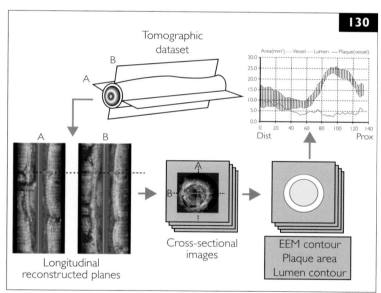

130 Figure to show the analysis path. The tomographic dataset is used to reconstruct a maximum of 72 so-called longitudinal planes (L-views). Two of these L-views, perpendicular to each other (indicated by A and B) are presented. In these planes the contours of the vessel (e.g. the boundary of the external elastic membrane, EEM), stent, and lumen are detected. These contours are mapped into control points on the acquired cross sectional ultrasound images and are used to find, with different algorithms, the three above named contours in each individual cross section. The advantage of this procedure is that the contours in many cross sectional images (>2250 when using PAL, 2700 frames with NTSC images present in a 1.5 minute pullback dataset) can be detected by only detecting a few contours in the L-view and thus saving time. After detection, area and volumetric calculations of the examined segment can be performed (area plot per cross section, **top right**). Dist: distal; Prox: proximal.

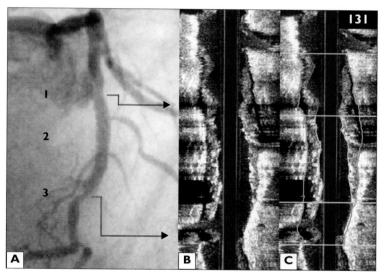

131 Angiogram (**A**) and a longitudinal reconstruction (L-view) of an electrocardiogram-gated pullback procedure (**B**, **C**) from the same patient data as in **126**. The investigated coronary segment is divided into three different segments separated by the yellow lines (**C**). These L-views are not only useful to get a comprehensive view of the segment, almost similar to the angiographic view in **A**, but also for quantitative analysis. The red lines in **C** indicate the detected luminal borders, the blue lines the stent borders, and the green lines the so-called total vessel borders. In this particular case in the target segment the stent and lumen borders are superimposed since there is no detectable intima hyperplasia. 1: proximal; 2: target; 3: distal.

THREE-DIMENSIONAL RECONSTRUCTION

Besides the above-described clinical usage of ICUS, other research applications based on ICUS imaging have been developed or are under development. Such an application is 3D reconstruction.

The tomographic ICUS image data set acquired during a motorized pullback, preferably ECG-gated (to avoid catheter motion artifacts and to produce dynamic reconstructed images), can also be used for 3D image reconstruction[12,13] (**132**). A gray level range is used to subtract the blood pool and background from the coronary wall structures in each cross sectional ICUS image (e.g. image segmentation). Volume rendering techniques are than applied to perform the 3D reconstructions. Rendering is a processing step, producing a spatial (3D) appearance on a planar monitor or hardcopy printout. A rendering technique called gradient shading is frequently used for these 3D reconstructions. This technique uses an illumination model. 'Light' emitted from the viewer's perspective is 'reflected' from the surface undulations of the reconstructed object. This type of rendering provides very realistic and detailed views, but is susceptible to artifacts in the image data. A special reconstruction technique makes it possible to create a simulated black-and-white angioscopic procedure (e.g. so-called 'fly-through').

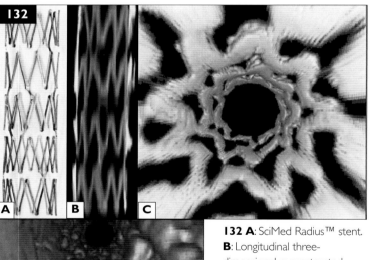

132 A: SciMed Radius™ stent. **B**: Longitudinal three-dimensional reconstructed ultrasound image of this stent *in vitro*. **C**: From a pullback procedure *in vitro*, a so-called fly-through reconstruction is produced. The strut geometry of this stent is not only clearly visible *in vitro* and but also *in vivo* (**D**).

CORONARY ANGIOSCOPY

YASUMI UCHIDA, MD

INTRODUCTION

Coronary angioscopy is routinely performed in selected institutes for diagnosis of the changes occurring in the coronary vessels[1-6], for selection of therapeutic modalities[6], for evaluation of medical[7], interventional[8-11], and surgical therapies[12], and for prediction of acute coronary syndromes (ACS)[13]. Hitherto, visible light has been used for coronary angioscopy. Recently however, dye image[6,14] and fluorescent image angioscopy[6,15] have been employed for more detailed evaluation of the changes and discrimination of the composition of the coronary vessels.

CORONARY ANGIOSCOPES

The angioscopy system is composed of an angioscope, illumination source, camera, image mixer, video recorder (tape or disc), and monitor. The monorail-type angioscope routinely used by the author is shown in **133A,B** and is shown schematically in **133C**. By using a mixer, both angioscopic and fluoroscopic images are simultaneously recorded and monitored for identification of the location of the observed target. At present, three types of angioscope are frequently used for observation of coronary arteries in the author's laboratories[6,16,17]. The angioscope is composed of a fiberscope, operating part, and guiding catheter with or without balloon. The fiberscope contains 3,000, 6,000 or 8,000 image guide quartz fibers and 25 or 50 light guide (illumination) fibers. The fiberscope also has a guide wire slider at its distal most tip which allows a 0.014 inch guide wire to pass through. By manipulating the fiberscope operation part, the fiberscope part can be advanced or pulled back over the wire for observation.

TECHNIQUE

After diagnostic coronary angiography with 5 or 6 F catheters, the sheath in the right femoral artery is replaced with a sheath. An 8 F guiding catheter for coronary interventions is introduced through the sheath into the aortic root so as to locate its tip in the ostium of the coronary artery. An angioscope is then introduced through the guiding catheter into the coronary artery. An angioscope and guiding catheter appropriate for observation of the given plaque are selected and angioscopy is performed.

In general, an Amplatz catheter is more suitable for the LCA. In the case of the RCA, the suitability of the catheter is dependent on the branching angle of the RCA to the aorta. A Judkins catheter is suitable for horizontal or downward branching and an Amplatz catheter for upright branching RCAs. A guiding catheter with side holes is recommended when the ostium is narrow.

The first choice for middle to distal segments is a monorail-type angioscope[6]. A 0.014 inch guide wire is advanced across the plaque. The angioscope is then advanced carefully over the guide wire so as to locate the tip of the fiberscope part just proximal to the target plaque and the balloon is located in the proximal segment and not in the left main trunk (LMT) (in the case of the LCA). Use of a guide wire with markers at every 1 cm is recommended for confirmation of the location of the plaque and the fiberscope tip. The tip of the fiberscope is easily identified by its metallic slider and the balloon by a marker. When the angioscope is suitably located, the balloon is inflated manually. Usually, 0.5 ml carbon dioxide is enough for complete occlusion. Then, heparinized and warmed saline is infused. Manual infusion of saline using a plastic syringe containing 20 ml heparinized saline is recommended because the infusion speed can be controlled during observation and excessive infusion can be prevented. Use of a power injector may be beneficial when there are fewer than three operators. However, special care should be taken not to infuse saline when the fiberscope part is in the completely pulled back position. In this situation, an excessive rise in pressure within the catheter part occurs and, accordingly, shaft perforation may occur. When blood is completely displaced with saline, clear visualization of the coronary interior will be obtained. An interval of 1–2 seconds is required for complete blood displacement. Then, the fiberscope part is slowly advanced over the wire, confirming the wall changes successively.

After observation by advancing the fiberscope part, the balloon is deflated and the saline infusion is topped up to prevent excessive ischemia and serious arrhythmias. When the ECG has returned to the control state, the balloon is again inflated and saline is infused to observe the same target by pulling back the fiberscope part.

INDICATIONS

Coronary angioscopy is indicated for plaque and thrombus characterization, selection of therapeutic modalities, evaluation of medical, interventional, and surgical therapies, and for prognosis. In the guidelines for coronary angioscopy of the Japanese Society of Cardioangioscopy, the operator of coronary angioscopy is limited to a cardiologist with experience of coronary intervention in at least 100 patients and after angioscopy experience in 50 patients directed by a coronary angioscopist who is authorized by the Society.

CONTRAINDICATIONS AND COMPLICATIONS

The patients contraindicated for CAG and coronary intervention are also contraindicated for coronary angioscopy. Angioscopy of LMT should not be performed by untrained operators. Use of conventional angioscopes is not recommended for small distal coronary segments with a diameter <0.5 mm since the procedure might cause serious damage to the segment.

During saline infusion, giant negative T, extreme elongation of QT segment, and elevation or depression of the ST segment of the ECG always occurs. When elongation of the QT segment and T inversion appear, the author immediately deflates the balloon and stops saline infusion. On deflation of the balloon and cessation of saline infusion, the ECG features disappear promptly. According to the author's experience, appearance of advanced ventricular arrhythmia is very rare when the patients are premedicated with xylocain. Serious complications experienced by the author in the management of 649 patients include: dissection in five, acute closure in three, acute MI in three, and death in one.

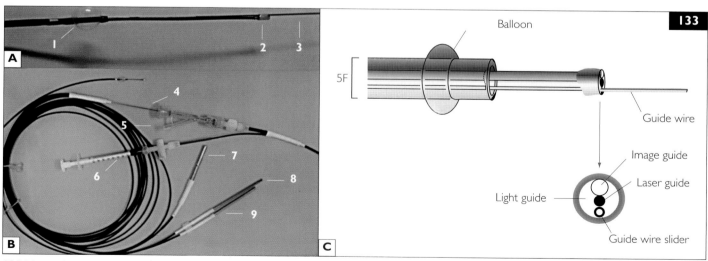

133 Monorail-type angioscope. **A**: Fiberscope part advanced: 1: balloon; 2: fiberscope-tip; 3: guidewire. **B**: Proximal control part: 4: control part for fiberscope; 5: saline flush channel; 6: balloon inflation syringe; 7: light guide; 8: image guide; 9: laser guide. **C**: Schematic representation of angioscope tip.

LIMITATIONS

Failure of complete visualization of the coronary plaques is not infrequent even in large coronary segments due to the coronary anatomy and the lack of flexibility of the angioscope. The changes behind the plaque are also difficult to visualize.

Plaque

134A,B show the angioscopic appearances of coronary plaques. Angioscopically, atherosclerotic masses protruding into the coronary lumen when observed longitudinally are called coronary plaques. They are classified from surface morphology into regular (smooth and without obvious disruption) (**134A,B**) and complex (irregularly surfaced, usually with disruption accompanied by any or none of hemorrhage, hematoma, and thrombus) plaques (**134B**).

Regular and complex plaques are called 'simple plaques' and 'complicated plaques' respectively, in some literature. The plaques are also classified from surface color into white, light yellow, yellow, brown, and white and yellow in mosaic fashion. Based on histologic and clinical studies, the author also classifies yellow regular plaques into nonglistening and glistening types, since the latter category is considered histologically to be more vulnerable than the others[6,18]. The plaques with frosty glass-like surface or uneven surface without obvious disruption are included in complex plaques. These minimal changes are hardly detectable by conventional angiography and IVUS. However, the author has found that these changes can be stained with Evans blue, indicating that the frosty-glass portions are composed of damaged endothelia and/or fibrin threads[6,14]. The plaques with smooth surface but accompanied by prestenotic or poststenotic thrombi are also included into complex plaques. Furthermore, regular plaques are classified into nonprotruded (lined) and protruded when observed coaxially, and concentric and eccentric when observed longitudinally[6]. The angioscopic classification system used by the author[6] is a modification of that described by den Heijer *et al.*[19].

Thrombus

Angioscopically, a predominantly mural mobile or nonmobile mass, adherent to the vessel surface but clearly a separate structure, is classified as a thrombus. Coronary thrombi are classified based on surface color into red, pink or purple, white, white and red in mosaic fashion, dark red, yellow, and brown (**135A,B**). The color of the thrombus is determined by its composition and age. In the case of a fresh thrombus, color is also influenced by the presence or absence of blood flow or by interventions. Red indicates the existence of abundant red blood cells in loose fibrin networks. Pink or purple indicates a reduced number of red blood cells and abundant fibrin and platelets. White indicates that at least the superficial layer is composed of fibrin and/or platelets. Dark red is probably a red blood cell-rich thrombus aged for a few days. According to animal experiments, yellow indicates an organized thrombus aged at least 2 weeks. Brown may indicate a mixture of atheromatous debris and thrombi, especially when glistening particles are also present.

The coronary thrombus is also classified, based on its morphology and localization, into amorphous, mural (lining or non-protruded), globular (protruded), band or web, and streamer-like. Red amorphous configuration indicates red blood cell stagnation in a very loose fibrin network. White amorphous configuration indicates a loose fibrin network with or without platelets aggregated on it. White band, web, and membranous configurations indicate residual fibrin after washout or autolysis of the thrombus. A streamer-like configuration indicates flow-dependent growth toward downstream or upstream[6].

Hemorrhage

Hemorrhage is also observed in the wall, which may apparently be intact by angiography and IVUS. It is usually clearly demarcated, not protruding and does not disappear with saline flush. It is either red or purple, respectively indicating arterial and venous bleeding. In the disrupted plaques, bleeding from the wall (red or purple in color) into the lumen can also be observed[6].

134 Coronary plaques. **A**: Regular plaques: a: normal coronary artery with smooth and milky-white luminal surface; arrow: guidewire; b: white plaque; c: light yellow plaque; d: yellow plaque; e: glistening yellow plaque. **B**: Complex plaques: a: fractured yellow plaque with globular red thrombus (white arrow); b: multiple flaps (white arrow) with mural thrombus; black arrow: guidewire; c: a large flap obstructing the lumen (white arrow); d: a pore (white arrow) in the fibrous cap connecting to the lipid core. (Reproduced with permission of the author, from Uchida [2000][6]. *Coronary Angioscopy*. Futura Publishing Co, Armonk.)

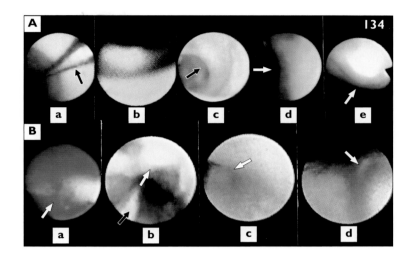

135 Coronary thrombi. **A**: Commonly observed globular (protruded) coronary thrombi (arrows in each picture): a: red thrombus; b: pink thrombus; c: thrombus in red and white in mosaic fashion; d: white thrombus; e: cotton candy-like white thrombus. **B**: Less commonly observed thrombi (arrows in each picture): a: amorphous red thrombus; b: membranous transparent thrombus; c: band or web-like thrombus; d: amorphous brown thrombus; e: brown (black arrow) and red (white arrow) thrombi. (Reproduced with permission of the author, from Uchida [2000][6]. *Coronary Angioscopy*. Futura Publishing Co, Armonk.)

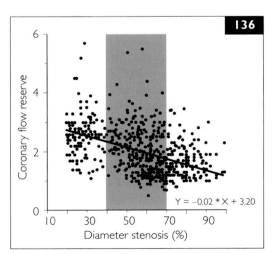

INTRACORONARY DOPPLER FLOW

M. VOSKUIL, MD, PhD AND J.J. PIEK, MD, PhD

INTRODUCTION

In clinical practice, noninvasive techniques such as ECG exercise testing, myocardial perfusion scintigraphy and stress echocardiography are frequently used in the diagnosis of CAD. Moreover, perfusion scintigraphy yields prognostic information relevant for risk stratification of patients with CAD[1]. Nevertheless, CAG is still considered the gold standard in the documentation of CAD. However, this technique is of limited value for the assessment of the functional severity of, in particular, intermediate coronary narrowings[2]. The poor correlation between the angiographical (reflected in the percentage diameter stenosis; %DS) and functional (reflected in the coronary flow reserve; CFR) severity of an arterial narrowing is generally acknowledged (**136**). Furthermore, the assignment of the 'culprit lesion' is particularly

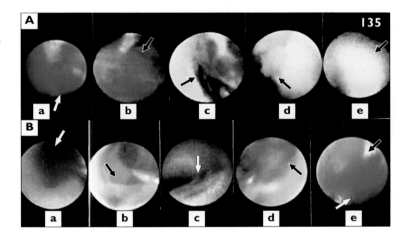

136 Plot to show the poor correlation between the angiographical severity of a stenosis and CFR. Particularly in the segment of the intermediate stenosis (DS 40–70%) a large range in values of CFR is observed, as depicted in the blue box. CFR: coronary flow reserve.

difficult in the presence of multiple lesions in different vascular territories. The functional severity of a stenosis is determined not only by its angiographical narrowing, but also by the capacity of the distal microvascular bed to dilate during stress conditions, ensuring sufficient blood flow to meet the myocardial oxygen demand[3]. Recent technical developments have made it possible to assess the physiologic severity of a stenosis during cardiac catheterization using guide wires that are equipped with Doppler sensors on the tip[4]. Using this technique, blood flow velocity can be assessed before and after administration of a vasodilator (simulation of exercise; hyperemia). Several parameters can be assessed using this method. The ratio between blood flow velocity during maximal vasodilatation (hyperemic average peak flow velocity) and the resting situation (baseline average peak flow velocity) is defined as CFR. In the absence of a severe epicardial stenosis, CFR may still be abnormal due to microvascular abnormalities. In this situation, the relative CFR (ratio between CFR of the culprit artery and an angiographically normal artery) can be useful in assessing the functional significance of an (intermediate) coronary lesion[3]. A normal reference vessel is a prerequisite for the assessment of relative CFR and, hence, this parameter cannot be used in patients with three-vessel disease. However, both parameters are important for diagnostic purposes and the direct evaluation of the result of a percutaneous intervention, while they also provide prognostic information on the clinical outcome following PTCA.

DIAGNOSTIC EVALUATION OF CORONARY ARTERY DISEASE

Validation studies have shown an excellent agreement between the results of Doppler flow parameters and noninvasive stress tests such as exercise ECG, stress echocardiography, and perfusion scintigraphy (*Table 21*)[5–16]. The selective assessment of the functional severity of a stenosis during cardiac catheterization is a major advantage of intracoronary derived parameters. This is, in particular, important for the assignment of the culprit lesion in patients with multi-vessel disease (**137**). These validation studies were performed to determine cut-off values of the different parameters for clinical decision making to perform PTCA or to defer from coronary intervention (i.e. pharmacologic treatment). The cut-off values of CFR and relative CFR that were determined in patients with single-vessel disease were similar to the cut-off values in patients with multi-vessel disease. For CFR, a cut-off value of 1.7–2.0 (i.e. that the blood flow velocity increases to 170–200% during pharmacologically induced vasodilatation) has been reported. For relative CFR, a cut-off value of 0.60–0.75 (i.e. CFR in the diseased artery varies between 60% and 75% of CFR in an angiographically normal artery) is used in clinical practice. A large multi-center study has been performed, the ILIAS study, in which the safety of deferral of execution of PTCA (cut-off value CFR 2.0) was examined in patients with an intermediate coronary narrowing (40–70% diameter stenosis)[17]. The results showed that patients with a CFR above 2.0 have a very low incidence of major adverse events during 1-year follow-up. It was concluded that deferral of PTCA is safe in

Table 21 Results of previous validation studies for coronary flow reserve (CFR) and relative CFR versus noninvasive stress testing

First author	Year	Number of patients	Noninvasive test	Agreement (%)	Cut-off value
CFR					
Miller[5]	1994	33	SPECT	89	2.0
Joye[6]	1994	30	SPECT	94	2.0
Deychak[7]	1995	17	SPECT	96	1.8
Tron[8]	1995	62	SPECT	84	2.0
Heller[9]	1997	55	SPECT	88	1.7
Danzi[10]	1998	30	DSE	87	2.0
Verberne[11]	1999	37	SPECT	85	1.9
Piek[12]	2000	225	X-ECG	76	2.1
Chamuleau[13]	2001	127	SPECT	75	1.7
Meuwissen[14]	2002	151	SPECT	80	1.7
Rel-CFR					
Verberne[11]	1999	37	SPECT	85	0.65
Duffy[15]	2001	28	DSE	81	0.75
El-Shafei[16]	2001	48	SPECT	75	0.75
Chamuleau[13]	2001	127	SPECT	75	0.60

DSE: dobutamine stress echocardiography; Rel-CFR: relative coronary flow reserve; SPECT: single photon emission computed tomography; X-ECG: exercise electrocardiography.

this subset of patients with multi-vessel disease. These results are in accordance with previously performed small sized single-center studies using the cut-off value for CFR of 2.0[18,19]. Moreover, the results of the ILIAS study showed that the predictive value of the CFR measurement for the occurrence of adverse events related to the intermediate lesion is better than the noninvasive assessment of myocardial perfusion using single photon emission computerized tomography (SPECT).

EVALUATION OF THE RESULT AFTER PERCUTANEOUS TRANSLUMINAL CORONARY ANGIOPLASTY

The described parameters can also be of use in the evaluation of the hemodynamic result after a percutaneous intervention. The results of the Doppler Endpoints Balloon Angioplasty Trial Europe (DEBATE) I study showed that patients with single-vessel disease and a good angiographical (DS 35%) result after balloon angioplasty, in combination with a good hemodynamic result (CFR >2.5) have a good clinical outcome at 6-month follow-up[20]. This finding was confirmed in the DESTINI, FROST, and DEBATE II trials, which showed that a strategy of provisional stent implantation (i.e. only perform stent implantation in case of a suboptimal result after balloon angioplasty) results in a similar outcome as compared to the patients who had an elective stent

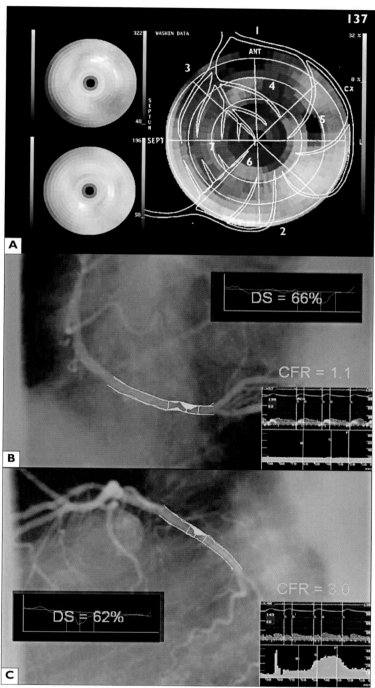

A

B

C

137 A: Results of myocardial perfusion scintigraphy. The 'bulls eye' reconstruction is presented with the global coronary anatomy. The stress picture (left upper panel) shows an infero-postero-lateral reversible perfusion defect. Coronary angiography showed a narrowing in the distal RCA (**B**) and mid LCx (**C**), both of approximately 60% (**B** 66%, **C** 62%). CFR appeared to be impaired in the RCA (1.1), while CFR was normal in the LCx (3.0). 1: Anterior; 2: Posterior; 3: Left Anterior Descending; 4: diagonal branches; 5: marginal branches; 6: posterior descending artery; 7: sceptal branches. CFR: coronary flow reserve; RCA: right coronary artery; LCx: left circumflex artery.

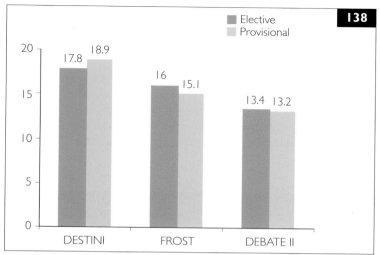

138 Chart to show the percentage of major adverse cardiac events (MACE) (death, myocardial infarction, target lesion revascularization) of three large multi-center trials comparing the strategies of provisional stent implantation guided by CFR (pink) and elective stent implantation (blue)[21–23]. CFR: coronary flow reserve.

implantation (**138**)[21–23]. Nevertheless, an impaired CFR is a frequent finding after PTCA and occurs in approximately 50% of the patients, despite a good angiographical result. Several mechanisms have been postulated for this finding such as temporary disturbed autoregulation, distal embolization of microparticles, or microvascular abnormalities due to diabetes mellitus, LV hypertrophy, or diffuse atherosclerotic disease[24].

Several additional treatment options (e.g. upsized balloon dilatation, stent implantation and/or pharmacologic intervention using IIb/IIIa inhibition, clopidogrel or statins) can be considered, depending on the origin of the impaired CFR. In the DEBATE II study, an aggressive approach was pursued to obtain an optimal angiographical result, as defined in the DEBATE I study (DS 35%), after balloon angioplasty. The results of this large multi-center study confirm the assumption that patients with a suboptimal result after balloon angioplasty (i.e. in case of a diameter stenosis >35% and/or a CFR >2.5), benefit from additional stent implantation in order to improve clinical outcome (**139**). In these patients, hyperemic blood flow velocity increased after stent implantation, suggesting the presence of a residual coronary stenosis after balloon angioplasty that could not be appreciated angiographically[25].

Although approximately 50% of the patients in the provisional stent arm of the DEBATE II study showed an unsatisfactory result after balloon angioplasty, this also indicates that the remaining 50% of the patients showed a good 'stent-like' clinical outcome after optimal balloon angioplasty. From a clinical point of view this is an essential observation, since a restenotic lesion after balloon angioplasty can be treated easily with a stent, while the treatment of in-stent restenosis is still cumbersome. The data from multi-center studies indicate that CFR and/or relative CFR is/are also useful for guidance of elective stent implantation, showing a 'drug-eluting' clinical outcome in cases of an optimal angiographal result in combination with a CFR >2.5 and/or a relative CFR >0.88, respectively (**140**)[26–28]. Therefore, it is concluded that despite the current clinical trend toward elective stenting because of its many benefits (i.e. ease of stent placement, more satisfying angiography), this treatment strategy is not supported by randomized clinical data. In contrast, the current studies show that intracoronary Doppler parameters provide information, beyond that obtained by the eyes of experienced angiographers, that is relevant for clinical decision-making during coronary interventions[29].

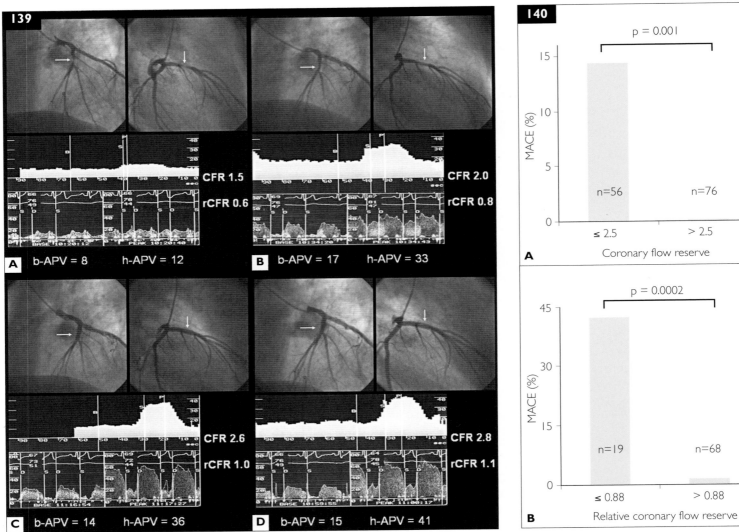

139 Hemodynamic measurements before (**A**) and after (**B**) balloon dilatation, additional stent implantation (**C**) and upsized postdilatation (**D**) in a patient. The angiogram shows a significant stenosis in the left anterior descending coronary artery in two orthogonal views (white arrow). Below the angiograms, the baseline (b-APV) and hyperemic blood flow velocity (h-APV) signals and the trend over time are depicted. rCFR: relative CFR.

140 Charts to show the percentage of major adverse cardiac events (MACE) during follow-up in the subgroup of patients with an optimal angiographical result (diameter stenosis ≤11%) after stent implantation, subdivided for the patients above or below the cut-off values for CFR (**A**: data derived from Voskuil et al. (2002). Optimized stent implantation according to intracoronary Doppler derived parameters. Am. J. Cardiol. **90**:1139–1142.) and relative CFR (**B**: data derived from Haude et al. (2001). Intracoronary Doppler- and quantitative coronary angiography-derived predictors of major adverse cardiac events after stent implantation. Circulation **103**:1212–1217.).

ENDOTHELIAL DYSFUNCTION

K.E. SØRENSEN, MD AND D.S. CELERMAJER, MBBS, MSC, PhD, FRACP

INTRODUCTION

The ability of the normal endothelium to release vasodilatory substances in response to physical and pharmacological stimuli remains the basis for the *in vivo* study of endothelial physiology. Endothelial function is traditionally assessed by contrasting the vasodilatory responses to endothelial-dependent vasodilators (e.g. acetylcholine, substance P, reactive hyperemia) with endothelial-independent vasodilators (e.g. nitroglycerin and nitroprusside). Whereas normal vessels respond to such stimuli with vaso-dilatation, vessels with injuried endothelium exhibit either attenuated dilatation or even paradoxical vasoconstriction.

Endothelial function can be studied invasively and noninvasively, in larger conductance arteries and in small resistance vessels. Vasodilatation of the large epicardial coronary arteries is normally evaluated angiographically, but can be assessed by IVUS (see Chapter 7, Intracoronary Ultrasound). Coronary microvascular responses can be determined by Doppler flow measurements (see Chapter 7, Intracoronary Doppler Flow) or with positron emission tomography (PET) (see Chapter 8, Position Emission Tomography).

Forearm venous occlusion plethysmography is the gold standard technique for assessment of resistance vessel function. Finally, a completely noninvasive US-based method for evaluation of flow-mediated dilatation of the brachial or radial artery has been extensively studied and has been used as a surrogate marker for endothelial function in the coronary circulation.

TECHNIQUE

For all the techniques, vasoactive medications are generally discontinued at least 18–24 hours prior to investigation, although non-nitrate vasoactive drugs seem to be without significant effect on (at least) brachial artery reactivity. Attention must also be paid to other potential factors that have been shown to influence vascular reactivity such as exercise, caffeine, high-fat foods, and vitamin C.

Epicardial coronary arteries

A study protocol on drugs, drug dosages, infusion times, and timing of angiograms must be available and followed accurately throughout the study. The left anterior descending artery (LAD) is the most commonly used target vessel, but the circumflex (Cx) and RCA can also be studied.

To guide the procedure, for choosing the target artery and to identify subjects at particular risk of vasoconstrictive complications, the coronary angiographic status must be delineated before contemplating a coronary endothelial study. For assessment of the LAD, an 8 F guiding catheter is placed in the left main coronary artery. Through this catheter, a small (2–3 F) infusion catheter is advanced into the proximal part of the LAD for administration of vasoactive agents. Alternatively, a Doppler catheter (usually 3 F) can be used for drug infusion as well as for flow velocity recordings. The set-up is illustrated in **141**. Vasodilatation of large epicardial arteries is usually assessed by repeated angiograms obtained at baseline and during stepwise serial intracoronary infusions of the selected vasodilators at incremental doses and control solutions. It is crucial to maintain stable position of the catheters throughout the study. Vasomotoric responses are evaluated off-line using QCA (see Chapter 7, Quantitative Coronary Arteriography). Typical vasomotoric responses of coronary arteries to acetylcholine and nitroglycerin in a subject with pathological endothelial responses are shown in **142**.

IVUS can be used as an alternative for measuring vessel size but cannot be combined with flow measurements. Whereas IVUS is restricted to imaging a small section of the target artery, the entire vessel can be interrogated angiographically.

Myocardial blood flow

Flow calculation requires combined angiographic (flow area) and Doppler flow velocity analysis but makes it possible also to explore endothelial function of the myocardial microvasculture. Similarly, PET can be used to assess endothelial function in the microvasculature.

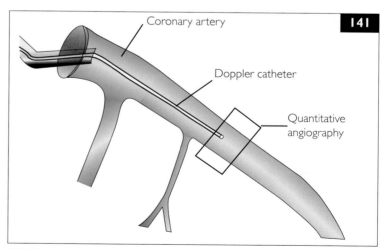

141 Schematic drawing of placement of guiding and Doppler flow velocity catheters for *in vivo* assessment of coronary endothelial function.

Forearm venous occlusion plethysmography

Forearm venous occlusion plethysmography measures total forearm blood flow using strain gauges (**143, 144**). The hand is usually excluded from the circulation by inflating a wrist cuff to suprasystolic pressure. Forearm venous return is stopped for 10 seconds by inflating a cuff around the upper arm to 40 mm Hg (5.3 kPa). The unobstructed arterial flow leads to a gradual increase in forearm circumferential swelling which is measured by the strain gauge, from which flow can be calculated in ml/100 ml forearm/minute.

Intrabrachial administration of vasoactive drugs (e.g. acetylcholine, metacholine, bradykinin, nitroprusside) can be used to assess endothelial/vascular reactivity, which is usually presented in a dose-response curve format.

Flow-mediated vasodilatation of the brachial artery

Flow-mediated vasodilatation of the brachial artery is endothelium-dependent and can be quantified noninvasively with high-resolution external US (**145**). The endothelial stimulus is reactive hyperemia induced by transient (usually 4–5 minutes) upper arm or forearm cuff occlusion. The endothelium-independent stimulus is 0.4 mg nitroglycerin (spray or sublingual tablet). The brachial artery is imaged longitudinally above (or just below) the antecubital fossa. Arterial diameter is measured at baseline, 45–60 seconds after induction of reactive hyperemia (cuff deflation), after 10 minutes rest (second baseline recording), and 3–4 minutes after nitroglycerin (**145**).

Interpretation is usually off-line from video recordings, either with USA cursors or automated edge detection systems. Due to the noninvasiveness of this technique, repeated analysis is easy and abundant data on vascular function in health and disease have now been published. This also includes technical aspects, not least the strengths and weaknesses of the test.

INDICATIONS

Assessment of endothelial function is rarely used clinically but remains an investigative tool for assessing vascular physiologic responses in research protocols. Recent studies, however, suggest that endothelial responses in the coronary arteries and brachial arteries may provide prognostic information.

CONTRAINDICATIONS

Due to the risks of severe paradoxical vasoconstriction caused by the endothelium-dependent 'vasodilator', coronary endothelial testing is not performed in coronary arteries with luminal narrowing >50%. Similarly, subjects with left main disease and those with ACS should not be investigated.

If vasoactive substances have been taken within the preceding 18 hours, responses may be modified and testing may therefore be unreliable. There are no contraindications to forearm plethysmography or brachial arterial testing.

LIMITATIONS

It is important to remember that vasoreactivity only constitutes one aspect of 'endothelial function'. Normal values are difficult to define, particularly for coronary testing. Similar uncertainties remain for the reproducibility of coronary evaluation and for venous occlusion plethysmography. Brachial imaging is often difficult in elderly people. Small arteries can be difficult to analyze. Large vessels dilate only minimally to flow, making it quite difficult to differentiate normal from abnormal responses. The brachial technique has clearly documented that multiple factors such as smoking, caffeine, vitamins, fatty foods, menstrual cycle, and exercise may influence vascular reactivity and thus influence data interpretation significantly.

There are no current noninvasive alternatives available for the assessment of endothelial function in the large coronary arteries. Improvements in USA, CT, and MRI of the large epicardial coronary arteries may, however, make noninvasive assessment feasible. MRI can be used as an alternative to USA for brachial artery imaging.

COMPLICATIONS

Complications are generally few and are the same as those described for CAG (see Chapter 7, Diagnostic Coronary Angiography), ICUS (see Chapter 7, Intracoronary Ultrasound) and coronary Doppler flow (see Chapter 7, Intracoronary Doppler Flow) studies. In some patients, endothelial-dependent stimuli can induce severe vasoconstriction which may require prompt intracoronary nitroglycerin administration. Systemic effects to the agents used are rare and negligible.

Venous occlusion pletysmography requires arterial cannulation but complications are exceedingly rare. Brachial artery studies are only associated with mild discomfort associated due to the cuff inflation.

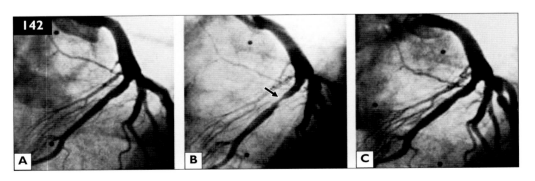

142 Baseline angiogram (**A**) showing paradoxical vasoconstriction to acetylcholine (**B**) and vasodilatation to nitroglycerin (**C**). (Reproduced with permission, Lippincott, Williams, and Wilkins, from Schächinger et al. [2000]. Prognostic impact of coronary vasodilator dysfunction on adverse long-term outcome of coronary heart disease. *Circulation* **101**:1899–1906.)

143 Schematic drawing of venous occlusion plethysmography. Arterial access is used for pressure recordings and infusion of vasoactive substances. Ach: acetylcholine; SNP: sodium nitroprusside. The low-pressure cuff is used to occlude transiently venous flow. The high-pressure cuff is inflated to exclude hand circulation.

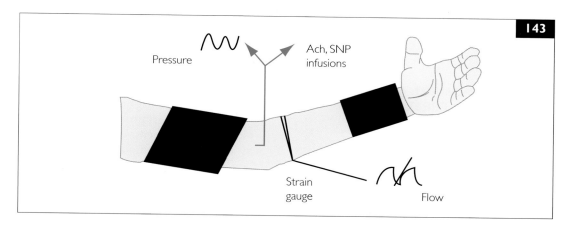

144 Venous occlusion plethysmography. (Courtesy of Dr. Christian Rask Madsen, Joslin Diabetes Center, Boston MA.)

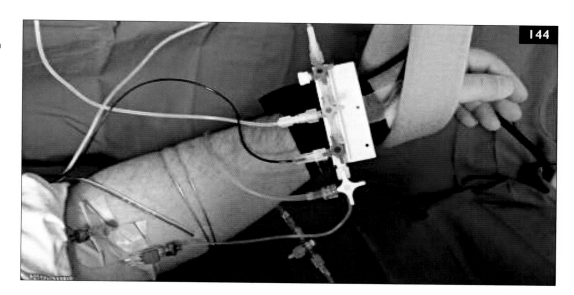

145 Noninvasive assessment of flow-mediated dilatation in the brachial artery. A high-frequency linear transducer is placed over the brachial artery. A cuff is placed distal to the artery and transiently inflated to suprasystolic pressure to induce reactive hyperemia. Flow-mediated, endothelium-dependent dilatation (11%) is measured 45–60 seconds after cuff deflation. Endothelium-independent vasodilatation to nitroglycerin is 18%.

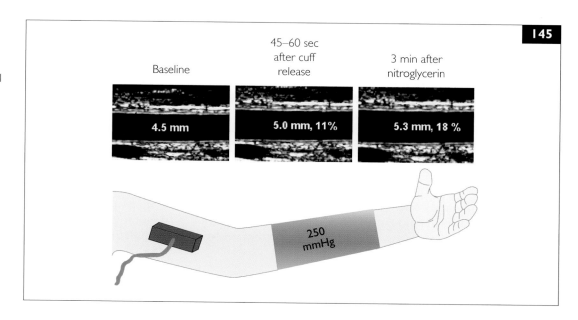

ELECTRON-BEAM COMPUTED TOMOGRAPHY: CORONARY CALCIUM

AXEL SCHMERMUND, MD, STEFAN MÖHLENKAMP, MD AND RAIMUND ERBEL, MD

INTRODUCTION

Electron-beam computed tomography (EBCT) was the first method to allow for direct, noninvasive assessment of the coronary arteries. Other noninvasive tests try, in principle, to detect perfusion abnormalities caused by high-grade coronary stenoses. EBCT is aimed at direct detection and quantification of coronary atherosclerosis and plaque development.

TECHNIQUE

The most important distinction between EBCT and other CT machines is that no mechanical parts are moved. Whereas the distance between cathode and anode is usually very short in CT, it measures approximately 9 feet (2.8 m) in EBCT. The electron-beam, which produces the X-rays by striking the anode, is steered over this distance by an electromagnetic deflection system. The latest generation of EBCT machines ('e-Speed', GE-Imatron) achieves an image acquisition time of only 33 ms, which is sufficient to freeze the motion of the heart.

Standardized methods for imaging, identification, and quantification of coronary calcium using EBCT have been established. Currently, EBCT scanners are usually operated in the high-resolution mode with continuous, nonoverlapping slices of 3 mm thickness and an acquisition time of 100 ms. Patients are positioned supine, and a sufficient number of slices is obtained to cover the complete heart through the apex (usually 36–40 slices). Electrocardiographic triggering is performed at a fixed point within the RR-interval, generally 40% or 80%. Coronary calcium is defined as a hyperattenuating lesion above the threshold of a CT density of 130 Hounsfield units (HU) in an area of two or more adjacent pixels. The 'calcium score' is a product of the area of calcium and a factor rated 1–4 dictated by the maximum CT density. The calcium score can be calculated for a given coronary segment, a specific coronary artery, or for the entire coronary system (**146**).

More recently, a volumetric score has been introduced, which uses isotropic interpolation and may thus be more reproducible. Further, calcium mass measurements have been suggested which should be the same irrespective of the CT technology in use (EBCT or spiral CT with different slice thickness).

INDICATIONS

Noncontrast-enhanced EBCT allows for direct, noninvasive visualization of calcified coronary plaques. The primary aim is not to diagnose coronary stenoses, but rather to detect and quantify coronary plaque burden. There is a relationship between the extent of calcified plaque burden and that of total plaque burden[1]. Of note, coronary calcium appears to indicate coronary disease activity. Calcium is a frequent feature of plaque rupture (found in 70–80%)[2]. Among all types of plaques which can be defined histologically, the extent of calcium is greatest in healed plaque rupture[2]. Further, calcium is associated with positive arterial remodeling[3]. The mechanisms leading to positive arterial remodeling appear to share common aspects with those ultimately leading to plaque rupture, and plaques displaying positive remodeling of the arterial segment are prone to rupture.

The design and main outcomes of a number of prospective studies in selected patient cohorts have been summarized[2,4]. These reports indicate that in seemingly healthy middle-aged and older adults, EBCT has a very high negative predictive value regarding cardiovascular hard endpoints. Also, high-risk persons can be identified whose risk exceeds an event rate of 2% per year. Actual guidelines include EBCT coronary calcium scanning as a diagnostic modality which can add useful prognostic information in adults with an indeterminate risk (**147**)[4,5].

Recently, results from population-based studies with unselected participants have begun to emerge. In the Rotterdam coronary calcification study, 2,013 persons from a suburb of Rotterdam, The Netherlands, participated. After a mean follow-up time of 2.7 years, there was a strong and graded relationship between the EBCT calcium score and cardiac death. The 15% of participants with the highest scores had a relative risk of 11 of dying from ischemic heart disease. The total yearly death rate due to CAD was 4% (**148**), with ischemic heart disease (IHD) accounting for almost 2%. In the approximately 50% of participants with low or zero calcium scores, these rates were 2% and 0.07%[6], respectively

In symptomatic patients who undergo CAG, it is consistently reported that the EBCT coronary calcium score provides prognostic information independent of CAG anatomy[7]. The event rate in symptomatic patients is dictated by arteriosclerotic plaque development and complications and not by the degree of stenosis itself. Indeed, EBCT appears to be superior to CAG in predicting events in these patients[7]. In particular, patients with very high calcium scores have an extremely elevated risk.

In patients presenting to the Emergency Department with atypical chest pain or findings not diagnostic for acute MI, EBCT coronary calcium scanning has a high negative predictive value for ruling out clinically relevant coronary artery disease. The risk of an event appears to be negligible if there is no or very little coronary calcium[8].

Indications for the use of EBCT coronary calcium scanning are given in *Table 22*. Apart from the calcium score, age and sex of the patient should be considered by using specific percentile values ('nomogram') such as those provided for adults in the general population with no history of coronary artery disease in one study[9]. An algorithm used by the authors for interpreting EBCT

146 Coronary calcium scans at the level of the left anterior descending coronary artery. **A**: No coronary calcium. **B**: Moderate coronary calcium, total calcium score 235, with typical localization of calcium in the proximal left coronary artery and near the bifurcation with the first diagonal branch. **C**: Extensive coronary calcium, total calcium score 2,001; in addition calcium is depicted in the wall of the descending aorta.

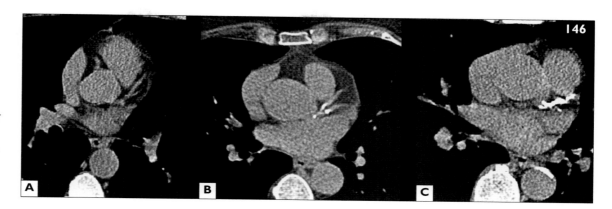

147 Algorithm for the use of electron-beam computed tomography coronary calcium scanning for advanced risk stratification. In patients in whom office-based risk assessment determines an intermediate risk level, calcium scanning can be used for advanced risk stratification (box). In the presence of a very high or a very low calcium score, the initial office-based risk estimate is corrected towards a high or a low risk. Even in the presence of an intermediate calcium score, the scan is useful. In this case, the probability of a truly intermediate risk is much greater than if determined by office-based risk assessment alone.

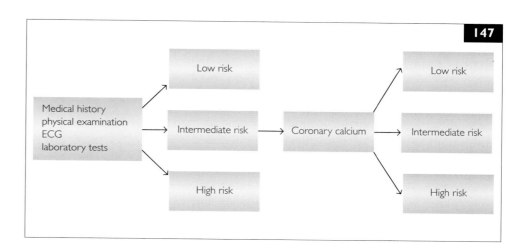

Table 22 Indications for the use of electron-beam computed tomography coronary calcium scanning

Asymptomatic patients:
- Persons with risk factors who cannot be determined by office-based risk assessment to have either a low or a high cardiovascular risk.
- Older persons in whom the established risk factors lose some of their predictive value and whose risk remains indeterminate.

Symptomatic patients:
- Patients in whom advanced risk stratification is useful, e.g. if extensive coronary plaque disease is suspected.
- Patients presenting to the emergency room with nonspecific chest pain ('rule out myocardial infarction').

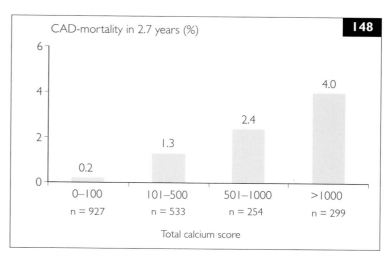

148 Chart to show the rate of coronary artery disease- (CAD) related deaths associated with elevated coronary calcium scores in the Rotterdam coronary calcification study, a population-based study. Mean follow-up was 2.7 years. (Data derived from Vliegenthart *et al.* [2002]. Coronary calcification is a strong predictor of all-cause and cardiovascular mortality in elderly (Abstract). *Circulation* **106**(Suppl.):II.743.)

coronary calcium scans is shown in **149**. The inter-scan variability of the scans is small enough to allow for follow-up studies of the progression of coronary calcium (**150**). Importantly, emerging data suggest that patients with an increased rate of progression of the coronary calcium score have an increased risk of clinical coronary events. However, randomized trials have not been able to demonstrate an effect of lipid-lowering therapy on the rate of progression of coronary calcium, so that the usefulness of serial studies in individual patients remains uncertain.

CONTRAINDICATIONS AND COMPLICATIONS

Contraindications are relative and relate to the use of ionizing radiation. Using an anthropomorphic phantom, effective radiation dose of an EBCT coronary calcium scan was determined to be approximately 1.0 mSv[10]. For comparison, a simple 2-plane chest X-ray is associated with approximately 0.1 mSv, selective CAG (only coronary anatomy) with 2–3 mSv, and environmental exposure during 1 year in most areas of the western world also within 2–3 mSv. Only persons selected by a knowledgeable physician to have a clear indication for advanced risk stratification should be scanned by using EBCT.

There are no known immediate or long-term complications. However, the issue of radiation must be kept in mind.

LIMITATIONS

For coronary calcium scanning, no contrast enhancement is used. Accordingly, noncalcified coronary plaques are not routinely visualized. Because of the simplicity of the test, the ability to quantify calcified plaque burden, the good interscan and interobserver reproducibility, and the excellent prognostic power, this does not appear to be a principal limitation.

149				
	Step I		Step II	
EBCT score (Agatston method)	Interpretation		Age- and sex-specific interpretation (EBCT score percentiles)	Risk assessment
0–10	No/minimal plaque		0–25	Small risk
11–100	Some plaque present		26–50	Moderate risk
101–400	Moderate plaque burden		51–75	Increased risk
401–1000	Severe plaque burden		76–90	High risk
>1000	Very severe plaque burden		>90	Very high risk

149 Algorithm used by the authors for interpreting electron-beam computed tomography coronary calcium scans. In a first step, the total calcium score is considered. Because of the relationship between coronary calcified and coronary total plaque burden, a high calcium score indicates a high coronary plaque burden. In a second step, the total calcium score is put in perspective regarding age and sex of the individual person. If the calcium score is greater than expected (above the median 'normal' value), cardiovascular risk is increasingly elevated.

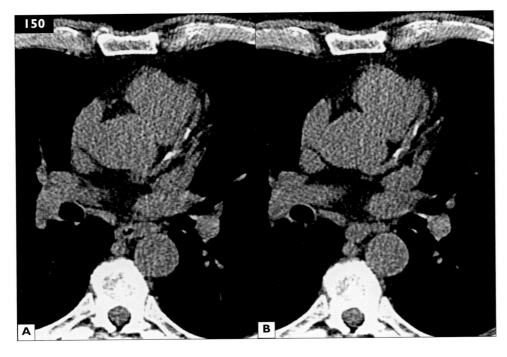

150 Stable calcified plaque in a 55-year-old male patient.
A: Baseline scan, total Agatston calcium score: 164.
B: Follow-up scan 14 months later, total Agatston calcium score: 171.

VULNERABLE ATHEROSCLEROTIC PLAQUES

ERLING FALK, MD, PhD, JOHANNES A. SCHAAR, MD AND MORTEZA NAGHAVI, MD

INTRODUCTION

Atherosclerosis is a chronic and multi-focal immunoinflammatory, fibroproliferative disease of medium-sized and large arteries driven by lipid. Atherosclerotic plaques may limit the flow of blood and give rise to stable angina pectoris. However, atherosclerosis is rarely fatal unless thrombosis supervenes, causing an ACS. Therefore, for event-free survival, the vital question is not why atherosclerosis develops but rather why atherosclerosis, after years of indolent growth, suddenly becomes complicated with luminal thrombosis.

DEFINITION

Coronary atherosclerotic plaques are very heterogeneous in structure and function, and even neighbouring plaques in the same artery may differ markedly. The great majority of coronary plaques are and will remain quiescent, at least from a clinical point of view. In fact, during a lifetime, none or only few coronary plaques become complicated by clinically significant thrombosis, and these rare but dangerous thrombosis-prone plaques are termed vulnerable. Thus, a vulnerable plaque is a plaque assumed to be at high short-term risk of thrombosis, causing an ACS (**151**).

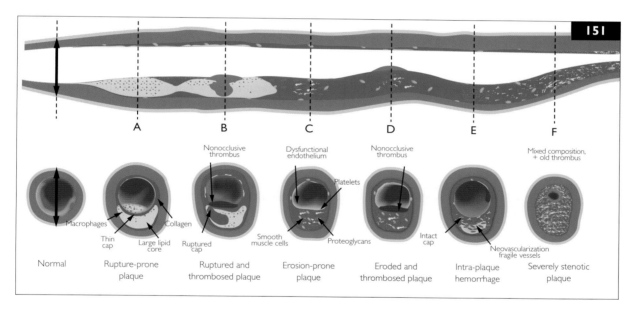

151 Diagram to show the different types of vulnerable and thrombosed plaques preceding or precipitating acute coronary syndromes. **A**: Rupture-prone plaque consisting of a large lipid-rich core covered by a thin and inflamed fibrous cap and associated with expansive remodeling of the artery. **B**: Ruptured plaque with nonocclusive thrombosis superimposed. **C**: Erosion-prone plaque rich in smooth muscle cells and proteoglycans (and often associated with constrictive remodeling). **D**: Eroded plaque with nonocclusive thrombosis superimposed. **E**: Intraplaque hemorrhage from fragile new vessels at the base of the plaque (neovascularization). **F**: Severely stenotic plaque where factors related to flow and blood rather than plaque may confer increased risk for thrombosis. (Modified from Naghavi *et al.* [2003]. From vulnerable plaque to vulnerable patient: a call for new definitions and risk assessment strategies (Parts I and II). *Circulation* **108**:1664–1672, 1772–1778. With permission.)

Thrombosed plaques

Approximately 75% of all coronary thrombi responsible for ACS are precipitated by a ruptured plaque. In plaque rupture, there is a structural defect, a gap, in the fibrous cap that separates the lipid-rich core of a plaque from the lumen of the artery (**54**). For unknown reason(s), plaque rupture is a more frequent cause of coronary thrombosis in men (about 80%) than in women (about 60%). Based on analysis of ruptured plaques, it is assumed that a rupture-prone plaque will possess the features outlined in *Table 23* and illustrated in **152** (see also **55**).

The term plaque erosion is generally used for intact plaques with superimposed thrombosis, i.e. there is no underlying plaque rupture but the endothelium is missing at the plaque–thrombus interface (**58**). These plaques have been identified as being relatively thrombogenic, but the precipitating factor or condition may, in fact, be found outside rather than inside the plaque (e.g. a hyper-thrombotic tendency or so-called vulnerable blood).

Multi-focal disease activity

After an ACS, the risk of a recurrent ischemic event is high during the following 3–6 months. Many of these 'new' events are probably caused by reactivation of the original culprit lesion (rethrombosis), but both postmortem and clinical observations indicate that patients with ACS often have many ruptured and/or 'active' plaques in the coronary arteries. Their role in subsequent ischemic events is unknown.

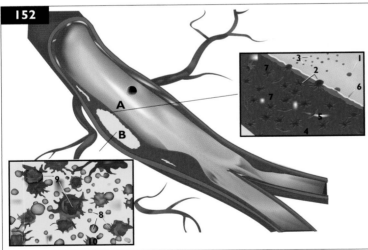

152 The most common type of vulnerable plaque, the plaque assumed to be rupture-prone, is characterized by a thin fibrous cap (**A**), a large lipid-rich core (**B**) with extensive macrophage infiltration and paucity of smooth muscle cells, and expansive arterial remodeling which mitigates luminal narrowing.

1: Monocyte; 2: infiltrating monocytes/macrophages; 3: red blood cells and platelets; 4: extracellular matrix; 5: smooth muscle cell; 6: endothelial cell; 7: MMPs; 8: Ox-LDL; 9: apoptotic macrophages; 10: T-cell. (Reproduced with permission from Naghavi *et al.* [2003]. From vulnerable plaque to vulnerable patient: a call for new definitions and risk assessment strategies (Parts I and II). *Circulation* **108**:1664–1672, 1772–1778.

IDENTIFICATION

The challenge for the clinician is to find the plaque(s) destined for the next thrombus-mediated heart attack(s) and treat, thus avoiding the heart attack(s). Because plaque rupture is the most frequent cause of coronary thrombosis, and ruptured plaques have many features in common, the identification of rupture-prone plaques has become a key issue. Many of the imaging techniques used to detect CAD and discussed in this section of the book are also able to detect different features of the rupture-prone type of vulnerable plaque (**152** and *Table 24*). This capability will now be discussed, but it should be stressed that the natural history of individual plaques (risk of thrombosis) is unknown and needs to be established.

Conventional invasive X-ray angiography

The lumen of the coronary arteries, but not their wall (unless calcified), is visualized after injection of radiopaque contrast media (see Chapter 7, Diagnostic Coronary Angiography). Of importance, most plaques that underlie an ACS are angiographically invisible or nonsignificant (<70% stenosed) and asymptomatic prior to the acute event (**57**), not because these plaques are small but rather because they tend to grow outward and thus prevent or mitigate luminal narrowing (expansive remodeling). Angiography may detect plaques that have already ruptured, with or without thrombosis superimposed, and the presence of such 'complex lesions' in unstable patients is associated with an increased risk of a new ischemic event in the near future. Nonruptured but vulnerable plaques will, however, often remain hidden in the vessel wall. Therefore, any imaging technique that only visualizes the lumen (luminography) is not likely to be useful in detecting vulnerable plaques.

Some coronary lesions retain the angiographic contrast for a few seconds after the dye column has passed down the artery (local staining of the vessel wall), called 'plaque blush' (**153**). It may reflect neovascularization caused by 'active' disease in the vessel wall and appears to be associated with subsequent rapid progression of the stenosis (vulnerable plaque).

Table 23 Features of ruptured plaques*

- Thrombus.
- Large lipid-rich core (>30–40% of plaque).
- Fibrous cap covering the lipid-rich core:
  - Thin (thickness <100 μm).
  - Many macrophages (inflammation).
  - Few smooth muscle cells (apoptosis).
- Outward remodeling preserving the lumen.
- Neovascularization from vasa vasorum?
- Adventitial/perivascular inflammation?

*By inference, the same features, except thrombus, are assumed to characterize rupture-prone (vulnerable) plaques.

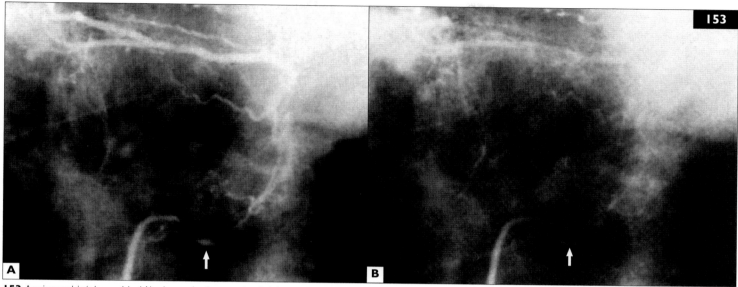

153 Angiographic 'plaque blush' is shown in the proximal right coronary artery (arrow) just after injection (**A**) and approximately 2 seconds later, when the main dye column has passed from the second portion of the artery to the bifurcation of the posterior descending artery and posterolateral left ventricular branches (**B**). Preinjection and late postinjection frames showed no opacity at the site, excluding calcium as the cause of the opacity. (Reproduced from Casscells *et al.* [2003]. Plaque blush, branch location, and calcification are angiographic predictors of progression of mild to moderate coronary stenoses. Am Heart J. **145**: 813–820, 2003, with permission from Elsevier)

Table 24 Imaging of coronary atherosclerosis and individual features of vulnerable plaques

Procedure	Lumen		Atherosclerotic plaque						Arterial wall		
	Sten	Thromb	Size	Cap	Inflamm	Core	Fibr	Ca	Thick	Remodel	Neovasc
Invasive											
• X-ray	+++	+	-	-	-	-	-	+	-	-	blush?
• IVUS	+++	+	+++	+	-	++	++	+++	+++	+++	-
• Elastography	-	-	-	+	+	+	+	+	-	-	-
• OCT	+++	+	+	+++	+	+++	++	+++	+	-	-
• Angioscopy	+	+++	-	+	-	++	-	-	-	-	-
• Thermography	-	-	-	-	+++	-	-	-	-	-	-
• Spectroscopy	-	-	-	+	++	++	+	++	-	-	-
Noninvasive											
• SPECT/PET	-	+	-	-	?	-	-	-	-	-	?
• EBCT/MSCT	++	+	+	-	-	-	-	+++	+	+	-
• MRI	++	+	+	-	-	-	-	+	+	+	-

Sten: stenosis; Thromb: thrombus; Inflamm: inflammation; Core: lipid-rich core; Fibr: fibrous tissue; Ca: calcium; Thick: thickness; Remodel: remodeling; Neovasc: neovascularization; X-ray: X-ray angiography; IVUS: intravascular ultrasound; OCT: optical coherence tomography; SPECT: single-photon emission computed tomography; PET: positron-emission tomography; EBCT: electron-beam computed tomography; MSCT: multi-slice computed tomography; MRI: magnetic resonance imaging.
- : useless; +: low sensitivity; ++: moderate sensitivity; +++ : high sensitivity; ?: unknown.

Intravascular ultrasound

IVUS is currently the only commercially available imaging modality that provides real-time, cross sectional images of the coronary artery (see Chapter 7, Intracoronary Ultrasound). Variations in arterial and plaque morphology along the artery can be studied with an axial resolution of 100 μm (40 MHz systems) to 200 μm (20 MHz). Detailed information about calcification, plaque size, vessel size, and mode of remodeling can be obtained; echolucent areas are assumed to represent lipid and/or thrombosis with a sensitivity of approximately 70% and a specificity of 30%. Ruptured plaques may be seen (**154**) but the resolution of standard IVUS is inadequate to detect the thin and fragile, but yet intact, fibrous cap assumed to confer vulnerability (cap thickness <100 μm).

Analysis of the IVUS radiofrequency signal may permit a more detailed prediction of plaque composition, called virtual histology, and integrated backscatter IVUS may improve the resolution to approximately 40 μm.

Intravascular elastography/palpography

Elastography is an US-based imaging technique that assesses the local mechanical properties of the arterial wall for deformations and displacements caused by the pulsating blood pressure. The image, called an elastogram, visualizes the radial strain in the vessel wall and the plaque. IVUS images acquired at two different levels of intraluminal pressure are cross correlated with the corresponding radiofrequency data, and strain images visualizing the local radial strain of the tissue (elasticity) are constructed. This technique adds potentially important mechanical information to the anatomic images provided by IVUS. High-strain regions superficially in plaques, which appear to colocalize with macrophage infiltration, are assumed to be rupture-prone.

Since plaque rupture is a surface-related phenomenon, a technique in which the mechanical properties of the plaque surface are visualized has also been developed, called palpography (**155**). These images, palpograms, are easier to interpret than elastograms, and with the development of 3D palpography, identification of high-strain spots over the full length of a coronary artery becomes possible. Elastography and palpography have a high sensitivity and specificity *in vitro* and are now being tested prospectively for their capability to identify vulnerable plaques in the coronary arteries *in vivo*.

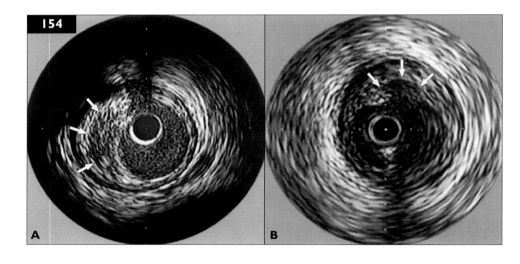

154 A: IVUS image showing an echolucent area (arrows) indicating a lipid-rich core. **B**: Direct communication between the lumen and the echolucent area (arrows) is identified, indicating plaque rupture. IVUS: intravascular ultrasound. (Courtesy of Dr. Paul Schoenhagen, MD, Cleveland.)

155 A: Coronary palpogram showing a clear high strain spot (yellow) next to a low strain (blue) calcified spot, indicating deformability change in the plaque. **B**: A complete low strain plaque in a calcified stenosis. **C**: Plaque with two deformable regions at the shoulders of the plaque. 1: media; 2: plaque; 3: calcification with shadowing; 4: palpogram.

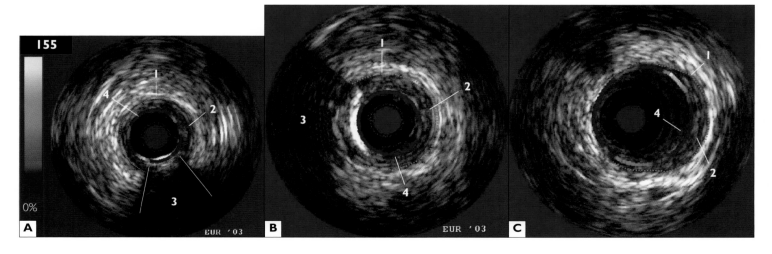

Coronary angioscopy

Using fiberoptics, angioscopy allows direct visualization of thrombi and surface features of plaques such as defects (rupture) and red discoloration (intraplaque hemorrhage), features that characterize culprit lesions causing ACS (see Chapter 7, Intracoronary Ultrasound). The presence of glistening yellow plaques, assumed to be lipid-rich, thin-capped, rupture-prone but still intact plaques, has been reported to be associated with adverse outcomes.

Angioscopy requires a blood-free field (proximal occluding balloon or flushing with saline during imaging), it is not in common use, easy or simple, and only the luminal surface is visualized. Because of these limitations, it will probably remain a research tool.

Intravascular optical coherence tomography

Optical coherence tomography (OCT) is a new light-based (optical) imaging modality. Fiberoptic technologies are used to measure backscattered light, or optical echoes, derived from an infrared laser light source directed at the arterial wall and, as such, OCT can be regarded as an analog of IVUS. OCT has been commercialized previously for use in ophthalmology, but to date no other commercial applications have been developed. In coronary arteries, OCT produces high-resolution, real-time, cross sectional, or 3D images of tissues at exceptionally high, near-histologic resolution (axial, 10 µm; transverse, 25 µm). The technique has been called 'optical biopsy' (**156**). In patients, OCT appears to be capable of visualizing plaque features assumed to confer vulnerability (thin cap, cap macrophages, lipid-rich core) with a much better resolution than IVUS.

The limitations of OCT for *in vivo* intravascular imaging are poor image quality when imaging through blood (saline injection with or without a proximal occlusion balloon is required to establish blood-free conditions) and a penetration depth of only 1–3 mm. Intravascular OCT is currently under clinical investigation.

Intravascular spectroscopy

Using fiberoptic technology, coronary plaques can be illuminated *in situ* and the reflected light can be collected and launched into a spectrometer. Spectroscopy is based on the fact that different chemical compounds absorb and scatter different amounts of energy at different wavelengths, leaving a unique chemical (molecular) fingerprint. Tissues of different chemical composition (lipid, collagen, calcium) and pH give rise to unique spectra.

Different approaches are under development such as Raman spectroscopy, which uses high-energy laser light (high molecular sensitivity but tissue penetration as low as 0.3 mm), and near-infrared spectroscopy (NIRS, wavelengths of 750–2500 nm), which has greater penetration (2 mm) but lower molecular sensitivity and, therefore, relies on pattern recognition for plaque typing.

Arterial wall thermography

Temperature (heat production) is one of the most sensitive markers of inflammation, and it is indeed possible to measure the temperature in coronary arteries with temperature-sensing catheters (thermistors with a temperature differentiation of 0.05°C). Measuring the local plaque temperature or mapping the 'thermographic burden' of the most important coronary segments is quite simple. Based on the fact that culprit plaques responsible for ACS (thrombosed plaques) are, in general, warmer that other plaques and the plaque-free vessel wall, it is assumed that inflamed, rupture-prone plaques produce measurable heat (hot lesions). Preliminary observations indicated that thermal heterogeneity was an independent predictor of adverse coronary events, but these results need to be confirmed. Thus, arterial wall thermography appears to be sensitive to blood flow and clinical settings. Different thermography catheters are currently under clinical investigation.

X-ray computed tomography

Noninvasive EBCT can visualize the lumen of coronary arteries (angiography after IV contrast) and detect coronary calcification, which reflects the overall plaque burden (see Chapters 7, Noninvasive Multi-Slice Spiral Computed Tomography and Electron-beam Computed Tomography: coronary calcium). Although subclinical plaque burden is an important prognostic determinant, it is not only the calcified plaques that mediate the associated risk because, if anything, calcification appears to confer stability on

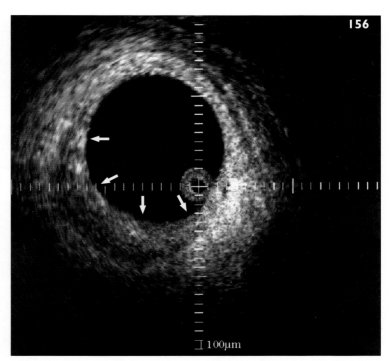

156 *In vivo* OCT showing coronary artery with eccentric lipid-rich plaque in 5–9 o'clock position, covered by a thick fibrous cap (arrows). OCT: optical coherence tomography. (Courtesy of Dr. Evelyn Regar, MD, Erasmus MC, Rotterdam.)

plaques. Calcium scores must be interpreted in light of a person's age since all will develop coronary calcification with time.

Noninvasive MSCT can provide high-quality imaging of the lumen (angiography), the wall (calcification and plaque burden), and the size (remodeling) of coronary arteries (**157**). Thus MSCT can detect subclinical coronary atherosclerosis but, except for expansive remodeling, the resolution does not (yet) permit visualization of specific features assumed to be associated with plaque vulnerability.

Nuclear imaging

Nuclear medicine has exquisite sensitivity for the detection of extremely small quantities of biologically important substances. Several radiolabeled tracers have been developed and used to visualize specific pathophysiologic changes associated with atherosclerosis in animals, such as low-density lipoprotein (LDL), annexin V (apoptotic cells), monocyte chemotactic protein-1 (MCP-1; receptors upregulated on activated monocytes/macrophages), thallium (neovascularization), and fluoro-deoxyglucose (FDG; uptake in macrophages). Imaging of vascular metabolic activity (e.g. active inflammation) with FDG PET has been tried in a few patients with encouraging results, but more data are needed to assess the potential to detect hypermetabolic hot spots (possible vulnerable plaques) in the coronary arteries.

Relatively few radiolabeled molecules are needed to obtain a positive signal (high sensitivity) but the spatial resolution is low.

This limitation is mitigated by combining PET and CT, creating PET/CT fusion images with improved anatomic localization of the emitted signal (hot spot) (**158**).

Magnetic resonance imaging

Noninvasive MRI is capable of providing information about the lumen (angiography), the wall (thickness), and the size (remodeling) of coronary arteries (see Chapter 7, Magnetic Resonance Coronary Angiography). The lack of sufficient resolution (currently about 0.4 mm in-plane) prevents, however, a more detailed plaque characterization. Higher resolution can be obtained with the use of catheter-based receiver coils (intravascular MRI). Functional information may be obtained by contrast agents, such as gadolinium (possible extravasation in neovascularized areas) and superparamagnetic iron oxide (SPIO) nanoparticles, either alone (taken up avidly by macrophages) or conjugated to tracers (apoptosis). Noninvasive MRI studies of coronary plaque composition are not available and the capability of MRI to detect vulnerable plaques has not (yet) been proven.

MANAGEMENT

There is currently no clinically available imaging technique capable of identifying rupture-prone or other vulnerable plaques. Prospective clinical trials are required to learn the natural history of plaques assumed to be vulnerable and to assess the benefit of local (e.g. stenting) and systemic treatments.

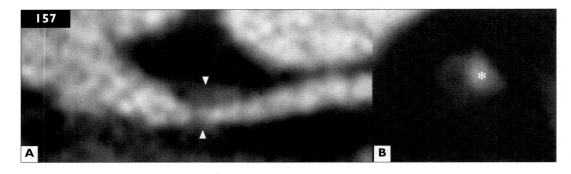

157 A: MSCT angiography showing significant stenosis proximal in the left anterior descending coronary artery caused by a noncalcified plaque (arrowheads). **B**: Cross sectional image of the narrowed lumen (*) and the noncalcified plaque. MSCT: multi-slice spiral computed tomography. (Courtesy of Dr. Nico Mollet, MD, Erasmus MC, Rotterdam.)

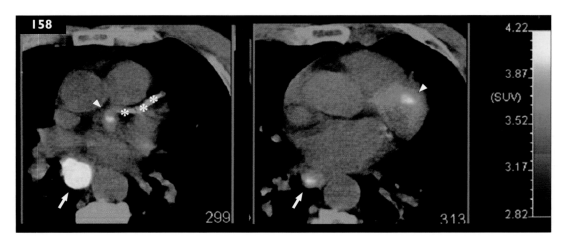

158 Transaxial [18F]FDG PET-CT fusion images showing tumor activity in esophagus (arrow). Additionally, FDG activity is seen proximal (arrowhead, left) and distal (arrowhead, right) in or near a calcified left anterior descending coronary artery (*), indicating high metabolic activity (inflamed plaques?). CT: computed tomography; FDG: fluorodeoxyglucose; PET: positron emission tomography. (Courtesy of Dr. Mark Dunphy et al., Memorial Sloan-Kettering Cancer Center, New York.)

Chapter Eight

Detection of Myocardial Ischemia and Infarction

ELECTROCARDIOGRAPHY

K.S. CHANNER, MD, FRCP

INTRODUCTION
Electrocardiography remains the most useful noninvasive test in cardiology today. This simple technique allows the clinician to evaluate the cause of symptoms of palpitation by assessing the cardiac rhythm and is an essential aid to the diagnosis of acute coronary syndromes.

TECHNIQUE
The heart is an electrically active organ and by using skin surface electrodes it is possible to record this activity. The standard 12-lead electrocardiogram (ECG) is recorded by attaching sticky electrodes to the legs, arms, and chest wall (159). In order to obtain good electrical contact it may be necessary to shave the area and gentle rubbing provides good skin attachment.

To maximize the quality of the recording it is necessary to have a relaxed patient. The atmosphere in the recording room should be appropriate with soft indirect lighting, warm temperature to prevent shivering, quiet, and private. The recording cables should not be moved during the recording since this would introduce artifact. Interference from mains alternating current (AC) is reduced by using a grounded electrical source for the equipment. Use of other electrical appliances in the immediate surroundings should be avoided.

With the electrodes attached to a recorder, the patient is asked to remain still and breath gently. This reduces movement artifact and provides a stable baseline (known as the isoelectric line). By convention, the 12-lead ECG is configured to produce a recording in a standard format with three bipolar leads (I, II, and III) recorded first, followed by nine unipolar leads (aVR, aVL, aVF, V1–V6).

Before recording begins it is necessary to calibrate the deflection so that 10 mm = 1 mV. By doing this it is possible to standardize recordings to allow comparison within and between individuals. This is important because the size of the deflection can be used to diagnose the presence of left or right ventricular hypertrophy (L/RVH).

The different lead positions allow the electrical activity of different parts of the heart to be studied. Thus, the inferior wall is best 'visualized' from leads II, III, and aVF, the interventricular septum from V1–V3, left ventricular anterior wall from V2–V6, and apex and lateral wall from V4–V6, I, and aVL. The ECG

signal represents a summation of activity from a complex 3D structure and precise localization is impossible. More accurate mapping of the ventricular myocardium can be provided by using an array of 35 lead positions over the anterior chest wall. However, this is reserved for use as a research tool.

ELECTROCARDIOGRAM DATA
The ECG is the technique which is used to assess the normal conducting system of the heart. Normal sinus rhythm occurs when the prime cardiac pacemaker is the sinoatrial node (SAN). This triggers atrial contraction which is manifest on the ECG as the P wave (160). After a short delay in the atrioventricular node (AVN), the P-R interval, the normal electrical impulse passes to

159

VI	Fourth intercostal space at right margin of sternum
V2	Fourth intercostal space at left margin of sternum
V3	Midway between position 2 and position 4
V4	Fifth intercostal space at junction of midclavicular line
V5	At horizontal level of position 4 at left anterior axillary line
V6	At horizontal level of position 4 at mid-axillary line

159 Chest positions of standard electrocardiogram leads.

160 Assessment of electrocardiogram waves, intervals, segments, and QRS complex.

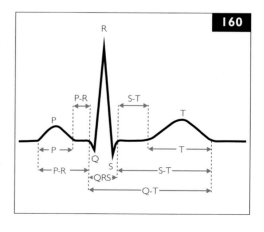

119

the His bundle and Purkinje fibers, causing the ventricular myocardium to depolarize from the apex upwards. Ventricular depolarization produces the QRS complex. By convention, the first negative deflection is called a q or Q wave, the first positive an r or R wave, and a negative deflection after a positive one an s or S wave. The shape and dominance of each component depend on the electrical vectors, which in turn depend on the position of the monitoring electrodes in relation to the main muscles masses of the right ventricle (RV), interventricular septum, and left ventricle (LV). Again, by convention, a small negative deflection is given the annotation q and a major negative deflection a Q.

The contribution of negative and positive deflections changes but the pattern in each lead is reproducible with time in any individual unless the heart muscle has been damaged. Thus, by comparing changes in the ECG over time it is possible to detect morphologic/pathologic changes in cardiac structure and function.

Atrial repolarization does not produce an independent electrical signal and any that is produced is lost in the QRS complex. Ventricular muscle repolarization produces a T wave after the QRS complex.

DIAGNOSIS OF ISCHEMIA
ST segment depression
During myocardial ischemia the ECG appearances change in the area overlying the ischemic territory, producing a downward shift of the ST segment. This change is not specific to ischemia and can also occur with hyperadrenergic syndrome in association with sinus tachycardia and with digoxin therapy, but is usually more widespread. Moreover, if the ST change is planar or down-sloping and >2 mm from the isoelectric line, it is more likely to be caused by ischemia (**161A**). The degree of shift of the ST segment is determined by the size of the preceding R wave, which is reduced by inspiration. ST depression is seen most commonly in leads V4–V6 because these leads have the largest R waves. ST segment depression during provocative exercise testing is used to diagnose angina. When there are ST segment changes at rest these may be due to unstable angina but, more commonly, they represent other myocardial abnormalities (especially LVH and cardiomyopathy).

T wave inversion
T wave inversion is normal in lead III and may be normal if it is also present in lead aVF, but only if it is accompanied by inversion in lead III. The T wave inversion in lead III can sometimes be reversed by deep inspiration, indicating that it reflects a change in the heart's electrical axis. It can also occur normally in lead V1 and less commonly in V2, but again only if accompanied by inversion in V1.

All T wave changes are nonspecific and none are pathognomonic of ischemia or infarction. T wave inversion in I or aVL is always abnormal when the preceding QRS is mainly positive (an upward deflection or qRs complex). T wave changes may be dynamic and sometimes may appear flat rather than frankly inverted. Biphasic T waves are usually due to myocardial ischemia and often develop into deep arrowhead T wave inversion, which is a feature of ischemia or subendocardial infarction (**161B**, **162**).

ST segment elevation
A degree of ST segment elevation is often present in healthy individuals, especially in young adults and in people of African

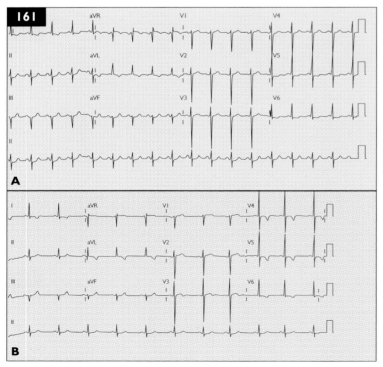

161 A: Electrocardiogram from a patient presenting with cardiac chest pain at rest (unstable angina). Note the planar ST depression (1 mm) in leads V5, V6 and down-sloping ST depression + T wave inversion in leads I, aVL. **B**: Four days later, a biphasic T wave is present in lead V3 and arrowhead T wave inversion in leads V4–V6, I, and aVL.

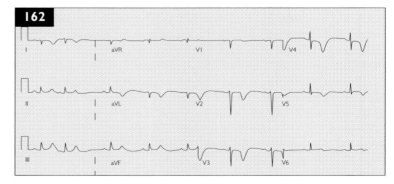

162 Electrocardiogram showing arrowhead T wave inversion 4 days after the patient presented with chest pain (negative troponin I).

descent. This ST segment elevation is most commonly seen in the precordial leads (V1–V6). The pattern of ST segment change may include elevation of the J point above the isoelectric line, with high take-off of the ST segment, a distinct notch at the junction of the R wave and the J point, an upward concavity of the ST segment, and symmetrical, upright T waves, often of large amplitude. It is essential when analyzing the ECG to have a good clinical history available. (For definition of J point see **166**.)

The hallmark of transmural ischemia is elevation of the ST segment. This may be transient and reversible when it is caused by coronary artery spasm. When it is caused by coronary thrombosis, the first change is hyperacute T wave where the ST segment elevation merges with the T wave. **163** shows the natural evolution of the ST changes during the course of an infarction. Reduction in the extent of ST elevation occurs normally with evolution of the infarction but is also a measure of successful reperfusion with a thrombolytic drug.

The pattern of changes of ST elevation provides some indication of the area of heart muscle damaged in the infarction. Changes in leads II, III, and aVF represent inferior wall infarction, whereas changes in the anterior chest leads V1–V2 represent anterior wall infarction. The number of leads affected is also a marker of the size of the damaged muscle mass. Posterior wall infarction is diagnosed by the development of dominant R waves in leads V1and V2, with marked ST segment depression in these leads which persists longer than expected in ischemia.

PROGNOSTIC SIGNIFICANCE

Transient ST depression that occurs with exercise is a measure of the severity of the underlying coronary artery disease (CAD). Adverse prognostic changes include:
- Early change with exercise.
- The larger the ST shift, the worse the prognosis.
- Prolonged ST shift persisting into the recovery period.

Changes on the resting ECG in patients presenting with unstable angina have also been demonstrated to have prognostic significance: 4-year survival of T wave inversion was 84% compared with 82% if there was 0.5 mm ST segment depression, 77% if 1–2 mm ST depression, and only 53% if >2 mm ST depression.

DIAGNOSIS OF OLD INFARCTION

The resting ECG may show changes of old infarction manifest by pathological Q waves, defined as an initial negative deflection of the QRS complex which is at least 1 mm wide and less than one-quarter of the depth of the ensuing R wave. Often the T wave inversion returns to normal after weeks or months. Q waves may become smaller with time.

Myocardial infarction (MI) but, more commonly, LVH can cause left bundle branch block (LBBB) which may be permanent or intermittent and rate related (i.e. develops on exercise testing). The presence of LBBB on the admission ECG of a patient with

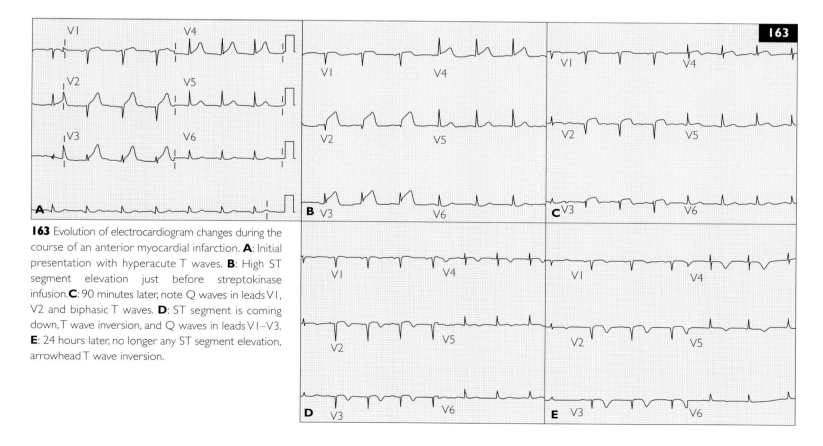

163 Evolution of electrocardiogram changes during the course of an anterior myocardial infarction. **A**: Initial presentation with hyperacute T waves. **B**: High ST segment elevation just before streptokinase infusion.**C**: 90 minutes later, note Q waves in leads V1, V2 and biphasic T waves. **D**: ST segment is coming down, T wave inversion, and Q waves in leads V1–V3. **E**: 24 hours later, no longer any ST segment elevation, arrowhead T wave inversion.

chest pain produces a diagnostic dilemma. Many criteria have been proposed in order to identify acute infarction in LBBB, but none are sensitive or specific enough to allow the diagnosis to be made with sufficient accuracy. However, some ECG features when present are specific indicators of acute ischemia. When ST segment elevation is present with a positive QRS complex, or ST segment depression in leads V1, V2, or V3 with predominantly negative QRS complexes, this is termed inappropriate concordance, which is highly indicative of acute ischemia. Extreme ST segment elevation in leads V1 and V2 (5 mm or more) is also suggestive of acute ischemia. Sometimes, the natural evolution of changes over time allows more precise analysis.

LIMITATIONS

The majority of patients with significant CAD and angina pectoris will have a normal resting 12-lead ECG. That is why provocative exercise testing is necessary. Similarly, about 10% of patients presenting with acute MI will have a normal ECG.

Careful attention to technique during recording minimizes errors and allows consistent and high quality recordings. However, poor technique can cause diagnostic difficulties from AC interference, tremor, and incorrectly connecting the ECG leads.

Knowledge of what the ECG should normally look like is necessary to ensure that it has been recorded correctly. It is possible to connect the ECG leads to the wrong electrodes and produce an abnormal ECG. The commonest mistake is to transpose the limb lead electrodes, which initially produces an abnormal configuration of aVR.

Lead aVR should always have a predominantly negative shaped QRS complex (**164**). Respiratory variation is most marked on the precordial electrodes (V1–V6) and may cause marked baseline wander. This may make interpretation of ST segment changes difficult or impossible. Patients should be encouraged to relax and either hold their breath or breathe gently. Patients with tremor (e.g. Parkinson's disease) have baseline shift that may mimic atrial fibrillation (AF) (**165**).

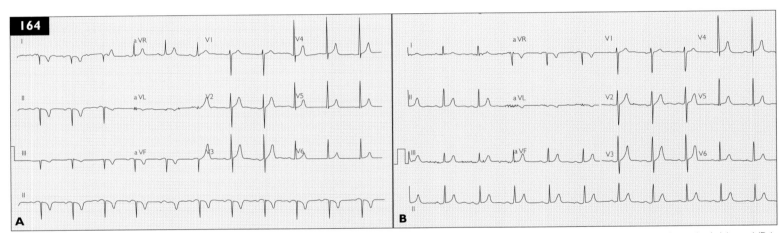

164A: Right arm and left leg leads are crossed giving the appearance of inferior myocardial infarction (Q wave in leads II, III, and aVF, T wave inversion). Note aVR is positive, T wave inversion in leads aVL and I. **B**: Correctly positioned leads. Note aVR is negative. The only abnormality is T wave inversion in aVL.

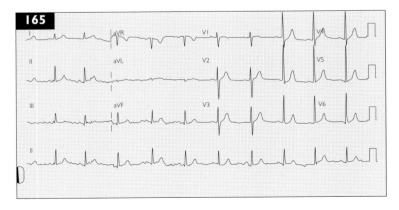

165 Electrodes not correctly prepared, resulting in baseline instability looking like atrial fibrillation in the limb leads.

EXERCISE TESTING

JONATHAN M. HILL, MD AND ADAM D. TIMMIS, MD

INTRODUCTION

Exercise testing is one of the most widely performed tests for the diagnostic and prognostic assessment of patients with ischemic heart disease. The basic principle underlying its value is that during exercise, coronary blood flow must increase to meet the increased energy/metabolic demands of the myocardium. This occurs in a reproducible fashion with comparable oxygen consumption between individuals. In the event of a limitation caused by an anatomic obstruction in the coronary circulation, this flow cannot increase sufficiently to meet the myocardial oxygen demand. This results in myocardial ischemia with detectable changes on a surface ECG.

TECHNIQUE

Beta blockade should be discontinued for 24 hours to ensure an adequate heart rate response and, ideally, digoxin should be stopped for 1 week because of its effect on ST segment/repolarization changes. The skin must be adequately prepared prior to electrode attachment. During the test the ECG machine needs to provide a continuous readout of a 12-lead ECG, with minimal interference from movement of the subject.

The Bruce protocol is the most widely adopted technique for exercise testing using a standardized method of graded increase in exercise over seven stages of 3 minutes. During the first stage, patients are required to walk at 1.7 mph up a slight incline of 10%. The estimated energy usage during this stage is 4.8 METS (metabolic equivalents) where 1 MET (3.5 ml O_2/kg per minute) is the oxygen consumption of an average individual at rest. The speed of the treadmill is increased with each stage.

Patients are rarely exercised beyond Stage 4. The aim is to reach the maximum predicted heart rate, which by convention is defined as 220 (210 for women) minus the patient's age. Reaching 85% of the maximum predicted heart rate is considered satisfactory and achievement of the maximum predicted rate is a good prognostic sign. Blood pressure must be measured at the start of the test and at the end of each stage. At the beginning of exercise, the blood pressure may fall slightly but then should increase throughout the course of the test. A systolic pressure up to 225 mmHg (30 kPa) is normal. Diastolic blood pressure tends to fall slightly. For the prognostic assessment of patients post-MI in whom revascularization is being considered, a less strenuous modified Bruce protocol is commonly used.

ELECTROCARDIOGRAM CHANGES DURING EXERCISE

ECG changes during exercise are shown in *Table 25*. Exercise-induced ST segment depression (horizontal or down-sloping) is the most reliable indicator of myocardial ischemia. Most modern exercise ECG machines have computerized analysis programs but these should not be a replacement for close clinical evaluation of the test results. The J point is the point of inflection of the S wave and the ST segment, and this point becomes depressed during normal exercise (**166**). ST segment changes are conventionally measured 80 ms after the J point and ST movement is measured relative to the isoelectric baseline.

Abnormal ECG changes

Horizontal or down-sloping depression of the ST segment relative to baseline is the hallmark of ischemia (**167**). Changes of >1 mm may be taken as significant, although if 0.5 mm is taken to be significant then the test increases in sensitivity but loses specificity. The test should be stopped if there is ST segment elevation without Q waves in any lead, or >3 mm of ST segment depression. New onset of arrhythmias such as multiple ventricular extrasystoles,

---

Table 25 Electrocardiogram changes during exercise

High probability of obstructive coronary artery disease
- Horizontal or downsloping ST segment depression of ≥ 2mm.
- Early positive response within 6 minutes of start of test.
- Persistence of ST segment depression more than 6 minutes after test stopped.

Normal changes during excercise
- Increased P wave height.
- Decreased R wave height.
- J-point depression.
- ST segment up-sloping.
- Shortened QT interval.
- T wave decreases in height.
- Increased blood pressure.

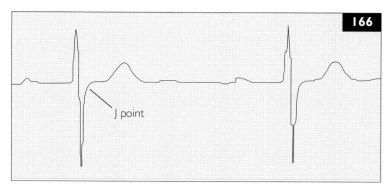

166 The J point is the point of inflection of the S wave and the ST segment on the electrocardiogram.

ventricular tachycardia, supraventricular tachycardia, AF, second or third degree heart block, and new LBBB are all indications for stopping the test.

INDICATIONS
Indications for exercise testing are shown in *Table 26*.

CONTRAINDICATIONS AND COMPLICATIONS
Contraindications to exercise testing are shown in *Table 27*.

Careful patient selection reduces the incidence of complications. Serious complications such as death or MI occur in approximately 1 in 10,000 tests. Ventricular tachycardia/ fibrillation occurs in approximately 1 in 5,000 tests. Staff supervising the test must be trained in cardiopulmonary resuscitation with immediate access to a defibrillator. Tests should be stopped immediately if the patient has severe chest pain, dyspnea, ataxia, or dizziness. A fall in blood pressure of >20 mmHg (2.7 kPa) or a rise in blood pressure to >300 mmHg (40 kPa) systolic or >130 mmHg (17.3 kPa) diastolic are also indications for stopping immediately.

LIMITATIONS
The sensitivity of exercise testing is approximately 75%, with a specificity of approximately 70% for detecting CAD. In patients with a low pretest probability such as young men (<30 years) and women (<40 years), the positive predictive value is low with a high rate of false positive tests. Similarly in patients with a high pretest probability of ischemic heart disease (IHD), a negative result does not definitively exclude significant obstructive CAD. ST segment change interpretation can be limited by the quality of recording but, in addition, the estimation of the inflection point of the ST segment change during repolarization at the J point and the level of ST segment change taken to be indicative of myocardial ischemia are arbitrary, and can greatly alter the sensitivity and specificity. ST segment depression can occur in up to 20% of normal individuals. If the resting ECG is abnormal, e.g. LBBB or LVH, the ST segment changes can be difficult or impossible to interpret.

According to Bayes' theorem, the predictive power of an abnormal exercise test is dependent on the pretest probability of obstructive CAD in the population under study. Thus exercise testing is most useful in patients with a moderate probability of CAD and is not suitable as a screening tool for those with a very low probability. Excercise testing adds little to the diagnostic process in those patients with a high pretest probability, where angina is the most reliable predictor of the need for further investigation.

Table 26 Indications for exercise testing in myocardial ischemia/infarction

- Diagnostic evaluation of chest pain in patients with intermediate probability for CAD.
- Prognostic assessment for risk stratification postmyocardial infarction.
- Assessment of revascularization or drug treatment.
- Assessment of cardiopulmonary function in patients with ischemic heart failure.
- Provocation of exercise- /ischemia-induced arrhythmia.

CAD: coronary artery disease.

Table 27 Contraindications for exercise testing

- Recent acute myocardial infarction (within 4–6 days).
- Recent history of unstable angina (pain at rest within 48 hours).
- Decompensated heart failure.
- Acute myocarditis.
- Acute pericarditis.
- Refractory or uncontrolled hypertension (systolic BP>220 mmHg [29.3 kPa], diastolic>120 mmHg [16 kPa]).
- Critical or symptomatic aortic stenosis.
- Deep venous thrombosis.
- Hypertrophic cardiomyopathy with outflow tract obstruction.
- Dissecting aneurysm.
- Recent aortic surgery including valve replacement.

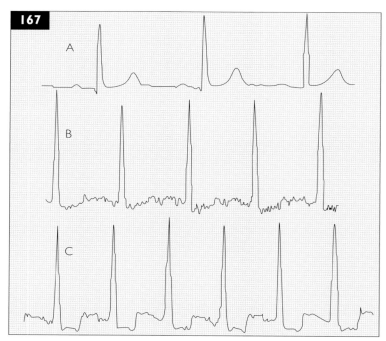

167 Abnormal ST segment changes on the electrocardiogram during exercise. **A**: At rest. **B**: After 3 minutes. **C**: After 6 minutes with down-sloping ST segment depression.

CONTINUOUS VECTORCARDIOGRAPHIC MONITORING

BJARNE LINDE NØRGAARD, MD, PhD

INTRODUCTION

Evidence of the prognostic value in patients with unstable coronary syndromes of transient ST episodes during ambulatory ECG (Holter) ST segment monitoring was first provided two decades ago. In addition, it was shown that approximately 70–90% of these ST episodes were not accompanied by angina. Holter monitoring, however, has no real-time analysis capacity; thus, technical problems during the recording may not be identified, and risk assessment cannot be performed until the recording has been completed. Also, there is an inherent risk of poor sensitivity in detecting myocardial ischemia due to the limited number of exploring electrodes. These shortcomings of the classic Holter ST segment monitoring technique led to the introduction of on-line multi-lead monitoring techniques during the late 1980s.

CONTINUOUS VECTORCARDIOGRAPHIC MONITORING

In vectorcardiographic monitoring, the ECG signals are continuously collected from eight conventional body surface electrodes (**168**). The signals are sampled via a bedside acquisition unit, and averaged into three orthogonal leads, X, Y, and Z (**168**). These vectorcardiographic complexes are continuously conveyed to a central computer for storage and analysis. During the first 10–20 seconds of the monitoring period, the dominant vectorcardiographic complex of the patient, i.e. the reference class, is established. Subsequent complexes with a different morphology from the reference class are discarded from further analyses; thus, all variables are calculated on analogous complexes. Since the complex may change over time, the template of the reference class is slightly updated according to the information from each incoming complex. Hereby, the system may adjust to small changes in complex morphology, i.e. due to ischemia or infarction. The process of averaging is performed for consecutive periods defined by the operator (10 seconds–4 minutes). The reference complex is the vectorcardiographic complex from the first averaging period. Relative vectorcardiographic variables are calculated as the difference between the current and the reference complexes. Following each averaging period, different vectorcardiographic variables are calculated and displayed as trend curves continuously updated during the recording period (**170–172**). In addition, a derived 12-lead ECG (**170** and **172**) as well as vector loops for the P, QRS, and T waves may be displayed at any given time.

Interpretation

The most useful vectorcardiographic monitoring variables are the QRS vector difference (QRS-VD), and ST vector magnitude (ST-VM) (**169**).

An ischemic episode in unstable myocardial ischemia is generally accepted as a transient ST-VM change >50 µV (over >1 minute) from the individual ST-VM baseline level (**170**). A decline in ST-VM >50% relative to the peak ST-VM level within 60 minutes after commencement of thrombolytic treatment in patients with ST elevation MI (STEMI) is indicative of successful reperfusion (**171**). An irreversible rise in QRS-VD >15 µV indicates a process of ongoing MI (**171**, **172**).

INDICATIONS

In unstable angina pectoris and non-ST elevation MI (NSTEMI), the presence of ST-VM episodes during 24 hours of continuous vectorcardiographic monitoring is associated with a high risk of subsequent death or acute MI (**170**). In addition, it has been shown that patients with transient ST episodes are those in whom antithrombotic treatment is most beneficial. In patients with STEMI, lack of ST segment resolution following revascularization therapy is a poor prognostic sign (**172**), irrespective of the angiographic findings. Continued vectorcardiographic monitoring for up to 24 hours after revascularization treatment may well be

168 Electrode positions in continuous vectorcardiographic monitoring. The orthogonal leads, X, Y, and Z are illustrated. 1: left arm; 2: left leg; 3: right arm; 4: right leg.

169 A: QRS-VD is the summated changes between the reference and current (ischemic) complex. **B**: ST-VM is the sum of ST deviations from the isoelectric level measured 20 msec after the J-point. QRS-VD: QRS vector difference; ST-VM: ST vector magnitude.

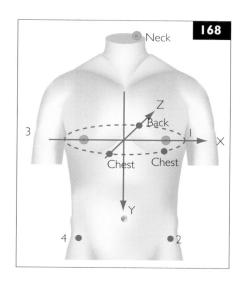

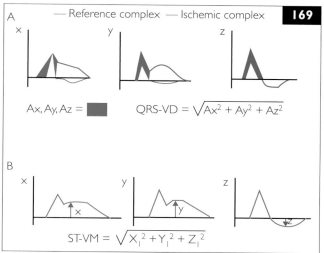

A — Reference complex — Ischemic complex

$Ax, Ay, Az = $ ▓ $QRS\text{-}VD = \sqrt{Ax^2 + Ay^2 + Az^2}$

B

$ST\text{-}VM = \sqrt{X_i^2 + Y_i^2 + Z_i^2}$

indicated, since occurrence of transient ST-VM episodes or ST-VM reelevation (indicative of reocclusion) indicates a very poor prognosis. If 50% or more ST-VM resolution is not achieved or signs of residual ischemia or even reocclusion occur, further therapeutic actions may need to be taken. The characteristic QRS-VD course in patients with STEMI is an increase from 0 V/second to a higher plateau (**171**, **172**). Just how fast this plateau is reached depends partly upon the time from onset of symptoms to commencement of monitoring and partly on the rate of infarct evolution. There is a positive association between the QRS-VD plateau level and infarct size evaluated by myocardial biochemical markers, LV function, and prognosis. In unstable angina, NSTEMI, and STEMI, the prognostic ability of vectorcardiographic monitoring is further enhanced when adding the information from biochemical markers of myocardial injury. Vectorcardiographic monitoring has been found useful in the evaluation of the anti-ischemic effect of various drugs, for detection of ischemia during coronary angioplasty, and in animal studies. Continuous vectorcardiographic monitoring is easily carried out in the clinical setting and data analysis has high interobserver reproducibility.

LIMITATIONS

The most important limitation of all electrocardiographic monitoring systems is the risk of technical problems and loss of data. The applicability of vectorcardiographic monitoring has been documented in supine, immobile patients only. The usefulness of ST-VM telemetry systems is yet to be determined. The value of vectorcardiographic monitoring among patients with BBB or pace rhythm has not yet been fully established, although preliminary results indicate that the technique may be useful in the detection of ischemia in patients with bundle branch block (BBB).

SUMMARY

Continuous vectorcardiographic monitoring noninvasively and instantaneously reflects the dynamic nature of myocardial ischemia and infarction. This technique yields important prognostic information when applied to patients with acute coronary syndromes (ACS). These features of the method are of great value regarding tailoring and targeting treatment for the individual patient suffering from unstable coronary disease.

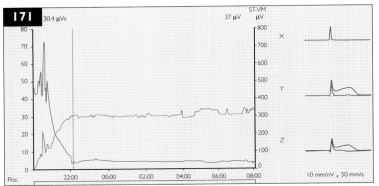

171 ST-VM (blue) and QRS-VD (yellow) trend curves and corresponding vectorcardiographic leads from a patient with an inferior-posterior ST elevation myocardial infarction treated with thrombolysis. Analysis of the ST-VM trend curve indicates successful reperfusion. ST changes in the vectorcardiographic leads at baseline (pink) and 60 minutes after the commencement of thrombolysis (yellow) are shown. Subsequently, no signs of residual myocardial ischemia were present. The QRS-VD plateu level (30 μV/second) indicated the development of a small to moderate sized infarction.

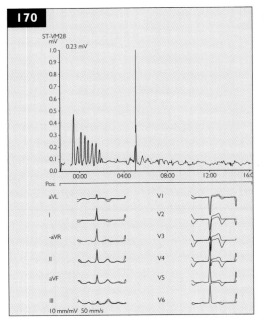

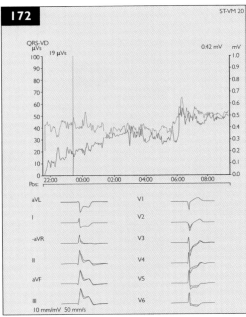

170 ST-VM trend curve and corresponding derived 12-lead electrocardiogram (ECG) from a patient with unstable angina. The patient evolved several asymptomatic ischemic episodes. The ECG revealed 'antero-septal' ST changes (pink: ECG at baseline; yellow: ECG at the time of the cursor). A subsequent coronary angiogram revealed significant proximal stenosis of the left anterior descending coronary artery.

172 ST-VM (blue) and QRS-VD (yellow) trend curves and corresponding derived 12-lead electrocardiogram (ECG) from a patient with an inferior ST elevation myocardial infarction treated with thrombolysis. Analysis of the ST-VM trend curve indicates nonsuccessful reperfusion. ST changes in the derived 12-lead ECG at baseline (pink) and 60 minutes after the commencement of thrombolysis (yellow) are shown.

ELECTROPHYSIOLOGY

ANDERS KIRSTEIN PEDERSEN, MD, DMSC

INTRODUCTION

Changes in the electrophysiological properties of the heart by acute or chronic ischemic heart disease (IHD) are secondary to either tissue ischemia or tissue destruction (infarction). Additionally, changes in the electrophysiology of the myocardium might be induced by drugs used in the therapy of ischemia or other aspects of ischemic heart disease.

An electrophysiologic (EP) study is not used in the primary diagnosis of IHD. It has a limited but valuable place as a tool in the evaluation of symptoms such as palpitations or syncope, and in the prognostic classification of patients with damage to the LV.

TECHNIQUE

The EP study is performed as a right heart catheterization with a femoral insertion of catheters into the right atrium (RA), the region of His, and the right ventricular apex. If necessary, catheters might be moved to the right ventricular outflow tract (RVOT), the coronary sinus, or to the LV.

By programmed introduction of paced beats a number of parameters are determined: the sinoatrial node recovery time, the atrioventricular (AV) conduction properties (the atrial paced rate at which Wencheback block is observed, decremental AV conduction), the atrial-His and the His-ventricle interval, the refractory periods in atrium, AVN, and ventricle, and the ability of the AVN or other structures to conduct retrogradely.

Standard electrophysiologic study

The standard EP study can confirm the presence of sinus node dysfunction and AV conduction abnormalities (abnormal supra- or infra-His block) only if they are present during the study. Unfortunately, both the positive and the negative predictive values of an EP study regarding bradyarrhythmia are quite low.

In the diagnosis of AF, the EP study is of very limited value. The EP study has a very high predictive value for the diagnosis of regular supraventricular tachycardias, if present, in IHD patients.

Programmed stimulation

The programmed ventricular stimulation has been introduced as an amendment to the standard EP study. Its focus is the induction of monomorphic ventricular tachycardia in patients with scars after infarctions (**173**). The induction is performed by a detailed sequence of stimulation sites, extrastimuli, and basic stimulation trains. If a clinical tachycardia is present, it can be induced by programmed stimulation in more than 95% of patients. Importantly, in patients with nonsustained ventricular tachycardia, an induction of either a monomorphic ventricular tachycardia or ventricular fibrillation (**174**) is an important prognostic marker of the risk for sudden cardiac death (SCD).

INDICATIONS

The indications for an EP study in IHD are limited to unexplained syncope, suspicion of intra- or infra-His conduction abnormality, and the evaluation of a clinical tachycardia of uncertain origin. The indication for programmed ventricular stimulation is either a need for a prognostic classification as 'inducible or noninducible' or as a tool in the closer study of a clinical ventricular tachycardia, e.g. for the purpose of catheter mapping and ablation.

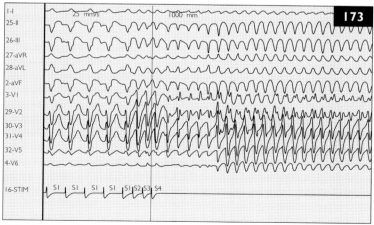

173 Electrocardiogram to show inducible monomorphic ventricular tachycardia by programmed electrical stimulation (three extrastimuli).

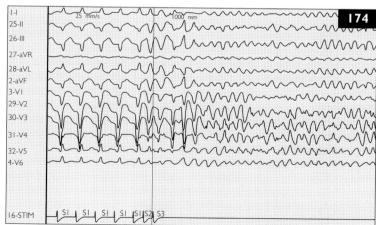

174 Electrocardiogram to show inducible ventricular fibrillation (two extrastimuli).

ECHOCARDIOGRAPHY

HENRIK EGEBLAD, MD, DMSC

INTRODUCTION

Echocardiography is an ultrasound (US) method that provides real-time tomographic images of the heart, visualizing the pericardium, myocardium, cavities, valves, and blood flow. Echocardiography is available day and night in every modern hospital and may be performed as a bedside examination, by means of small portable equipment. These features explain why echocardiography is the most commonly used imaging technique in heart disease, including in patients with known or suspected myocardial ischemia.

Occlusion of a coronary artery branch gradually leads to akinesia of the related myocardium over approximately 1 minute. This is well known from animal experiments. In the clinical setting, similar findings can be made, e.g. when echocardiography is performed during balloon dilatation of a coronary artery or immediately after some cases of STEMI. Ischemia caused by coronary artery stenoses may present as hypokinesia. However, even in cases of severe stenoses, decreased wall motion or wall thickening may not be revealed until stress echocardiography is performed (see below). Dyskinesia (paradoxical systolic bulging) is commonly seen in thin scar tissue and often in anterior wall Q wave infarction. Thus, the distinctive echocardiographic feature of myocardial ischemia is decreased or absent contraction appearing as a regional change matching with the diseased coronary artery.

2D ECHOCARDIOGRAPHY

2D echocardiography presents tomographic black and white sector images. With the transducer at the apex, the standard views for examination of the LV are the apical four- and two-chamber views and the apical long-axis view (**175**). With the transducer in the 3rd or 4th left intercostal space close to the sternum, the parasternal long- and short-axis views are visualized (**176**). For practical purposes the lungs are not penetrated by diagnostic US, and in patients with emphysema subcostal views may be of value.

In clinical practice all LV walls are carefully examined for ischemia using the views mentioned above. A digital or videotape recording is performed for documentation.

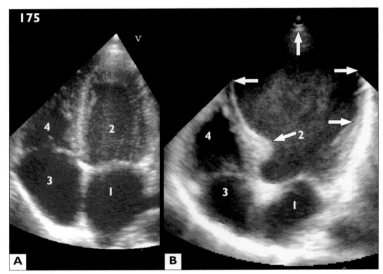

175 Apical four-chamber echocardiography views obtained in systole. **A**: Normal heart. **B**: Ultimate ischemic myocardial lesion, a huge anterior aneurysm (arrows). Slow swirling blood flow in the aneurysm induces the formation of unstable aggregates of red blood cells. These aggregates are large enough to be reflected by ultrasound and present as swirling, smoke-like faint echoes. 1: left atrium; 2: left ventricle; 3: right atrium; 4: right ventricle.

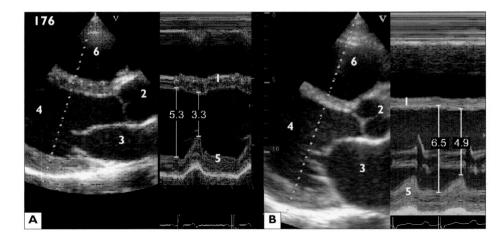

176 Parasternal views with corresponding standard M-mode echocardiograms. **A**: Normal heart. **B**: Earlier large anteroseptal Q wave AMI. The M-mode echocardiogram records the echoes along the 1D dot-and-dash lines as function of time. The interventricular septum (1) is thin and akinetic in **B** and the end-diastolic dimension is enlarged (measurements are given in cm and the approximate normal upper limit is 5.5 cm). In **A** the fractional shortening ([end-diastolic dimension − end-systolic dimension]/end-diastolic dimension) is (5.3 − 3.3)/5.3 or 38% (normal range approximately 25–40%). In **B** the fractional shortening is only 25%. Although signs of ischemia clearly may appear in an M-mode echocardiogram if the interrogated walls are affected (here 1), myocardial ischemia outside the ice-pick view will be missed. 2: aortic root; 3: left atrium; 4: left ventricle; 5: posterior wall of the left ventricle (in **A** & **B** with normal systolic thickening but in B with moderate hypertrophy); 6: right ventricle.

The ejection fraction (EF), i.e. the stroke volume divided by the end-diastolic volume, is an expression of the overall LV systolic function. The endocardial border of the LV is outlined by a cursor on images frozen in end-diastole and end-systole. From these markings and by means of specific geometric assumptions, the equipment is capable of computing the cavity volumes and thus the stroke volume and EF. The normal range of EF is 55–75%. Several studies have documented that EF is an important prognostic determinant, with low EF values related to a poor prognosis. In randomized studies, it has also been shown that patients with EF of 40% or less will benefit from treatment with angiotensin-converting enzyme (ACE) inhibitors and beta blockers.

M-MODE ECHOCARDIOGRAPHY

M-mode (motion-mode) echocardiography records the echoes along a 1D direction as a function of time. This modality provides very high time resolution and high resolution regarding distance. It is used for measurement of LV wall thickness, cavity dimensions, and fractional shortening (**176**).

COLOR-DOPPLER ECHOCARDIOGRAPHY

Color-Doppler echocardiography visualizes the blood flow in the frame of a black and white real-time 2D echocardiogram. Laminar flow toward the transducer is coded red, while laminar blood flow in the opposite direction is blue on the image screen. Turbulence is presented in yellow and green colors. In the setting of IHD, color-Doppler echocardiography is particularly useful for documenting turbulence reflecting mitral incompetence or ventricular septal rupture (see Chapter 11, Mechanical Complications).

Indications, contraindications, and limitations

The above mentioned modalities are performed for diagnosing the localization and extent of an acute myocardial infarction (AMI) or chronic ischemia and the potential morphological sequelae to these conditions, e.g. aneurysms. EF is either measured or merely estimated. There is no discomfort associated with the examination and no contraindications. Poor image quality in patients with large body mass or emphysema may impede image interpretation. This problem may require supplementary transesophageal echocardiography (TEE) or contrast echocardiography.

TRANSESOPHAGEAL ECHOCARDIOGRAPHY

TEE is performed by an endoscope constructed similarly to a gastroscope. However, the optic lenses at the tip are replaced by a small US transducer that can be rotated in any plane by means of a wheel in the handle. TEE provides very clear images because there is very little tissue attenuating the US waves between the transducer and the heart.

Indications, contraindications, and limitations

In ischemic heart disease, TEE is of value in cases of a poor transthoracic image quality, in particular in patients on a ventilator in intensive care. In addition, TEE is useful for monitoring high-risk patients during a coronary artery bypass operation or major vascular surgery. However, the transducer is very close to the heart and it is often impossible to include the entire LV in one image field.

In patients with dysphagia or known esophageal disease, esophageal gastroscopy must precede TEE. This precaution reduces the minimal risk of inadvertent perforation of the esophagus.

STRESS ECHOCARDIOGRAPHY

Myocardial ischemia may be induced by physical exercise or, more commonly, during pharmacologic provocation. Ischemia is diagnosed if decreasing systolic wall motion or wall thickening is observed during increasing doses of dobutamine (commonly 0,5,10,20,40 µg/kg/minute with a dose increment every 3 minutes), often supplemented by atropine (0.25 mg) to obtain target heart rate. Real-time 2D images are stored digitally at each dobutamine dose. Analysis for new wall motion abnormalities takes place off-line by comparison of the various digital image loops on a divided computer screen.

Viability, i.e. hibernation and stunning can also be revealed by stress echocardiography using lower doses of dobutamine (often 5–20 µg/kg/minute). Hibernation or stunning is diagnosed when dobutamine provokes improvement of the wall motion in a region showing hypo- or akinesia at rest or, in some cases, if hypokinesia immediately turns into akinesia.

Indications, contraindications, and limitations

Stress echocardiography is used for the diagnosis of inducible myocardial ischemia or viability. The contraindications and precautions are the same as for other stress tests applied to patients with suspected myocardial ischemia. Malignant arrhythmia is very rare.

Although the result relies on subjective reading of a change in wall motion or wall thickening, stress echocardiography is far more accurate than exercise ECG for the diagnosis or exclusion of inducible ischemia. In experienced hands, it is as reliable as myocardial scintigraphy. For the diagnosis of hibernation or stunning, stress echocardiography seems to be less sensitive but more specific than positron emission tomography (PET) scanning.

CONTRAST ECHOCARDIOGRAPHY

Microbubbles invisible to the naked eye are present in any fluid that is injected or infused intravenously. The bubbles reflect the US, waves and give rise to echoes in the right heart cavities. The bubbles are too large to pass through the capillary bed of the lungs; instead, the bubbles are eliminated and the air expired. Commercially manufactured microbubbles of erythrocyte size pass through the pulmonary circulation and opacify both right and left sided cavities after IV injection (**177**). Recent technical development has even made it possible to enhance echoes from microbubbles in the microcirculation (**178**).

Indications and contraindications

Contrast echocardiography may contribute to the identification of vaguely defined endocardial borders. It is also a promising method for the demonstration of decreased regional myocardial perfusion. However, the technique is hardly ready for widespread clinical perfusion studies, e.g. for deciding whether an intervention has resulted in satisfactory reflow in a patient with AMI.

There are no contraindications but mild local irritation and warmth may occur at the injection site. Otherwise the instructions and precautions advised by the individual manufacturers should be followed.

TISSUE DOPPLER ECHOCARDIOGRAPHY

Tissue Doppler echocardiography is another promising modality. It is obtained by suppression of the low-intensity, high-velocity Doppler signals from the blood, while the high-intensity, low-velocity echoes from the myocardium are enhanced. By means of tissue Doppler the regional myocardial velocity toward and away from the transducer can be recorded in every pixel of the image of the myocardium and presented in a color-coded format or as graphs (**179**).

One of the more promising tissue Doppler presentations is 2D strain imaging. In systole, the AV plane moves toward the apex, that remains almost fixed. Thus, in the normal heart the myocardial velocity decreases gradually from the AV plane to the apex. In contrast, an infarcted region is passively moved or even stretched in systole by the adjacent myocardium. The strain rate is the difference between the velocities at two points on a straight line along a myocardial wall, e.g. from the AV plane to the apex, divided by the distance between the two points. Negative strain rate indicates contraction, while positive strain rate reflects stretching (**179**). Strain is computed as the integral of the strain rate. At the same time, strain denotes regional contraction or stretching (%) and it can be presented in a color-coded format (**180**).

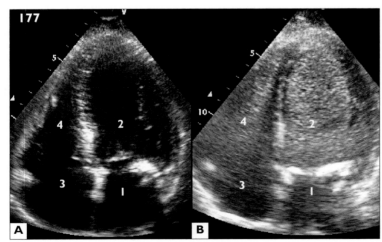

177 Contrast echocardiography recorded in the apical four-chamber view. **A**: Standard 2D echocardiogram. **B**: Bolus of a commercially available echocardiographic contrast medium is injected intravenously, and opacifies both right and left heart cavities and gives an improved outline of the left ventricular cavity as compared with the standard 2D echocardiogram. The patient was admitted the night before the recordings with AMI and an occluded circumflex coronary artery branch of the left coronary artery. According to a control coronary arteriography, satisfactory reopening of the occluded branch was performed by means of percutaneous coronary intervention within 2 hours of the onset of symptoms. Echocardiography with and without IV contrast medium showed no hypo- or akinesia and a normal ejection fraction. 1: left atrium; 2: left ventricle; 3: right atrium; 4: right ventricle. (See also **178**, **180**.)

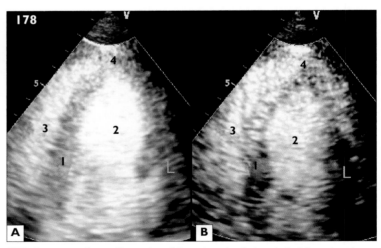

178 Contrast echocardiography of the microcirculation. Apical four-chamber views focusing on the left ventricular myocardium visualized by a recently developed imaging technique. **A**: Normal heart. **B**: Same patient as in **177**. Although this patient had satisfactory reflow after PCI according to coronary arteriography and normal wall motion and ejection fraction, contrast echocardiography indicated a perfusion defect in the lateral wall (L) the day after PCI. 1: interventricular septum; 2: left ventricle; 3: right ventricle; 4: apex; PCI: percutaneous coronary intervention.

Indications, contraindications, and limitations

The motion of the AV plane from basis to apex in systole is supposed mainly to be caused by contraction of the longitudinal fibers. These are located in the subepicardium and in the subendocardium. Thus apical tissue Doppler and, maybe in particular strain scanning, seem very promising for the demonstration of subtle changes caused by myocardial ischemia (**180**).

There are no contraindications but most tissue Doppler techniques including strain scanning need more scientific evaluation before they can be considered ready for use in everyday clinical practice for diagnosis and exclusion of myocardial ischemia.

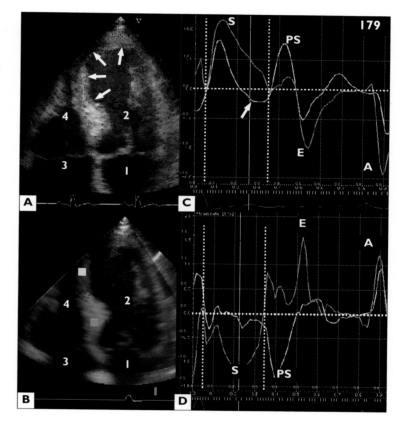

179 Tissue Doppler echocardiography. **A**: Apical four-chamber view recorded in systole 2 days after the onset of AMI caused by proximal occlusion of the left anterior descending branch of the left coronary artery. Despite PCI, a large anterior Q wave infarction with akinesia developed (arrows). The corresponding color-coded tissue-Doppler echocardiogram (**B**) shows that most of the left ventricle moves towards the apex in systole (red color). However, the infarcted septum exhibits abnormal motion in the opposite direction (blue). The green sample point is localized in normal myocardium, the yellow sample in the infarct area. **C**: Corresponding tissue velocity curves. The green sample point exhibits systolic motion (S) of normal direction and duration, but in diastole there is inversed E to A ratio (the E-point velocity being less than the A-point velocity), indicating diastolic dysfunction. The yellow sample point also shows anterior motion at the beginning of systole while there is paradoxical motion later in systole with a velocity below 0 cm/second (horizontal dot-and-dash line). A postsystolic motion (PS) towards the apex is observed in the yellow curve. **D**: Corresponding strain rate curves, showing that the myocardium at the yellow sample point is passive during systole (the strain rate is almost at the zero-line), while there is negative strain rate in the green sample point reflecting contraction. The postsystolic motion of the yellow sample point exhibits negative strain rate indicating true contraction. This finding is considered to reflect viability. 1: left atrium; 2: left ventricle; 3: right atrium; 4: right ventricle.

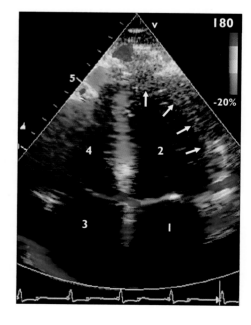

180 Strain imaging recorded in systole in the apical four-chamber view. Same patient as in **177** and **178**. According to the scale in the upper right corner, negative strain (shortening or contraction [%]) is coded red while stretching is coded blue. Only the basal part of the lateral wall shows normal contraction while either no strain or paradoxical stretching is present in the remaining part of the wall in systole (arrows). There is not complete agreement with the contrast echocardiogram in **178** but both methods revealed subtle abnormalities in the lateral wall that were detectable by neither coronary arteriography after PCI of the related artery, nor by conventional 2D echocardiography. 1: left atrium; 2: left ventricle; 3: right atrium; 4: right ventricle; PCI: percutaneous coronary intervention.

MYOCARDIAL SCINTIGRAPHY

ANNE KALTOFT, MD, PhD AND MORTEN BØTTCHER, MD, PhD

INTRODUCTION
Myocardial scintigraphy is increasingly used to diagnose noninvasively the occurrence of stress-induced reversible myocardial ischemia. The method has replaced or supplemented traditional exercise testing because of superior sensitivity and specificity and because of its ability to provide optimal prognostic information. In patients with established CAD, the method provides information about the net perfusion effect of often complex coronary lesions.

TECHNIQUE
Myocardial scintigraphy is a noninvasive imaging method, used to visualize the relative distribution of left ventricular perfusion. A radioactive tracer is injected into a peripheral vein and within 1–2 minutes it will be taken up by the myocytes. Once inside the myocytes the tracer is 'trapped' and the image acquisition can be performed at a later time point and still reflect the perfusion at the time of injection. The most common tracers are labeled with [99m]technetium, a gamma-emitting isotope. Images are acquired with a tomographic technique known as single photon emission computed tomography (SPECT). The camera rotates around the patient and 64 images are taken. The images are reconstructed to yield both 3D and short-, vertical- and horizontal-axis scintigrams (**181, 182**).

The most common setup consists of two image acquisitions, the first during rest and the second after either exercise testing or pharmacologic stress. The stress images reveal areas in which a coronary stenosis will reduce the stress-induced hyperemia (**182**). The exercise test is performed as a routine treadmill or bicycle test and the tracer is injected at peak exercise. Pharmacologic stress is achieved by infusion of adenosine or dipyridamole, often combined with low level exercise. Adenosine will induce microvascular dilatation and thereby increase epicardial flow. Resting perfusion is visualized following 30 minutes of supine rest and the acquisition of data takes 15–25 minutes.

The scintigrams are primarily evaluated visually by a direct comparison between the rest and stress images. Perfusion defects can be reversible, that is only present during stress, or permanent, that is present during rest (**183–185**). The location, the relation to the coronary branches, the extent, and the severity of defects can be evaluated.

INDICATIONS
Suspected coronary artery disease
Patients suspected of CAD have traditionally been evaluated with a treadmill or bicycle exercise ECG. However, only two-thirds of the patients referred to an outpatient clinic are actually able to perform a sufficient test, which requires achieving 85% of maximal heart rate. Several reasons such as claudication, joint disease, pulmonary disease,

and beta blockade can account for this. Furthermore, to be able to diagnose induced ischemia, it requires a rest ECG without LBBB, Q waves, and abnormal T wave configuration and pace rhythm. Unfortunately, very often stress ECGs are misinterpreted and described as negative, when they do not show ischemia. This is only true in cases where the patient has completed the test and achieved the expected heart rate. Otherwise the results should be described as inconclusive. Such patients should undergo a perfusion scan to rule out ischemic heart disease.

Angiographically verified coronary artery disease
Patients with established heart disease can also benefit from perfusion scintigraphy. The hemodynamic significance of a coronary stenosis is often difficult to evaluate, particularly if multiple stenoses are present or the stenoses occur as serial stenosis. Perfusion scintigraphy can define the culprit lesion in these types of patients. Patients already revascularized are candidates for scintigraphy, if a restenosis is suspected or if disease progression indicates further attempts at revascularization. In patients previously revascularized, the sensitivity of traditional stress testing with exercise ECG is lower. Myocardial scintigraphy can be used in this context because it not only enables an evaluation of whether there is a problem, but also indicates the location and the perfusion-related impact of the stenosis.

CONTRAINDICATIONS
Contraindications for adenosine stress are primarily severe asthma and greater than first degree AV block. Regarding stress testing, see Chapters 8, Exercise Testing and 6, Stress Echocardiography.

CLINICAL INTERPRETATION
A normal stress myocardial scintigram indicates a very favorable prognosis, very similar to a member of the general population. Several large-scale studies have independently confirmed this using several different approaches. In a recent investigation including almost 5,000 patients 89% had a normal scintigram; after 7 years of follow-up, 98.5% of these were alive[1]. In a similar investigation of 5,000 patients with an occurrence of a normal scintigram of 57%, the annual mortality rate was 0.5% for the 2-year follow-up period as opposed to 4.2% in the group of patients with abnormal scintigraphy[2].

FUTURE DEVELOPMENTS
With the newer gamma cameras additional features will be likely to improve further the diagnostic capability and sensitivity of SPECT. Image acquisition can now be performed in such a short time period that several images can be achieved during the cardiac cycle. These so-called gated images are recorded, triggered by the ECG, and can be reconstructed to yield not only ventricular volumes but also information on LV function globally and regionally (**186**). This is particularly important in cases with borderline abnormalities, where reductions in regional wall motion will provide further evidence of stress-induced changes.

With the newest cameras the possibility of acquiring images with positron-emitting isotopes has become available. These tracers are used in the evaluation of patients with severely depressed LV function, to distinguish between viable and nonviable tissue (see Chapter 8, Positron Emission Tomography). The use of high-energy PET isotopes requires compromise regarding image acquisition, and the image quality is not quite as high as with the dedicated PET cameras. However, the availability and the easy linkage to the high-quality gated perfusion images yield a diagnostic sensitivity that has turned out to be very similar to that of the dedicated PET cameras.

181 3D single photon emission computerized tomography image of the left ventricle from a patient with normal perfusion. **Right column**: Short-vertical and long-axis cuts. 1: Base; 2: Anterior; 3: Apex; 4: Inferior.

182 Dual headed gamma camera.

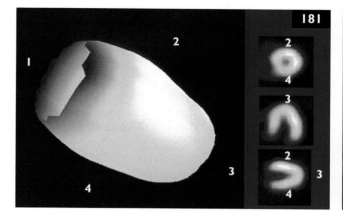
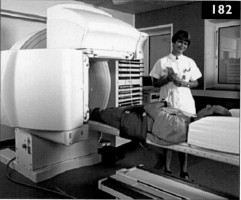

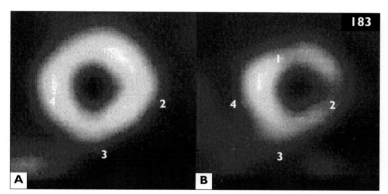

183 Single photon emission computerized tomography of a reversible perfusion defect in the lateral wall. **A**: Rest perfusion; **B**: Stress perfusion. 1: Anterior; 2: Lateral; 3: Inferior; 4: Septal.

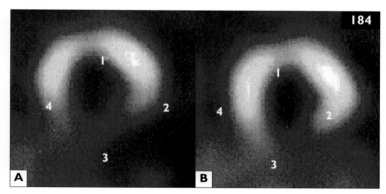

184 Single photon emission computerized tomography of a irreversible perfusion defect in the inferior wall. **A**: Rest perfusion; **B**: Stress perfusion. 1: Anterior; 2: Lateral; 3: Inferior; 4: Septal.

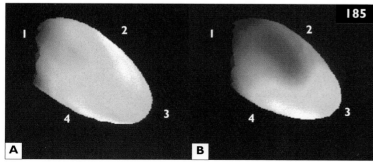

185 3D single photon emission computerized tomography view of a reversible perfusion defect in the anterior wall. **A**: Rest perfusion; **B**: Stress perfusion. 1: Base; 2: Lateral; 3: Apex; 4: Septal.

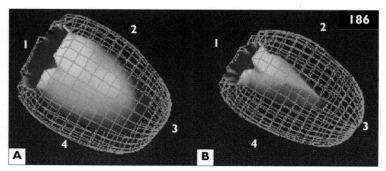

186 Gated single photon emission computerized tomography image from a patient with normal left ventricular contraction. **A**: Rest perfusion; **B**: Stress perfusion. 1: Base; 2: Anterior; 3: Apex; 4: Inferior.

POSITRON EMISSION TOMOGRAPHY

MORTEN BØTTCHER, MD, PhD

INTRODUCTION
PET is a technique used primarily in clinical cardiology for detecting viable myocardium in patients with severe congestive heart failure on the basis of IHD. In combination with other noninvasive techniques and coronary angiography (CAG) it enables identification of patients who will benefit both symptomatically and prognostically by undergoing surgical revascularization. PET scanning can be performed on both dedicated PET scanners and on modified SPECT scanners.

PET scanning was originally developed for research purposes in order to quantify perfusion and metabolic processes. This capability is only used in a very limited number of patients, e.g. patients with syndrome X in whom the quantitative perfusion reserve can be measured.

Positron-emitting isotopes are produced in a cyclotron and are chemically processed before injection. A positron-emitting isotope is characterized by a surplus of protons in its nucleus. The unstable structure results in the conversion of a proton to a neutron and the charge thereby released is emitted as a positron. The positron, which is an elementary particle, will only travel a few millimeters before it is 'captured' by an electron in a process known as annihilation. This annihilation results in the emission of two high-energy gamma quanta in opposite directions. By applying a system of coupling detectors positioned opposite each other in the scanner, the location of the event can be determined and a high-resolution image of the heart can be achieved.

TECHNIQUE
The patient is placed in the scanner with the thorax centered in the scanner (**187**). The isotope is injected into a peripheral vein and the image acquisition is started (**188**). The duration of the acquisition depends on the type of investigation and ranges from 2 minutes in investigations of perfusion using ^{15}O water, to 70 minutes in metabolic investigations using 2-deoxy-2-[^{18}F]fluoro-D-glucose (FDG). A routine clinical investigation will typically include a perfusion scan with ^{13}N ammonia (**189**) and a metabolic scan with FDG. The total imaging time is approximately 2 hours.

ISCHEMIC DYSFUNCTION AND (MIS)MATCH
Patients with reduced LV function include both those with irreversible dysfunction and reversible dysfunction. Reversible dysfunction has traditionally been subdivided into patients with chronic ischemia 'hibernation' or repetitive ischemia 'stunning'. Irreversible dysfunction can occur based in scar tissue after an MI or mechanical dysfunction. It is important to determine the cause of the LV dysfunction because revascularization with coronary artery bypass graft (CABG) or percutaneous coronary intervention (PCI)

not only relieves angina but also improves long-term prognosis in patients with reversible dysfunction.

The evaluation of reversibility with PET is a combined evaluation of perfusion and metabolic conditions reflected by the regional glucose uptake. Myocardial perfusion is reflected by the uptake of tracers like ^{13}N ammonia, while glucose uptake can be evaluated by the uptake of the glucose analog FDG. Three fundamentally different patterns of perfusion and glucose uptake can be recognized. A homogeneous uptake of both tracers will occur in normal tissue. In areas with reduced contractility, the regional perfusion can be reduced while the glucose uptake can be normal or increased. This condition is referred to as perfusion-metabolic 'mismatch' (**190**). The condition reflects a reduced perfusion with preserved glucose uptake and potentially reversible dysfunction. Finally, a combined pattern of reduced perfusion and glucose uptake can be seen in areas with reduced contractility. Such a pattern represents perfusion-metabolic 'match' (**191**) and characterizes irreversible dysfunctional myocardium, often representing scar tissue. Often, patients will display several of these patterns and the decision for revascularization should be based not only on the occurrence of these patterns but also on the location and extent and the ability to perform revasularization effectively.

The predictive value of identifying reversible dysfunctional regions and the ability to regain or improve contractility after revascularization have been evaluated in different series and are reported to be between 70% and 90%, while the predictive value for irreversible areas in which contractility is not improved after revascularization is >85%. Reversible dysfunction does not seem to be related to any of the obtainable clinical parameters such as the occurrence of Q waves in the ECG.

RESEARCH APPLICATIONS
Quantitation of myocardial perfusion and glucose uptake is a validated method using dynamic PET. Mathematical models enable quantification based on dynamically acquired data (**192**). The short half-life of the tracers enables repeated measurements to be made, e.g. under different physiologic conditions.

COMBINED TOMOGRAPHY
PET scanning is increasingly used in combination with SPECT isotopes and conventional gamma cameras (see Chapter 8, Myocardial Scintigraphy). New developments have enabled detection of the high-energy photons emitted by the PET isotopes in gamma cameras. This will allow the combination of a traditional SPECT perfusion tracer such as ^{99m}Tc-sestamibi and PET isotopes such as FDG. The capacity for viability detection will thereby increase due to the increased availability of traditional SPECT cameras.

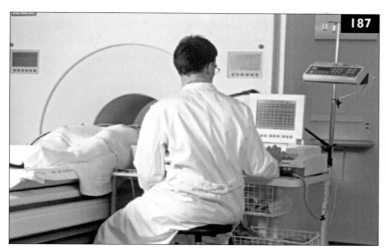

187 A dedicated positron emission tomography scanner.

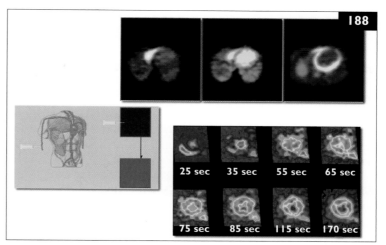

188 The radioactive tracer is injected into a peripheral vein and first reaches the right ventricular cavity. After a passage through the pulmonary circulation it reaches the left ventricle and is taken up by the myocytes through the coronary circulation.

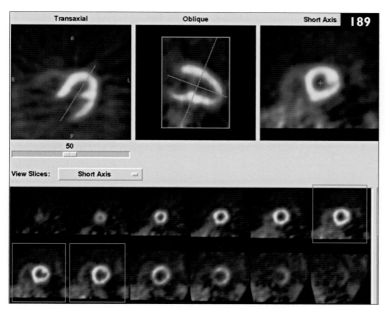

189 Positron emission tomography scanning of a normal volunteer with perfusion tracer ^{13}N ammonia. The images are a matrix and can be reoriented. Lower panel shows short-axis images with the apex in the top row to the left.

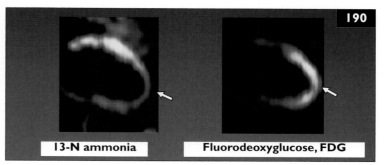

190 Positron emission tomography scanning of a patient with apical mismatch (arrows). **A**: ^{13}-N-ammonia perfusion image with low perfusion in the apical area. **B**: Glucose uptake (fluorodeoxyglucose) which is high in the hypoperfused region indicating 'mismatch'. The inferior wall displays a pattern of 'match'.

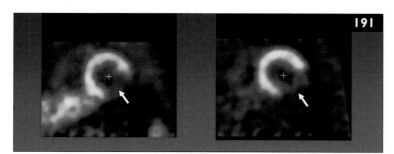

191 Positron emission tomography scanning of a patient with an infero-lateral infarct (arrows). **A**: Perfusion pattern (^{13}-N-ammonia). **B**: Similarly reduced glucose uptake (fluorodeoxyglucose), a 'match'.

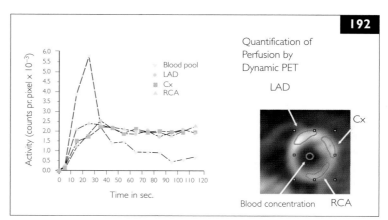

192 Analysis of quantitative perfusion values is achieved in each of the distribution areas of the main three coronary branches using positron emission tomography (PET). LAD: left anterior descending coronary artery; Cx: circumflex artery; RCA: right coronary artery.

MAGNETIC RESONANCE IMAGING

WON YONG KIM, MD, PhD AND EIKE NAGEL, MD

INTRODUCTION
Cardiovascular magnetic resonance imaging (CMRI) has emerged as a comprehensive noninvasive method for the assessment of reversible LV myocardial ischemia and visualization of necrotic/infarcted myocardium.

MAGNETIC RESONANCE STRESS IMAGING
Technique
Cine-CMRI is obtained by gradient echo- (GE) based sequences and in particular 3D steady-state free precession sequences, resulting in a bright appearance of blood compared with the ventricular wall. ECG triggering and patient breath holding compensate for intrinsic cardiac and respiratory motion during data acquisition.

CMRI is typically performed in standard echocardiographic views including three short-axis views, a two- and a four-chamber projection (**193**, top). Left ventricular wall motion is evaluated at rest and at incremental doses (10, 20, 30, and 40 µg/kg/minute) of dobutamine infusion until ≥85% of the age-predicted maximum heart rate is achieved (220 minus age in years). Wall motion is evaluated on a segmental basis using a 17-segment model according to guidelines from the American Heart Association (**193**, top). Stress testing is terminated on the occurrence of new wall motion abnormalities (**193**, bottom) or other clinical manifestations of manifest myocardial ischemia.

Indications
In a direct comparison of stress CMRI and stress echocardiography in a study of 179 patients, Nagel et al.[1] showed that stress CMRI had a significantly higher diagnostic accuracy due to superior image quality. With stress CMRI, sensitivity was increased from 74% to 86% and specificity from 70% to 86% compared to stress echocardiography. In a subsequent study by Hundley et al.[2], which specifically included 153 patients with a nondiagnostic stress echocardiography (due to poor acoustic windows), stress CMRI had a sensitivity and specificity of 79% and 83%, respectively. These results have encouraged an increasing use of stress CMRI for the detection of reversible myocardial ischemia in patients with moderate or poor echocardiographic image quality.

Contraindications
Contraindications are related to the magnetic field itself (e.g. interference from aneurysm clips, pacemakers, and electronic implants), or from practical problems such as pregnancy, severe claustrophobia and the use of pharmacologic stressor agents.

Limitations and complications
During stress examinations with high-dose dobutamine, monitoring of the patient is obligatory to immediately detect and treat possible adverse side-effects. Even though monitoring is more difficult inside the MRI environment (no ST segment evaluation, distance to patient), the stress test can be performed safely. Implementation of vector ECG and real-time monitoring of wall motion have greatly facilitated patient monitoring.

MYOCARDIAL PERFUSION IMAGING
Technique
The imaging sequence for assessment of myocardial perfusion employs a T1-weighted (saturation prepulse), segmented k-space, GE technique. A series of short-axis slices through the LV is acquired during the first passage of an IV bolus injection of gadolinium contrast agent (0.05 mmol/kg body weight) at rest and during pharmacologic stress (most commonly either adenosine

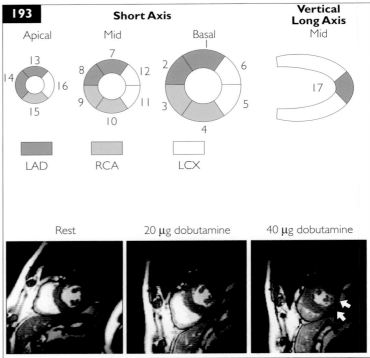

193 Cardiovascular magnetic resonance dobutamine stress imaging. **Top panel:** Left ventricular segmentation according to the Guidelines of the American Heart Association/American College of Cardiology. Usually three short-axis views, a four-chamber view and a two-chamber view are acquired. Blue: left anterior descending coronary artery; Pink: right coronary artery; White: left circumflex coronary artery. **Bottom panel:** End-systolic short-axis images at rest (left), intermediate stress (middle), and maximal stress (right). At rest and intermediate stress no wall motion abnormality can be seen, whereas reduced end-systolic wall thickness and endocardial motion can be seen at maximal stress (arrows).

or dipyridamole) (**194A**). The relative changes in signal intensity over time are analyzed qualitatively and semi-quantitatively (**194B–194D**). Due to the T1-shortening characteristics of the contrast agent, the signal intensity within the myocardium depends on the amount of contrast agent passing through the myocardium. Areas of normally perfused myocardium have a more rapid and steep increase in signal intensity under stress as compared to rest conditions. Areas of myocardium with reversible ischemia show a less pronounced rise in signal intensity during pharmacologic stress (**194B**).

Indications
CMRI first-pass perfusion measurements have demonstrated a diagnostic accuracy in the detection of CAD which compares favorably with nuclear techniques. In a prospective semi-quantitative analysis of myocardial perfusion reserve by Al-Saadi et al.[3], sensitivity, specificity, and diagnostic accuracy for detection of significant CAD (≥75% coronary artery stenosis) were 90%, 83%, and 87%, respectively. Schwitter et al.[4] using a multi-slice approach for CMRI myocardial perfusion imaging, showed a sensitivity and specificity of 91% and 94%, respectively, for the detection of CAD as defined by PET.

Contraindications
Contraindications are related to the CMRI examination itself (see above), the contrast agents (prior adverse effects to gadolinium derivatives), and the pharmacologic stressor agents (e.g. AV-block, obstructive lung disease).

Limitations
The need for real-time imaging has hitherto limited the spatial coverage of the LV myocardium. Faster gradient systems and further optimization in CMRI sequence designs has allowed for more extensive myocardial coverage. Automated algorithms would facilitate routine use by reducing the analysis time to derive indices for myocardial perfusion reserve. Currently, only data from selected patient populations are available.

MAGNETIC RESONANCE DELAYED CONTRAST-ENHANCEMENT TECHNIQUE
Technique
Contrast-enhanced CMRI can identify reversible myocardial dysfunction or 'viability' by selectively imaging scar tissue within the myocardium. Following an IV injection of gadolinium contrast agent (0.2 mmol/kg body weight), inversion-recovery prepared, T1-weighted GE images are acquired at mid diastole in standard short-axis and long-axis projections after a delay of 10–15 min. The inversion time, which is determined interactively for each patient to null normal myocardium after contrast injection, is of critical importance for accurate assessment of scar tissue. Typically, the inversion time is chosen from 200–300 ms. As a result of optimizing the inversion time, the late-enhancement images depict nonviable tissue as a bright structure due to increased amounts of

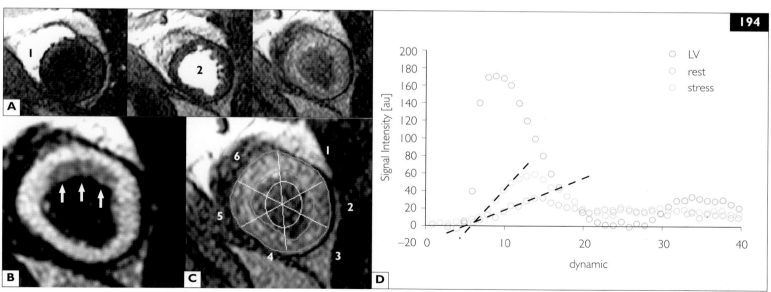

194 Cardiovascular magnetic resonance myocardial perfusion imaging. **A**: The first-pass effect of a bolus injection of gadolinium contrast agent through the right ventricle (RV, 1) (left image), the left ventricle (LV, 2) (middle image), and the myocardium (right image). **B**: Visualization of a hypoperfusion defect in the subendocardium of the anterior left ventricular wall (arrows). **C**: For semiquantitative analysis, each short-axis view is divided into six equiangular segments (1–6) beginning at the anterior septal insertion of the RV. Signal intensity–time curves are plotted for each segment, showing the arrival of the contrast agent bolus into the myocardium. **D**: A myocardial perfusion reserve index is calculated from the signal intensity–time curves as the ratio of the up-slope during stress (orange) and at rest (yellow), and corrected by the LV input function (green).

residual gadolinium (**195**). The normal or viable myocardium appears dark.

Indications

Contrast-enhanced CMRI assessment of chronic reversible ischemia allows for the distinction between subendocardial and transmural infarctions, due to the high spatial resolution of the technique (**195**). With the use of hyperenhancement of 25% of tissue as the cut-off value for regions with any degree of dysfunction, the positive predictive value (71%) and the negative predictive value (79%) of the method are similar to those reported for other noninvasive techniques[5]. These values, however, increase to 88% and 89%, respectively, for segments with akinesia or dyskinesia, which are often the most problematic to evaluate. Delayed enhancement CMRI is therefore a technique that is expected to have a significant clinical impact in the very near future, guiding therapeutic strategies in patients with CAD and congestive heart failure.

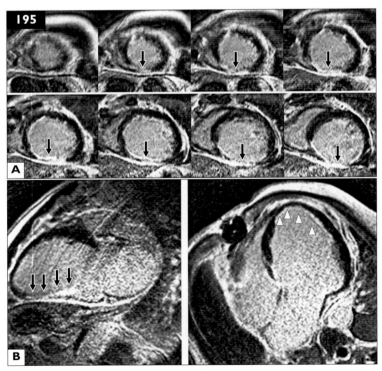

195 3D contrast-enhanced cardiovascular magnetic resonance imaging in a patient with chronic occlusion of the proximal right coronary artery. **A**: Left ventricular short-axis slices (from apex to base of heart) reveal thinned myocardial tissue with bright signal intensity of the posterior wall (arrows), indicating chronic transmural infarction. **B**: Corresponding two-chamber view (left panel) confirms the transmural hyperenhancement of the left ventricular posterior wall (arrows) while the four-chamber view (right panel) reveals subendocardial scarring of the apex (arrow heads).

COMPUTED TOMOGRAPHY

SRIRAM PADMANABHAN, MD, MS, MATTHEW J. BUDOFF, MD, FACC AND PREDIMAN K. SHAH, MD, FACC

INTRODUCTION

Computed tomography (CT) is a robust methodology to evaluate coronary anatomy, vessel patency, atherosclerotic burden, and EF, both pre- and postinfarction.

Electron-beam computed tomography (EB[C]T) is a fourth-generation CT imaging process, able to obtain thin slices of the heart and coronaries. Rapid image acquisition allows approximately five times greater imaging speed than conventional multi-slice computed tomography (MSCT), limiting the respiratory and cardiac motion artifacts inherent in cardiac imaging.

TECHNIQUE

In CT, 30–40 axial images are usually obtained to include the entire myocardium. Coronary arteries are imaged during a single 20–30 second breath-hold. In EBT, instead of rotating the X-ray tube around the patient as in conventional scanners, the patient is positioned inside the X-ray tube, obviating the need to move any part of the scanner during image acquisition.

The cine scanning mode is designed to assess cardiac function. Scanning frequency of 17 scans/second is sufficient to study systolic and diastolic function. The spatial resolution adequately defines the endocardium of both ventricles. Precise measurements of cardiac volumes, mass, and EF are feasible. Quantitative measurement of wall motion and thickening can be performed, particularly useful for evaluating CAD patients. Bicycle exercise can be coupled with EBT to detect exercise-induced ischemia. Both a fall in EF, and development of a new wall motion abnormality, have been shown to be accurate for detection of ischemia, with data indicating that exercise CT may be at least as sensitive and more specific than 99[m]technetium sestamibi stress testing[1].

INDICATIONS
Coronary artery calcification and atherosclerosis

Calcific deposits in coronary arteries are pathognomonic of atherosclerosis (**196**; see also Chapter 7, Electron-Beam Computed Tomography: Coronary Calcium). Histopathologic and intravascular US studies confirm the close correlation between atherosclerotic plaque burden and extent of coronary artery calcification (CAC). EBT can noninvasively quantify the amount of CAC (r >0.90)[2], which has been demonstrated to be highly sensitive for the presence of significant CAD. A recent report of 1,764 persons undergoing angiography and EBT showed a very high sensitivity and negative predictive value in both sexes (>99%)[3]. Thus, a score of 0 can virtually exclude those patients with obstructive CAD. While the presence of CAC is nearly 100% specific for atheromatous plaque[4], it is not specific for obstruction due to remodeling. EBT is comparable to nuclear exercise testing in the detection of obstructive CAD[5].

CAC scoring has been shown to be useful in monitoring therapy with statins (**197**). The progression rate of coronary calcium under the influence of no therapy, mild therapy, and aggressive therapy (low density lipoprotein [LDL] value <100 mg/dl [2.6 mmol/l] on treatment) is depicted in the figure. Those with 'tight' control of their LDL cholesterol had, on average, no progression of their coronary calcium.

Studies have documented that EBT is a rapid and efficient screening tool for patients admitted to the emergency department with chest pain to rule out MI[6,7]. These studies demonstrate sensitivities of 98–100% for identifying patients with acute MI, and very low subsequent event rates for persons with negative tests[1]. The high sensitivity and negative predictive value may allow early discharge of those patients with nondiagnostic ECG and negative EBT scans (scores = 0). Exclusion of coronary calcium may therefore be used as an effective filter prior to invasive diagnostic procedures or hospital admission.

The most powerful data for this modality relate to its ability to predict future coronary events in both symptomatic and asymptomatic persons. A meta-analysis of five studies (4,348 subjects) found that a calcium score above a median was associated with an increased risk of a combined outcome of nonfatal infarction, death, or revascularization (risk ratio 8.7, 95% CI 2.7–28.1), and of a hard event, i.e. death or infarction (risk ratio 4.2, 95% CI 1.6–11.3)[8]. A recent meta-analysis (**198**) of seven prospective trials involving EBT, including more than 10,000

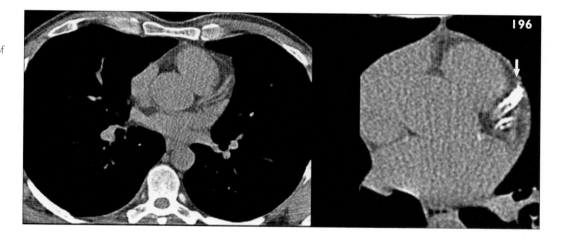

196 Coronary artery calcium. The left image reveals no coronary calcium, while the right image reveals a patient with significant calcium of the left anterior descending artery (arrow).

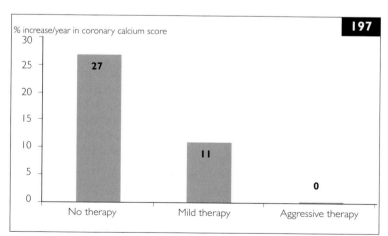

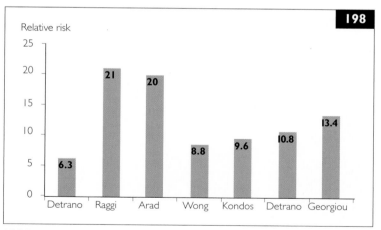

197 The progression rate of coronary calcium (% increase per year) under the influence of no therapy (**left**), the median of the entire treated cohort, and those patients achieving an LDL value <100 mg/dl on treatment. Those with 'tight' control of their LDL cholesterol had, on average, no progression of their coronary calcium. (Adapted with permission from Achenbach et al. [2002].) Influence of lipid-lowering therapy on the progression of coronary artery calcification: a prospective evaluation. Circulation **106**:1077–1082.

198 Prognostic value of coronary artery calcium from seven prospective trials involving electron-beam computed tomography, including more than 10,000 patients, followed for an average of 4 years. In each study, a high calcium score in an age-adjusted cohort was highly predictive of future cardiac events. (Modified from Budoff and Raggi [2001]. Coronary artery disease progression assessed by electron-beam computed tomography. Am J. Cardiol **88**: 46E–50E.)

patients followed for an average of 4 years, showed that a high calcium score in an age-adjusted cohort was highly predictive of future cardiac events (for a representative study see[3]). Population-based studies are now under way to evaluate the prognostic power in larger cohorts.

Evaluation of systolic and diastolic function

CT has been utilized to evaluate systolic and diastolic performance of the LV (**199**). Diastolic filling variables (as those measured by blood pool scintigraphy) can be determined. Application of this technique may prove useful for detecting subtle changes in LV function induced by myocardial ischemia, accurately diagnosing EF postinfarction, and patency of blood vessels using noninvasive angiography.

Myocardial blood flow/perfusion

Noninvasive quantification of myocardial blood flow is possible by evaluating flow patterns of iodinated contrast. Flow is proportional to the peak iodine concentration in the myocardium after intravenous injection of contrast medium. The technique is accurate for myocardial flow up to 2 ml/min/g. Technical factors related to Compton scatter and beam hardening may cause inaccuracies. Further research is necessary, but work in progress looks promising for the development of clinically useful methods for accurate quantification of flow. Colorization methodology has also been developed, which should simplify analysis of regional flow differences (**200**)[9].

Since iodine concentration is proportional to blood flow, acute MI can be imaged by CT as a region of little or no iodine (low density) during contrast infusion. This technique has also been used to quantify the infarct size and detect patency of the infarct vessel, using flow and 3D techniques. Complications of MI, including ventricular septal defects, thrombi (**201**), aneurysms, and pericardial effusions can be easily visualized.

Noninvasive angiography

Electron-beam angiography (EBA) has the potential for obtaining essentially noninvasive coronary arteriograms (**202**, **203**; see also Chapter 7, Noninvasive Multi-Slice Spiral Computed Tomography). This procedure requires IV contrast to opacify the lumen, and is completed within 20–30 minutes. Recent studies have reported that this modality could be used to identify significant coronary lumen narrowing (>50% stenosis) with sensitivity of 78–92% and specificity of 79–100% as compared to invasive coronary angiography[10,11]. Selective use of EBA might prove cost effective and provide a safer, less-invasive method to assess for luminal stenosis.

Using EBA in patients post-CABG (**203**) or poststent, demonstrated sensitivities of 92–100% and specificities of 91–100% for establishing patency as compared to conventional coronary angiography[12,13].

CONTRAINDICATIONS

There are no specific contraindications for noncontrast studies. Neither claustrophobia nor metal objects have any impact on scanning with CT. Contrast studies (perfusion, EF, angiograms) require iodinated contrast, which would be contraindicated in patients with significant renal dysfunction or allergies to iodine. The radiation dose with EBT is modest (approximately one-quarter that of a cardiac catheterization).

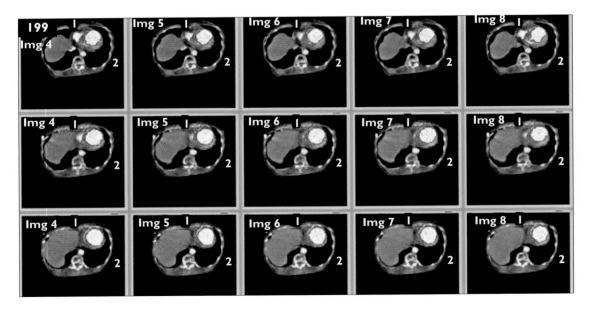

199 Systolic and diastolic function. Images are obtained every 50 milliseconds, and images are automatically traced for left ventricular endocardium and epicardium (red lines). From this image set (on each level of the heart), measurements are taken of myocardial mass, ejection fraction, and wall thickening. 1: anterior; 2: left.

LIMITATIONS

EBT is not widely available and the high cost of equipment prohibits its widespread use. MSCT has been shown to have some of the capabilities of EBT, with promise of wider availability. Unfortunately, the speed of acquisition (temporal resolution) greatly differentiates EBT from the slower images from MSCT. The only studies demonstrating similar results between EBT and spiral CT consisted of elderly symptomatic men with very high plaque burdens. A recent comparison study of EBT and MSCT concluded that 'spiral CT has not yet proved to be a feasible alternative to electron-beam CT for CAC quantification'[14]. Since there is no improvement of temporal resolution with newer MSCT scanners (each slice is still obtained in 250–330 msec), it is unlikely that closer correlations with EBT will be obtained with more slices. Furthermore, with images obtained over a longer time, the radiation doses to the patient with MSCT are 6–38-fold greater than with EBT[15].

Overall, CT (both EBT and MSCT) is a rapidly developing modality for the comprehensive analysis of CAD.

200 Myocardial blood flow. A single level is imaged, and the brightness of contrast (Hounsfield Units) for each pixel is measured. A color perfusion map is inlaid over the myocardium, where red is the brightest density (most blood flow) and blue is the least. This patient suffered an anteroseptal infarction, and the dark blue area reflects that decreased perfusion.

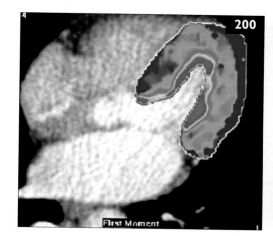

201 Apical thrombus and infarction. A patient status postmyocardial infarction with a resultant large anteroapical aneurysm and thrombus. The thrombus is easily visualized (black arrow) and the infarcted tissue is both thinned and darker (less perfusion with contrast enhanced blood, white arrows).

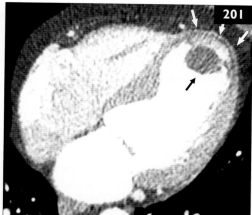

202 Electron beam angiogram of a patient with a large anterior infarction after thrombolytic therapy. The left anterior descending (black arrows) and diagonals (white arrow heads) are easily seen, and are patent. The circumflex (black arrow head) has mild nonobstructive disease. This three dimensional image would have to be rotated to see the right coronary artery (white arrows) and distal vessels.

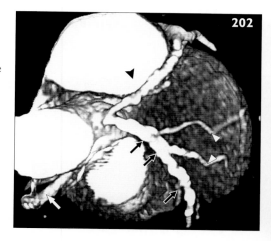

203 Electron beam angiogram of a patient 9 years after bypass surgery, now returning with an inferior infarction. The right coronary artery (black arrow) is completely occluded, and the three saphenous vein grafts to the right coronary and circumflex are all proximally occluded (arrow heads). The left anterior descending has an 80% stenosis in its midportion (white arrow) and is successfully bypassed with a patent saphenous vein graft.

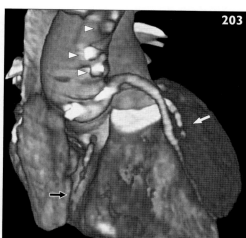

ELECTROMECHANICAL MAPPING

HANS ERIK BØTKER, MD, PhD

INTRODUCTION
Cardiac mapping implies registration of electrical activation by recording of electrograms. The principle was initially used for electrophysiologic analysis of cardiac arrhythmias, by navigation of electrophysiologic catheters in the cardiac chambers guided by multi-planar fluoroscopy. Recent developments using magnetic technology allow generation of 3D cardiac maps that yield information not only about local electrical but also about local mechanical function of the heart, without use of fluoroscopy.

TECHNIQUE
Acquisition, analysis, and display of electromechanical maps are only of clinical relevance in the LV and can be obtained with the commercially available NOGA™ system (Biosense, Haifa, Israel). Dysfunctional but yet viable ('hibernating' or 'reversibly dysfunctional') myocardium can be identified by demonstration of electromechanical uncoupling; electrical activity is preserved in reversibly dysfunctional regions, and separates from nonviable tissue (scar or 'irreversibly dysfunctional myocardium'), which displays electromechanical coupling, because both mechanical and electrical activity are equally reduced. The maps are constructed by combining and integrating information from the intracardiac electrograms with the respective endocardial locations. Catheters designed for use with the NOGA™ system are equipped with a miniature location sensor (**204**). Ultra-low magnetic fields are radiated from three discrete radiators placed under the operating table. The location and orientation of the sensor are determined by comparing the sensed magnetic fields with a set of known radiated fields. The location sensor thereby provides information not only about the location but also about movement of the sensor, such that local and global mechanical function can be assessed.

The NOGA™ system is equipped with a mapping screen that displays in real time the position of the catheter tip superimposed on the cardiac map being constructed (**205**). The catheter is

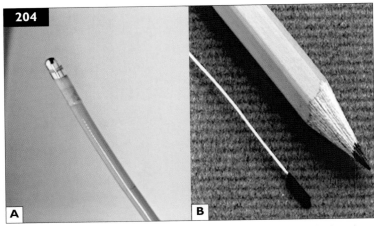

204 NOGA diagnostic catheter (NOGA Star™) (**A**) containing the location sensor (**B**).

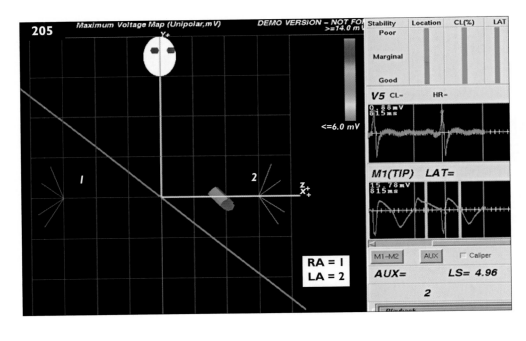

205 NOGA™ mapping screen. 1: right atrium; 2: left atrium.

advanced retrogradely from the femoral artery to the LV and as it moves on the endocardium, the amplitudes of local electrical signals and catheter tip position are reported simultaneously to the system. With specified software dedicated for the NOGA™ system, this information is used to construct a 3D color-coded electromechanical map (**206**). Nominal values of electrical voltage amplitudes and mechanical local shortening values are also obtainable on a polar map, as well as electromechanical cine with global parameters of end-diastolic, end-systolic, and stroke volumes and EF.

A total of 55 points or more are necessary to secure sensitivity and specificity above 70%. To obtain this goal, procedural time varies

between 25 and 45 minutes. Visual inspection of the color-coded electromechanical map allows identification of dysfunctional regions with preserved or reduced electrical activity, and enables distinction between viable and nonviable dysfunctional myocardium (**206**, **207**). Nominal values form the basis for the color-coded maps and allow a similar distinction. However, the exact nominal value for mechanical function in terms of a specific local shortening value has been difficult to establish but is considered to be 10%. The exact value for unipolar voltage that distinguishes between viable and nonviable myocardium is 6.8 mV, but there is a considerable overlap such that the use of exact nominal values on a segmental basis has no major advantage over visual inspection of the color-coded map.

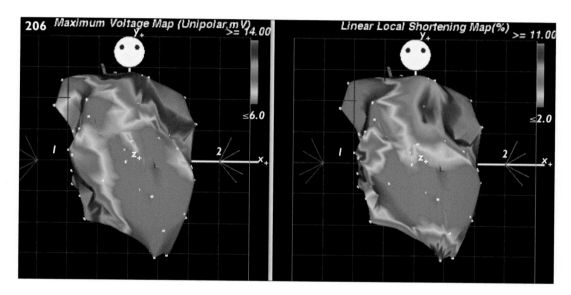

206 Anterior view of accompanying left ventricular voltage (left) and mechanical maps (right) in a patient with previous anterior myocardial infarction and reduced left ventricular function (ejection fraction 25%). Colors represent peak-to-peak amplitudes of intracardiac voltages and linear local shortening, ranging from ≤6 (red) to ≥14 (purple) mV and ≤2 (red) to ≥11 (purple) %, respectively. Infarct causes matched reduction of electrical and mechanical activity in the anterior wall. 1: right atrium; 2: left atrium.

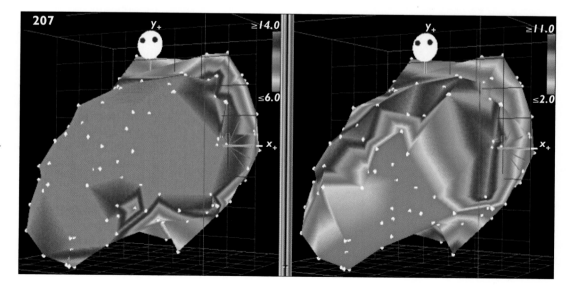

207 Left anterior oblique view of accompanying left ventricular voltage (left) and mechanical maps (right) in a patient with congestive heart failure (ejection fraction 25%) and a proximal 99% stenosis of the left anterior descending artery supplying a collateral dependent anterior wall. Colors represent peak-to-peak amplitudes of intracardiac voltages and linear local shortening, ranging from ≤6 (red) to ≥14 (purple) mV and ≤2 (red) to ≥11 (purple) %, respectively. Reduced perfusion in a dysfunctional but still viable myocardium causes reduced mechanical but preserved electrical activity in the anterior wall.

INDICATIONS

On-line detection of myocardial viability in patients with impaired LV function in the catheterization laboratory is indicated, in relation to subsequent therapeutic procedures.

CONTRAINDICATIONS, LIMITATIONS, AND COMPLICATIONS

Mural thrombus in the left ventricle. Consequently, echocardiography must precede electromechanical mapping.

The major limitation is the invasive nature of the methodology. Stroke, transient cerebral ischemia, hematoma, and other well-known complications that are related to invasive catheter-based diagnostic procedures are not seen with increased frequency during electromechanical mapping with the NOGA™ system. However, electromechanical mapping may cause hemorrhagic pericardial effusion and tamponade.

Electromechanical mapping with the NOGA™ system does not seem to have superior diagnostic accuracy for the detection of viability in dysfunctional myocardial segments compared to noninvasive procedures like SPECT, PET, and stress echocardiography. Because of its invasive nature and potentially serious complications, the procedure should only be carried out for diagnostic purposes in selected cases. However, the methodology has a unique therapeutic potential, because the catheters containing location sensors may also be equipped with needles (**208**). Distinction between viable and nonviable dysfunctional myocardium on a regional basis has decisive significance for local treatment with vascular growth factors and stem cells in patients with no established treatment options.

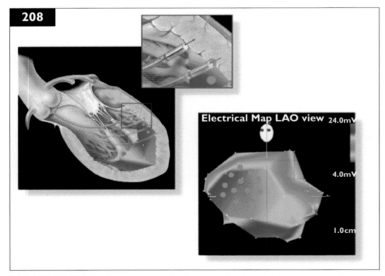

208 NOGA™ injection catheter for local application of treatment in the heart.

INVASIVE HEMODYNAMIC MONITORING

ERIK SLOTH, MD, PhD AND CHRISTIAN LINDSKOV CHRISTIANSEN, MD

INTRODUCTION

The invasive techniques most often used for hemodynamic monitoring are arterial cannulation and insertion of central venous (CVC) and pulmonary artery catheters (PAC). The information obtained by either of these techniques is neither sensitive nor specific for myocardial ischemia or infarction, and is solely used to guide the treatment in the hemodynamically unstable patient.

ARTERIAL CANNULATION
Technique

Allen's test should be used to ensure sufficient collateral ulnar artery blood supply. If sufficient supply is obtained, the radial artery of the nondominant hand can be cannulated. If cannulation fails, the femoral, brachial or axillary artery can be used instead.

The radial artery can be cannulated by different techniques, of which the direct and transfixation approaches are most widely used. The wrist is dorsiflexed over a towel, the skin disinfected, and local analgesia applied (**209**). In the direct approach, a 20 G arterial catheter-over-needle is directed proximally at an angle of 30° toward the skin (**210**). When the artery is punctured and blood flows through the needle, the angle should be reduced to 5–10° and the catheter gently advanced (**211**). In the transfixation approach, both the anterior and posterior arterial walls are punctured, and the needle retracted 1–2 cm before reducing the angle between the needle and the skin. The catheter is slowly withdrawn until pulsatile blood flow appears. Thereafter the catheter can be advanced. A correct cannulation can be validated by a pulsatile pressure trace on the monitor or by the testing of an arterial blood gas sample.

Indications

Intra-arterial blood pressure (IAP) monitoring provides a continuous measurement of blood pressure and access to multiple arterial blood samples. The upstroke, size, range, and respiratory changes of the pulse pressure roughly reflect global myocardial contractility and hypovolemia.

Thus, IAP measurement is essential to guide hemodynamic optimization, especially when inotropic and vasodilating therapy are being applied.

Contraindications

Local infection is an absolute contraindication. Relative contraindications include coagulopathy due to risk of hematoma. Patients with Raynaud's syndrome or trombangiitis obliterans should only be cannulated if it is strongly necessary.

Limitations

The quality of the IAP curve depends on the entire measurement system, including catheter, tubes, stopcocks, transducers, and monitor. Damping due to air bubbles, inappropriate fixation, and improper zeroing of the arterial cannula, are important sources of error.

Complications

Complications include infection, hematoma, thrombosis, and embolism. Severe vascular occlusion occurs in approximately 0.01% of patients cannulated.

CENTRAL VENOUS CANNULATION
Technique

A central venous catheter is inserted by the Seldinger technique, with either a catheter-over-needle or a catheter-in-needle. The internal jugular, external jugular, and subclavian veins can be used and single or more lumen catheters inserted.

The right internal jugular vein offers direct access to the superior caval vein and right side of the heart. Before puncture, the patient is placed supine in a 20–30° Trendelenburg position with the head turned 30° to the left. The internal jugular vein is punctured in the top of the triangle between the medial and lateral heads of the sternocleidomastoid muscles at the level of the cricoid cartilage (**212**). The needle is directed towards the ipsilateral nipple. The common carotid artery runs just medial to the vein.

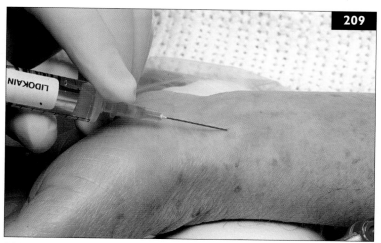

209 Central arterial cannulation. The wrist position during application of local analgesia.

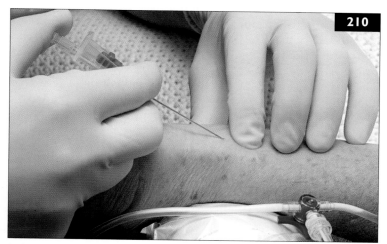

210 Central arterial cannulation. Needle is angled toward the skin during arterial cannulation.

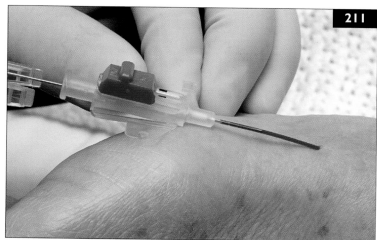

211 Central arterial cannulation. Reducing the needle angle towards the skin during cannula advancement.

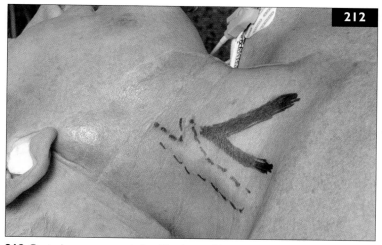

212 Central venous cannulation. The internal jugular vein is located in the top of the triangle between the medial and lateral heads of the sternocleidomastoid muscles.

After disinfection, local analgesia is applied. In the Seldinger technique, a 5 ml syringe is attached to a 22 G finder cannula, which is inserted at an angle of 45° toward the skin (**213**). A slight vacuum is applied on the syringe when the needle is advanced. Often the needle must be redirected to achieve vascular access. When blood is aspirated, the syringe is removed while venous blood flows freely through the cannula. An identical procedure is then performed with an 18 G cannula, through which the guide wire can be advanced into the vessel without any resistance (**214**). The needle is removed and the puncture site dilated. The CVC is advanced into the vein by means of the guide. The guide wire is removed when the CVC is in place.

Indications
Central venous pressure (CVP) indicates RA pressure, and therefore central volume state. A normal CVP trace should have three upward deflections (A,C,V) and two downward deflections (X and Y descents). The A wave reflects the atrial contraction, and the C wave the tricuspid valve closure. The c wave is followed by the X descent, as the tricuspid valve moves away from the atria. The V wave is caused by the rapid atrial filling during late systole and the Y descent is caused by the opening of the tricuspid valve[1]. CVC is essential as IV lines for drug therapy and for the collection of blood samples.

Contraindications
Infection of the cannulation site is an absolute contraindication. Relative contraindications include coagulopathy and active bleeding. Under such conditions the external jugular vein should be chosen.

Limitations
In general, the CVP reflects the LV filling pressure in patients with LV EF >0.40. However, in surgical patients undergoing myocardial revascularization with LV EF <0.40, the CVP was not found to reflect pulmonary artery occlusion pressure (PAOP), unless biventricular failure was present[2]. In patients with reduced LV function and scheduled for CABG, a CVP increase of 5 mmHg (0.7 kPa) had sensitivity/specificity 11%/93% for detecting myocardial ischemia compared to myocardial lactate production[3].

Complications
Arterial puncture occurs in approximately 2% of patients and may cause hematoma and airway obstruction in extreme cases. The use of a finder needle may reduce the severity of this complication. Pneumothorax (0.5%), hydrothorax, chylothorax and pericardial effusion are all reported complications, and occur most frequently during subclavian access.

More seldom nerve lesions of the brachial plexus, the stellate ganglion, or the phrenic nerve may occur during cannulation attempts. Venous air embolism is a potential risk, especially if the CVP is negative. The use of the Trendelenburg position usually prevents this. Cardiac arrhythmias are common when the guide wire is deeply advanced.

PULMONARY ARTERY CATHETERIZATION
Technique
The PAC (**215**) is inserted through a sheath by means of the Seldinger technique. The sheath and the dilator are advanced over the guide wire in a one-step procedure after sharp skin incision (**216**). All PAC ports should be filled with saline and connected to separate transducer lines, and an antiseptic contamination shield should be applied. The floating PAC is advanced 15–20 cm through the sheath while pointing the tip at the 10 o'clock direction to promote the insertion (**217**). When the CVP trace appears on the monitor, the 1.5 ml balloon at the tip of the PAC is inflated with air before further advancement. Guided by the pressure waveforms, the PAC will float along the blood stream through the RA, RV, and pulmonary artery (PA) until a PAOP trace which resembles a CVP trace is reached (**218–220**). The balloon is then deflated. In adults, the cardiac chambers should be reached by: RA 30±5 cm, RV 40±5 cm, PA 50 ±5 cm, and PAOP 55±5 cm.

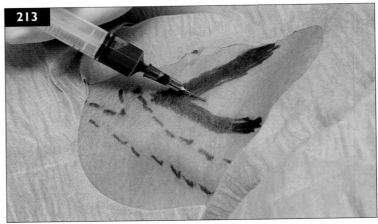

213 Central venous cannulation. The needle angle toward the skin is approximately 45° during cannulation.

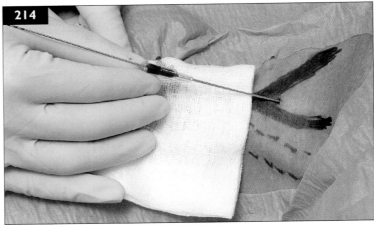

214 Central venous cannulation. The guide wire should be advanced approximately 20 cm without any resistance.

215 A pulmonary artery catheter to measure continuous cardiac output and mixed venous oxygen saturation.

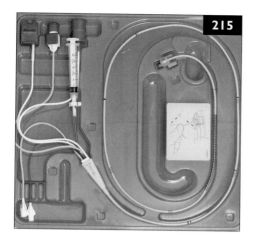

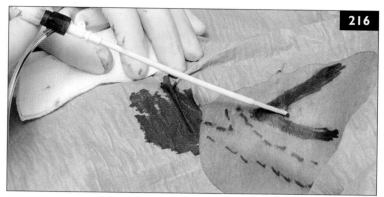

216 Pulmonary artery sheath and the dilator are advanced over the guide wire in a one-step procedure.

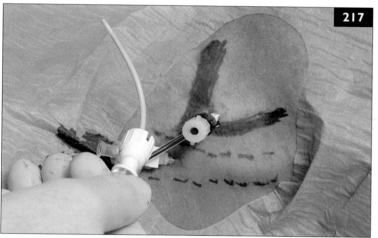

217 Curved pulmonary artery catheter tip should point at 10 o'clock during insertion through the sheath.

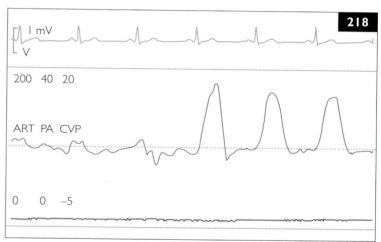

218 Pressure trace as the pulmonary catheter floats from the right atrium to the right ventricle.

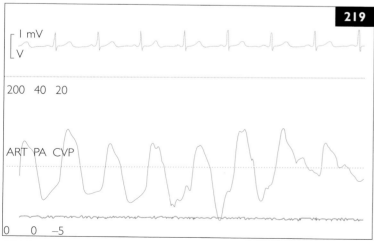

219 Pressure trace as the pulmonary catheter passes the pulmonary valve into the pulmonary artery.

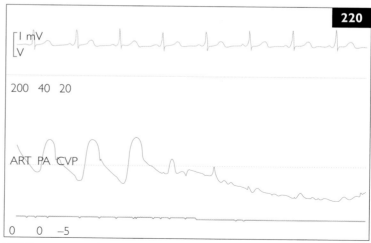

220 Pressure trace in pulmonary artery occlusion pressure.

Indications

From the PAC, blood pressure can be measured in the superior caval vein, RA, RV, PA, and PAOP. Some PACs provide measures of cardiac output and mixed venous oxygen saturation. PAOP reflects left atrial pressure (LAP). Based on these measurements, a number of hemodynamic parameters can be calculated. The PAC is therefore very useful in the diagnosis of severe hemodynamic deterioration. Ischemic impairment of LV systolic and diastolic function will increase left ventricular end-diastolic pressure (LVEDP), LAP and, consequently, PAOP. When papillary muscle dysfunction causes mitral valve regurgitation, an increased V wave is seen on the PAP curve. PAC has been recommended as a method to monitor myocardial ischemia[4], but the major indications for PAC in patients with ischemic heart disease are: (1) MI complicated by progressive hypotension or cardiogenic shock, (2) mechanical complication to MI, and (3) RV infarction[5].

Contraindications

Absolute contraindications include RA or RV thrombus or tumor masses. A tricuspid or pulmonary valvular stenosis may be increased during PAC monitoring. Relative contraindications are as for central venous cannulation.

Limitations

The interpretation of PAC data is difficult, and the pitfalls numerous, especially for PAOP measurement. A questionnaire has shown that only 50% of intensive care physicians were able to identify the correct value PAOP from a clear hard copy printout[6]. A correct pressure recording requires a continuous column of fluid from the transducer to the LA, which is seldom fulfilled[7]. A PAOP increase above 5 mmHg (0.7 kPa) has a sensitivity of 2–25% and a specificity of 92–99% in detecting myocardial ischemia[8]. The American Society of Anesthesiologists' Task force on pulmonary artery catheterization does not recommend PAC for detection of myocardial ischemia because of poor sensitivity and specificity[9].

Complications

In addition to those described during CVP monitoring, PAC has numerous complications itself. In a review of PA catheterization in 6,245 patients, transient ventricular arrhythmias were reported in 68% and supraventricular arrhythmias in 1%. Persistent ventricular arrhythmias occurred in 3% after readjusting the PAC but they responded to medical treatment. Transient right BBB developed in 0.05% of the patients. Endobronchial hemorrhage was seen in four patients (0.06%), of whom one died. Another four patients had pulmonary infarction. The following risk factors for endobronchial hemorrhage were observed: age, female, pulmonary hypertension, coagulopathy, and hyperinflation of the PAC balloon[10]. Catheter knotting, thrombocytopenia, and valvular damage have been reported.

BIOCHEMICAL MARKERS

JAN RAVKILDE, MD, DMSC, FESC, FACC

INTRODUCTION

Biochemical markers are essential as a diagnostic tool in ischemic heart disease, especially in ACS, i.e. acute MI (AMI) and unstable angina pectoris (UAP). In particular, biochemical markers, while missing from the the first WHO report on diagnosis of AMI in 1959 and not represented until the early 1970s, have become the most important tool in the triad of diagnosing AMI (clinical symptoms, ECG, and biochemical markers).

REQUIREMENTS TO BIOCHEMICAL MARKERS

Before using a biochemical marker, the purpose of use must be decided, e.g. for diagnosis (early and/or late, rule-in, rule-out, definitive for AMI), for prognosis (importance of increased level at admission, peak value, risk stratification), to detect reperfusion, and/or for therapeutic guidance. Additionally, there are five important characteristics of a biochemical marker: (1) the type of biochemical marker, (2) the immunoassay to be used, (3) the discrimination limit (if any), (4) consideration of the diagnostic time-window, and (5) setting (Emergency Room, Chest Pain Unit, Cardiac Care Unit).

Creatine kinase (CK), in particular the MB isoenzymes (CKMB) and isoforms (CKMB-1, CKMB-2, CKMM-1, CKMM-2, and CKMM-3) and lactate dehydrogenase (LD), including LD-1 isoenzyme, have been the mostly used biochemical markers, but they have limited diagnostic power. Therefore, cardiac troponins I (cTnI) and T (cTnT), components of the contractile apparatus of the myocyte, have increased in importance as a diagnostic tool within the last decade.

The troponins possess characteristics that make them suitable as a biochemical marker for necrosis, being sensitive for cardiac injury and specific for cardiac tissue. More than 15 commercially available cTnI immunoassays and one cTnT immunoassay (fourth generation) are currently available. The immunoassays are continually being improved in subsequent generations. The recent description of the degradation with several fragments/complexes of the troponins is of great importance, not only for understanding the differences between the numerous cTnI immunoassays, but also for the potential different use of assays in the early phase of ischemia, their probable time setting for irreversible ischemia, and to differentiate early versus late processes in evolving AMI and cardiac related pathologies.

Further, a new and very interesting marker called ischemia modified albumin has recently been introduced. It is based on the principle that ischemia alters the ability of albumin to bind cobalt, probably through a mechanism involving free radicals. This marker may be able to separate reversible and irreversible ischemia and thereby be an even earlier marker than the present fastest markers, i.e. myoglobin and fatty acid binding protein (FABP).

DISCRIMINATION LIMIT AND DIAGNOSTIC TIME-WINDOW

A chosen discrimination limit for myocardial injury is often based on values from a normal population without cardiac disease. However, the discrimination limit chosen is not consistent as it depends on whether the upper limit of normal (>1, >2 or higher), the 97.5 or 99th percentile of normal, or a value based on the coefficient of variation of an immunoassay is used. For the troponin immunoassays, a coefficient of variation of 10% at the 99th percentile reference limit is needed to obtain acceptable imprecision.

Knowledge of the diagnostic time-window of the biochemical marker is necessary, when preparing blood sampling schedules. In ACS, a simple and reliable time schedule has been evolved by international working groups (see below), with blood sampling at admission, at 6–9 hours, and optionally at 12–24 hours if the first two samples are negative. For practical purposes all three blood samples should be collected. The dissimilarity in time curves of the most common biochemical markers used in ACS is shown in **221A, B**.

221 A: Biochemical marker release in a patient with acute myocardial infarction. Individual time courses with relative concentrations, i.e. 1 = upper limit of normal. cTnI is not illustrated based on the numerous different assays measuring different complexes of cTnI (see text). **B**: Similar figure to **A** but with changed abscissa and ordinate to highlight the marker time-curves in the early period. m-ASAT is omitted in this figure. CK: creatine kinase; CKMB: creatine kinase MB fraction ; LC1: light chain isotype 1; LD1: lactate dehydrogenase isoenzyme 1; m-ASAT: mitochondrial aspartate aminotransferase.

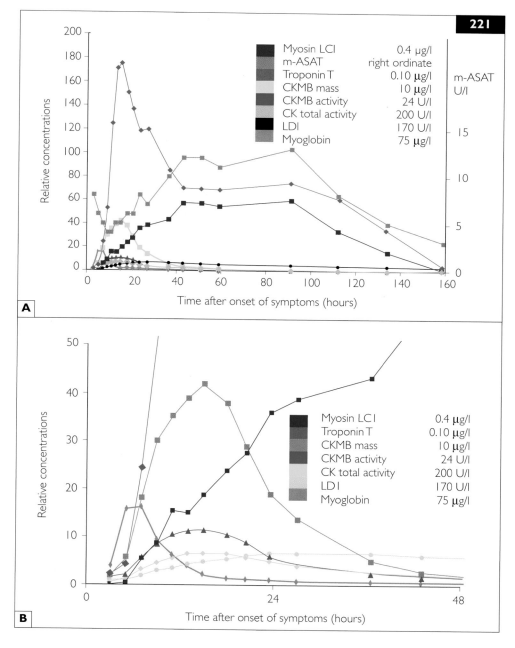

DIAGNOSTIC AND PROGNOSTIC SIGNIFICANCE

A gray zone has always existed between UAP and definite AMI. Over the years, isoenzymes of already existing biochemical markers or improved immunoassays have been introduced and integrated into the diagnosis of AMI without common guidelines. This has resulted in an astounding diversity in the diagnosis of AMI between, and even within, countries. However, not much attention has been paid to these changes in diagnosis internationally until the introduction of the troponins in the early 1990s. Numerous publications between 1992 and the millennium have been important in altering the concept of diagnosis of AMI today. These studies demonstrated the potential of the troponins to detect a subgroup of around one-third of the patients suspected of AMI or UAP with increased troponin levels, and subsequently showed these patients to have a three- to fivefold increased risk of a short-term cardiac event (**222, 223**).

The integration of novel biochemical markers of myocardial damage to the routine diagnosis of ACS is not without difficulty. However, the working groups of the International Federation of Clinical Chemistry (IFCC) in Europe and the National Academy of Clinical Biochemistry (NACB) in the USA, coupled with the consensus report of the European Society of Cardiology and the American College of Cardiology have supported the use of troponins. There still remain unclarified issues with regard to standardization of assays and decision limits. The definition of AMI in 2004 is still based on the WHO triad, with the main focus on a combination of ECG changes and biochemical markers, especially the troponins. These are today used on an operational and confirming basis; an early diagnosis made within minutes to the first hour after admission is based on ST-segment elevation, non-ST segment elevation, or is judged clinically as UAP. This early diagnosis is named the operational diagnosis (evolving MI). A later diagnosis is made within hours to the first days, and is based on the possible development of Q waves in the ECG (Q wave or non-Q wave MI), as well as elevated biochemical markers used to confirm the diagnosis (healing or healed MI).

SOURCES OF ERROR

Although the troponins are highly cardiac specific, increases of troponin are seen in a proportion of patients in certain clinical conditions. Congestive heart failure, ventricular and supraventricular tachycardia, hemodynamic conditions (e.g. shock), pulmonary embolism, aortic dissection, myocarditis, renal failure (in particular hemodialysis), stroke, drug toxicity (e.g. certain types of antineoplastic agents) can all increase troponin levels above normal values. This can lead to diagnostic confusion as the increased troponin is often assumed to be as a result of infarction. Troponin is a marker of *injury*, not only a marker of infarction, thus all causes of cardiac injury need to be considered. Although these novel biomarkers have improved the diagnostic capability, they are only tools to be used in conjunction with clinical judgement.

SURGERY AND PERCUTANEOUS CORONARY INTERVENTION

The troponins can be used as markers of myocardial injury in noncardiac surgery, similarly to their use in ACS patients. In cardiac surgery and after PCI, the current guideline suggests that a level greater than fivefold (the upper limit of normal after cardiac surgery) and greater than threefold (the upper limit of normal in post-PCI patients) is indicative of myocardial injury. However, in ACS patients undergoing cardiac surgery or PCI the case is much more complex, and further studies are still needed to refine the application for these populations.

NEW MARKERS OF RISK

The clinical application of cardiac biomarkers in ACS is no longer limited to establishing or refuting the diagnosis of myocardial necrosis. New markers associated with worse clinical outcomes include C-reactive protein (CRP, high-sensitivity testing) and other systemic markers of inflammation (e.g. transcription factor nuclear factor kappa B, interleukin 6, serum amyloid A protein, and whole blood choline [marker of phospholipase D]), soluble CD40 ligand (sCD40L), brain natriuretic peptide (BNP), and pregnancy-associated plasma protein A (PAPP-A). Although these markers are nonspecific for myocardial ischemia/necrosis, their elevation in ACS indicates the presence of a high-risk state. Thus, clinical observations indicate that besides troponins, CRP, sCD40L, and BNP each provides unique prognostic information in patients with ACS.

222 Individual time courses with relative concentrations of biochemical markers in a patient with unstable angina pectoris and subsequent acute myocardial infarction. CKMB: creatine kinase MB fraction.

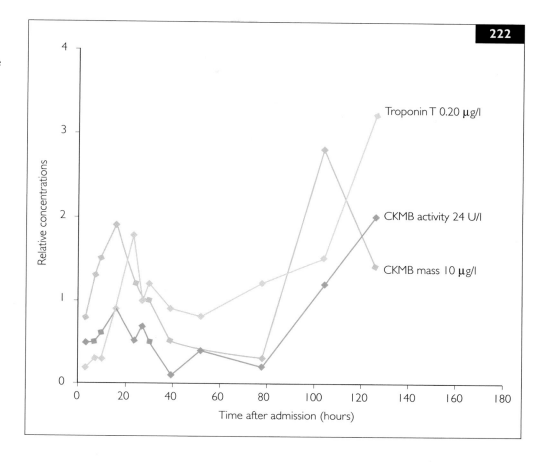

223 Histogram showing the proportion of cTn positive (Tn pos) and cTn negative (Tn neg) patients in suspected acute myocardial infarction or unstable angina pectoris based on the peak cTn value after serial blood sampling (red bars). The prognostic value of these subgroups is indicated in the blue bars and shows the events (cardiac death, acute myocardial infarction). (Based on combined results from 17 studies from the years 1992–1999 comprising 3194 patients.)

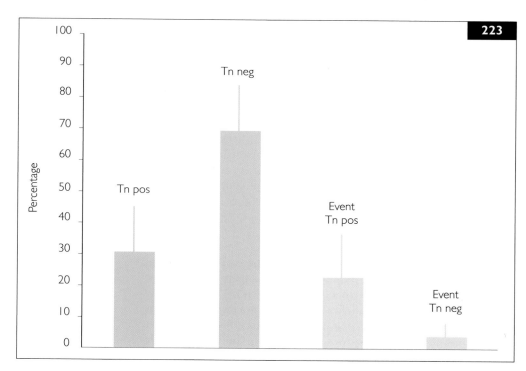

Chapter Nine

Stable Ischemic Syndromes

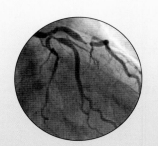

STABLE ANGINA PECTORIS

JENS ERIK NIELSEN-KUDSK, MD, DMSC

DEFINITION

Angina pectoris is defined as discomfort in the chest or adjacent areas caused by myocardial ischemia. In the syndrome of chronic stable angina it occurs in a predictable manner, typically with physical exertion or mental stress, and is relieved by rest or nitroglycerin.

EPIDEMIOLOGY

Chronic stable angina is the initial manifestation of ischemic heart disease (IHD) in appoximately 50% of patients. The prevalence is 30,000–40,000 per million. It increases markedly with age and is more prevalent in men than women until the age of 75 years.

PATHOGENESIS

Angina pectoris results from myocardial ischemia that occurs when there is an imbalance in myocardial oxygen supply and demand. Most patients with stable angina have underlying obstructive coronary atherosclerotic lesions that limit myocardial blood flow during periods of increased demand. Paradoxic vasoconstriction of atherosclerotic epicardial coronary arteries with exercise due to endothelial dysfunction is likely to contribute to the limitation of coronary blood flow (CBF). Some patients with severe left ventricular hypertrophy (LVH) (aortic stenosis or hypertrophic cardiomyopathy [HCM]) may suffer from angina pectoris even in the presence of normal coronary arteries due to increased myocardial oxygen demand.

CLINICAL PRESENTATION

Patients with stable angina most often have a typical history of chest discomfort brought on by physical activity, emotional stress, heavy meals, or exposure to cold weather. The patients may experience a feeling of strangling and discomfort in the chest, as if someone was sitting on it or a band was put tightly around it. It is often a pressure-like, squeezing, or heavy feeling that only infrequently is described as pain. The discomfort is most often retrosternal and may radiate to the ulnar site of the left arm, left shoulder, neck, jaw, right arm, upper arms, back, or epigastrium (**224**). Sometimes it is primarily felt in the areas adjacent to the chest. In some patients (often diabetics), angina is a more vague feeling of fatigue or dyspnea ('angina equivalents'). The duration of an anginal episode is usually only a few minutes. It is relieved by cessation of exertion or quickly ceases (0.5–3 min) after nitroglycerin. Although the threshold for angina is variable, the frequency of anginal episodes is quite stable over months in this syndrome.

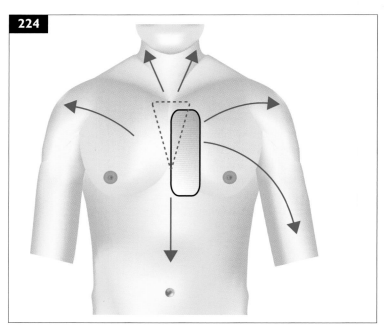

224 Schematic diagram to show the pattern of discomfort in angina pectoris. Discomfort is typically located behind the sternum towards the left side of the chest. It may radiate to the left arm, left shoulder, neck, jaw, right shoulder, upper arms, epigastrium, or the back.

DIAGNOSIS

A detailed history is the most important step in the diagnosis of stable angina. Chest discomfort should be characterized according to quality, location, duration, and factors that provoke and relieve it. This will allow a grouping into typical angina, atypical angina, or noncardiac chest pain (*Table 28*). The severity of angina should be assessed according to the Canadian Cardiovascular Society (CCS) clasification of angina (*Table 29*). Information about risk factors such as smoking, hyperlipidemia, diabetes, hypertension, and a family history of premature IHD are important. Resting electrocardiogram (ECG) is abnormal in 50% of patients showing ST/T changes and/or Q waves. Possible associated conditions such as valvular heart disease or anemia should be identified.

Noninvasive cardiac stress testing (exercise-ECG, radionuclide perfusion imaging, or stress echocardiography) may provide additional diagnostic information in the group of patients with atypical angina (**225**). Negative test results indicate a very low likelihood of IHD and a good prognosis. Coronary angiography

---

Table 28 Classification of chest discomfort

Typical angina:
- Retrosternal chest discomfort with a characteristic quality and duration.
- Provoked by exertion or emotional stress.
- Relieved by rest or nitroglycerin.

Atypical angina:
- Two out of three characteristics of typical angina.

Noncardiac chest pain:
- None of the characteristics of typical angina.

Table 29 Classification of the severity of angina (Canadian Cardiovascular Society; CCS)

CCS-class I: Ordinary physical activity does not cause angina, e.g. walking, climbing stairs. Angina occurs with strenuous, rapid, or prolonged exertion at work or recreation.

CCS-class II: Slight limitation of ordinary activity. Angina occurs on walking or climbing stairs rapidly; walking uphill; walking or stair climbing after meals, in cold, in wind, or under emotional stress; or only during the few hours after awakening. Angina occurs on walking more than two blocks on the level and climbing more than one flight of ordinary stairs at a normal pace and in normal conditions.

CCS-class III: Marked limitations of ordinary physical activity. Angina occurs on walking one or two blocks on the level, and on climbing one flight of stairs in normal conditions and at a normal pace.

CCS-class IV: Inability to carry on any physical activity without discomfort; anginal symptoms may be present at rest.

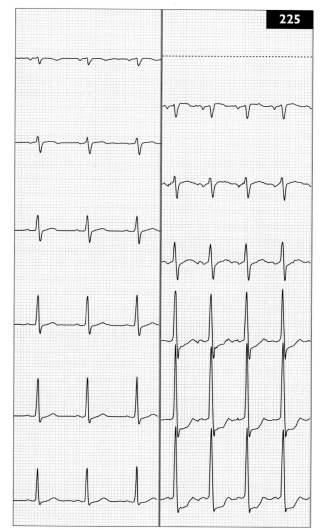

225 Electrocardiogram tracings (V_1–V_6) taken from a 70-year-old male with stable angina pectoris (CCS-class III) at rest (**A**) and during bicycle exercise test at a load of 50 W (**B**). There is marked ST segment depression in V_4–V_6 during exercise. The coronary angiogram is shown in **226**.

(CAG) should be performed in patients with positive test results (**226**). Patients with typical angina have a very high likelihood of IHD and should be evaluated by CAG. CAG plays a pivotal role in the management of patients with stable angina. It accurately determines the extent, severity, and localization of atherosclerotic coronary artery lesions, gives important information on prognosis, and is required for therapeutic decisions about myocardial revascularization. Noninvasive CAG by multi-slice computed tomography (CT) scanning or magnetic resonance imaging (MRI) is expected to be incorporated into clinical practice in the near future.

DIFFERENTIAL DIAGNOSIS

Acute myocardial infarction (AMI) is typically associated with severe and prolonged angina-like chest pain that occurs at rest. Acute aortic dissection produces severe chest pain which is sharp in character and radiates to the back. Acute pericarditis and pleuritis produce chest pain that is synchronous with respiration. Angina can be provoked in severe pulmonary arterial hypertension due to right ventricular ischemia. Also, gastrointestinal disorders (esophageal reflux or spasm, peptic ulcer, pancreatitis, cholelithiasis) and musculoskeletal disorders in the chest wall or back should be considered.

MANAGEMENT

The aim of treatment in stable chronic angina is to reduce symptoms, inhibit the progression of coronary atherosclerosis, and reduce the risk of acute coronary syndromes (ACS) or death. The treatment contains five main elements (*Table 30*).

Modification of risk factors

Cessation of smoking, proper control of hypertension and diabetes, physical activity, low-fat Mediterranean-like diet and correction of overweight are all important factors in the general management of stable chronic angina. Large clinical trials have shown that cholesterol-lowering statins reduce mortality and the risk of acute myocardial infarction (MI). In the 'Heart Protection Study' involving more than 20,000 patients, these beneficial prognostic effects were found irrespective of initial cholesterol concentrations even in those patients with plasma cholesterol <5 mmol/l (193 mg/dl).

Antiplatelet therapy

Treatment with low-dose aspirin (75–150 mg daily) reduces the risk of MI and death and should be given to all patients with ischemic heart disease. Clopidogrel is used in patients who do not tolerate aspirin.

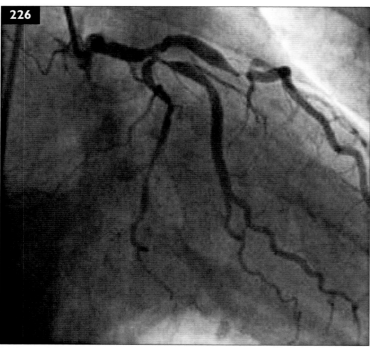

226 Coronary angiogram from a 70-year-old male with stable angina pectoris (CCS-class III). Exercise electrocardiogram was positive, showing marked ST segment depression in V_4–V_6 (**225**). There is a severe proximal left anterior descending coronary artery stenosis and a proximal stenosis on a large, obtuse, marginal branch.

Table 30 Treatment of stable angina pectoris

Modification of risk factors:
- Cessation of smoking.
- Control of hypertension and diabetes.
- Low-fat Mediterranean-like diet.
- Correction of overweight.
- Physical activity.
- Cholesterol-lowering statins.

Antiplatelet therapy:
- Aspirin.
- Clopidogrel.

Anti-ischemic drugs:
- Nitrates.
- Beta blockers.
- Calcium channel blockers.
- Nicorandil.

Angiotensin-converting enzyme inhibitors

Myocardial revascularization:
- Percutaneous coronary intervention (PCI).
- Coronary artery bypass grafting (CABG).

Anti-ischemic drugs

Nitrates are NO-donors that dilate epicardial coronary arteries and collaterals, and reduce cardiac preload by venodilation. Nitroglycerin is highly effective for the treatment of acute angina episodes. The effect of long-acting nitrates is limited by the development of tolerance. Beta blockers reduce myocardial oxygen demand by a reduction in heart rate and contractility. They increase myocardial blood flow by prolonging diastole. Beta blockers reduce mortality in post-MI patients and also have antiarrhythmic effects. Calcium channel blockers are coronary vasodilators that also reduce afterload by peripheral vasodilatation. Some of these drugs additionally slow heart rate.

Nicorandil is an opener of ATP-sensitive potassium channels and is also a NO-donor. It dilates coronary arteries and reduces cardiac preload and afterload. It reduces the risk of ACS.

Angiotensin-converting enzyme inhibitors

It is well established that angiotensin-converting enzyme (ACE) inhibitors improve prognosis in patients with left ventricular systolic dysfunction. In the HOPE study, ramipril reduced cardiovascular death, MI, and stroke in patients who were at high risk for, or had, vascular disease in the absence of heart failure. In the EUROPA trial, perindopril reduced the risk of cardiovascular death, MI, or cardiac arrest in a low-risk population with stable coronary heart disease and no apparent heart failure. However, in the PEACE trial, trandolapril failed to reduce cardiovascular death, MI, and revascularization in a large low-risk population of patients with coronary artery disease (CAD) and preserved left ventricular function. In this study, the patients received a more aggressive risk factor management (70% on statins) than did those in HOPE and EUROPA. In CAD with preserved left ventricular function, ACE inhibitors should not be routinely used but considered when diabetes or a poor risk factor status is present.

Myocardial revascularization

Treatment of angina by percutaneous coronary intervention (PCI) or coronary artery bypass grafting (CABG) produces better relief of symptoms, higher exercise capacity, and higher quality of life compared with medical treatment. In patients with left main stem stenosis, three-vessel disease, or proximal left anterior descending coronary artery (LAD) stenosis, myocardial revascularization improves prognosis. Drugs that prolong life in stable chronic angina should be continued after successful revascularization.

PROGNOSIS

The over-all prognosis in stable angina is good, with a mortality of 2–3% and a risk of acute MI of 2–3% per year. Patients with reduced left ventricular function, heart failure, left main stem stenosis, proximal LAD stenosis, or three-vessel disease have a higher risk of death.

PRINZMETAL'S VARIANT ANGINA

JOSEPH ARAGON, MD AND PREDIMAN K. SHAH, MD

INTRODUCTION

Prinzmetal's angina, also known as variant angina pectoris, is an uncommon clinical syndrome that was first identified as a distinct clinical entity by Myron Prinzmetal and Rexford Kennamer of Cedars Sinai Medical Center in the early 1950s. This syndrome is characterized by recurrent episodes of chest pain at rest that are associated with transient elevations of ST segment on the ECG (227). This syndrome is most often caused by epicardial coronary artery spasm, leading to transient reduction in epicardial coronary artery lumen size and reduction in blood flow. Coronary spasm may be focal (most often) or diffuse (228), and may be localized to one artery (most often) or may occur in multiple arteries. CAG reveals minimal to no fixed coronary luminal stenosis in about 30–40% of cases, whereas fixed stenosis is present in 60–70% of cases. Recent studies using intravascular ultrasound (IVUS) have helped to confirm the presence of atherosclerotic changes at sites of coronary vasospasm, and have also suggested that the process(es) of coronary spasm is/are associated with a high incidence of negative coronary remodeling at the site of the spasm. Continuous ECG monitoring frequently reveals a relatively high frequency of asymptomatic ST segment elevation in these patients.

Ventricular arrhythmias, sinoatrial node and atrioventricular node (AVN) dysfunction may occur during ischemic episodes or soon after resolution of ischemic episodes. Ischemic episodes often cluster around evenings and early mornings and may be trigerred by exposure to cold, hyperventilation, vasoconstrictor agents, and alcohol. In premenopausal women with Prinzmetal angina, clustering of ischemic episodes during times of low circulating estrogen levels has also been demonstrated.

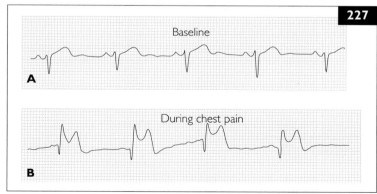

227 Baseline (**A**) and spontaneous transient ST segment elevation (**B**) on an electrocardiogram recording during an episode of rest angina in a patient with Prinzmetal's angina. The patient was later shown to have no angiographic evidence of fixed coronary stenosis.

DIAGNOSIS

In suspected cases, diagnosis may be established during CAG using ergonovine or acetylcholine to unmask the tendency for coronary spasm (**229**). Provocative testing with ergonovine is not recommended when the diagnosis is clear or when severe fixed coronary stenosis coexists. Noninvasive provocative testing using hyperventilation to induce transient ST segment elevation has also been advocated.

PROGNOSIS

Cardiac mortality or morbidity in the patient with Prinzmetal's angina is infrequent but can occur, depending on the presence and severity of associated coronary atherosclerosis. Patients without angiographic signs of fixed luminal obstruction generally have an excellent prognosis. A higher risk of cardiac events is observed in patients with associated severe multi-vessel stenosis, those who develop ventricular arrhythmias during or following ischemic episodes, and when increased QT interval dispersion is present on a 12-lead ECG.

MECHANISMS OF CORONARY SPASM

The precise mechanisms of coronary spasm remain unclear but endothelial dysfunction related to underlying atherosclerosis, as well as abnormalities of vasomotor autonomic tone and hypersensitivity of the vascular smooth muscle cells to vasomotor stimuli have been implicated (**230**). Recently, abnormalities of cardiac membrane potassium channels have been suggested, based on experimental studies in murine models of coronary vasospam (**231, 232**).

MANAGEMENT

Management of Prinzmetal's angina includes elimination of provocative agents. Cigarette smoking, cocaine use or withdrawal, unneeded cold exposure, hyperventilation, alcohol withdrawal, and use of vasoconstrictive agents have been shown to precipitate coronary spasm. Drug therapy includes the use of long-acting nitrates and calcium channel blockers, either as monotherapy or as combination therapy. In patients unable to take nitrates and calcium blockers, or when these agents are not effective, anecdotal reports of the benefits from vitamin E (as an antioxidant), cyproheptidine, and percutaneous transluminal coronary angioplasty (PTCA)/stenting have appeared, but their precise role remains unclear. Recent evaluation of a cohort of patients with Prinzmetal's angina associated with a severe epicardial coronary stenosis treated with PCI revealed that spasm could be frequently induced at other coronary sites, despite good angiographic results

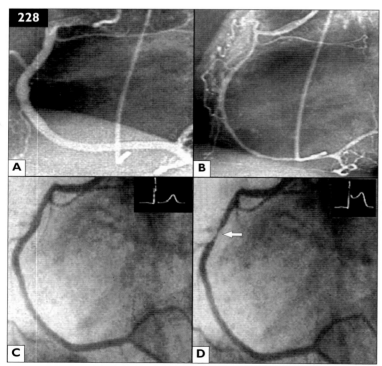

228 Right coronary angiograms of two patients with Prinzmetal's angina showing two different patterns of spontaneous coronary spasm: diffuse spasm (**A**: baseline; **B**: spasm) and focal spasm (**C**: baseline; **D**: focal spasm; insets show corresponding electrocardiogram trace).

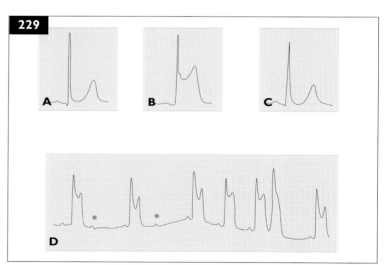

229 Electrocardiogram from a patient with Prinzmetal's angina. **A**: Pain-free state. **B**: Transient ST segment elevation. **C**: Following sublingual nitroglycerin administration, chest pain and ST segment elevation have resolved. Angiography demonstrated no evidence of fixed coronary stenosis, and spasm of the right coronary artery was induced by ergonovine administration. During this induced coronary spasm, 2nd degree atrioventricular block was noted along with ST segment elevation (**D**: non-conducted p waves are marked with an asterisk).

post-PCI and the absence of significant restenosis. This suggests that calcium antagonists and/or nitrates should be continued in patients treated with PCI. When it can be demonstrated that the distal part of the artery is not involved in spasm (by angiography)

CABG surgery has been successful. This is particularly the case when spasm is well localized to a proximal site with associated atherosclerotic obstruction.

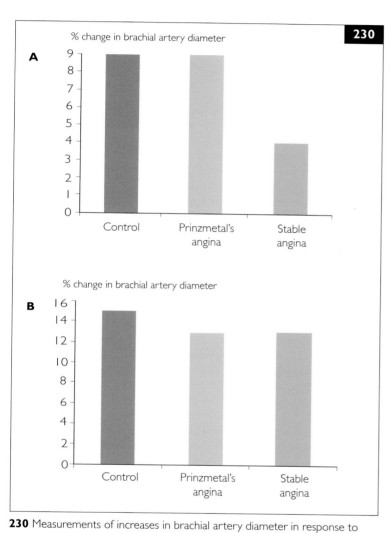

230 Measurements of increases in brachial artery diameter in response to increased flow (**A**, endothelium-dependent) and nitroglycerin (**B**, endothelium-independent) are shown in normal control subjects (blue), in patients with Prinzmetal's angina (pink), and in patients with coronary artery disease with exercise-induced angina (green). Patients with the usual form of coronary artery disease with exercise-induced angina have reduced endothelium-dependent vasodilator response compared to normal controls and patients with Prinzmetal's angina. Nonendothelium-dependent direct vasodilator responses are similar in all three groups of subjects. (Modified from Ito *et al.* [1999]. Systemic endothelial function is preserved in men with both active and inactive variant angina pectoris. *Am. J. Cardiol.* **84**:1347–1349.)

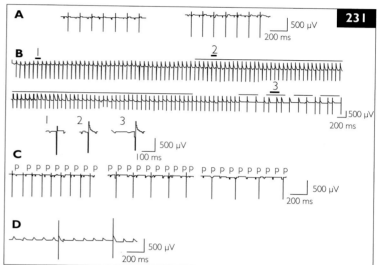

231 Representative electrocardiograms (ECG) from wild-type and Kir6.1-null mice using radio telemetry. **A**: Normal ECGs from wild-type (left) and Kir6.1-null (right) mice. **B**: Spontaneous ST elevations and atrioventricular (AV) block in ECG recorded from Kir6.1-null mouse. A longer period of recording (16 seconds), including ST elevation (solid line) and AV block (dotted line), is shown. Typical waveforms at time points indicated in the chart (1, 2, and 3) are shown in greater detail. ST elevation appears in all Kir6.1-null mice examined (*n* = 4). The elevation lasted for a short time, and then returned to baseline. After a short latency period, the ST elevation was followed by AV blocks of various degrees as shown in **C**. **C**: ECGs of first (left), second (middle), and third (right) AV block in Kir6.1-null mice. P: P wave. **D**: Bradycardia in Kir6.1-null mouse. The chart is a representative ECG of marked bradycardia in 1 of the 2 Kir6.1-null mice that died during ECG monitoring (Modified from Miki *et al.* [2002]. Mouse model of Prinzmetal angina by disruption of the inward rectifier Kir6.1. *Nature Medicine* **8**:466–472.)

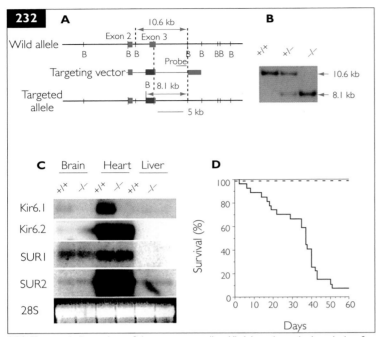

232 Targeted disruption of the gene encoding Kir6.1 and survival analysis of Kir6.1-null mice. **A**: Maps of the Kir6.1 locus, targeting vector and the resulting targeted locus. The open, shaded, filled, and gray boxes indicate untranslated exon, coding exon, neomycin-resistant gene, and thymidine kinase gene, respectively. B: *Bam*HI site. **B**: Southern-blot analysis of genomic DNA digested with *Bam*HI from wild-type (+/+), Kir6.1-heterozygous (+/-) and Kir6.1-null (-/-) mice. **C**: Northern-blot analysis of RNAs from wild-type and Kir6.1-null mice. **D**: Survival of wild-type (thin line, n = 36), Kir6.1-heterozygous (dotted line, n = 67), and Kir6.1-null (thick line, n = 27) mice after birth. (Modified from Miki et al. [2002]. Mouse model of Prinzmetal angina by disruption of the inward rectifier Kir6.1. *Nature Medicine* **8**:466–472.)

CARDIAC SYNDROME X

HANS ERIK BØTKER, MD, PhD

DEFINITION
Cardiac syndrome X is defined as a syndrome comprising angina pectoris, ≥ 0.1 mV ST segment depression during exercise stress testing, and normal CAGs in patients without other specific cardiac or vascular disease.

EPIDEMIOLOGY
Between 10 and 30% of patients who undergo CAG because of angina pectoris have normal-appearing epicardial coronary arteries on angiogram. The majority have specific cardiac and vascular disease such as arterial hypertension, cardiomyopathy, valvular disease, and others (see Chapter 5, Microvascular disease) that may compromise microvascular function and lead to myocardial ischemia. After exclusion of specific disorders, patients with syndrome X constitute 0.5–1% of the patients, the majority (70–80%) being women. The age of onset is similar in patients with syndrome X and patients with coronary atherosclerosis.

PATHOGENESIS
The pathophysiology of cardiac syndrome X has not been established. The syndrome is heterogeneous by nature and contains cardiac and noncardiac components, without a unifying mechanism. Even though the coronary arteries appear smooth on the CAG, up to 60% of the patients reveal atheromatous disease and intimal thickening, which may affect coronary vasomotion.

Approximately 40% of patients with syndrome X have an abnormally reduced capacity to increase coronary perfusion. The evidence for myocardial ischemia in terms of metabolic and functional consequences of the reduced coronary flow reserve is not demonstrable in the majority of patients, indicating that heterogeneity of perfusion may lead to patchily distributed ischemia (**233**) or subendocardial ischemia (**234**). However,

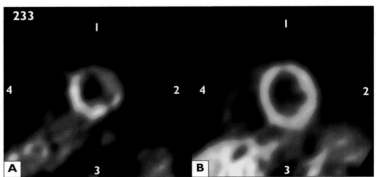

233 Heterogeneity of myocardial perfusion in a patient with syndrome X; studies with positron emission tomography and ^{13}N ammonia as perfusion tracer. **A**: Syndrome X. **B**: Healthy control. 1: anterior; 2: left; 3: posterior; 4: right.

mechanisms other than ischemia may be responsible for the symptoms in a considerable number of cases (*Table 31*). A patchy prearteriolar constriction may lead to compensatory release of adenosine, which mediates dilatation of the coronary arterioles by stimulating adenosine A_2 receptors, in order to assure adequate perfusion in these areas. Because adenosine also acts as a pain messenger, the resulting increase in adenosine concentrations in the myocardial interstitium causes pain by stimulation of adenosine A_1 receptors.

Interstitial accumulation of potassium caused by abnormalities in potassium metabolism may also provoke pain. Potassium modifies systemic and coronary vasoreactivity. Myocardial accumulation of potassium may account for all of the features of cardiac syndrome X, including angina pectoris, ST segment changes, and reduced coronary flow reserve (CFR). Abnormal handling of afferent messages from the heart by the central nervous system has also been recognized in some patients with syndrome X.

CLINICAL PRESENTATION
Anginal attacks may be of prolonged duration and with a poor response to sublingual nitrates. Traditional prophylactic antianginal

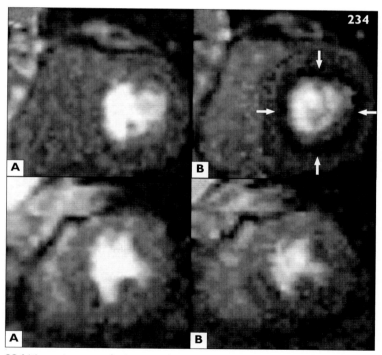

234 Magnetic resonance images of myocardial perfusion with gadolinium at rest (**A**) and during exercise (**B**). **Upper**: Delayed subendocardial perfusion during exercise in a patient with syndrome X. **Lower**: Uniform myocardial perfusion at rest and during exercise in a healthy control subject. (From Panting *et al.* [2002]. Abnormal subendocardial perfusion in cardiac syndrome X detected by cardiovascular magnetic resonance imaging. *N. Engl. J. Med.* **346**:1948–1953. With permission. Copyright 2002 Massachusetts Medical Society. All rights reserved.)

medication is often insufficient in syndrome X. In addition to angina pectoris, many patients suffer from generalized fatigue in skeletal muscles. The symptoms are similar to those seen in patients who have fibromyalgia.

DIAGNOSIS
The combination of angina pectoris, a normal coronary angiogram and ischemic ST segment depression of at least 0.1 mV during an exercise stress test occurs in syndrome X. However, in order to diagnose syndrome X, it is necessary to exclude other causes for the symptoms, such as a cardiac or other generalized disorder for which specific therapy is obtainable. A thorough medical history and clinical examination often uncover the presence of a generalized disorder, which may affect the coronary micro-circulation. If appropriate, serological markers must be measured. Echocardiography can clarify whether specific cardiac diseases such as valvular disease, cardiomyopathies, deposit diseases, and pericardial diseases are present. Epicardial spasms are excluded by a provocative spasm test.

To clarify whether syndrome X is caused by microvascular dysfunction requires measurement of the CFR by positron emission tomography (PET) and perfusion markers such as ^{13}N-ammonia and ^{15}O-water at rest and after maximum vasodilatation achieved with papaverine, dipyridamole, or adenosine. The result rarely has therapeutic consequences, but may be helpful for exclusion of differential diseases in some patients. PET and single photon emission computerized tomography (SPECT) can be used for semiquantitative purposes to clarify whether a patient has a heterogeneous distribution of blood flow in the heart (**233**).

DIFFERENTIAL DIAGNOSIS
The differential diagnosis includes epicardial spasm ('variant angina') and myocardial ischemia caused by microvascular dysfunction due to specific cardiac diseases.

Table 31 Mechanisms that contribute to a reduced coronary flow reserve in cardiac syndrome X

- Microvascular spasm.
- Endothelial dysfunction.
- Capillary rarefaction.
- Coronary artery hyperreactivity.
- Increased circulating endogenous vasoconstrictor peptides.
- Estrogen deficiency.
- Increased adrenergic tone.
- Prearteriolar constriction and patchy release of adenosine.
- Abnormal interstitial release of potassium.
- Increased pain perception.

MANAGEMENT

Since the prognosis is good, the goal of therapy is a reduction in the frequency and the severity of pain. The cornerstone of therapy remains reassurance, but many patients need medical therapy. Because treatment is empiric and efficacy is lower than in classic CAD, the goal may be difficult to accomplish. Thus, treatment of patients with syndrome X must be based on a good doctor–patient relationship and requires patience.

Nitrates influence microvasculature to a limited extent. Patients who have pain relief by sublingual nitroglycerin usually benefit from nitrate preparations with prolonged duration. Beta blockers produce improvement in exercise-induced angina pectoris in patients who have evidence of enhanced sympathetic tone, which can be detected by a rapid increase in rate–pressure product during exercise stress testing.

Calcium channel blockers may reduce anginal attacks. Aminophylline is a rational treatment for patients who have abnormal adenosine metabolism and has beneficial effects on angina pectoris in some patients with syndrome X. Unfortunately, no specific test allows identification of this subgroup.

Estrogen (β_{17}-estradiol) has beneficial influence on exercise-induced angina pectoris and may be recommended for postmenopausal women who have syndrome X.

Imipramine reduces anginal episodes in patients who have normal coronary angiograms, but is only recommended for patients for whom other agents are not applicable due to side-effects. Nonnarcotic analgesics may be used in patients who have cardiac syndrome X. Narcotic analgesic agents should be used infrequently for pronounced anginal attacks that are not relieved by other treatment. Spinal cord stimulation reduces exercise-induced angina in selected patients with syndrome X.

PROGNOSIS

The prognosis of patients who have cardiac syndrome X is good with regard to mortality and incidence of MI. The social prognosis is poor in patients with persistent anginal symptoms and an insufficient response to medical therapy.

A small subgroup of patients, initially classified as having syndrome X, may experience deterioration in left ventricular function over time. These patients present with left bundle branch block (LBBB) at rest or during exercise stress testing, and are considered to be suffering from cardiomyopathy.

Chapter Ten

Acute Coronary Syndromes

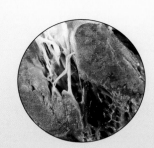

NON-ST ELEVATION ACUTE CORONARY SYNDROMES

R.J. DE WINTER, MD, PhD, FESC

DEFINITION

Patients presenting with progressive chest pain at rest or with minimal exertion, caused by myocardial ischemia, potentially have what is now called an acute coronary syndrome (ACS). The admission electrocardiogram (ECG) will distinguish between patients with ST elevation, who may be candidates for reperfusion therapy, and patients without ST elevation. The latter group then either has evidence of myocardial necrosis (non-ST elevation myocardial infarction, NSTEMI) or no myocardial necrosis (unstable angina pectoris, UAP).

EPIDEMIOLOGY

In the United States, over 5 million visits to the emergency department each year are for the evaluation of chest pain and related symptoms. Typically, about 10% of patients are diagnosed with an ACS. Thus, both the initial triage and subsequent treatment of chest pain patients signify an important burden on health care resources.

PATHOGENESIS

UAP and NSTEMI often, but not always, result from rupture or denudation of a vulnerable plaque, with subsequent superimposed platelet-rich thrombus formation. Typically, an occlusive thrombus in a large epicardial coronary artery will lead to transmural myocardial ischemia and ST elevation on the standard 12-lead surface ECG. In contrast, a nonocclusive thrombus with cyclic growth and disintegration of platelet aggregates, often accompanied by distal vasospasm, leads to intermittent flow impairment and subendocardial or nontransmural myocardial ischemia. This in turn will be visible on the standard 12-lead ECG as ST segment depression or T wave changes (**235**). Long-standing subendocardial ischemia will eventually result in subendocardial or nontransmural infarction, which will not be represented by Q waves on the standard 12-lead ECG (**236**).

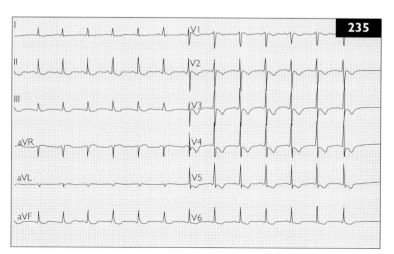

235 Standard 12-lead electrocardiogram of an 80-year-old male patient presenting with chest pain at rest. There is widespread ST segment depression in leads II, III, aVF, and V5–V6 and T wave inversion in leads V2–V6, signifying diffuse subendocardial ischemia. On subsequent angiography, the patient was diagnosed with severe diffuse three-vessel coronary artery disease.

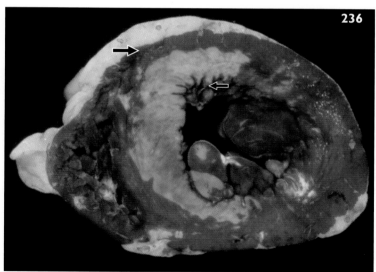

236 Postmortem section of the mid-portion of the heart from the patient in **235**, showing the demarcated infarct zone several months after the occurrence of a non-Q wave acute myocardial infarction. The 2 mm subendocardial layer (small arrow) and the 6 mm epicardial zone of myocardial tissue that survived the infarct (large arrow) are clearly visible. (Courtesy of Dr. A. van der Wal and Prof. A.E. Becker, Department of Cardiovascular Pathology, Academic Medical Center, Amsterdam.)

In recent years it has become apparent that not only does inflammation play an important role in the pathogenesis of the gradual and insidious process of atherosclerotic coronary disease, but that the onset of instability and plaque rupture is due to inflammatory activation. Infiltration of activated T-lymphocytes and macrophages can be observed in the shoulder region of the fibrous cap where plaque rupture occurs. Atherectomy specimens of coronary lesions with complex angiographic morphology from patients presenting with an ACS show T-lymphocyte and macrophage infiltration (**237**). In contrast, plaques from patients with stable angina and simple lesion morphology predominantly show smooth muscle cells.

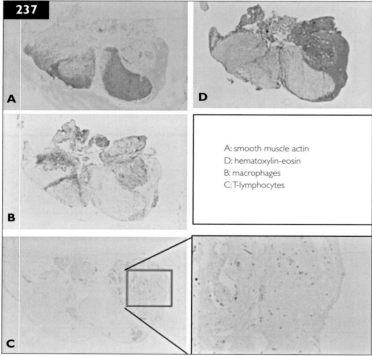

237 Atherectomy specimen from a patient presenting with severe unstable angina, Braunwald class IIIb, and a complex lesion with irregular contours and rough edges on the coronary angiogram. Immunohistochemistry was performed with Mabs against smooth muscle α-actin (**A**), CD-68 for macrophages (**B**), and CD-3 for T-cells (**C**), Hematoxylin-eosin (**D**). There is a significant positive association between the extent of atherosclerotic plaque inflammation and angiographic grading of coronary lesion complexity according to Ambrose (Meuwissen *et al.* [2001]. Coronary plaque inflammation in relation to angiographic appearance of coronary narrowings. *JACC* **37**(Suppl.A):242A).

DIFFERENTIAL DIAGNOSIS

It is important to recognize several (not uncommon) clinical conditions that can mimic non-ST elevation ACS:

- Occlusive thrombosis in a large epicardial coronary artery supplying the postero-lateral myocardium with transmural ischemia but without ST elevation on the 12-lead standard ECG. This can be detected by recording lateral leads V7–V12 or documenting wall motion abnormalities on the echocardiogram.
- Occlusive thrombosis in a large epicardial coronary artery supplying an area of myocardium that has collateral vessel residual perfusion, preventing transmural ischemia.
- Supply/demand mismatch due to increased myocardial work load or tachyarrhythmias with a fixed coronary artery stenosis.
- Prinzmetal or variant angina.
- Subendocardial ischemia in the setting of left ventricular hypertrophy (LVH) due to other cardiac conditions such as severe aortic stenosis or hypertrophic cardiomyopathy, or noncardiac conditions such as hypertension.
- Right ventricular ischemia due to sudden pressure overload with acute pulmonary embolism.
- Pericarditis and myocarditis.

CLINICAL PRESENTATION
Risk stratification

Early risk stratification in patients with non-ST elevation ACS consists of two parts: (1) assessing the likelihood of the disease, obstructive coronary artery disease due to arterial thrombosis, being present, and (2) assessing the likelihood of adverse clinical outcome, or the risk of short-term or long-term occurrence of death, nonfatal acute myocardial infarction (AMI), stroke, congestive heart failure, recurrent ischemia, or serious arrhythmia.

Patients are considered to have either a low, intermediate, or high risk of short-term complications according to the history (prior myocardial infarction [MI], coronary artery bypass graft [CABG]), rapidity of onset of symptoms, characteristics of chest discomfort, clinical findings such as age, gender, hemodynamic, or rhythmic instability, ECG changes, and the presence or absence of elevated cardiac markers that signify myocardial necrosis.

The distal embolization of platelet aggregates and components of the ruptured plaque may lead to downstream patchy obstruction of the microcirculation and myocardial necrosis that is detectable with sensitive myocardial necrosis markers such as the cardiac troponins or creatine kinase-MB ($CKMB_{mass}$).

Additional risk stratification may be based on other biological markers such as C-reactive protein (CRP), a marker of systemic activation of inflammation, and serum brain natriuretic peptide (BNP), a marker of left ventricular dysfunction and congestive heart failure.

ACS may present without any prior clinical sign or symptom, and indeed the majority of plaque ruptures occur at lesions that, prior to the rupture, did not obstruct coronary blood flow. As a consequence, after dissolving the platelet-rich intracoronary thrombus, a hemodynamically significant lesion is often absent (**238**).

MANAGEMENT

Recent data from the GRACE registry reveal substantial differences in the management of patients with ACS based on hospital type and geographic location. Whether these differences translate into differences in clinical outcome remains to be determined. Several aspects of the early treatment of patients with non-ST elevation ACS are generally accepted:

- Patients with an ACS should receive antithrombotic treatment, anti-ischemic treatment and, if considered high risk on the basis of early risk assessment, timely coronary angiography (CAG) and revascularization.
- Patients should be treated with aspirin and heparin, preferably low molecular weight heparin, which have been shown to reduce significantly the risk of short-term complications by approximately 50%.

Recent evidence suggests that the addition of clopidogrel is associated with a 20% reduction in the incidence of the combination of death, MI, or stroke. The addition of clopidogrel was associated with an increase in bleeding complications, especially in the setting of bypass surgery. In addition to aspirin, heparin, and clopidogrel, treatment with glycoprotein IIb/IIIa inhibitors has been shown to be of clinical benefit, particularly in the setting of percutaneous coronary intervention. In addition, secondary prevention in the form of life-long aspirin and the lowering of low density lipoprotein- (LDL) cholesterol through life-style changes in combination with treatment with statins, are important.

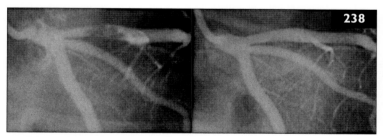

238 Right anterior oblique angiogram image of the left coronary artery of a 38-year-old male patient presenting with non-ST elevation acute coronary syndrome. **Left**: Large irregular filling defect in the proximal left anterior descending coronary artery (LAD) that corresponds to a large intraluminal thrombus. A percutaneous coronary intervention was deferred. **Right**: Image of the left coronary artery one week later after treatment with Reopro, aspirin, and low molecular weight heparin. A small irregularly shaped lower edge of the LAD is visible where the plaque rupture has taken place. A residual lesion causing impairment of flow in the LAD is clearly not present, and subsequent percutaneous intervention was not performed.

ACUTE MYOCARDIAL INFARCTION WITH ST SEGMENT ELEVATION

JOHN K. FRENCH, MB, PhD, FRACP AND HARVEY D. WHITE, MB, DSC, FCSANZ

DEFINITION

Patients are defined[1] as having AMI if they have either: a typical rise and gradual fall in troponin T or troponin I level, or a more rapid rise and fall in creatine kinase-MB levels, with at least one of the following:

- Ischemic symptoms.
- Development of pathologic Q waves on the ECG.
- Electrocardiographic changes indicative of ischemia (ST segment elevation or depression).
- Coronary artery intervention.

or : pathologic findings of acute myocardial infarction.

ST elevation myocardial infarction (STEMI) is associated with ST segment elevation of ≥1 mm in two contiguous leads, or ≥2 mm in chest leads V_1–V_3 (**239, 240**).

EPIDEMIOLOGY

The incidence of STEMI varies by country and by region, and parallels the prevalence of coronary heart disease. Over the last few decades there has been a reduction in the relative rate of STEMI compared with non-ST elevation ACS. The incidence of MI is rising in Eastern Europe and in developing countries, and is likely to increase worldwide with the aging of populations and the growing prevalences of diabetes and obesity.

PATHOGENESIS

STEMI is usually due to a ruptured atherosclerotic plaque or, less frequently, plaque fissuring, which is more common in women than in men. Platelet aggregation and initiation of the coagulation cascade lead to thrombus formation, shown angiographically in **239**. Myocardial necrosis may also occur without symptoms, and may be detected by ECG, cardiac imaging, or other investigations such as autopsy (**241, 242**). Other less common pathogenic mechanisms include coronary embolism of thrombi from the left atrium or ventricle, vegetations from infective endocarditis on the mitral or aortic valves, intense coronary vasospasm, subacute stent thrombosis following percutaneous coronary intervention (PCI), and aortic or coronary dissection.

CLINICAL PRESENTATION

Ischemic symptoms typically manifest as central retrosternal chest discomfort, usually of a dull or constricting nature, which may radiate to the arms, neck, or jaw, and less commonly to the epigastrium or to the back. Alternatively, the discomfort may occur in the epigastrium (which is often confused with indigestion) or in the arm, shoulder, wrist, jaw, or back without being felt in the chest, but such patterns are atypical. The discomfort is not usually

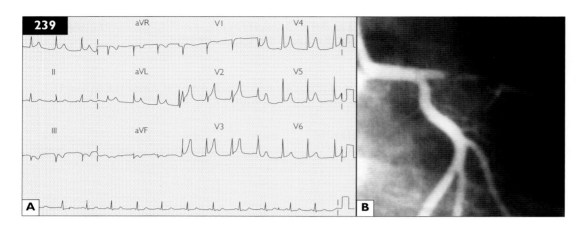

239 Anterior ST elevation myocardial infarction. **A**: Electrocardiogram of a 32-year-old male smoker (with a strong family history of premature death from heart disease) who presented 80 minutes after symptom onset. **B**: Left coronary angiogram showing thrombus in the proximal left anterior descending coronary artery.

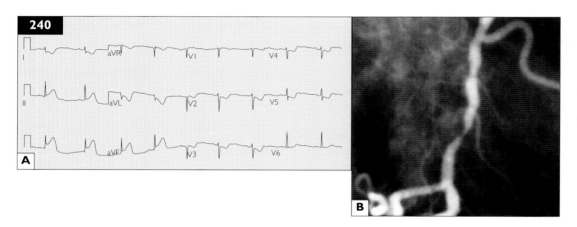

240 Infero-posterior ST elevation myocardial infarction. **A**: Electrocardiogram of a hypertensive 54-year-old female smoker who presented within 90 minutes of symptom onset. **B**: Right coronary angiogram showing a stenosis with thrombus and normal distal flow 3 days after fibrinolysis.

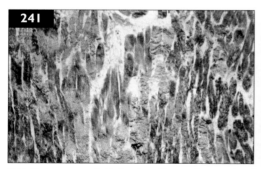

241 Early myocardial infarction. Photomicrograph of a histology section stained with phosphotungstic acid hematoxylin, showing contraction band necrosis in the myocardial cells of a patient who had undergone fibrinolysis 12 hours after symptom onset. (Courtesy of Dr Lois Armiger, Green Lane Hospital, Auckland, New Zealand.)

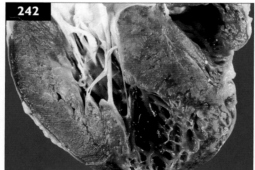

242 Anterio-apical myocardial infarction. Autopsy specimen showing left ventricular hypertrophy and thinning of the apex, with overlying left ventricular thrombus. (Courtesy of Dr Timothy Koelmeyer, Auckland Hospital, Auckland, New Zealand.)

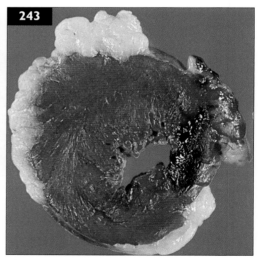

243 Cardiac rupture. Autopsy specimen showing rupture of the left ventricle with blood in the myocardium and pericardium. (Courtesy of Dr Timothy Koelmeyer, Auckland Hospital, Auckland, New Zealand.)

sharp or highly localized, and may be associated with breathlessness, sweating, nausea, vomiting, or light-headedness.

DIAGNOSIS

An ECG should be recorded as soon as possible, and will typically show ST segment elevation of ≥1 mm in two contiguous leads, or ≥2 mm in chest leads V_1–V_3. Cardiac troponin levels should be measured at presentation and at 12 and 24 hours after symptom onset[1]. It should be noted, however, that the release of troponins from the myocardial contractile apparatus into the blood occurs slowly, and so troponin levels in the blood can take at least 6 hours to reach the discrimination threshold. Thus patients who present very early after symptom onset may initially test negative for troponins.

Since 2–6% of patients suffer reinfarction while in hospital, creatine kinase (CK) or CKMB levels should be measured at 24–36 hours to provide a baseline for the detection of subsequent reinfarction by reelevation of these markers. Cardiac troponin levels may remain elevated for 10–14 days after the index infarction, and so troponin testing cannot be reliably used to identify reinfarction within this timeframe. In situations where left bundle branch block (LBBB) is present on the initial ECG, measurement of a more rapidly released biomarker, such as myoglobin, may aid diagnosis[2].

DIFFERENTIAL DIAGNOSIS

Other possible causes of chest discomfort include musculoskeletal causes, costochondritis, pneumothorax, pericarditis, aortic dissection, pain of upper gastrointestinal origin, pleurisy, and pulmonary embolus.

MANAGEMENT

Acute management is based on pain relief and administration of reperfusion therapies[3], aimed at early restoration of normal blood flow in the epicardial infarct-related artery and, hence, minimization of myocardial necrosis. Early ST segment recovery (i.e. return of the elevated ST segments toward normal on the ECG) and preservation of left ventricular function correlate with successful reperfusion[4], and are associated with increased early and late survival rates[2].

Clinical trials of fibrinolytic therapies have shown that the mortality risk is reduced if patients receive treatment within 12 hours after symptom onset[3]. The earlier reperfusion therapies are administered after symptom onset, the greater the survival benefit. In the comparison of primary angioplasty and prehospital thrombolysis in the acute phase of myocardial infarction (CAPTIM) trial[5] of 840 patients, those given fibrinolytic therapy within 2 hours had a 30-day mortality rate of only 2.2%, compared with 5.7% for those treated with primary angioplasty. p=0.05.

Approximately 8–10% of patients meeting the ECG criteria for reperfusion therapy are subsequently found to have contra-indications against fibrinolysis, and these patients should be considered for primary PCI[6]. PCI has been compared with fibrinolytic therapy, and has been shown to reduce the risks of reinfarction, intracranial hemorrhage, and mortality as compared

with fibrinolytic therapy. For patients presenting within 3 hours either fibrinolysis or primary PCI are appropriate as long as time from first medical contact to balloon inflation is expected to be <90 minutes[7].

All patients undergoing reperfusion therapies should be given adjunctive therapy with aspirin (150–325 mg), a loading dose of clopidogrel, and either enoxaparin or unfractionated heparin. It should be noted that some guidelines recommend the use of adjunctive heparin with streptokinase only in patients at high risk of systemic or venous embolism[8,9]. The standard dose of unfractionated heparin has recently been reduced because of concerns about the risk of intracranial hemorrhage with fibrinolytic therapy, and so it is currently recommended that a bolus of 60 IU/kg (maximum 4,000 IU) be administered, followed by an infusion of 12 IU/kg/hour (maximum 1,000 IU/hour), adjusted according to the activated partial thromboplastin time at 3 hours[8,9]. Enoxaparin has been shown to reduce the risk of death and MI by 17%, p<0.0001.[10]

The use of IV beta blockers is recommended in patients in Killip Class I and II followed by long-term oral beta blocker therapy[8]. Angiotensin-converting enzyme (ACE) inhibitor therapy should be commenced as early as 2 hours after presentation in patients without cardiogenic shock. Both classes of agent enhance the chance of survival[8]. Statin therapy, cessation of smoking, and control of hypertension should also be initiated in hospital, and all patients should be enrolled in a rehabilitation program. Other adjunctive therapies such as adenosine, and systemic cooling have shown promise in small randomized trials, but these findings are yet to be confirmed in large trials with clinical outcome endpoints.

PROGNOSIS

The overall mortality rate within 30 days after acute STEMI is still around 40–50%, accounted for mainly by sudden cardiac death before the patients reach hospital. Unselected patients hospitalized with STEMI have a mortality rate of 10–15%, due predominantly to cardiogenic shock or left ventricular (LV) failure. Other causes of early mortality include ventricular arrhythmias and mechanical complications such as cardiac rupture (**243**), mitral regurgitation, or ventricular septal defect[6]. From 6 months onwards, the annual mortality rate is 2–3%.

OUT-OF-HOSPITAL CARDIAC ARREST AND SUDDEN CARDIAC DEATH

R.W. KOSTER, MD, PhD

DEFINITION

Sudden cardiac death (SCD) can be defined in several ways, which influences the reported cause and characteristics of SCD. The currently accepted maximum time interval between onset of symptoms and collapse is 1 hour, with instantaneous death as a special situation, when the collapse is not preceded by any symptom. Since an autopsy is not performed in many patients who die instantaneously without expressing symptoms or who die unwitnessed, the cardiac origin of death cannot be established with certainty. Noncardiac causes such as embolism in the main pulmonary trunk or a ruptured aortic aneurysm are possible and sudden death, rather than SCD, may be a preferred term.

EPIDEMIOLOGY

The incidence of SCD in the population is estimated at 1–2/1000/year. SCD may occur at any age. There is a peak in the first year of life associated with sudden infant death syndrome, of which a cardiac origin is unclear, a low rate of SCD up to the age of 30–40 years, and a gradual increase thereafter. SCD occurs at home in 70–80% of cases, in public places in10–15% of cases, and in the workplace in the remainder. SCD is seen slightly more frequently in men than in women, maybe associated with earlier development of coronary artery disease (CAD) in men.

PATHOGENESIS

Seventy to 80% of patients die of ventricular tachycardia (VT), deteriorating into ventricular fibrillation as the immediate cause of cardiac arrest. It becomes of increasingly lower amplitude and ends in asystole. The remainder of cases are caused by primary bradycardia and asystole or have electromechanical dissociation (EMD), also called pulseless electrical activity (PEA). The underlying pathology is CAD leading to ischemia, but not always AMI, in 80% of cases. Myocardial scarring and especially aneurysm formation may contribute greatly to the risk of arrhythmic SCD. In 10–15% of cases, hypertrophic or dilated cardiomyopathy of nonischemic origin causes the arrhythmia. More rarely, lethal arrhythmia can be caused by congenital heart disease, aortic stenosis, coronary artery abnormalities, and primary electrical causes (<5%) such as long QT syndromes, Brugada syndrome, and Wolff–Parkinson–White syndrome, especially in younger patients.

CLINICAL PRESENTATION

In about 50% of cases, SCD is the first manifestation of CAD and causes instantaneous collapse or death without symptoms or warning. Less frequently, patients experience symptoms of chest pain suggesting AMI, dyspnea, palpitations, or dizzyness minutes prior to collapse. Some may have alerted an ambulance for these symptoms, collapsing in the presence of the ambulance personnel and benefiting from a subsequent better immediate outcome.

Symptoms of patients with known heart disease are of variable severity, from mild angina pectoris to old MI with depressed LV function, congestive heart failure, and nonsustained ventricular arrhythmia. These findings may be helpful to some extent in estimating the risk of future SCD. Low (<30–35%) ejection fraction (EF), particularly when associated with VT and congestive heart failure, poses the highest risk, yet is the cause of SCD in only a small minority of patients compared with the largest group of SCD victims with no or mild prior disease (**244**).

DIAGNOSIS

Diagnosis of a circulatory arrest as the cause of an unexpected collapse may be simple for professionals, yet is difficult for the lay person who is usually the witness. For most witnesses, even when trained in cardiopulmonary resuscitation (CPR), it is usually a first experience, and is very stressful, especially when it concerns a close relative. Until recently, confirming loss of consciousness and absence of a palpable carotid pulse were considered sufficient for the diagnosis, activating the Emergency Medical System (EMS) and instituting basic life support (BLS). The predictive value of the absence of the carotid pulse for confirmation of circulatory arrest by lay persons was found to be limited and was initially replaced by looking for 'signs of a circulation'. However, agonal breathing proved confusing and resulted in inappropriately withholding CPR when needed. Therefore, in the recently published Guidelines for Resuscitation 2005, unconsciousness in combination with absence of normal breathing was adopted as the indicator for need of CPR for lay rescuers[1,2].

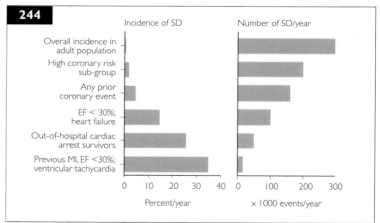

244 The epidemiologic paradox. Patients at high risk for sudden death (SD) can be identified by history of previous cardiac arrest, myocardial infarction, severely depressed left ventricular function and/or manifestation of ventricular tachycardia, yet they consitute only a small portion of all SD patients in the community. (Modified from Myerburg et al. [1993]. Sudden cardiac death: epidemiology, transient risk, and intervention assessment. *Ann. Intern. Med.* **119**:1187–1197.)

For professionals with a monitor, confirmation of ventricular fibrillation or asystole is simple and points to further action. The automated external defibrillator (AED) employs an algorithm, which differentiates with almost 100% accuracy between 'shockable rhythm' ventricular fibrillation (VF) or rapid VT and 'non shockable rhythm' asystole or organized rhythms (**245**).

DIFFERENTIAL DIAGNOSIS

Sudden loss of consciousness without circulatory arrest may occur in fainting, seizures, shock from massive hemorrhage (external or internal), nonocclusive pulmonary embolism, cerebrovascular bleeding, or hypoglycemic coma and are usually differentiated by their clinical presentation. However, when such conditions are erroneously believed to be the cause of loss of consciousness, resuscitation can be fatally delayed. Straddling pulmonary embolism or tension pneumothorax are rare but important causes of noncardiac circulatory arrest; treatment for these conditions is only possible when they are immediately recognized.

MANAGEMENT

Resuscitation from imminent SCD is possible with a rapid response of recognition, institution of BLS, defibrillation, and advanced life support (ALS). These components constitute the 'chain of survival' (**246**). Identification of the weakest link is key to improvements in the outcome of resuscitation.

Immediate outcome of resuscitation is improved when VF is found to be present rather than any other rhythm, but the emergency services generally arrive too late for defibrillation. Therefore, the recently developed AED may play a major role in improving outcome when distributed in the community, and is currently being investigated in large-scale community studies. AEDs will probably not replace but rather are an adjunct to the EMS, whose improvement in performance remains important.

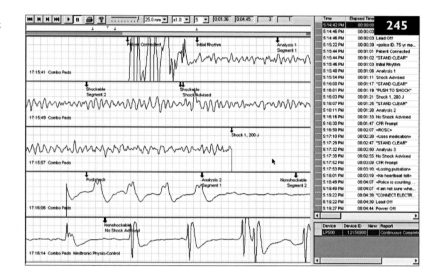

245 Electrocardiogram showing use of an automatic external defibrillator. After download into a computer documentation of the initial rhythm, rhythm analysis, shock delivery, and reanalysis are useful for clinical decisions and quality control. In the right panel all timed events after power-on of the device and annotations are displayed.

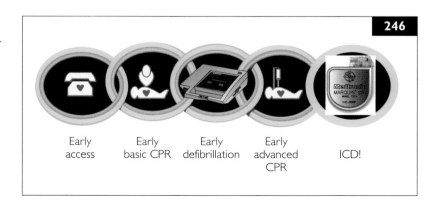

246 The chain of survival. The rapid activation of each of the first four components is critical for survival from out-of-hospital cardiac arrest. After recovery from the event, while still in hospital, all patients must be evaluated and many should receive an ICD in order to reduce the risk of death from recurrence of ventricular fibrillation, adding a fifth link to the chain. CPR: cardiopulmonary resuscitation; ICD: implantable cardioverter defibrillator.

Early access | Early basic CPR | Early defibrillation | Early advanced CPR | ICD!

PROGNOSIS

Immediate outcome of resuscitation is critically dependent on the execution of the chain of survival (**247**). At least 60–70% of cases die before hospital admission when restoration of circulation is not possible, and a further 50% of those admitted die in hospital, mainly from cerebral ischemia during the arrest. As a result, survival to discharge is 2–20%. Mental and social functioning after discharge is good or only slight impaired in 70–80% of patients, moderately impaired in 10–15% and poor in the remaining 5–15%.

Long-term prognosis is good when the cause of the cardiac arrest is transient or treatable, such as AMI or ischemia suitable for revascularization. Otherwise, the yearly recurrence rate of lethal arrhythmias is 30–40%. The treatment of choice is implantation of an implantable cardioverter defibrillator (ICD), with or without antiarrythmic medication, with proven improved survival (**246**).

247

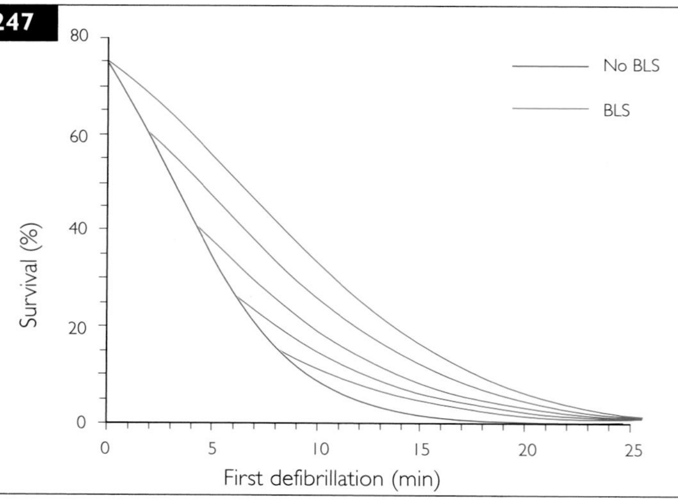

247 Graph to show the survival to discharge as a function of the delay between collapse (presumed onset of ventricular fibrillation) and defibrillation. Without basic life support (BLS) the probability of survival decreases by 10–15% per minute delay. Institution of BLS will buy some time and generally doubles chance of survival. However, delay in start of BLS greatly reduces its potential benefit. (Adapted from Waalewijn *et al.* [2001]. Survival models for out-of-hospital cardiopulmonary resuscitation from the perspectives of the bystander, the first responder, and the paramedic. *Resuscitation* **51**:113–122.)

TRIGGERING OF ACUTE CORONARY SYNDROMES

CHRISTIAN J. MUSSAP, MBBS, PhD, JAMES E. MULLER, MD AND GEOFFREY H. TOFLER MBBS, MD

INTRODUCTION

The past two decades have witnessed a rapid growth in the understanding of the pathophysiology of ACS. It is recognized that inflammation undermines plaque stability, predisposing to rupture and coronary thrombosis[1–4].

Concomitant with these advances has been a greater insight into the triggering of plaque rupture. A trigger may be defined as an activity of the patient, or specific environmental factor, that results in acute plaque disruption with sudden diminution of coronary artery blood flow (**248**)[5]. Evidence to support triggering comes from several sources: (1) acute MI frequently occurs at the site of a lesion with <50% stenosis, (2) the frequent absence of symptoms prior to disease onset suggests that an acute transformation has occurred, and (3) demonstration of a circadian variation in cardiovascular events precludes a random distribution.

CIRCADIAN VARIATION OF ACUTE CORONARY SYNDROMES

Studies have shown a morning peak in cardiovascular events, often with a smaller secondary evening peak[6–8]. The commencement of morning physical activity may be more critical than the time of day itself[9]. The morning correlates with a synchronization of adverse hemodynamic, hematologic, and humoral parameters[10]. A 20–30 mmHg (2.7–4.0 kPa) rise in systolic blood pressure, together with increases in heart rate and sympathetic activity, may precipitate plaque fissuring. Elevated cortisol levels may sensitize coronary arteries to the vasoconstrictor effects of catecholamines. Thrombogenicity is increased upon waking due to enhanced blood viscosity, increased platelet adhesiveness and aggregation, and reduced fibrinolytic activity[5]. In the Physicians' Health Study, aspirin conferred most benefit in the morning, coincident with peak platelet aggregability [5].

The rapid eye movement (REM) phase of sleep, most prevalent just prior to waking, may also contribute to the morning peak of MI. Dreams occur almost exclusively during REM sleep and are often characterized by strong emotions, sympathetic surges, and ventricular arrhythmia. There is an increased rate of infarction during the colder winter months[11], which in part may reflect more respiratory tract infections.

TRIGGERS OF MYOCARDIAL INFARCTION

Physical exertion

A triggering role for heavy physical activity is supported by descriptive studies reinforced by more recent case-crossover designed studies. In the Onset Study, there was a relative risk of 5.9 of infarction in the first hour after heavy exercise >6 metabolic equivalents (METS)[12]. Among sedentary individuals, there was a

100-fold relative risk of infarction but only a doubling in risk among those exercising regularly (>5 times per week; see **249**). The relative risk of sudden death at high workloads is markedly greater among those who exercise sporadically[13]. Physical exertion during competition correlates with a heightened risk of cardiac death. Of note, MI during exertion is associated with less severe coronary atherosclerosis[6], and incurs a lower mortality risk than infarcts occuring at rest or nocturnally.

Anger and emotional stress

Patients often blame psychological stress for their MI, although until recently the association was predominantly anecdotal. A strong association between acute emotional stress and SCD is a feature of the long QT syndrome. The Stockholm Heart Epidemiology Program (SHEEP) found a 9-fold increased MI risk in the hour following an episode of anger[14]. In the Onset Study, the risk of infarction doubled in the 2 hours following anger.

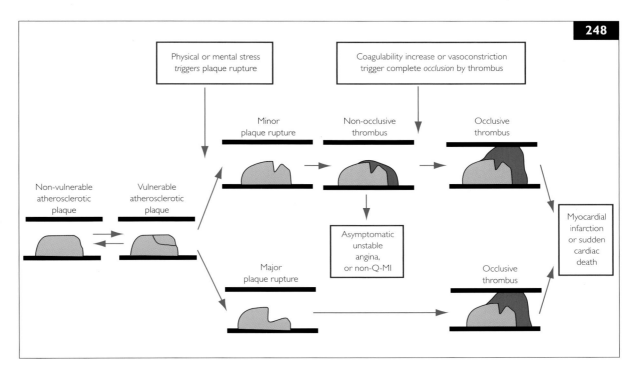

248 Illustration of a hypothetical method by which activities such as heavy physical exertion and emotional stress may trigger acute coronary syndromes. MI: myocardial infarction. (Adopted from Müller *et al.* [1994]. Triggers, acute risk factors and vulnerable plaques: the lexicon of a new frontier. *J. Am. Coll. Cardiol.* **23**:809–813.)

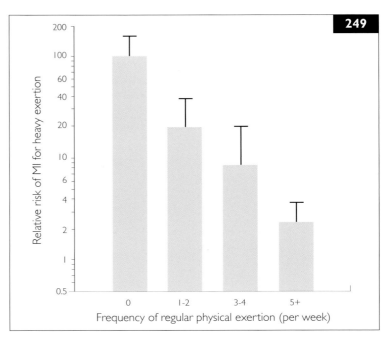

249 Modification of the relative risk of myocardial infarction (MI) by usual frequency of heavy exertion (defined as ≥6 METS). The relative risks are shown for patient subgroups relative to frequency of heavy exertion. Note the logarithmic scale and see text. METS: metabolic equivalents. (From Mittleman *et al.* [1993]. Triggering of acute myocardial infarction by heavy physical exertion. Protection against triggering by regular exertion. Determinants of myocardial infarction onset study investigators. *N. Engl. J. Med.* **329**:1677–1683. Copyright 1993 Massachusetts Medical Society. All right reserved.)

A lifetime tendency towards high-level anger responsiveness predisposes to early-onset coronary disease and particularly MI (relative risk 3.1–3.5). Similar asociations were observed in the ARIC study.

Earthquakes and the threat of missile attacks have been linked to transient increases in cardiac events, especially sudden death (**250**). Mental stress can lead to increased catecholamine levels and ischemia manifest by ventricular arrhythmias and T wave alternans[15]. Cultural factors may modulate cardiovascular risk. In Chinese and Japanese high-risk cohorts, cardiac mortality was shown to peak on the fourth day of each month (odds ratio 1.5), possibly because of increased apprehension caused by the phonetic similarity between the words 'four' and 'death'[16].

Melancholia and depression resulting from bereavement, divorce, or unemployment, lead to increased cardiovascular risk. Middle-aged widowers suffer a 40% higher mortality rate compared to controls in the 6 months after the death of their spouse[17]. Social isolation and lack of a support network have a negative effect on mortality post-MI[18].

Data support the implementation of stress management programs, including behavioral therapy, for the prevention of stress-induced cardiac events[19]. Stress management courses have led to 34% and 29% reductions in cardiac mortality and reinfarction, respectively[20].

Recommencement of sexual activity following MI is often disconcerting since sex involves the perceived triggers of physical exertion and emotional excitement. In the ONSET group of postinfarct patients, sexual activity was associated with a relative risk of 2.5[21]. Prior ischemic heart disease did not increase the relative risk of sex-induced cardiac events, and the risk was less in individuals who exercised regularly. Couples can in general be reassured that the absolute risk associated with sexual activity is low.

MI has been documented following recreational cocaine use. In ONSET there was a relative risk of >20-fold[22]. Cocaine elevates heart rate (by 30 beats/minute) and blood pressure (by 20/10 mmHg [2.7/1.3 kPa]), and can cause coronary vasoconstriction (up to 30%), platelet activation, and accelerated atherosclerosis.

There is an increased awareness of the risk posed by long-haul air travel to coronary patients[23]. Prolonged exposure to decreased cabin pressure and poorer quality recycled air can represent a significant hypoxic stress. Additional considerations include dehydration and immobility predisposing to thrombosis, and heightened anxiety (especially post-September 11) increasing hemodynamic stress on vulnerable plaques.

MANAGEMENT

Since triggers such as physical exertion and anger are mostly unavoidable, interventions should seek to protect at-risk individuals through pharmacologic and nonpharmacologic measures. The principal aims are to enhance coronary plaque wall stability, minimize hemodynamic shear stress, and inhibit thrombogenicity. Antiplatelet agents, beta blockers, ACE inhibitors, and lipid-lowering statin medications are efficacious in this regard. The use of longer-acting formulations to cover the high-risk morning period may confer additional benefit. Where appropriate, this may be complemented by a regular exercise regimen and/or stress management courses to attenuate the stress of heavy exertion and anger. A better knowledge of the mechanisms underlying triggering will provide an important therapeutic focus for ACS in the future.

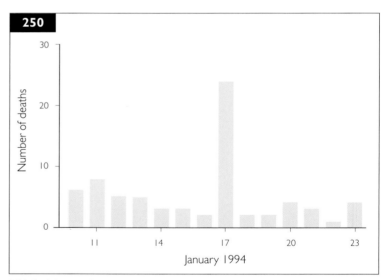

250 Sudden cardiac death triggered by the Northridge Earthquake. (From Leor et al. [1996]. *N. Engl. J. Med.* **334**:413–419. Copyright 1996 Massachusetts Medical Society. All rights reserved.)

Chapter Eleven

Acute Myocardial Infarction: Complications

CARDIOGENIC SHOCK

SØREN BOESGAARD, MD, PhD, AND JAN ALDERSHVILE, MD, PhD (deceased)

DEFINITION

Cardiogenic shock remains the leading cause of death in patients hospitalized with myocardial infarction. A primary cardiac dysfunction resulting in inadequate tissue perfusion is the underlying prerequisite. Clinically, cardiogenic shock is defined as: (1) sustained systolic blood pressure <90 mmHg (12 kPa) without hypovolemia, in combination with (2) signs of organ hypoperfusion (e.g. oliguria, impaired consciousness) and (3) signs of sympathetic activation (e.g. cool extremities, sweating). Diagnostic specificity is improved by the finding of low cardiac index (<2.2 l/minute) despite elevated left ventricular filling pressure (>15 mmHg [2 kPa]).

EPIDEMIOLOGY

Cardiogenic shock occurs in 7–10% of acute myocardial infarction (AMI). Risk factors include older age, diabetes, prior infarction, and female gender. Although large infarctions and anterior infarctions are predominant, shock can result from an infarct in any location. In fact, almost one-third of cardiogenic shocks are complications to a non-Q wave infarction. Median delay from onset of symptoms is 7 hours with a trend towards later shock development in non-ST elevation AMI. The majority of shocks therefore develop after hospital admission, 60–75% within the first 24 hours. Short-term mortality exceeds 60–70% (**251**) and is even higher in older patients and patients who develop shock more than 48 hours after AMI.

PATHOGENESIS

Left ventricular failure is the most common cause of cardiogenic shock, accounting for 75–80% of cases. Isolated right ventricular failure occurs in 3%, while mechanical complications such as severe mitral regurgitation, ventricular septal rupture, or cardiac tamponade account for 10–15% of cases of cardiogenic shock (see Chapter 11, Mechanical Complications). Ventricular dysfunction results in low stroke volume reducing cardiac output. Myocardial perfusion is compromised by systemic hypotension and increased left ventricular end-diastolic pressure (LVEDP). In some patients, hypotension and myocardial depression may be further aggravated by a systemic inflammatory response. Together with neuro-hormonal activation, these changes contribute to a cycle of worsening ischemia and organ perfusion.

CLINICAL PRESENTATION

The typical patient with cardiogenic shock presents with hypotension, sinus tachycardia, cool extremities, oliguria, pulmonary rales, and respiratory distress due to pulmonary congestion. While the clinical appearance of this syndrome is often easily recognizable, it must be emphasized that shock can be

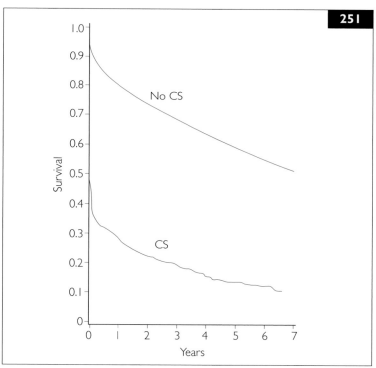

251 Kaplan–Meier survival curves for consecutive patients with acute myocardial infarction with (n=444) and without (n=6226) cardiogenic shock (CS). (From Lindholm MG *et al.* [2003]. Cardiogenic shock complicating acute myocardial infarction: Prognostic impact of early and late shock development. *Eur. Heart J.* **24**:258–265. With permission from the publisher, WB Saunders.)

present or emerging without the presence of these classic features (e.g. a significant proportion of patients with left ventricular failure show no signs of pulmonary congestion). Similarly, hypotension, which traditionally has been considered the hallmark of circulatory failure, may not necessarily be the dominating problem in the early phases of shock because blood pressure may be maintained initially by a high sympathetic drive. This early phase is termed preshock and the majority of patients with fully developed shock have passed through this preshock period. Thus, the presence of AMI, sinus tachycardia, cool extremities, and low urine output, indicative of a low cardiac output state, should be considered important warning signals of evolving cardiogenic shock even in patients with normal systemic blood pressure.

DIAGNOSIS AND DIFFERENTIAL DIAGNOSIS

Cardiogenic shock is an emergency condition. Consequently, diagnostic verification, initial hemodynamic stabilization, and plans for definitive therapy must be dealt with simultaneously (**252**). A medical history, electrocardiogram (ECG), physical examination, and echocardiography constitute the initial diagnostic procedures. Echocardiography is necessary to confirm the diagnosis of primary ventricular failure as opposed to mechanical complications or other noncardiac causes of shock (e.g. septic shock, aortic dissection, pulmonary emboli) needing a different treatment strategy (**253**). Invasive hemodynamic monitoring is used to confirm the presence

of low cardiac output, to exclude volume depletion and primary right ventricular infarction, and to estimate filling pressures and treatment response.

MANAGEMENT

Multiple data suggest that an aggressive hemodynamic- and revascularization-based approach is associated with improved outcome in cardiogenic shock. Initial therapy of cardiogenic shock therefore optimally includes: (1) early identification, (2) intensive care monitoring including a low threshold towards mechanical ventilation, (3) circulatory support with sympathomimetic inotropic and vasopressor agents, (4) coronary reperfusion (**254**), and (5) general measures including correction of acidosis and significant arrhythmias and discontinuation of negative inotropes, anti-hypertensive, or nephrotoxic agents. Mechanical circulatory support with an intra-aortic balloon pump (IABP) is usually indicated and should routinely be performed before attempting coronary reperfusion (**255**).

In normovolemic, hypotensive patients, dopamine or norepinephrine are the initial drugs of choice. Due to their vasodilatory properties, inotropes such as dobutamine or the phosphodiesterase inhibitor milrinone should await correction of overt hypotension. Peripheral vasodilators such as nitroglycerin or nitroprusside may be combined with inotropes in patients with high filling pressures. IABP improves coronary perfusion, reduces

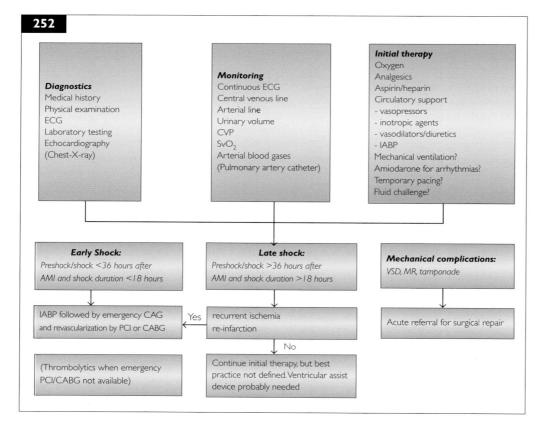

252 Management of cardiogenic shock complicating acute myocardial infarction. AMI: acute myocardial infarction; CABG: coronary artery bypass grafting; CAG: coronary angiography; CVP: central venous pressure; IABP: intra-aortic balloon pump; MR: mitral regurgitation; PCI: percutaneous intervention; SvO$_2$: central venous oxygen saturation; VSD: ventricular septal defect.

253 Left: Echocardiographic four-chamber view showing a large ventricular septal defect (1) complicating an acute myocardial infarction. 2: left atrium; 3: left ventricle; 4: right atrium; 5: right ventricle. **Right**: Doppler image of the same patient showing a large left-to-right shunt.

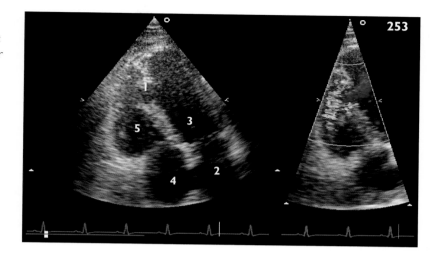

254 A 75-year-old female was admitted with severe chest pain. At arrival she was pale with cool extremities and an arterial oxygen saturation of 84%. The arterial blood pressure was 82/53 mmHg (10.9/7.1 kPa), heart rate 102 bpm, and electrocardiogram showed an anterior ST elevation acute myocardial infarction. After initial respiratory/circulatory stabilization, emergency coronary angiography was performed within 3 hours of start of symptoms. The angiography shows an occluded left main coronary artery (left). The lesion was immediately managed by percutaneous transluminal coronary angioplasty and stenting of the left main artery (right).

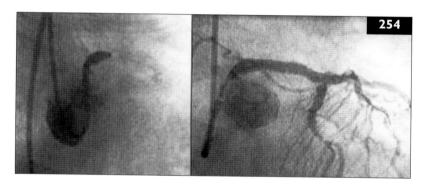

255 The principle of intra-aortic balloon pump. Initiation of balloon inflation is timed to the arterial dicrotic notch, producing an augmentation in proximal aortic diastolic pressure. Deflation of the balloon is timed to begin just before the onset of the next ventricular systole, which produces the systolic unloading effect (presystolic dip). LV: left ventricle. (Modified from Cercek and Shah [2001]. In: *Cardiology*. MH Crawford, JP Di Marco, WJ Paulus (eds). Mosby, London.)

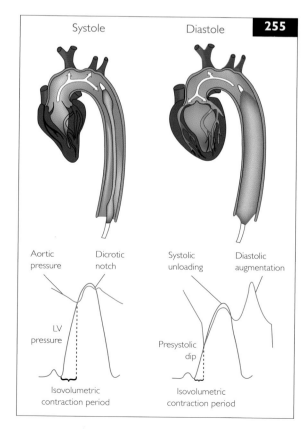

afterload, increases cardiac output without increasing oxygen demand, and may allow reduction in pharmacologic vasopressor therapy. In addition, IABP insertion reduces the incidence of serious complications during invasive procedures.

These initial treatment measures have not been shown to improve prognosis in cardiogenic shock and should only be regarded as temporary means to establish adequate tissue perfusion while awaiting the effect of a coronary reperfusion. Therefore, in most patients with early shock due to ventricular failure and short shock duration, the next treatment goal is myocardial revascularization. In clinical practice this condition may be defined as shock duration <18 hours and onset of shock <36 hours after AMI. This strategy is supported by data from the randomized SHOCK trial, where emergency invasive revascularization tended to reduce 30-day mortality and significantly reduced 6-month and 12-month mortality (**256**). In particular, patients <75 years old seem to benefit from invasive therapy, with a 12-month mortality of 48% as compared to 77% in medically treated patients. Since the effect of thrombolysis is reduced in cardiogenic shock, thrombolytic therapy should be reserved for patients who cannot rapidly be transferred for emergency coronary revascularization with coronary angioplasty or bypass surgery. To improve the chances of reperfusion, thrombolytics should then be administered on top of proper pharmacologic and mechanical (IABP) circulatory support.

PROGNOSIS

Cardiogenic shock complicating AMI continues to be a very serious condition (*Table 32*). Thirty-day mortality in medically treated patients is at least 60–70%. With best practice therapy, including mechanical circulatory support and early revascularization, 30-day mortality is still >30–40%. For the few patients surviving 30 days, the long-term mortality rate is slightly higher than in patients with myocardial infarction and an in-hospital diagnosis of heart failure without cardiogenic shock. The majority of these patients are classified in NYHA functional class I/II.

SUMMARY

Several sets of data suggest that if cardiogenic shock is recognized early and managed with rapid initiation of up-to-date supportive measures and emergency invasive revascularization, outcome can be improved. On the other hand, it is likely that there are groups of older patients, and patients with long lasting cardiogenic shock and fully developed multi-organ failure, where invasive therapy is futile. Therefore, management of cardiogenic shock needs to be individualized and treatment strategy carefully selected.

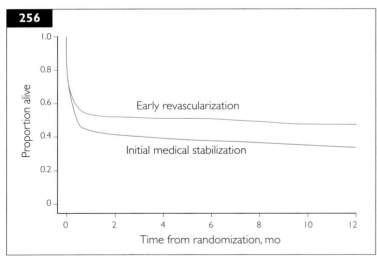

256 One year Kaplan–Meier survival curve for patients randomized to early emergency revascularization (n=152) and initial medical stabilization (n=149)(p<0.04). Data from the SHOCK trial. (From Hochman *et al.* [2001]. One-year survival following early revascularization for cardiogenic shock. *JAMA* **285**:190–192. Copyrighted 2001, American Medical Association.)

Table 32 principles in cardiogenic shock complicating acute myocardial infarction

- Cardiogenic shock is an emergency.
- Most shock patients slowly slide into shock after admission to hospital.
- Act immediately on signs of organ hypoperfusion.
- Echocardiography and intensive care monitoring/therapy are standard.
- Pharmacological and mechanical circulatory support are generally both needed.
- Use IABP/dopamine as first-line therapy in hypotensive patients.
- Add inodilators/vasodilators when mean arterial pressure >65 mmHg (8.7 kPa).
- Every patient with early shock should be evaluated for emergency invasive revascularization.
- Insert IABP before initiation of CAG/PCI.
- In the initial clinical setting, left ventricular ejection fraction carries little prognostic information.

MECHANICAL COMPLICATIONS

HENRIK EGEBLAD, MD, DMSC

DEFINITION

Ruptures or tears in infarcted, necrotic myocardium are denoted together as mechanical AMI complications (*Table 33*). Most of these complications have a mortality rate close to 100% unless the condition is treated surgically. Despite surgical treatment the average mortality is still high, around 50%, although considerably lower in the case of an easily accessible anterior pseudoaneurysm with a narrow communication to the left ventricle (LV). Mechanical complications may occur early after AMI and during the following few weeks, usually from day 1–4.

Hypertension, first-time AMI, age >60 years, delayed thrombolysis, and absent collaterals are considered to predispose to rupture. Most mechanical complications are accompanied by the sudden onset of a new attack of pain, severe discomfort, dyspnea, sweating, and heart failure with low blood pressure and pulmonary congestion.

Ventricular septal rupture and papillary muscle rupture are usually recognized by a loud systolic murmur but the key diagnostic method is echocardiography. In any patient with sudden worsening during the course of AMI, auscultation of the heart and echocardiography should immediately be carried out.

EXTERNAL RUPTURE

External rupture accounts for at least 10% of in-hospital deaths in AMI. A complete external rupture results in hemopericardium and nearly always in cardiac tamponade, shock, electromechanical dissociation, and death. Slow oozing of blood through a partial or incomplete rupture may result in localized pericarditis that may limit later bleeding. The patient often experiences pericardial pain and a friction rub is often present. Echocardiography reveals a more or less localized pericardial effusion and, with newer techniques, it may even be possible to reveal the incomplete rupture (**257**). In the author's experience in the past few years, findings indicating incomplete rupture are regularly present in cases of more severe pericarditis in AMI. Sometimes the diagnosis may be supported by a small decrease in blood hemoglobin.

An incomplete external rupture may heal over weeks or, in the case of a new rupture, may result in more limited hemopericardium. The latter condition will often lead to the formation of a pseudoaneurysm, a sac connected to the LV cavity through a narrow neck (**258**). In rare cases a to-and-fro murmur may occur from turbulence of the blood flow through the neck of the pseudoaneurysm. As it is formed by pericardium, the wall of the pseudoaneurysm is weak and expansion develops over weeks and months, and sometimes years (**259**). Heart failure may then develop and sometimes discomfort, with a sensation of a burden in the chest.

Table 33 Mechanical complications of acute myocardial infarction

External rupture
- Complete: Immediate cardiac tamponade, survival rare.
- Incomplete/partial: Pericardial pain/pericarditis/risk of secondary rupture/pseudoaneurysm: beta-blocking, ACE inhibition/surgery?
- Pseudoaneurysm
  Pericardial pain, late development of heart failure/secondary rupture: Surgical closure and extirpation.

Ventricular septal rupture
- Transient pain, sudden onset of dyspnea, hypotension.
- Almost always loud systolic murmur.
- Afterload reduction, pressure support, surgery.

Papillary muscle rupture
- Sudden onset of hypotension, pulmonary edema.
- Often loud systolic murmur (sometimes absent).
- Afterload reduction, pressure support, surgery.

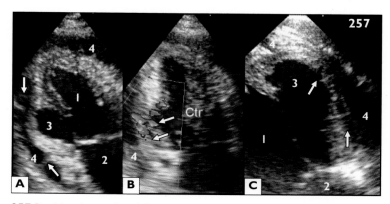

257 Partial or incomplete left ventricular (LV, 1) rupture to the pericardium. Two days after the onset of inferior acute myocardial infarction, secondary pain and a pericardial friction rub developed in a 50-year-old male. **A**: Apical 2-chamber view demonstrating the left atrium (2) and ventricle (1) with a posterior aneurysm (AN, 3). In addition, pericardial effusion (4) with small bridges of fibrin are seen (arrow). **B**: IV injection of echocardiographic contrast medium (Ctr) results in opacification of LV and powerful color-Doppler echoes in a communication between AN and a subepicardial hematoma (arrow). **C**: Transesophageal echocardiography provides a close-up view of the AN showing a thin, bulging and dilacerated wall with small fissures (upper arrow) towards the pericardium and the subepicardial hematoma (lower arrow). At coronary artery by-pass, bloody pericardial effusion and hematoma in the wall of the AN were documented. The wall of the AN was reinforced by duplication and a patch.

Management

Complete external rupture is usually resistant to resuscitation. However, life saving urgent surgery is occasionally reported and, very rarely, patients may even recover spontaneously from the shock and survive on medical treatment alone.

It is generally advocated that patients with a pseudoaneurysm should be treated surgically, at least if expansion is observed. A permanent risk of rupture of the thin wall is also possible. Surgery is rewarding in cases of a large anterior pseudoaneurysm with a narrow neck, where constriction of the neck with subsequent extirpation of the pseudoaneurysm can be performed (**259**). The perioperative risk is much higher in cases of posterior pseudoaneurysm that have distorted the mitral valve apparatus.

It is unknown whether an incomplete rupture with localized pericardial effusion should be left to heal spontaneously or be treated surgically with reinforcement of the wall; surgical treatment is considered if by-pass surgery is otherwise indicated (**257**). In other cases, medical treatment with beta blockers and angiotensin-converting enzyme (ACE) inhibitors may suffice together with close echocardiographic control.

VENTRICULAR SEPTAL RUPTURE

Rupture of the interventricular septum occurs in <1% of AMI patients. It is commonly a catastrophic event with sudden onset of breathlessness, hypotension, and pulmonary congestion caused by the left-to-right shunt. At auscultation a loud holosystolic murmur is heard. Typically the murmur has its maximum at the left sternal border but in many cases auscultation does not permit differentiation between ventricular septal rupture and papillary muscle rupture. Echocardiography nearly always enables demonstration of the rupture (**260**), not unusually as an irregular valve-like tear in a smaller septal aneurysm. The noninfarcted part of the LV is usually hyperkinetic because of the shunt. Measurement of the blood flow velocity through the rupture by means of the echocardiograph makes it possible to calculate the pressure in the right ventricle (**260**). Thus, echocardiography provides information on the severity of the rupture not only from anatomy but also from hemodynamics.

Management

Systemic arterial output is facilitated by afterload reduction of the LV by means of nitroglycerin infusion. Dobutamine and dopamine infusion are added to maintain cardiac output and renal function. Insertion of an IABP also facilitates systemic arterial output and is required in most cases until the rupture can be closed at open-heart operation. Coronary arteriography is performed early after hemodynamic stabilization to decide the need for simultaneous by-pass surgery. Closure of the rupture seems to be more successful if the operation is postponed for a couple of weeks. However, while the surgeons are awaiting tissue consolidation,

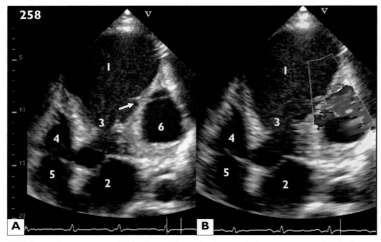

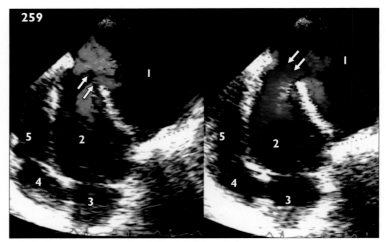

258 Pseudoaneurysm (PSA, 6) and large left ventricular aneurysm (AN, 1). During the first week of extensive Q wave acute myocardial infarction, heart failure, persistent pain synchronous with the respiration, and a friction rub developed in a 55-year-old male. **A**: The apical four-chamber view shows spontaneous echo contrast in AN. A communication (arrow) between the left ventricle (LV, 3) and the PSA is present at the border between normal and infarcted myocardium. **B**: Color-Doppler reveals turbulent blood flow from LV into the PSA in systole and facilitates the demonstration of their communication. Because of severe heart failure and a massively injured LV, the patient (successfully) underwent heart transplantation within 1 week. 2: left atrium; 5: right atrium; 4: right ventricle.

259 Fully developed pseudoaneurysm (PSA, 1) in a 48-year-old female seen 1.5 years after anterior Q wave acute myocardial infarction. She was readmitted because of heart failure and chest discomfort. The PSA is at least as large as the left ventricle (LV, 2). The arrows indicate the communication with flow from LV to PSA in systole (left panel) and *vice versa* in diastole (right panel). There was no turbulent blood flow within the PSA or communication and accordingly no murmur on auscultation. The patient underwent uneventful extirpation of PSA after constriction of the communication. 3: left atrium; 4: right atrium; 5: right ventricle.

many patients may die from the hemodynamic burden of the defect. Early operation is currently generally recommended, soon after the establishment of medical treatment and pressure support. Closure of ventricular septal ruptures by means of catheter-introduced devices has been reported and is likely to be a future treatment possibility.

PAPILLARY MUSCLE RUPTURE

Papillary muscle rupture is a complication of inferior or posterior infarction. It is more rare than rupture of the septum. The infarct area is seldom extensive and sometimes is limited to the papillary muscle itself. If the lesion is a complete transverse rupture of the body of the papillary muscle, free mitral valve regurgitation and pulmonary edema immediately develop. The mitral insufficiency may be less severe in incomplete ruptures with detachment of a part of the tip of the muscle and its associated chordae. A loud holosystolic murmur is usually heard but the murmur may be more faint or even absent if severe heart failure and hypotension develop. The diagnosis is made by echocardiography (**261**). Transesophageal echocardiography (TEE) may be necessary in these very ill patients who are either suffering from severe dyspnea or are treated on a ventilator.

Management

Treatment includes immediate afterload reduction and pressure support with subsequent urgent insertion of a prosthetic valve or, if possible, mitral valve repair. If time permits, coronary arteriography precedes the operation.

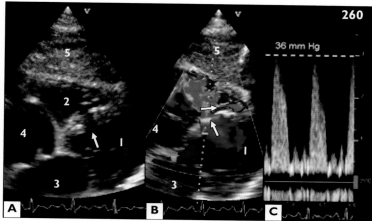

260 Ventricular septal rupture in a 60-year-old male with onset of inferior Q wave acute myocardial infarction 1 week earlier. **A**: Subcostal four-chamber view showing the rupture (arrow). **B**: Color-Doppler examination visualizes turbulent blood flow from the left to the right ventricle (LV, 1; RV, 2 respectively). The main direction of the blood flow is perpendicularly to the septum but there is also flow through a longer tear within and along the septum (arrows). **C**: Continuous-wave Doppler measurement of the flow velocity through the septum shows a peak systolic velocity of 3 m/second. The simplified Bernoulli equation (pressure difference in mmHg = 4 $\times$ velocity^2) permits translation of the blood flow velocity into a pressure gradient of 36 mmHg (4.8 kPa). As the systemic systolic arterial blood pressure was 90 mmHg (12 kPa), the systolic pressure in RV was (90-36) mmHg or 54 mmHg (7.2 kPa), indicating that the shunt had resulted in considerable pulmonary hypertension. Surgical closure of the defect was successfully performed by means of a patch. 3: left atrium; 4: right atrium; 5: liver.

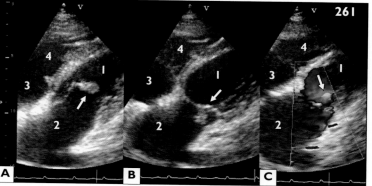

261 Papillary muscle rupture in a 75-year-old male with a small inferior Q wave acute myocardial infarction 2 days earlier. The patient suddenly developed severe dyspnea and the systolic blood pressure fell from 120 mmHg (16 kPa) to 60 mmHg (8 kPa). No murmur was noticed on auscultation. Subcostal echocardiography shows a large fragment of a papillary muscle prolapsing from the left ventricle (1) in diastole to the left atrium (2) in systole (arrows in **A**, **B**). This finding indicating very severe mitral insufficiency was considerably more spectacular than the modest eccentric regurgitant jet by color-Doppler examination (arrow in **C**). Mitral valve repair or substitution was omitted because of known coexistent lung cancer and the patient died soon after the examination. 3: right atrium; 4: right ventricle.

ARRHYTHMIAS COMPLICATING ACUTE MYOCARDIAL INFARCTION

MIGUEL VALDERRÁBANO, MD AND C. THOMAS PETER, MD

BRADYARRHYTHMIAS

Bradyarrhythmias occur in 25–30% of patients with AMI, resulting from abnormalities of impulse formation or impulse conduction. Ischemia results in various alterations in myocardial cellular electrophysiology (**262**). Besides ischemia of tissues in the specialized conduction system, vagal autonomic influences and concomitant metabolic disorders (hypoxia, electrolyte disturbances, local increases in adenosine or potassium concentrations) contribute to the generation of bradyarrhythmias. There are distinct pathophysiologic processes leading to bradyarrhythmias depending on infarct location.

Inferior and inferoposterior myocardial infarction

Infarctions involving these territories have frequent bradyarrhythmias that are thought to result from enhanced parasympathetic tone (Bezold–Jarisch reflex). Such infarctions mostly, but not always, arise from occlusion of the right coronary artery (RCA). Bradyarrhythmias tend to develop early in the course of the infarction (within the first 6 hours) and their spectrum of severity ranges from mild sinus bradycardia or first degree atrioventricular (AV) block, to second and third degree AV blocks with relatively slow ventricular rates. There is usually a rapid response to atropine or isoproterenol. Ischemia of the sinoatrial node (SAN), leading to sinus bradycardia or sinus arrest may also occur when the sinus node artery is compromised from an ostial occlusion of the artery from which the sinus node artery

originates (RCA = 60% and circumflex = 40%). AV node (AVN) ischemia can complicate RCA or left circumflex (LCx) occlusions, which can cause similar bradyarrhythmias; however, these tend to occur later (after 6 hours) and do not respond to medical therapy. AV block from inferoposterior MI tends to develop proximal to the His bundle.

Anterior and anteroseptal myocardial infarction

MIs due to occlusion of the left anterior descending (LAD) artery and its septal branches can result in AV and intraventricular blocks due to ischemia of the infraHisian conduction system. These do not respond to medical therapy, may require transvenous pacing, and have a poor prognosis due to the extent of myocardium involved.

Sinus bradycardia

Sinus bradycardia is the most common bradyarrhythmia complicating AMI (about 40% of all bradyarrhythmias), frequently in the setting of inferior or inferoposterior MI (**263**).

First degree atrioventricular block

First degree atrioventricular block frequently accompanies sinus bradycardia. It is usually of no clinical significance by itself but may progress to a higher degree of AV block in 13% of patients.

Mobitz type I second degree atrioventricular block (Wenckebach)

Mobitz type I second degree AV block is identified electrocardiographically by progressive PR prolongation until the dropped beat, progressive RR interval shortening (in typical cases, about 55%), group beating, and RR interval of the dropped beat being shorter than twice the shortest RR interval (**264**). It usually occurs in inferior or inferoposterior MIs and consequently is supraHisian in nature; it is secondary to increased vagal tone or reversible AVN ischemia, responds to atropine, and escape beats have narrow QRS. Such blocks rarely occur in anterior MIs, but are then infraHisian, carry a higher risk of progression to higher-grade AV block, and do not respond to atropine.

Mobitz type II second degree atrioventricular block

Mobitz type II second degree AV block is identified by a fixed PR interval until nonconducted P waves occur (**265**). It reflects infraHisian disease, and is usually secondary to extensive anteroseptal

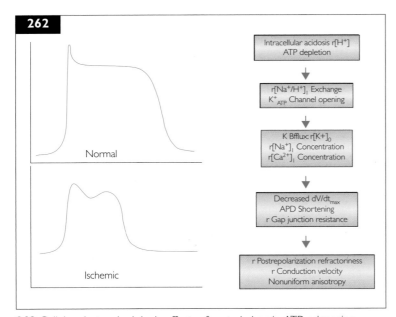

262 Cellular electrophysiologic effects of acute ischemia. ATP: adenosine triphosphate; APD: action potential duration.

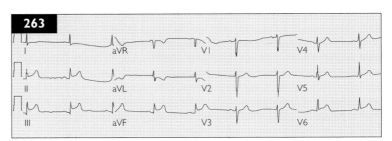

263 Electrocardiogram showing sinus bradycardia during an inferior myocardial infarction.

MIs. The ventricular escape rhythm, if present, tends to have a wide QRS and relatively low rates. It tends to progress to higher-grade AV block and, therefore, it is usually treated by transvenous pacing. Atropine may worsen type II second degree AV block by increasing the sinus rate and is therefore contraindicated.

Complete heart block

Abolition of AV conduction is diagnosed electrocardiographically by the absence of any relationship between P waves and QRS complexes. The clinical impact depends on the rate of the ventricular escape rhythm. Large (cannon) *a* waves may be present on examination (jugular venous pulse), as well as variable S1 intensity. As for other bradyarrhythmias, the MI site is a determining factor in the clinical significance and prognosis of complete heart block (CHB). MI-associated CHB is due to inferior or inferoposterior MIs in 60% of cases. In these, it is usually the result of gradual progression from first or second degree AV block, does not cause hemodynamic compromise, and has a narrow, relatively rapid (40–60 bpm) ventricular escape rhythm. It tends to resolve within 3–7 days. Therapy with transvenous pacing is determined by the individual clinical status of each patient. Conversely, CHB complicating anteroseptal MIs carries a poor prognosis due to extensive myocardial damage. In these cases, therapy with transvenous pacing is warranted due to the slow, wide QRS ventricular escape rhythm.

Intraventricular conduction defects
Left bundle branch block

Left bundle branch block (LBBB) occurs in <5% of patients with AMI, usually in large anterior MIs with extensive damage. About 11% of patients progress to CHB. It commonly posits a clinical dilemma since new onset LBBB in the appropriate clinical setting is an indication for thrombolytic therapy, and the presence of LBBB interferes with the electrocardiographic detection of myocardial injury. The criteria for MI in the presence of LBBB include ST elevation concordant with the QRS vector, and ST elevation >7 mm (**266**).

Left anterior fascicular block

As opposed to the right bundle and the left posterior fascicle (which receive dual blood supply from the LAD and RCA), the left anterior fascicle is only supplied by septal perforators from the LAD. Isolated left anterior fascicular block (LAFB) occurs in 3% of patients with AMI and seldom progresses to CHB. In an additional 5%, LAFB occurs in association with right bundle branch block (RBBB) (see below).

Left posterior fascicular block

Left posterior fascicular block (LPFB) is rare (1–2%) and does not tend to progress to CHB. The larger size of the posterior compared to the anterior fascicle requires a larger infarct to impact on its function. Therefore, its presence markedly increases mortality since it reflects a larger MI.

Right bundle branch block

RBBB occurs in approximately 2% of patients with MI, usually with large anteroseptal MIs (**265**, complicated with Mobitz II AV block). It carries a risk of about 20% of progression to CHB. Its presence markedly increases mortality, even in the absence of CHB.

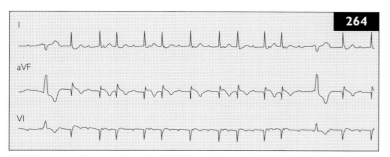

264 Electrocardiogram showing Mobitz type I second degree atrioventricular (AV) block (Wenckebach) in a patient with an inferior myocardial infarction. Periods of 3:1 and 2:1 Wenckebach can be seen. A ventricular escape beat follows an episode of high-grade AV block.

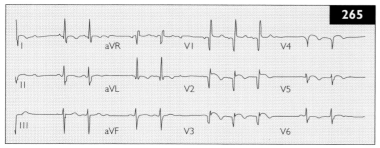

265 Electrocardiogram showing anteroseptal myocardial infarction complicated with right bundle branch block and Mobitz type II second degree atrioventricular block.

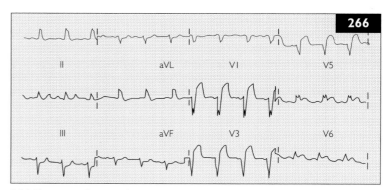

266 Electrocardiogram showing acute anterolateral myocardial infarction in the presence of left bundle branch block. Injury current can still be diagnosed despite left bundle branch block as ST segment elevation is >7 mm in V2 and V3, and concordant with the QRS axis in V5 and V6.

Bifascicular block
The combination RBBB–LAFB (**267**) in MI is much more common (8–10%) than RBBB–LPFB. The presence of bifascicular block carries a risk of 25% of developing CHB, which increases to up to 40% if first degree AV block is also present. Although reperfusion may revert these conduction defects, a transvenous pacemaker is recommended.

VENTRICULAR TACHYARRHYTHMIAS

The cellular and tissue level electrophysiologic effects of ischemia are summarized in **262**. In addition, sympathetic activation is equally relevant since it may enhance automaticity of ischemic Purkinje fibers. The combination of altered cellular electrophysiology in ischemic zones, systemic and local catecholamine release, and tissue heterogeneity with close apposition of normal myocardium (the 'border zone') set the stage for electrical instability and re-entry during MI.

Premature ventricular complexes

Premature ventricular complexes (PVCs) are an almost ubiquitous finding in patients with acute MI. In the era of reperfusion they do not predict further arrhythmogenic complications and do not warrant specific therapy by themselves.

Ventricular tachycardia

Ventricular tachycardia (VT) can present as monomorphic (likely due to a myocardial scar) or polymorphic (likely to respond to treatment of ischemia) VT. Nonsustained VT (three or more consecutive PVCs faster than 100 bpm and lasting <30 seconds) occurs in up to 67% of MI patients in the first 12 hours and is not associated with increased mortality (**268**). Conversely, sustained VT (>30 seconds or causing hemodynamic compromise requiring intervention) during the first 48 hours is often polymorphic and is associated with an in-hospital mortality of 20%. Those who survive to discharge, however, do not have increased mortality at 1 year. Management is directed by hemodynamic tolerability: unstable VT requires immediate cardioversion. Beta blockade use should be universal in MI patients unless hemodynamically compromised. Appropriate antiarrhythmic drugs include amiodarone, lidocaine, and procainamide.

Ventricular fibrillation

Primary ventricular fibrillation (VF) refers to VF occurring during the early stages of MI without overt left ventricular failure (**269**). Eighty percent of episodes occur within 12 hours of the onset of symptoms. Secondary VF occurs as a final deterioration in patients with left ventricular failure and cardiogenic shock. Late VF develops >48 hours after MI and tends to occur in patients with large MIs and left ventricular dysfunction. Other predictors include intraventricular conduction defects and anterior MI, persistent sinus tachycardia, atrial flutter or fibrillation, and right ventricular infarction requiring pacing. Prompt electrical cardioversion is the only effective treatment.

Accelerated idioventricular rhythm

Accelerated idioventricular rhythm is likely to be the result of enhanced automaticity in the Purkinje fibers. It is a well-tolerated ventricular rhythm at rates of 60–125 bpm, and is usually self-terminating. It has been associated with reperfusion, but it also occurs in nonreperfused patients. Accelerated idioventricular rhythm does not have prognostic significance or require therapy.

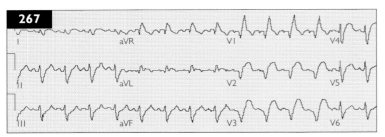

267 Electrocardiogram showing acute anteroseptal myocardial infarction complicated with right bundle branch block and left anterior fascicular block.

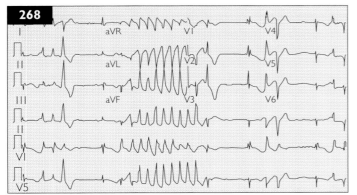

268 Electrocardiogram showing acute myocardial infarction complicated with QT prolongation and polymorphic ventricular tachycardia.

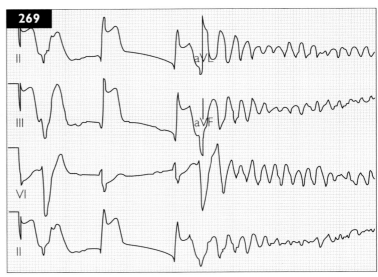

269 Electrocardiogram showing acute inferior myocardial infarction complicated with primary ventricular fibrillation.

OTHER COMPLICATIONS

IRA PERRY, MD AND SAIBAL KAR, MD

INTRODUCTION

In addition to major contractile, mechanical, and electrical complications, other complications following AMI include recurrent ischemia, pericarditis, Dressler's syndrome, and thromboembolic events. These complications often increase morbidity and mortality as well as hospitalization and length of hospital stay.

RECURRENT ISCHEMIA/REINFARCTION

Recurrent chest pain secondary to myocardial ischemia is a serious development and needs immediate attention. The discomfort is often similar to the original discomfort and comes on at rest or with minimal exertion. The pain may be associated with ST segment elevation, depression, or pseudonormalization of inverted T waves. Patients at risk for development of recurrent ischemia include those with non-ST elevation myocardial infarction (NSTEMI) who have received thrombolysis, or with multiple risk factors and significant multi-vessel disease. Postinfarction angina is associated with a twofold increase in reinfarction if not treated appropriately. Recurrent ischemia within a few weeks after MI is generally related to the same coronary artery that led to the index MI, but at times can be due to another lesion separate from the acute culprit vessel. Recent studies have documented a high prevalence of multiple complex plaques in the coronary arteries of patients presenting with an acute coronary syndrome (ACS).

Reinfarction should be suspected if there is a recurrence of prolonged ischemic chest discomfort with significant ST segment changes and re-elevation of cardiac enzymes. Once recurrent ischemia/infarction is suspected, the patient should be considered for urgent coronary angiography (CAG) followed by appropriate revascularization.

PERICARDITIS

Chest pain after AMI may also be due to postinfarct pericarditis. Pericarditis is more likely to occur with large transmural infarcts. Transmural infarction tends to occur more frequently when AMI patients do not receive prompt reperfusion therapy. Thus, the incidence has decreased with early and routine use of thrombolytics and percutaneous coronary intervention (PCI). Pericarditis is now seen in 6–12% of patients. It usually occurs within the first week following an AMI. In rare cases, acute pericarditis may be the manifestation of subacute or acute free wall rupture, in which case it carries a very sinister prognosis unless prompt surgical intervention is undertaken.

Pericarditis should be suspected if the pain is pleuritic, the physical examination shows a to-and-fro pericardial rub, and the ECG shows diffuse ST segment elevation (**270**). Postinfarct pericarditis, however, may be difficult to diagnose on the ECG because the underlying infarct pattern may obscure superimposed changes of pericarditis. Two types of atypical T wave evolution have been reported in regional postinfarct pericarditis: a persistently positive T wave for 48 hours or more, or premature reversal of initially inverted T waves to positive deflections. An echocardiogram should be performed to detect evidence of pericardial fluid and signs of early tamponade and to rule out cardiac rupture as a potential basis for pericarditis. Pericarditis not related to cardiac rupture is managed with symptomatic therapy using nonsteroidal anti-inflammatory agents; however, high doses and prolonged therapy should be avoided to prevent impaired healing of the infarct.

POSTMYOCARDIAL INFARCTION SYNDROME (DRESSLER'S SYNDROME)

Dressler's syndrome is a delayed form of postinfarct pericarditis associated with systemic manifestations including fever, elevated sedimentation rate, pleuritis, and malaise. In rare instances, it may appear weeks to months later with recurrences and remissions. The syndrome is believed to reflect an autoimmune response; however, it is so rare now that its very existence is being questioned.

Treatment is similar to that of early postinfarction pericarditis. However, in view of the recurrent nature of this syndrome, a course of gradually tapered oral corticosteroids may be required.

LEFT VENTRICULAR ANEURYSM AND THROMBUS

Aneurysms occur in the anterior or apical regions with an incidence of 5–10% of all patients with an AMI. Pathologically, the aneurysmal area is characterized by a thinned-out transmural scar that has completely lost its trabecular pattern. One half of aneurysms are

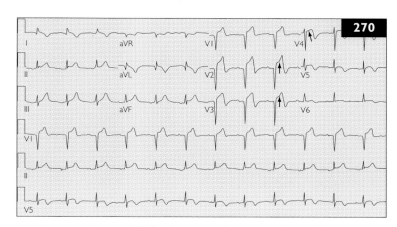

270 Electrocardiogram (ECG) of a patient showing persistent ST segment elevation (arrows) days after a successful reperfusion. At the time of ECG, the patient had symptoms of pericarditis.

lined by a laminated thrombus (**271**). The scar may eventually calcify and is clearly delineated from surrounding ventricular muscle.

Complications of a true ventricular aneurysm include formation of mural thrombus with subsequent thromboembolic events (e.g. stroke), congestive heart failure, and ventricular arrhythmias. Unlike pseudoaneurysms that form from contained rupture of the infarct, true ventricular aneurysms rarely rupture. Mural thrombi are associated with a 5–10% incidence of embolization. These thrombi often develop within the first week. The endomyocardial necrosis and inflammation are a nidus for layered mural thrombi. The risk of embolization is increased in cases with mobile or protruding thrombi and in areas of akinesis next to a hyperkinetic segment. The bulging noncontractile segment of the left ventricular wall can decrease the ejection fraction and increase the left ventricular end-diastolic volume, leading to chronic heart failure. Aneurysms are also associated with increased risk of ventricular tachycardia as a result of the development of multiple re-entry circuits in the peri-infarct zone.

If an aneurysm is suspected clinically by a demonstrated dyskinetic apical impulse, a conclusive diagnosis can be made by echocardiography, magnetic resonance imaging, radionuclide ventriculography, or left ventriculography. Early reperfusion with PCI or thrombolysis can limit the extent of necrosis and reduce the risk of aneurysm formation. Once an aneurysm does form, long-term progressive ventricular remodeling and enlargement can be attenuated using angiotensin-converting enzyme inhibitors and beta blockers. An aneurysectomy may be considered in cases of refractory congestive heart failure, refractory VT, and recurrent emboli. Warfarin should strongly be considered for 3–6 months in cases of documented mural thrombi.

PULMONARY EMBOLISM
The prevalence of deep vein thrombosis (DVT) following an AMI is 12–38%. Patients with large infarcts, congestive heart failure, and complicated infarctions are at relatively high risk. Associated reduced cardiac output and immobilization are additional risk factors. Venous thrombosis is often benign, but can lead to a pulmonary embolism which may be life threatening (**272**).

Early mobilization combined with therapy directed towards improving cardiac output is the most effective means of preventing pulmonary emboli. Prophylactic anticoagulant therapy is recommended for patients at high risk of development of DVT.

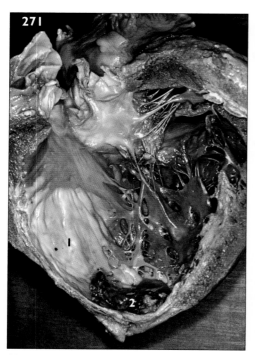
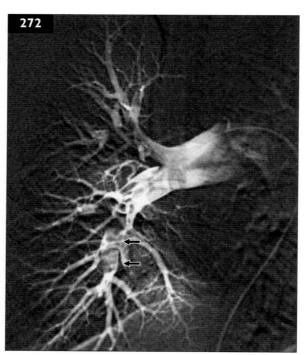

271 Autopsy specimen of a heart from a patient with a history of myocardial infarction, demonstrating a large left ventricular aneurysm (1). Note the thrombus in the aneurysm (2). (Courtesy of Prof. Michael Fishbein, Department of Pathology, UCLA School of Medicine.)

272 Right pulmonary arteriogram in an antero-posterior view showing two large filling defects in the right lower branches (double arrows), suggestive of pulmonary embolism, in a patient with a recent history of myocardial infarction and persistent shortness of breath.

3

183

Chapter Twelve

Acute Myocardial Infarction: Special Problems

RIGHT VENTRICULAR ACUTE MYOCARDIAL INFARCTION

HENNING RUD ANDERSEN, MD, PhD

INTRODUCTION

Right ventricular infarction occurs when the coronary blood supply to the right ventricular myocardium is interrupted. In anterior infarction, the infarct-related coronary artery is the left anterior descending artery (LAD), that supplies a small amount of the right ventricle (RV) near the septum, particular in the apical region (**273**). In posterior infarction, about 90% of RV infarcts are caused by occlusion of the right coronary artery (RCA), and 10% by occlusion of the left circumflex coronary artery (LCx). In patients with a right dominant coronary anatomy, the RCA supplies the lateral and posterior right ventricular wall, together with a variable amount of the posterior left ventricular wall. In patients with a left dominant coronary anatomy, the LCx supplies a small part of the posterior right ventricular wall near the septum. Consequently, RV infarction large enough to cause RV dysfunction is caused by occlusion in the proximal RCA, and is normally associated with some posterior left ventricular (LV) infarction (combined LV and RV infarction) (**273**).

EPIDEMIOLOGY

From autopsy studies in patients with acute myocardial infarction (AMI), isolated RV fibrosis is reported in 2–3% of cases, all due to occlusion of a right marginal branch. Combined LV and RV infarcts are found in 70–80%, and isolated LV infarcts in 20–30% of cases. Consequently, RV involvement should be considered in about two-thirds of all patients with anterior or inferior/posterior infarction, but is rare in patients with left lateral infarcts.

LOCATION AND SIZE

RV involvement is much larger in inferior/posterior than in anterior infarction. Consequently, when total infarct size (left plus right ventricular components) is similar in anterior and inferior/posterior infarction, a different infarct distribution exists between the two ventricles (**274**). This may explain the better prognosis after inferior/posterior than after anterior infarcts of apparently equal size (measured enzymatically), because preserved

LV function is a major determinant of postinfarct survival. Furthermore, severe RV dysfunction caused by extensive RV infarction is often present in patients with inferior/posterior infarction, but is very rarely seen in patients with other infarct locations.

CLINICAL PRESENTATION

Patients with hemodynamically important RV infarction usually present with an ST elevation, inferior/posterior myocardial infarction (MI). Increased jugular venous pressure and concomitant arterial hypotension (with or without shock) are often present, together with signs of low cardiac output. In contrast to

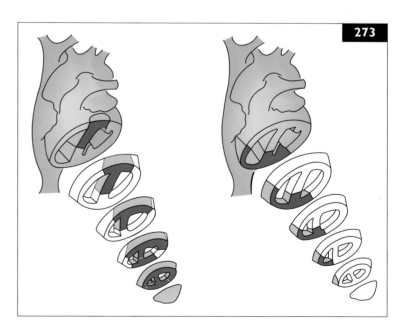

273 Diagram illustrating the topography of right ventricular involvement in anterior and posterior infarction due to proximal occlusion of the left anterior descending coronary artery and the right coronary artery, respectively. Both anterior and posterior right ventricular infarcts have a triangular shape but anterior right ventricular infarcts are small, and mainly located near the apex of the heart, whereas posterior right ventricular infarcts are larger and are predominantly located near the atrioventricular groove at the base of the heart.

predominant LV infarction with evidence of LV dysfunction, the lungs are usually clear at auscultation, and the chest X-ray is without signs of pulmonary edema.

DIAGNOSIS

Most patients with RV infarction have ST segment elevation ≥0.1 mV in one or more right chest leads V3R–V7R (**275**). Therefore, in patients with inferior MI, the right chest leads may provide the first clue that RV involvement is present. However,

the right chest leads do not add much to the overall diagnostic accuracy of the 12-lead electrocardiogram (ECG). Therefore, the risk of missing a diagnosis of AMI if the right chest leads are not examined is very small, but they are useful to diagnose the involvement of the RV in inferior/posterior infarction. In patients with ECG inferior/posterior infarction, the right chest leads can differentiate those patients with extensive infarction of the RV and minor infarction of the LV (ST elevation in right chest leads V3R–V7R) from patients with predominantly LV infarction (**274**). This ECG finding may guide the treatment in the acute phase.

Echocardiography in the acute phase is of utmost importance. Abnormal wall motion and/or RV dilatation may indicate RV infarction. Furthermore, M-mode echocardiographic demonstration of early opening of the pulmonary valve due to atrial contraction indicates severe RV dysfunction and highly increased RV diastolic pressure.

DIFFERENTIAL DIAGNOSIS

Hypotension caused by LV MI, pericardial tamponade, and pulmonary embolism are the most frequent differential diagnoses. Echocardiography is the most important tool to differentiate between these conditions.

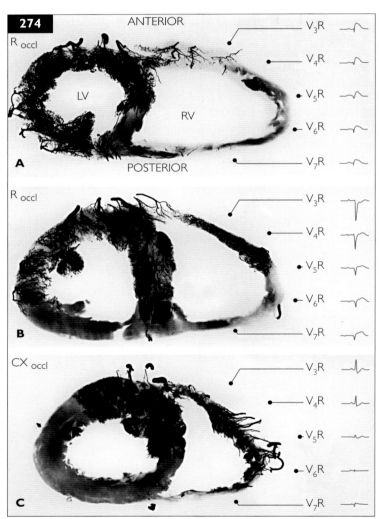

274 Inferior/posterior infarction. Right chest electrocardiogram (V3R–V7R) with corresponding necropsy angiograms of 1 cm thick transventricular slices, showing poor contrast filling in infarcted myocardium. **A**, **B**: Posterior infarction caused by occluded right coronary artery (R) with extensive right ventricular (1) infarction and concomitant minor (**A**) and larger (**B**) left ventricular (2) infarction. **C**: Posterolateral infarct caused by occluded circumflex coronary artery (CX) with extensive left ventricular infarction and minor right ventricular infarction. Corresponding electrocardiograms show ST segment elevation in five leads (**A**), three leads (**B**), and one lead (**C**).

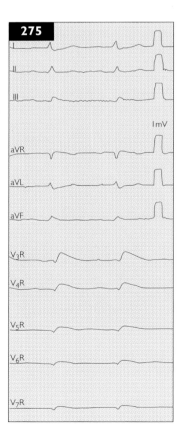

275 Electrocardiogram showing the three standard leads, I, II, III, the three unipolar extremity leads, aVR, aVL, aVF, and five right chest leads, V3R–V7R, from a patient with inferior myocardial infarction. Despite almost normal ST-T pattern in leads I, II, and aVL, ST segment elevation is observed in V3R–V7R.

MANAGEMENT

The etiology of shock in patients with extensive RV infarction is caused by severe dysfunction of the RV, that is unable to generate sufficient pressure to propel blood through the pulmonary circulation and into the LV. These patients suffer from a low-output syndrome despite a nearly intact LV. The treatment of such patients is related not only to instituting appropriate therapy for severe pump failure but also to avoiding inappropriate therapy. The goal of therapy is to increase LV output. Therefore, a greater blood flow must be propelled into the LV. This can be achieved by: (1) minimizing the pulmonary vascular resistance (by good oxygenation), (2) increasing the pressure gradient favoring passive flow through the lungs (saline or plasma infusion), and (3) increasing the contractile power in the RV and atrium (dobutamine infusion). In mild cases, cautiously infusing saline may reverse hypotensive episodes.

Patients who have refractory hypotension or shock should be considered for invasive monitoring. Treatment may be guided by measuring the LV filling pressure, which is often relatively low in the untreated patient with RV infarction and shock due to severe RV dysfunction. In contrast, measuring a high RV filling pressure (venous engorgement and high central venous pressure) does not guide treatment because it does not reflect LV dysfunction in such patients, and it may even lead the physician to choose inappropriate therapy (diuretics or nitroglycerin) which further lowers LV filling pressure.

PROGNOSIS

In the acute phase, extensive RV infarction is associated with a high frequency of atrioventricular (AV) block, ventricular fibrillation (VF), transient hypotension, and even shock. If these complications are treated successfully, the long-term prognosis for those patients who survive the initial days after infarction is good, mainly because of a preserved LV function in many of them.

THROMBOLYSIS OR PRIMARY ANGIOPLASTY?

HENNING RUD ANDERSEN, MD, PhD

INTRODUCTION

In myocardial infarction with ST segment elevation (STEMI), occlusive and persistent thrombosis prevails. Most cases are precipitated by sudden rupture of a vulnerable plaque followed by superimposed thrombus formation. Reperfusion therapy, whether catheter-based or pharmacologic, is critically needed to restore antegrade flow through the infarct-related artery, and thus arrest the propagating wave of necrosis. To preserve myocardium and reduce morbidity and mortality reperfusion must be rapid, complete, and sustained.

Traditionally, pharmacologic and catheter-based reperfusion therapies have been considered distinct and mutually exclusive strategies. Each strategy has its own advantages and shortcomings. Fibrinolytic therapy is widely available and can be given rapidly in emergency departments. Even with the most efficacious fibrinolytic agents, however, normal (Thrombolysis In Myocardial Infarction [TIMI] grade 3) flow at 90 minutes is achieved in only 50–60% of patients. Intracranial hemorrhage occurs in approximately 1% of patients treated with fibrinolytic therapy, and is fatal in >50% of patients. Almost 90% of patients with patent infarct-related arterie at 90 minutes after fibrinolytic therapy have a residual stenosis >50% at the culprit lesion, leaving the vessel more prone to reocclusion. Reinfarction occurs in 5–6% of patients within the first weeks after treatment.

In contrast, primary angioplasty results in TIMI grade 3 flow in more than 70% of patients, and patency (TIMI 2 or 3 flow) in >90% of patients, without the hemorrhagic risk of fibrinolytic therapy. It also significantly reduces the risk of reinfarction because primary angioplasty not only restores brisk antegrade flow but also treats (eliminates) the underlying stenosis.

PRIMARY ANGIOPLASTY VERSUS FIBRINOLYSIS

A meta-analysis of 23 randomized trials including 7,739 patients assigned to primary angioplasty (n=3,872) or fibrinolytic therapy (n=3,867) clearly demonstrated the superiority of primary angioplasty[1]. Streptokinase was used in 8 trials (n=1,837) and fibrin-specific agents in 15 (n=5,902). Primary angioplasty was better than fibrinolysis at reducing overall short-term mortality, nonfatal reinfarction, stroke, and the combined endpoint of death, nonfatal reinfarction, and stroke, irrespective of the fibrinolytic regimen used (streptokinase or fibrin-specific) (**276**). Also, during long-term follow-up after 6–18 months, a better outcome was seen with primary angioplasty. Thus, based on these trials, primary angioplasty is considered a superior strategy both for efficacy and safety.

For primary angioplasty, clinical trials have already defined the benefit of adjunctive stenting and use of platelet glycoprotein (GP)

IIb/IIIa blockade. Unanswered questions remain about the role of 'upstream' combination therapy before primary angioplasty, defining the role of intra-aortic balloon pumping in improving outcome, avoiding and treating no-reflow, clarifying the roles of thrombectomy and distal protection devices, and improving myocardial salvage.

For fibrinolysis, GP IIb/IIIa inhibition combined with reduced-dose fibrinolytic therapy was expected to improve mortality but did not improve outcome in recent randomized trials.

Therefore, primary angioplasty should be made available to many more patients with STEMI. Recently, two strategies have been tested: (1) primary angioplasty in hospitals without on-site cardiac surgical facilities and (2) transfer for primary angioplasty.

PRIMARY ANGIOPLASTY IN HOSPITALS WITHOUT ON-SITE CARDIAC SURGICAL FACILITIES

Traditionally, primary angioplasty has not been performed in hospitals without on-site surgical backup due to the (small) risk of complications in the primary angioplasty procedure. In the Atlantic C-PORT trial, 11 hospitals with cardiac catheterization facilities but without on-site cardiac surgery, adopted a training program and established 24-hour acute angioplasty services 7 days a week[2]. Patients were randomized to primary angioplasty versus thrombolysis; the outcome was better for angioplasty with similar results as in the meta-analysis. Among the patients randomized to angioplasty, none required emergency cardiac surgery for a catheterization-related or angioplasty-related complication, including abrupt closure, dissection, or coronary perforation due to a complication at the index hospital. Thus, the trial demonstrated that if an extensive development program is established primary angioplasty can be performed safely in hospitals without on-site cardiac surgery. Such a strategy can extend the reach of primary angioplasty to more patients.

TRANSFER FOR PRIMARY ANGIOPLASTY

The major limitation on a more widespread use of primary angioplasty as first-line therapy has been that most patients with AMI are admitted to a hospital without facilities for primary angioplasty. Until recently there has been a lack of documentation on the feasibility and safety of transporting patients with AMI to tertiary centers for primary angioplasty, and of the effect of treatment delay caused by interhospital transportation versus on-site fibrinolysis.

Most of the patients included in the meta-analysis were initially admitted directly to hospitals with cardiac catheterization facilities. When a patient presents at a hospital without interventional capabilities, a decision needs to be made regarding appropriate treatment. The principal therapeutic options in such a situation are either on-site fibrinolysis or transfer to a facility with a cardiac catheterization laboratory. Currently, data are available on 2,466 patients randomized between primary angioplasty after interhospital transportation (n=1,242) and on-site fibrinolysis (n=1,224). Even with the longer time delay inherent in transportation with transfer time up to 2 hours, primary angioplasty is superior to fibrinolysis in reducing overall mortality and the combination of death, nonfatal reinfarction, and stroke[3] (**277**). In the largest of these trials, the DANAMI-2 study, the time from admission to the first hospital until transport was started towards the invasive

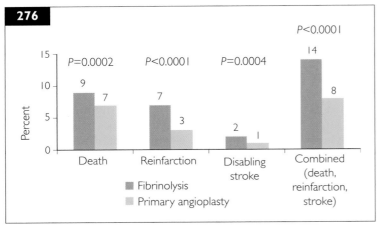

276 Short-term (4–6 weeks) clinical outcome of death, reinfarction, stroke, and the combined endpoint of death, reinfarction, and stroke in a meta-analysis of 23 randomized trials with 7,739 patients. Primary angioplasty was better than fibrinolysis in reducing all endpoints. (Data from Keeley *et al.* [2003]. Primary angioplasty versus intravenous thrombolytic therapy for acute myocardial infarction: a quantitative review of 23 randomized trials. *Lancet* **361**:13–20.)

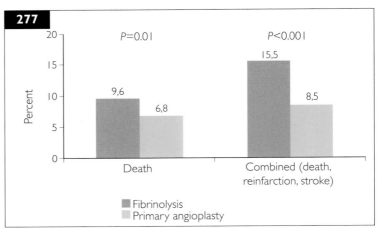

277 Short-term (30 days) clinical outcome of death and the combined endpoint of death, reinfarction, and stroke in a pooled analysis of 5 trials with 2,466 patients randomized between primary angioplasty after interhospital transportation versus on-site fibrinolysis. Primary angioplasty was better than fibrinolysis even with the longer time treatment delay. (Data from Zijlstra [2003]. Angioplasty versus thrombolysis for acute myocardial infarction: a quantitative overview of the effects of interhospital transportation. *Eur. Heart J.* **24**:21–23.)

hospital was 50 minutes, whereas the interhospital transport time lasted only a median of 30–35 min. (**278**).

The positive data on transfer of patients for primary angioplasty together with the long delay at the first hospital strongly suggest that it may be time to change the approach of the emergency medical response system for AMI. One approach could be to obtain ECG in the field followed by direct transfer to a hospital with primary angioplasty facilities, thus bypassing hospitals without such capability. This would further shorten the treatment delay and could improve outcome. Thus, transfer of patients directly to hospitals with established primary angioplasty facilities (with or without cardiac surgery) has the potential to further expand the availability of primary angioplasty to many patients.

SUMMARY

Primary angioplasty is superior to fibrinolysis as initial reperfusion strategy for patients with STEMI. The major task for the future is to reorganize services in the community to provide this treatment to the majority of patients.

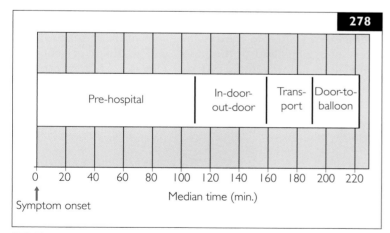

278 Time delays from the onset of symptoms to first balloon inflation in 559 patients transferred from referral hospitals to angioplasty centers for treatment with primary angioplasty in the DANAMI-2 trial. Patients arrived at the referral hospital after 107 minutes (pre-hospital time). It took 50 minutes before the ambulance left the hospital again (In-door-out-door time). The interhospital transport time (Transport) was 32 minutes (median distance 50 km [31 miles]) and the time from arrival at the angioplasty center until first balloon inflation (Door-to-balloon time) was 26 minutes. Thus, the interhospital transfer time by ambulance constituted only 15% of the total time from onset of symptoms to first balloon inflation.

REPERFUSION INJURY

MIGUEL VALDERRÁBANO, MD AND WILLIAM GANZ, MD

DEFINITION

Ischemia induces cellular processes that lead to cell death, both by necrosis as well as apoptosis. Restoration of blood flow can result in recovery of cells if they are reversibly injured, or not affect the outcome if irreversible cell damage has occurred. Cell death occurring after restoration of blood flow is referred to as lethal reperfusion injury. The term does not necessarily imply a pathogenic role of flow restoration *per se*, but rather defines the chronological relationship of cell death with flow restoration. The wealth of laboratory experimental data supporting various mechanisms of reperfusion injury is paralleled by a lack of data supporting clinical relevance of these hypothesized mechanisms of reperfusion injury.

PATHOGENESIS AND PATHOLOGY
Cellular processes

It is controversial whether reperfusion elicits new damage, or simply accelerates death in cells that are structurally intact yet biochemically compromised. New damage may be initiated during reoxygenation by increased generation of oxygen free radicals by parenchymal and endothelial cells and infiltrating leukocytes (*Table 34*). Superoxide anions can be produced in reperfused tissue as a result of incomplete and vicarious reduction of oxygen by damaged mitochondria, or because of the action of oxidases derived from leukocytes, endothelial cells, or parenchymal cells. Cellular antioxidant defense mechanisms may also be compromised by ischemia, favoring the accumulation of radicals. Reactive oxygen species can further promote the mitochondrial permeability transition, which, when it occurs, precludes mitochondrial energization and cellular adenosine triphosphate (ATP) recovery and leads to cell death. Ischemic injury is associated with the production of cytokines and increased expression of adhesion molecules by hypoxic parenchymal and endothelial cells. These agents recruit circulating polymorphonuclear leukocytes to reperfused tissue; the ensuing inflammation causes additional injury. The importance of neutrophil

Table 34 Proposed mechanisms of reperfusion injury

- Oxygen free radicals.
- Induction of mitochondrial permeability transition.
- Cytokines and adhesion molecules.
- Intracellular calcium overload.
- Polymorphonuclear leukocyte activation and migration.

influx in reperfusion injury has been demonstrated by experimental studies that have used anti-inflammatory interventions, such as antibodies to either cytokines or adhesion molecules, to reduce the extent of the injury.

Myocardial reperfusion

Reperfusion of myocardium within 15–20 minutes after onset of ischemia may prevent all necrosis. Conversely, reperfusion after a longer interval may not prevent necrosis but can salvage at least some myocytes that otherwise would have died. A partially completed then reperfused infarct is hemorrhagic because some vasculature injured during the period of ischemia becomes leaky on restoration of flow (**279**). Moreover, disintegration of myocytes that were critically damaged by the preceding ischemia is accentuated or accelerated by reperfusion. Microscopic examination reveals that myocytes already irreversibly injured at the time of reflow often have necrosis with contraction bands (**280**). Contraction bands are intensely eosinophilic transverse bands composed of closely packed hypercontracted sarcomeres. They are most likely produced by exaggerated contraction of myofibrils at the instant perfusion is re-established. After reperfusion, mitochondria in nonviable myocytes develop deposits of calcium phosphate and, ultimately, a large fraction of the cells may calcify. Reperfusion of infarcted myocardium also accelerates the washout of intracellular proteins producing an exaggerated and early peak value of substances such as the MB isoenzyme of creatine kinase (CKMB) and cardiac-specific troponin T and I.

Vascular reperfusion injury

Vascular reperfusion injury refers to progressive damage to the microvasculature that prevents restoration of normal blood flow to the cardiac myocytes (no reflow), and causes loss of coronary vasodilatory reserve. Microscopy studies have shown damage and swelling of the capillary endothelium, as well as intravascular plugging by fibrin or platelets, leukocytes, and microemboli of atherosclerotic debris.

CLINICAL IMPLICATIONS

The role of the cellular processes described above in extending myocardial necrosis has been questioned. Multiple studies have shown that reperfusion *per se* does not extend the necrotic areas beyond those already compromised before reperfusion. Furthermore, therapeutic strategies directed against processes alleged to mediate reperfusion-related cell death have been ineffective. There are, however, a few clinically relevant issues related to reperfusion.

Reperfusion arrhythmias

Premature ventricular contractions, accelerated idioventricular rhythm, and nonsustained ventricular tachycardia (VT) are seen commonly after successful reperfusion. Although reperfusion arrhythmias have a high sensitivity for detecting successful reperfusion, the high incidence of identical rhythm disturbances in patients without successful coronary artery reperfusion limits their specificity.

Myocardial stunning

Although most of the viable myocardium existing at the time of reflow ultimately recovers after alleviation of ischemia, critical abnormalities in cellular biochemistry and function of myocytes salvaged by reperfusion may persist for several days, referred to as stunned myocardium.

No reflow

No reflow is most commonly diagnosed during coronary angiography (CAG) as contrast stagnates in the distal coronary artery after angioplasty or thrombolysis. The clinical presentation is that of a nonreperfused MI (see Chapter 12, Downstream (micro)Embolization, Slow Flow, and No Reflow).

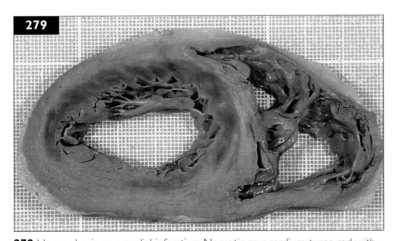

279 Hemorrhagic myocardial infarction. Necrotic myocardium turns red with reperfusion because of vascular dilatation and interstitial hemorrhage. This autopsy specimen of a reperfused infarct is from a 47-year-old man who received reperfusion therapy (primary stenting of an occlusion proximal in the left anterior descending coronary artery) 3 hours after onset of severe chest pain, and he died 30 hours later in circulatory failure. Autopsy revealed extensive hemorrhagic infarction involving most of the left ventricle.

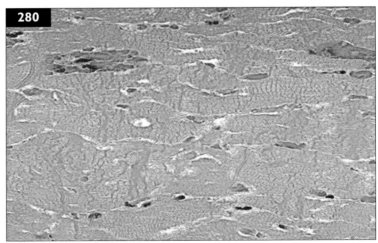

280 Reperfused myocardial tissue. Islets of hemorrhage are present between swollen myocardial fibers. Note the presence of contraction bands. (Hematoxylin-eosin stain.)

DOWNSTREAM (MICRO)EMBOLIZATION, SLOW FLOW, AND NO REFLOW

ERLING FALK, MD, PhD AND LEIF THUESEN, MD, PhD

INTRODUCTION

Coronary plaques responsible for ischemic heart disease contain a variable mix of chronic atherosclerosis and acute thrombosis. The exact nature of the mix is unknown in the individual patient but, in general, fibrous atherosclerotic plaques predominate in stable angina, whereas thrombosed plaques predominate in acute coronary syndromes (ACS). The nature of the culprit lesion is a major determinant for the risk of acute vascular occlusion, not only locally (epicardial artery) but also downstream. Particulate material (thrombus and plaque) may embolize and active substances (e.g. vasoconstrictors, tissue factor) may also be carried downstream and cause obstruction of peripheral branches and/or the microcirculation[1]. This phenomenon may occur spontaneously (see **61**) but is particularly frequent during percutaneous coronary intervention (PCI) in severely diseased aortocoronary saphenous vein grafts (SVGs) or infarct-related arterie. Thus, mechanical crushing and fragmentation of atherothrombotic lesion during PCI has emerged as a major cause of intracoronary (micro)embolization[2].

The risk of PCI-induced distal embolization depends on the atherothrombotic burden and the invasiveness of the procedure[3]. Consequently, it is relatively common in two clinical settings: PCI in symptomatic SVG disease (bulky and friable plaques, **281**) and in AMI (thrombosed plaques, see **54**); atherectomy and stenting cause more plaque fragmentation and distal embolization than balloon angioplasty[3]. Thus, despite otherwise successful recanalization, PCI-induced distal (micro)embolization and (micro)vascular obstruction may lead to inadequate myocardial perfusion and the so-called no or slow (re)flow phenomenon.

SPONTANEOUS INTRACORONARY (MICRO)EMBOLIZATION

Atherosclerotic plaques responsible for ACS are, in general, larger (hidden in positively remodeled arterie) and softer (contain more lipid and less calcification) than angina producing lesions (see Chapter 5, Atherothrombosis). Such plaques have a relatively high embolic potential. In plaque rupture, not only superimposed thrombosis but also plaque components may embolize downstream (**282, 283**). Postmortem studies of patients who died after an acute

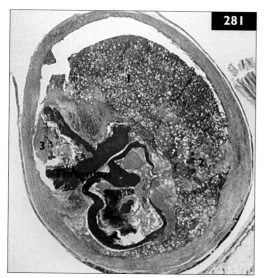

281 Cross-section of a 4-year-old saphenous vein graft, showing a ruptured and thrombosed plaque filled with lipid-rich and soft atheromatous gruel (1). Such a bulky and friable atherothrombotic lesion has a high embolic potential, particularly when crushed and fragmented during percutaneous coronary intervention. Thrombus and erythrocytes are red and collagen is blue (2) in this trichrome stain. 3: lumen.

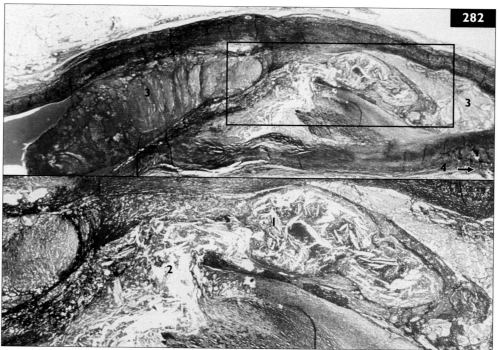

282 Spontaneous plaque disaster. Longitudinal section of a coronary artery occluded by atheromatous plaque material (rich in cholesterol crystals, 1) that has been displaced into the lumen through a large gap (rupture, 2) in the plaque surface. Such a 'plaque disaster' probably has a high atheroembolic potential. An erythrocyte-rich stagnation thrombus (3) has formed proximally and distally to the occluding atheromatous material. Thrombus and erythrocytes are red and collagen is blue in this trichrome stain. 4: downstream.

heart attack have revealed thromboemboli and, more rarely, atheroemboli impacted downstream in small intramyocardial arterie in a high proportion of cases[2].

The overall magnitude and significance of spontaneous intracoronary microembolization are, however, unknown. It is generally assumed that troponin elevations in ACS without ST elevation indicate (micro)infarction of thromboembolic origin[1], but it is not necessarily so. Thus, a dynamic atherothrombotic culprit lesion may cause subendocardial ischemia and necrosis by reducing the blood flow subcritically and/or temporarily without implicating microembolization.

PERCUTANEOUS CORONARY INTERVENTION IN SAPHENOUS VEIN GRAFT, (MICRO)EMBOLIZATION, AND SLOW FLOW

Atherogenesis is notably accelerated in SVGs, and fatal atherothrombosis may develop within a few years after grafting (**281**)[2,4]. Symptomatic plaques in SVGs are generally much larger and contain more lipid, inflammation (foam cells), and thrombus and less calcification, regardless of clinical presentation[4]. Consequently, the atherothrombotic burden is larger in SVG disease, and downstream embolization and (micro)vascular obstruction are frequent, particularly when these bulky and friable atherothrombotic plaques are crushed and fragmented mechanically during surgery or PCI.

PCI of stenotic SVGs is associated with an exceptionally high risk of macroembolization (angiographic distal cut-off) and slow flow through myocardium that was perfused normally before PCI[5]. The most obvious explanation is PCI-induced distal embolization, confirmed by the pronounced reduction in procedure-related slow flow and MI with the use of a distal embolic protection device during stenting[5,6]. In contrast, disappointing results have been obtained with catheter-based thrombectomy before stenting and with membrane-covered stents (to seal the lesion)[7-9]. The lack of a consistent benefit with the use of potent antiplatelet agents during PCI in SVGs may indicate that embolized atheromatous debris rather than platelet-mediated thromboembolism is responsible for the detrimental effects associated with stenting of stenotic SVG lesions[5,10].

PRIMARY PERCUTANEOUS CORONARY INTERVENTION, (MICRO)EMBOLIZATION, AND NO REFLOW

Timely, complete and sustained reperfusion may save myocardium at risk of undergoing necrosis in patients with evolving STEMI. Such infarcts nearly always remain anemic and pale if not reperfused. Therapeutic reperfusion is, however, associated with extravasation of erythrocytes in the ischemic tissues that already have passed the point of no return, giving rise acutely to a hemorrhagic and red infarct (**284**). In addition, reperfusion is not homogeneous and, in particular, 'no reflow' may be a cause and/or a consequence of infarction. In this

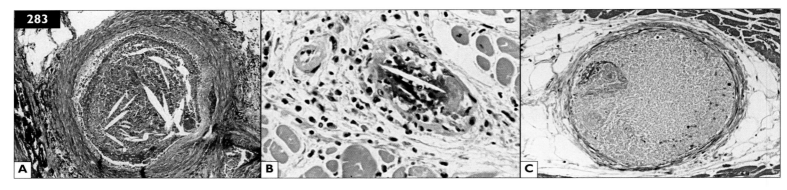

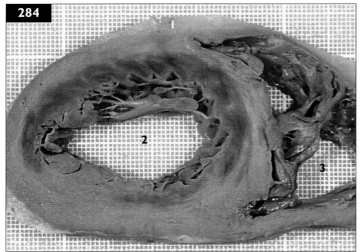

283 Spontaneous distal embolization. In plaque rupture, atheromatous plaque material may embolize distally and occlude side branches (**A**) and smaller intramyocardial arteries (**B**). Platelet-rich microemboli are frequently found impacted in myocardial microcirculation (**C**) downstream from a thrombotic culprit lesion in the supplying artery.

284 Hemorrhagic reperfusion myocardial infarction. Transventricular section of the heart from a patient who died 30 hours after primary stenting of a thrombosed left anterior descending (1) coronary artery. Although reperfusion may save myocardium at risk of undergoing necrosis, it is also associated with extravasation of erythrocytes (interstitial hemorrhage) into already necrotic tissues. 2: left ventricle; 3: right ventricle.

context it is important to realize that the pathogenesis of no reflow after primary PCI differs significantly from the 'classic' no reflow phenomenon seen after temporary occlusion of normal coronary arteries in animals[11].

Classic no reflow in animals

After coronary occlusion in dogs, myocytes begin to die in the subendocardial myocardium after ~20 minutes, and ischemic cell death progresses from the subendocardium to the subepicardium as a wavefront in a time-dependent fashion[11]. About 6 hours of ischemia are required to complete the wavefront of necrosis. Although myocardial necrosis averaging 28% of the vascular bed has developed after 40 minutes of ischemia, myocardial reperfusion is still homogeneous without any defect if coronary flow is restored. However, if coronary flow is not restored until after 90 minutes of ischemia, myocardial perfusion defects (no reflow) are now present in myocardium that was necrotic at an earlier time point, first in the subendocardial zone[11]. No reflow, or more correctly 'no reperfusion', appears to be confined to myocardium that is already necrotic and thus follows necrosis and not *vice versa*. To date, no study of 'pure' coronary occlusion (that is, without microembolization) has demonstrated myocardial no reperfusion preceding myocardial necrosis[11]. The no reperfusion areas enlarge both with the degree and duration of ischemia and with the duration of reperfusion (combined ischemia and reperfusion injury)[11,12].

The inability to reperfuse necrotic myocardium is caused by progressive microvascular occlusion. Many different obstructive mechanisms have been proposed such as endothelial swelling, neutrophil plugging, vascular 'squeezing' by ischemic contracture (intracellular calcium overload), or compression from the surrounding necrotic and swollen myocytes[11]. Microvessels plugged by platelets and fibrin are also seen, but microembolism does not occur in experimental coronary ligation and fibrinolytic treatment is ineffective in this model.

No reflow after primary percutaneous coronary intervention

No reflow in human MI is even more complex and multi-factorial than that seen after coronary ligation in animals, because the clinical setting involves an atherothrombotic dynamic occlusion with its innate risk of distal embolization when crushed or fragmented mechanically during PCI. Thus, coronary no reflow and myocardial hypoperfusion after otherwise successful recanalization of infarct-related artery probably involve more than just classic no reperfusion confined to myocardium that is already dead. No reflow may also result from PCI-induced (micro)vascular obstruction caused by distal (micro)embolization and/or microvascular spasm[1]. Because emboli necessarily stream preferentially to well perfused and viable myocardium, potentially salvageable myocardium may vanish. PCI-induced (micro)embolization may, in fact, not only prevent optimal reperfusion, it may worsen the ischemia if distal branches receiving collateral flow get closed. Thus, the vital question is, of course: how much of the coronary no reflow and myocardial hypoperfusion seen after primary PCI reflects the classic no reflow phenomenon caused by necrosis, and how much reflects PCI-induced distal microembolization (and possibly microvascular spasm) causing more necrosis? The thrombotic burden may prove to be critical, indicated by the beneficial effect of platelet glycoprotein (GP) IIb/IIIa receptor inhibition before stenting for AMI[13]. Whether thrombectomy before PCI or distal embolic protection devices during PCI (**285–288**) will improve myocardial perfusion and clinical outcomes remains to be documented by ongoing clinical trials [7,14–16].

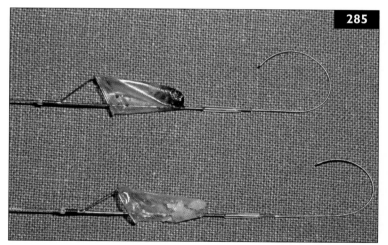

285 Distal embolic protection filter catches during primary percutaneous coronary intervention (PCI) (mixed [**upper**] and white [**lower**] thromboemboli). Retrieval of embolic material by distal protection devices (balloon occlusion/aspiration or filter) documents that distal (micro)embolization does occur during PCI.

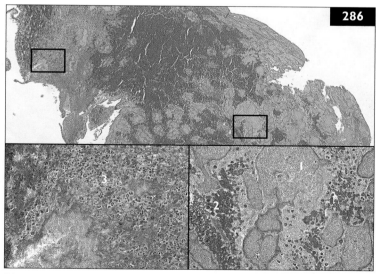

286 Percutaneous coronary intervention-induced thromboembolism. Filter-retrieved thromboembolus containing platelets (1), erythrocytes (2) and, in this case, also a lot of inflammatory cells (mainly neutrophils, 3).

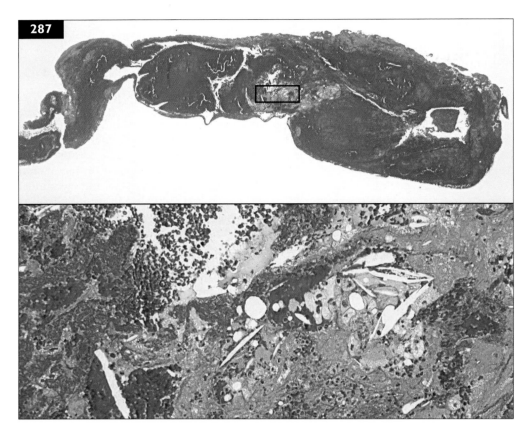

287 Percutaneous coronary intervention-induced atheroembolism. Filter-retrieved thromboembolus containing atheromatous plaque material (cholesterol crystals and foam cells).

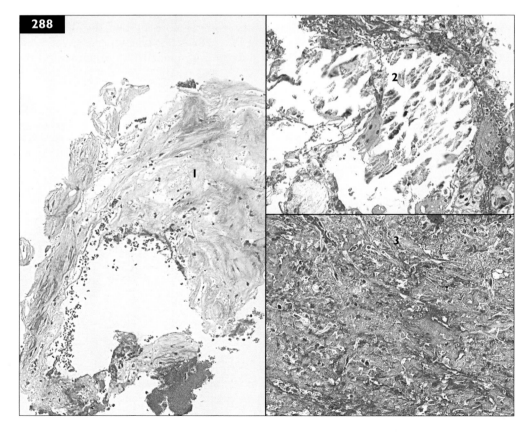

288 Percutaneous coronary intervention (PCI)-induced embolism. Embolized fragments of fibrous plaque (1), calcified plaque (2), and old thrombus (partly organized) (3) captured by distal protection devices during PCI.

AGE AND ACUTE MYOCARDIAL INFARCTION

WILBERT S. ARONOW, MD, FACC

INTRODUCTION

Although persons >65 years of age account for 12% of the USA population, this age group accounts for 61% of patients hospitalized with AMI and for 80% of all deaths attributable to AMI[1]. Older age is associated with increased mortality and morbidity during and after MI[2]. *Table 35* shows the age-related increase in mortality during hospitalization of 9,720 patients hospitalized with first MI treated with thrombolysis in the trial conducted by the Gruppo Italiano per lo Studio della Sopravvivenza nell' Infarto Myocardico (GISSI-2)[3].

Table 35 Mortality during hospitalization for first myocardial infarction in 9,720 patients treated with thrombolysis

Age (years)	Mortality (%)
≤40	1.9
41–45	2.2
45–50	2.1
51–55	3.1
56–60	3.5
61–65	5.8
66–70	10.1
71–75	14.7
76–80	18.9
>80	31.9

(Modified from Maggioni et al. [1993][3]. Age-related increase in mortality among patients with first myocardial infarctions treated in thrombolysis. *N. Engl. J. Med.* **329**: 1442–1448.)

Table 36 Mortality during interval from hospital discharge to 6 months follow-up for first myocardial infarction in 9,720 patients treated with thrombolysis

Age (years)	Mortality (%)
≤40	0.8
41–45	1.0
46–50	1.5
51–55	0.9
56–60	1.6
61–65	2.6
66–70	3.5
71–75	5.3
76–80	8.6
>80	11.6

(Modified from Maggioni et al. [1993][3]. Age-related increase in mortality among patients with first myocardial infarctions treated in thrombolysis. *N. Engl. J. Med.* **329**: 1442–1448.)

In this study, an age >80 years increased the odds ratio of mortality during hospitalization 18.8 times (95% CI, 5.3–66.8)[3]. *Table 36* shows the age-related increase in mortality during the interval from hospital discharge to 6 months after hospital discharge for first MI treated with thrombolysis in the GISSI-2 study[3]. An age >80 years also increased the odds ratio of mortality from hospital discharge to 6 months after hospital discharge 9.0 times (95% CI, 2.64–30.92)[3].

AGE-RELATED CHANGES CONTRIBUTING TO MORTALITY

Numerous factors contribute to the increased mortality and morbidity in elderly patients with MI. *Table 37* lists age-related changes contributing to increased mortality and morbidity in elderly patients with MI[4]. *Table 38* lists other age-related factors contributing to increased mortality and morbidity in elderly patients with MI. Compared to patients <75 years of age, patients aged 75 years and older in the Global Utilization of Streptokinase and Tissue Plasminogen Activator for Occluded Coronary Arteries (GUSTO) angiographic trial, had a higher prevalence of multi-vessel coronary artery disease (CAD), prior MI, anterior MI, hypertension, diabetes mellitus, congestive heart failure (CHF), abnormal LV ejection fraction, and shock[5]. In the Cooperative Cardiovascular Project, atrial fibrillation was present in 22% of 106,780 patients aged 65 years or older with acute MI[6]. Compared with sinus rhythm, patients with atrial fibrillation had a higher in-hospital mortality (25% versus 16%), 30-day mortality (29% versus 19%), and 1-year mortality (48% versus 33%)[6].

Elderly persons have a higher prevalence of unrecognized MI than younger persons, with 21% to 68% of MIs being unrecognized or silent in elderly persons[7–11]. The incidence of new coronary

Table 37 Age-related changes contributing to increased mortality and morbidity in elderly patients with acute myocardial infarction

- Increased vascular stiffness with rise in systolic blood pressure and pulse pressure.
- Reduced arterial compliance.
- Reduced LV early diastolic filling.
- Prolonged duration of LV contraction and relaxation.
- LV diastolic dysfunction predisposes to heart failure and atrial fibrillation, increasing mortality.
- Age-associated decreases in maximal heart rate and in LV contractility during maximal exercise are manifestations of reduced beta-adrenergic responsiveness.
- Reduction in number of myocytes due to apoptosis.
- Impaired production of ATP by mitochrondria of older myocytes.
- Reduction in pulmonary reserve and renal function.
- Impaired autoregulatory ability of central nervous system to maintain cerebral perfusion.
- Impaired neurohormonal responsiveness increases risk of hypotension and lability of blood pressure.

ATP: adenosine triphosphate; LV: left ventricle.

events in elderly persons with unrecognized or recognized MI is similar[9–12]. Some studies have also shown a higher incidence of dyspnea and of neurological symptoms than of chest pain in elderly persons with AMI[8,13,14].

In addition, elderly persons delay longer in seeking medical assistance after the onset of chest pain than younger persons[15,16]. In 102,339 persons aged >65 years with confirmed AMI in the Cooperative Cardiovascular Project, 29.4% arrived at the hospital ≥6 hours after symptom onset[16].

NON-ST ELEVATION MYOCARDIAL INFARCTION

The prevalence of non-ST elevation MI (NSTEMI) is also higher in elderly persons than in younger persons[15,17]. In a prospective study of 177 consecutive unselected patients aged ≥70 years (91 women, mean age 79 years, and 86 men, mean age 77 years) hospitalized for ACS, all patients had CAG[17]. Of the 177 patients, 95 (54%) had unstable angina pectoris (UAP), 61 (34%) had NSTEMI, and 21 (12%) had STEMI[17]. Regardless of the type of MI, elderly persons with AMI demonstrate more LV dysfunction than younger persons upon hospital admission and have a more complicated hospital course[15].

MANAGEMENT

Table 39 shows American College of Cardiology/American Heart Association Class I indications for treatment of acute MI[18]. All of these therapeutic interventions are underutilized in elderly patients with MI.

Thrombolysis

Thrombolytic therapy should be considered in patients <75 years of age with STEMI[18]. Pooling long-term data after thrombolytic therapy for MI from three studies showed that thrombolysis caused an 18% relative reduction in mortality in younger patients versus a 10% relative reduction in mortality in older patients, and a 2% absolute reduction in mortality in younger patients versus a

3% absolute reduction in mortality in older patients[19–21]. The Fibrinolytic Therapy Trialists' Collaborative Group summarized randomized, placebo-controlled data in 5,754 patients with AMI aged ≥75 years treated with thrombolytic therapy[22]. At 35-day follow-up, there was an insignificant difference in mortality in patients treated with thrombolysis (24.3%) versus placebo (25.3%). However, thrombolysis caused an absolute reduction of 10 deaths per 1,000 treated patients[22].

Older patients with AMI at increased risk for hemorrhagic stroke should not be treated with thrombolysis. Thrombolytic therapy is also not effective in the treatment of NSTEMI[22].

Table 39 American College of Cardiology/American Heart Association Class I indications for management of acute myocardial infarction

Intervention	Class I indication
Thrombolysis	Ischemic symptoms with ST elevation or LBBB =12 hours from onset of symptoms in patients <75 years.
Primary PTCA	PTCA with or without stenting is an alternative to thrombolysis when performed by experienced personnel within 90–120 minutes of hospital arrival for all age groups; cardiogenic shock within 36 hours of onset of MI in patients <75 years.
Aspirin	For all age groups beginning on day 1 of MI.
Unfractionated heparin	For all age groups undergoing PTCA or surgical revascularization.
Low-molecular weight heparin	For all age groups with NSTEMI.
Platelet glycoprotein II_b/ III_a inhibitors	For all age groups with NSTEMI with continuing ischemia, hemodynamic instability, or planned PTCA.
Beta blockers	For all age groups within 12 hours of onset of MI; for all age groups with continuing or recurrent ischemic chest pain; for all age groups with tachyarrhythmias.
ACE inhibitors	For all age groups with anterior MI within 24 hours; for all age groups with heart failure; for all age groups with left ventricular ejection fraction <40%.
Nitrates	First 24–48 hours for large MI, heart failure, or persistent ischemia in all age groups; after 48 hours for persistent ischemia or heart failure in all age groups.
Calcium channel blockers	None
Magnesium	None

ACE: angiotensin-converting enzyme; LBBB: left bundle branch block; MI: myocardial infarction; NSTEMI: non-ST elevation MI; PTCA: percutaneous transluminal coronary angioplasty. (Modified from Ryan *et al.* [1999][18]. ACC/AHA guidelines for the management of patients with acute myocardial infarction: executive summary and recommendations. *Circulation* **100**: 1016–1030.)

Table 38 Other age-related factors contributing to increased mortality and morbidity in elderly patients with acute myocardial infarction

- Higher prevalence of left main and multi-vessel coronary artery disease.
- Higher prevalence of prior myocardial infarction.
- Higher prevalence of congestive heart failure and of abnormal left ventricular ejection fraction.
- Higher prevalence of atrial fibrillation.
- Higher prevalence of hypertension and diabetes mellitus.
- Higher prevalence of valvular heart disease such as aortic stenosis.
- Higher prevalence of peripheral arterial disease and cerebrovascular disease.
- Higher prevalence of chronic obstructive pulmonary disease and renal insufficiency.
- Atypical symptoms with delayed presentation.
- Underutilization of established therapies.

PRIMARY CORONARY ANGIOPLASTY

Data favor the use of primary coronary angioplasty when available rather than thrombolysis in the treatment of elderly patients with AMI who are poor candidates for thrombolysis[23]. In such patients, coronary angioplasty was associated with a reduction in mortality of 26% at 30 days and of 12% at 1 year, compared with thrombolysis, after adjustment for baseline cardiac risk factors and admission and hospital characteristics[23].

Aspirin

Aspirin reduces mortality in elderly patients with acute MI[24,25] and should be administered on day 1 for an AMI and continued indefinitely[18]. In an observational prospective study of 1,410 patients, mean age 81 years, with prior MI and hypercholesterolemia, 59% of patients were treated with aspirin[26]. At 36-month follow-up, use of aspirin was associated with a 52% reduction in new coronary events (risk ratio = 0.48; 95% CI, 0.42–0.55)[26].

Low-molecular weight heparin

Data from the Thrombolysis in Myocardial Infarction II B trial[27,28] and the Enoxaparin in Unstable Angina and Non-Q-Wave Myocardial Infarction trial[28,29] showed that enoxaparin should replace unfractionated heparin as the antithrombin for the acute phase of treatment of patients with NSTEMI and be administered with aspirin in the treatment of these patients.

Beta blockers

Pooled data from the Goteborg Trial[30], the Metoprolol in Acute Myocardial Infarction Trial[31], and the First International Study of Infarct Survival[32] showed that early IV beta blockade caused a 23% reduction in mortality in elderly patients. Propranolol caused a 33% reduction in mortality at 25-month follow-up of elderly postinfarction patients[33]. Timolol caused a 43% reduction in mortality at 17-month follow-up of elderly postinfarction patients[34].

Angiotensin-converting enzyme inhibitors

Angiotensin-converting-enzyme (ACE) inhibitors administered within 24 hours of infarction to elderly patients reduce mortality[35–37]. In postinfarction patients aged ≥65 years with an LV ejection fraction ≤40%, captopril reduced mortality by 25% at 42-month follow-up[38]. Ramipril reduced mortality by 36% at 15-month follow-up in patients aged ≥65 years with MI and CHF[39]. In postinfarction patients, mean age 68 years, with an LV ejection fraction ≤35%, trandolapril reduced mortality by 33% in patients with anterior MI and 14% in patients without anterior MI[40]. On the basis of data from the Heart Outcomes Prevention Evaluation Study[41], all postinfarction patients should be treated with ACE inhibitors.

Statins

All elderly postinfarction patients with hypercholesterolemia should be treated with statins to reduce mortality, recurrent MI, stroke, CHF, and peripheral arterial disease[42–49]. On the basis of data from the Heart Protection Study[50], all elderly postinfarction patients should be treated with statins, regardless of their initial serum lipids.

GENDER DIFFERENCES IN ACUTE MYOCARDIAL INFARCTION

JOHAN HERLITZ, MD, PhD

INTRODUCTION

During the last few decades, many studies have been performed trying to explore differences between women and men suffering from AMI. One of the major limitations of many of these studies was that they only included patients hospitalized due to AMI and often only patients admitted to the Coronary Care Unit (CCU), thus studying selected cohorts, since only a subset of patients suffering from AMI will survive to hospital admission and an even smaller subset will be admitted to the CCU. With these limitations in mind, this section will try to compare women with men in terms of various aspects of AMI.

AGE AND PREVIOUS HISTORY

Many studies have shown that women who suffer from AMI are older than men. In terms of their previous history, women more frequently suffer from a history of hypertension, diabetes mellitus, and CHF even when correcting for dissimilarities in age. On the other hand, they less frequently suffer from a history of AMI (**289**).

SYMPTOMS AND DELAY TO SEEK MEDICAL CARE

Women seem to suffer more frequently from warning or prodromal symptoms other than chest pain prior to AMI. When suffering from AMI, the intensity and the occcurrence of chest pain do not differ markedly between sexes, although women require less morphine than men. However, such information has not been related to body weight.

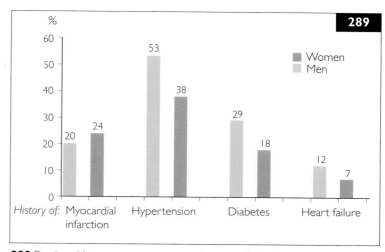

289 Previous history among women and men suffering from myocardial infarction (mean values from 24 reports comparing women and men suffering from acute myocardial infarction).

Women can localize their pain slightly differently from men (more often in their back, neck, and jaw). Furthermore, they have been reported to use some words when describing their pain more frequently than men (tearing, terrifying, tiring, and intolerable) and other words less frequently than men (grinding and frightening). Women more often suffer from nausea, vomiting, abdominal complaints, fatigue, and dyspnea and less often from cold sweat as compared with men. Whether these differences in symptoms explain the fact that women wait longer than men until they seek medical care after onset of AMI is not known. However, although there are many minor differences between women and men in terms of symptom presentation, the differences are not substantial enough to recommend that women should be treated differently from men in the early phase of a suspected AMI.

CLINICAL PRESENTATION
Among patients with ST elevation infarction, women have been reported to have less substantial ST elevation than men, but this was not confirmed by others. No clear differences between women and men have been found in terms of other ECG variables.

COMPLICATIONS IN HOSPITAL
As shown in **290**, women more frequently suffer from CHF than men, whereas ventricular fibrillation (VF) occurs with a similar frequency regardless of sex.

TREATMENT IN HOSPITAL
It has been suggested that women suffering from AMI are treated less aggressively than men. However, this has not been confirmed by others. Many studies have shown that women are more often treated with diuretics than men. This may be explained by a higher prevalence of hypertension and CHF in women. It has also been

reported that women are given less morphine than men, but the results were not adjusted for differences in body weight. Furthermore, women have repeatedly been shown to receive thrombolytic agents less frequently, and less frequently undergo coronary artery bypass grafting(CABG) and percutaneous transluminal coronary angioplasty (PTCA) than men (**291**). This may to some extent be explained by a difference in age.

EFFECT OF INTERVENTIONS ON MORTALITY
Results from large randomized trials indicate that treatment with thrombolysis is associated with a more marked reduction in mortality among men than among women, and the opposite has been found with regard to beta blockers. However, it is not clear in what way these results were influenced by differences in age. Furthermore, there was no significant relationship between treatment effect and gender.

SHORT-TERM MORTALITY
Women hospitalized for AMI have nearly double the short-term mortality than men (**290**). When correcting for dissimilarities between women and men in age and comorbidity much of the difference is eliminated. However, some studies still report a higher mortality in women. Among patients aged >50 years, this is explained by a higher pre-hospital mortality in men. Thus, among patients aged >50 years the overall mortality in AMI, including both the pre-hospital and the hospital phases, appears to be the same in women and men. However, among patients <50 years old, the overall mortality has been reported to be higher among women than men. Much of the excess mortality in young women seems to be associated with diabetes.

With regard to mortality among patients being hospitalized due to AMI there is a relationship between age and the difference

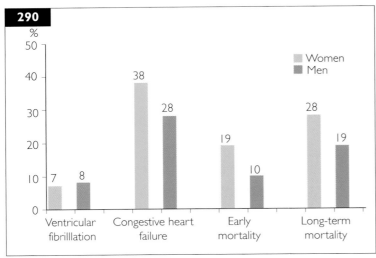

290 Occurrence of complications while in hospital and early mortality (mean values from 24 reports comparing women and men suffering from acute myocardial infarction).

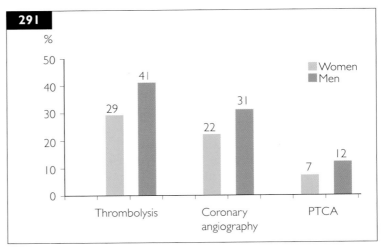

291 Use of revascularization (mean values from 24 reports comparing women and men suffering from acute myocardial infarction). PTCA: percutaneous transluminal coronary angioplasty.

in prognosis among women and men. Thus, the increased mortality in women is particularly observed among younger patients whereas no such difference is observed among the elderly.

MEDICATION AT DISCHARGE
There are no major differences in medication at discharge, but some studies suggest that beta blockers and aspirin are prescribed less frequently to women. This may be explained to some extent by a difference in age. Women have been reported to be more frequently prescribed diuretics than men.

LONG-TERM MORTALITY
As shown in **290**, women have a higher long-term mortality than men. However, the magnitude of the difference is the same as for short-term mortality, indicating that the survival curves do not deviate any further during the long term.

QUALITY OF LIFE
Women have repeatedly been shown to have an inferior health related quality of life after AMI than men. Whether this is explained by insufficient rehabilitation, less aggressive revascularization and medication, or simply that women have an inferior quality of life both among healthy and diseased persons is not clear.

SUMMARY
Among patients hospitalized due to AMI there are differences between women and men in terms of age, previous history, symptoms, delay to seeking medical care, clinical presentation, complications in hospital, treatment in hospital, prognosis, and quality of life after discharge from hospital. In many aspects these differences are small and of minor clinical significance. At present there is no reason to recommend that treatment of women with AMI should differ from the treatment of men.

DIABETES AND ACUTE MYOCARDIAL INFARCTION

JOSEPH ARAGON, MD AND PREDIMAN K. SHAH, MD

INTRODUCTION
'With an excess of fat diabetes begins and from an excess of fat diabetics die.'
E.P. Joslin 1927

The prevalence of type 2 diabetes has been steadily increasing in the USA and some Asian countries, in part related to increased prevalence of obesity and physical inactivity (**292**).

In the United States:
- 17 million have diabetes
  - 11.1 million have known diabetes
  - 5.9 million have undiagnosed diabetes
  - 90% to 95% have type 2 diabetes
- 114,400 new cases diagnosed per year
- CVD is the leading cause of diabetes-related deaths. Adults with diabetes have CVD death rates 2 to 4 times higher than adults without diabetes.

Obesity, in particular abdominal (visceral) fat accumulation, is associated with the development of the metabolic syndrome including insulin resistance, hyperinsulinemia, atherogenic dyslipidemia (see Chapter 19, Diabetic Atherogenic Dyslipidemaias), hypertension, reduced fibrinolytic potential (high plasminogen activator inhibitor 1 [PAI-1]), and eventually hyperglycemia and overt type 2 diabetes (**293**).

The spectrum of lipoprotein abnormalities commonly observed in diabetic patients includes:
- Hypertriglyceridemia (VLDL, intermediate-density lipoprotein, remnants)
- ↓ HDL cholesterol
- Lipoprotein composition
  - ↑ TG
  - ↑ Cholesterol/lecithin

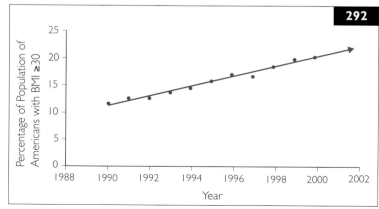

292 Graph to show the increasing prevalence of obesity in the USA from 1988–2002. This trend parallels the rising prevalence of type 2 diabetes.

- Glycation/oxidation
- ↑ LP(a) (renal disease)

HDL: high-density lipoprotein; Lp(a): Lipoprotein a; TG: triglyceride; VLDL: very low-density lipoprotein.

Diabetes mellitus, especially type 2 diabetes, is an important risk factor for athero-thrombotic cardiovascular disease (**294**). Diabetes also confers an adverse prognosis during all stages of coronary heart disease. Cardiovascular complications are the leading cause of death in diabetics. Approximately 18–25% of patients with AMI tend to have diabetes. Compared to individuals without diabetes, diabetics

face a 2–4-fold higher risk of coronary heart disease (**294**). Diabetic patients also experience a twofold higher risk of short-term and, in some studies, long-term death, following an AMI despite adjustments for other confounding covariates (**295**).

Diabetics without a history of coronary heart disease have similar long-term mortality to nondiabetics with prior MI, giving rise to the notion that diabetes is a coronary heart disease risk equivalent (**296**). Coronary angioplasty and stenting, with bare metal or drug-eluting stents, are associated with a higher risk of restenosis in diabetics compared to nondiabetics.

MECHANISMS OF ADVERSE CARDIOVASCULAR PROGNOSIS IN DIABETES

There are several potential mechanisms by which diabetes may confer an increased risk of adverse outcomes in patients with AMI. These include:

- High prevalence of unrecognized or silent MI, in part related to extensive coronary atherosclerosis.
- Autonomic neuropathy and cardiomyopathy related to diabetes may be associated with systolic and diastolic LV dysfunction and increased risk of heart failure.
- Increased cardiac fibrosis that has been observed in hypertensive patients with diabetes.
- Metabolic derangements may alter myocardial energetics i.e. depressed ATP production.
- Increased oxidative stress and generation of glycosylated end-products may increase and enhance arterial and myocardial stiffness, induce inflammation, and impair endothelial function.
- Abnormal sympatho-adrenal autonomic balance increasing the risk of arrhythmia and sudden death.
- Impaired fibrinolysis, elevated fibrinogen levels and enhanced platelet aggregability contributing to enhanced vaso-occlusive complications.

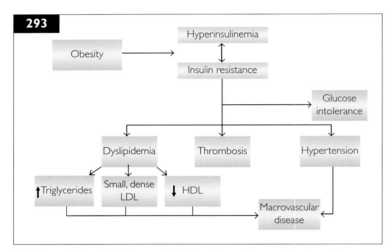

293 The relationship between obesity, insulin resistance, diabetes, and subsequent cardiovascular complications. Insulin resistance and relative insulin deficiency are believed to antedate the development of overt type 2 diabetes. HDL: high-density lipoprotein; LDL: low-density lipoprotein. (Adapted from Bloomgarden ZT. [1998]. Insulin resistance, current concepts. *Clin Ther* **20**:216–231; DeFronzo RA, Ferrannini E. [1991]. Insulin resistance. A multifaceted syndrome responsible for NIDDM, obesity, hypertension, dyslipidemia, and atherosclerotic cardiovascular disease. *Diabetes Care* **14**:173–194.

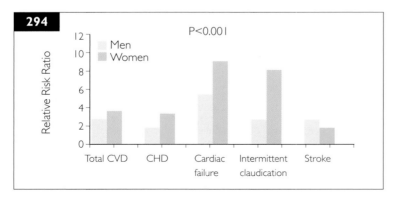

294 The increased relative risk of combined morbidity and mortality in diabetics is shown in comparison to nondiabetics from the Framingham cohort. CHD: coronary heart disease; CVD: cardiovascular disease. (Adapted from Wilson PWF, Kannnel WB [1992] Epidemiology of hyperglycemia and atherosclerosis. In: *Hyperglycemia, Diabetes and Vascular Disease*. N Ruderman et al., (eds.) Oxford University Press).

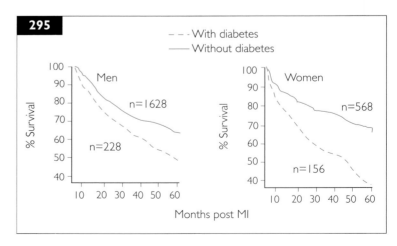

295 The adverse prognostic impact of diabetes in patients with acute myocardial infarction (MI) regardless of gender. (Adapted from Sprafka JM *et al* [1991]. Trends in prevalence of diabetes mellitus in patients with myocardial infarction and effect of diabetes on survival. The Minnesota Heart Survey. *Diabetes Care* **14**:537–543).

IMPROVING THE CARDIOVASCULAR PROGNOSIS OF DIABETICS

Several studies have demonstrated that effective control of hyperglycemia in diabetes reduces the risk of microvascular complications of diabetes (retinopathy, nephropathy, and neuropathy) with a modest beneficial effect on macrovascular complications (cardiovascular events) (**297**). Intensive glycemic control with insulin has been shown to reduce short-term and long-term mortality in diabetic patients with AMI (DIGAMI Study). Secondary prevention

measures including rigorous control of hypertension (preferably with renoprotective agents such as ACE inhibitors), use of antiplatelet agents such as aspirin, clopidogrel, and GP IIb/IIIa inhibitors during endovascular intervention, statins to modify dyslipidemia, and beta blockers to reduce ischemic complications have all been shown to reduce cardiovascular morbidity and mortality in diabetics (*Table 40*).

Preventive strategies for cardiovascular risk reduction in diabetes includes:
- Improved glycemic control.
- Lifestyle modification.
- Blood pressure reduction.
  Preferred agents.
  - angiotensin-converting enzyme (ACE) inhibitor.
  - angiotensin II receptor blocker (ARB).
- Antiplatelet therapy.
  - Asprin.
  - Clopidogrel.
- Lipid modification.
  - statin.
  - fibrate.
  - niacin.

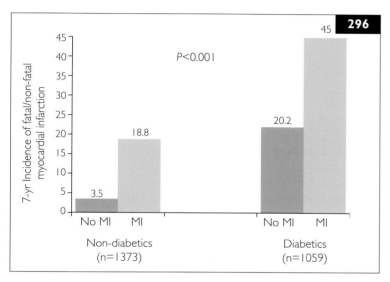

296 The adverse prognostic implications of diabetes, with or without a history of prior myocardial infarction (MI) are shown from the East-West study. Note that even in the absence of a history of MI, diabetics face a high risk which is comparable to that of a nondiabetic with prior MI. (Adapted from Haffner SM et al. [1998]. Mortality from coronary heart disease in subjects with type 2 diabetes and in nondiabetic subjects with and without prior myocardial infarction. *N Engl J Med* **339**:229–234.)

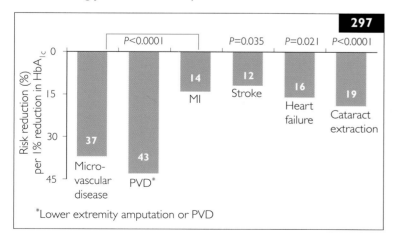

297 The benefits of tight glycemic control on microvascular and macrovascular complications of diabetes are shown from the UKPDS trial. MI: myocardial infarction; PVD: peripheral vascular disease. (Adapted from Stratton IM et al. [2000]. Association of glycemia with macrovascular and microvascular complications of type 2 diabetes for the UK PDS Group (UKPDS 35): prospective observational study. *BMJ* **321**:405–412.)

Table 40 Statin trials in diabetes

Study	Drug(dose)	n	CHD Risk Reduction (overall)	CHD Risk Reduction (diabetes)
1⁰ Prevention				
AFCAPS/TexCAPS[1]	Lovastatin	155	-37%	-43% (NS)
HPS[2]	Simvastatin	3985	-24%	-26% (P<.00001)†
2⁰ Prevention				
CARE[3]	Pravastatin	586	-23%	-25% (P=0.05)
4S[4]	Simvastatin	202	-32%	-55% (P=0.002)
LIPID[5]	Pravastatin	782	-25%	-19% (NS)
4S Reanalysis[6]	Simvastatin	483	-32%	-42% (P=0.001)
HPS[2]	Simvastatin	1978	-24%	-26% (P<.00001)†

*Subgroup analysis; †overall results for diabetic subgroup.
[1]Downs JR et al. Primary prevention of acute coronary events with lovastatin in men and women with average cholesterol levels: results of AFCAPS/TexCAPS. *JAMA* 1998;**279**:1615-1622; [2]HPS Investigators, MRC/BHF Heart Protection Study of cholesterol lowering with simvastatin in 20,536 high-risk individuals: a randomised placebo-controlled trial. *Lancet*. 2002;**360**:7-22; [3]Goldberg RB et al. Cardiovascular events and their reduction with pravastatin in diabetic and glucose-intolerant myocardial infarction survivors with average cholesterol levels: subgroup analyses in the cholesterol and recurrent events (CARE) trial. *Circulation* 1998;**98**:2513-2519; [4]Pyorala K et al. Cholesterol lowering with simvastatin improves prognosis of diabetic patients with coronary heart disease. A subgroup analysis of the Scandinavian Simvastatin Survival Study (4S). *Diabetes Care* 1997;**20**:614-620; [5]LIPID Study Group. Prevention of cardiovascular events and death with pravastatin in patients with coronary heart disease and a broad range of initial cholesterol levels. The Long-Term Intervention with Pravastatin in Ischaemic Disease (LIPID) Study. *N Engl J MED* 1998;**339**:1349-1357; [6]Haffner SM et al. Reduced coronary events in simvastatin-treated patients with coronary heart disease and diabetes or impaired fasting glucose levels: subgroup analyses in the Scandinavian Simvastatin Survival Study. *Arch Int Med* 1999;**159**:2661-2667.

CHD: coronary heart disease.

SMOKING

MORTEN BØTTCHER, MD, PhD

INTRODUCTION
Epidemiological data indicate that smoking is a risk factor for both myocardial infarction and sudden death[1]. In the Framingham study, male smokers had a 10-fold higher risk of sudden death and a 3.6 times higher risk of suffering an MI compared to nonsmokers[2]. Regarding stable angina pectoris, however, no increased risk could be detected. In both MI and sudden death, thrombosis and acute ischemia rather than the slow process of isolated atherosclerosis is believed to be the proximate cause. This would indicate that increased thrombogenetic factors which respond rapidly, rather than the slower processes of accelerated atherosclerotic factors, are the main determinants of the increased risk in smokers. Further evidence is provided by other studies in which the effect of smoking cessation has been evaluated. In these studies a rapid risk reduction is observed (3–6 months). This rapid risk reduction is different from the risk reduction seen in, for example, cholesterol-lowering trials such as LIPID, CARE, and 4S, in which the focus of treatment is the atherosclerotic process. In these trials, years of treatment are necessary to document any effect.

THROMBOSIS WITH LESS ATHEROSCLEROSIS
After successful thrombolysis for MI, less residual atherosclerosis has been documented in smokers[1]. This means that smokers develop a thrombus with less pre-existing disease than nonsmokers (**298**). It has been considered a paradox that after MI, smokers have a more favorable outcome with a relatively low short-term mortality. An explanation for this apparent paradox has been provided by recent large clinical trials looking at thrombolytic therapy. It was documented that although the patency rate was similar, smokers had more complete reperfusion, less residual stenosis, less multi-vessel disease, better ejection fraction and, perhaps most importantly, were much younger[1]. In the GUSTO-1 trial, smokers were on average 11 years younger than nonsmokers when suffering their first MI[3]. Therefore, the apparent paradox of smokers having a better survival after an MI is explained by a much lower age and by the fact that the occlusion causing the MI seems to contain much more thrombus and therefore responds much better to thrombolytic therapy. The same findings will no doubt be supported by recent trials of PCI for MI.

THROMBOGENIC RISK FACTORS
Smoking is associated with increased levels of thrombogenic factors[1]. Plasma fibrinogen is elevated in smokers, and both thrombin generation and platelet activation are seen after smoking just one cigarette. In patients with CAD, smoking has been shown to increase platelet thrombus formation even in patients taking aspirin. The mechanism of action is believed to be increased release of catecholamines.

ENDOTHELIAL DYSFUNCTION AND VASOMOTION
Chronic smoking is associated with both peripheral and coronary vascular endothelial dysfunction and an abnormal perfusion response to cold, suggesting an altered coronary vasomotor response. Acute smoking seemed to lower the coronary vasodilatory capacity while long-term chronic smoking did not affect the myocardial flow reserve[4] (**299**). Regarding endothelial independent vasodilatation, a similar degree of coronary vasodilatation following IV nitroglycerin in smokers and nonsmokers has been documented. Similarly, the hyperemic myocardial blood flow response to dipyridamole (which dilates the coronary microcirculation) was not significantly reduced in the smokers. These data add further support to the notion that smoking does not accelerate the atherosclerotic process, since a decreased dipyridamole response is used clinically in myocardial scintigraphy to detect the occurrence of flow-limiting atherosclerotic lesions. Several studies have documented that exposure to adrenergic stimuli such as smoking causes coronary segments with lesions to constrict. It has not been documented, however, whether smoking *per se* causes vasoconstriction.

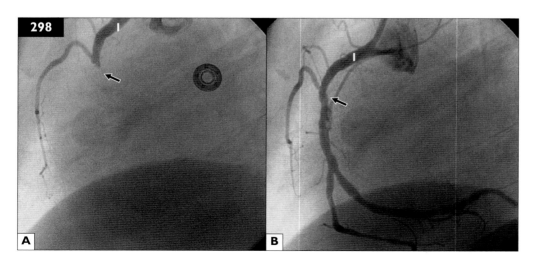

298 A 50-year-old male with no risk factors for ischemic heart disease other than smoking presented with acute onset of chest pain and electrocardiogram changes indicating inferior myocardial infarction. **A**: Acute coronary angiography revealed total occlusion (arrow) of the right coronary artery (1). **B**: The occlusion was penetrated with a guidewire and the thrombus disappeared (without angioplasty or stenting), leaving a nearly normal artery without any residual stenosis or other significant lesions.

AUTOPSY FINDINGS

The association between risk factors and the atherosclerotic process itself has been studied in five prospective epidemiologic trials with autopsy follow-up[1]. The trials were undertaken in five geographically different regions, and the findings are listed in *Table 41*. In all but the smallest study, serum cholesterol and blood pressure were found to correlate significantly with the total plaque burden. Smoking, however, did not correlate with plaque burden in the coronary arteries in any of the five studies. Other studies have confirmed these findings[5].

MYOCARDIAL OXYGEN DEMAND

Smoking causes the rate–pressure product to increase by approximately 20% and, correspondingly, myocardial perfusion increases[1]. Nicotine has been shown to be the causative agent of the adrenergic response, since smoking of nicotine-free cigarettes did not increase norepinephrine levels. It has been speculated that the increased wall stress and perhaps vasoconstriction in coronary segments with plaques might precipitate the occurrence of a plaque rupture.

ACUTE CORONARY OCCLUSION

Sudden cardiac death (SCD) may result from both plaque rupture with thrombus formation and from malignant arrhythmias arising from ischemic tissue. Regarding plaque rupture, there seems to be no good evidence to suggest that smoking changes the plaque composition, but the increased release of catecholamines and the resultant increase in hemodynamic variables may increase the mechanical strain on the plaque and cause it to rupture. Furthermore, increased adrenergic stress has the ability to constrict coronary artery segments with lesions. This might contribute to plaque rupture or at least to the requirement of a smaller thrombus to occlude a stenotic artery. Increased catecholamine stress also promotes thrombogenesis if a ruptured plaque is present in the coronary arteries. In combination with the unfavorable vasomotion effects of smoking, namely the decreased endothelial function which causes the coronary artery to diminish the dilatation response to the increased catecholamine levels, it forms the basis for an acute coronary occlusion. The documented increase in microvascular resistance during smoking may reduce the coronary flow and increase thrombus formation. The occlusion might be tightened by vasospasm at the pre-existing plaque in response to the increased adrenergic drive.

Table 41 Correlation between coronary plaque burden by autopsy and risk factors

Autopsy studies in five different geographical locations with indications of whether (+) or not (−) multi-variate analysis found the parameter to be a predictor of autopsy-verified coronary atherosclerosis, assessed as intimal area covered by plaques.

Study Location	n	Serum cholesterol	Blood pressure	Smoking
Oslo	129	+	+	−
Puerto Rico	139	+	+	−
Honolulu	258	+	+	−
Hisayama	281	+	+	−
Framingham				
Male	73	+	−	
Female	54	−	−	

Multivariate analyses: + = significant;   − = nonsignificant

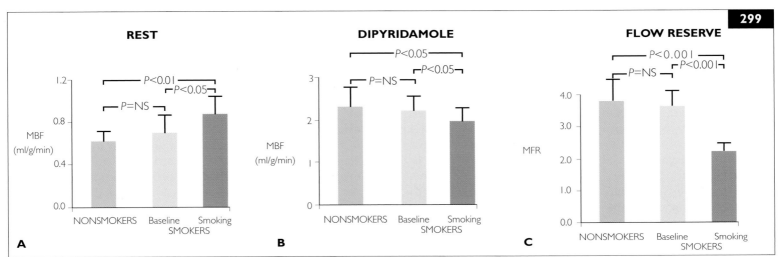

299 Bar graphs to show rest and hyperemic blood flow in study and control groups. **A**: Myocardial blood flow (MBF) at rest did not differ between smokers and nonsmokers under baseline conditions. Short-term smoking induced a significant increase in MBF in proportion to the increase in rate–pressure product.
B: MBF during intravenous dipyridamole did not differ between smokers and nonsmokers under baseline conditions. Short-term smoking induced a significant decrease in hyperemic MBF (*P*<0.05 versus baseline and control). **C**: The increase in resting blood flow together with the decline in hyperemic blood flow resulted in a marked reduction in the myocardial flow reserve (MFR) during short-term smoking (*P*<0.0001 versus nonsmokers; *P*<0.01 versus baseline). (Modified from Czernin et al. [1995]. Effect of acute and long-term smoking on myocardial blood flow and flow reserve. *Circulation* **91**:2891–2897.)

ACUTE MYOCARDIAL INFARCTION IN NORMAL CORONARY ARTERIES

IRA PERRY, MD AND SAIBAL KAR, MD

INTRODUCTION
An AMI is most often seen in the setting of atherosclerosis of the coronary arteries. However, the occurrence of an AMI in the setting of 'normal coronary arteries' has been well documented. However, the term 'normal coronarie' needs to be defined. In the literature, it is used to mean both angiographically normal and without evidence of atherosclerosis.

EPIDEMIOLOGY
The incidence reported ranges from 1% to 12%. The range can be explained by the differing definitions as well as the patient populations studied. The studies with a higher incidence allow for a higher level of angiographic irregularity. Some studies included patients with <25% stenosis as normal. Other studies have a selection or population bias, which can similarly alter the incidence. In younger populations, the incidence of AMI with angiographically normal coronary arteries is even higher than 12%. However, by all standards, while the percentage of AMI occurring in normal coronary arteries is low, it does occur.

ETIOLOGIES
The patient population is predominantly younger. Most studies report a strong smoking history. Given the diverse potential etiologies, it is not surprising that some studies show a lower cardiac risk profile when compared to patients with significant coronary stenosis, while others have not found a difference. Possible mechanisms of infarction include spasm, thrombus formation, embolization, and plaque rupture in a positively remodeled coronary, dissection, and myocarditis.

Vasospasm
The theory of MI caused by vasospasm with thrombus formation has been well described as a mechanism in atherosclerotic coronaries. It can also play a role in the occlusion of arterie without plaque. Spasm with evidence of thrombus has been documented angiographically, where intravascular ultrasound (IVUS) has confirmed the absence of atherosclerosis. The spasm may be due to a vasospastic syndrome such as Raynaud's phenomenon or migraine headaches. It can also be seen with cocaine, amphetamine, and tobacco use. Thrombus formation is felt to be due to hemostasis or the release of thrombogenic material with or without endothelial damage. In patients with a history of cocaine and amphetamine abuse, there is the additional factor of increased platelet aggregability. Tobacco can also cause increased platelet aggregability, endothelial damage, and inhibition of fibrinolysis. These factors greatly increase the formation of thrombus.

AMI with angiographically normal coronary arteries has also been reported in critically sick patients in intensive care units (see Case record and **300**). Hypovolemia, hypotension, and intense spasm due to endogenous catecholamines, or exogenous inotropic agents, or a systemic prothrombotic state, may collective or individually be responsible for the AMI. These patients may have significant LV dysfunction, which often resolves once the patient recovers from the systemic disease.

Prothrombotic states
Other proposed factors for thrombus formation include prothrombotic states such as antiphospholipid syndromes, protein C or S deficiency, antithrombin III deficiency, and factor V Leiden deficiency. Oral contraceptives and estrogen hormone replacement have also been indicted in studies. The incidence of prothrombotic states in normal coronary artery infarcts accounts for only between 0% and 20%, which makes screening for such etiologies controversial.

Embolus
Embolization from a noncoronary source can be a cause of coronary occlusion. The sources of emboli include valvular disease, prosthetic valve thrombus, intracardiac thrombi, emboli from a cardiac tumor or, very rarely, paradoxical emboli from a venous site in the setting of a patent foramen ovale. The most common valve sources are prosthetic valve thrombi, infective endocarditis, and nonbacterial thrombotic endocarditis. Clues which would suggest noncoronary emboli as a cause of AMI include distal occlusions in an otherwise normal appearing vessel, with the angiographic cut-off sign, and evidence of multiple occlusions.

Invisible atherosclerosis
Arterie that appear normal by angiography may in fact have atherosclerosis. There is often a compensatory enlargement of coronary arteries in relation to plaque burden in pathologic specimens. The vessels expand outward with an increase in the elastic lamina with preservation of the arterial lumen. In arterie with this type of positive remodeling, the classic concept of plaque disruption leading to thrombotic occlusion can still apply. With lysis of the thrombus the artery may once again show no lumenal encroachment. The use of IVUS may be the only way to discern between a normal coronary artery and an angiographically normal appearing coronary artery with an atheromatous plaque.

Arterial dissection
Dissection of a coronary artery has also been included in the mechanisms of AMI in normal coronary arteries. It can occur spontaneously or as a result of an aortic dissection, blunt chest trauma, or as a result of an iatrogenic complication during coronary catheterization and coronary artery surgery. Spontaneous coronary dissections often occur in young women, particularly in the peripartum period. The left coronary artery (LCA) appears to be a more common site, but this may be a selective bias from studies identifying patients at autopsy. Aortic wall weakening, with cystic medial necrosis and inflammation secondary to increased reproductive hormones, is thought to be the cause of spontaneous dissection in the peripartum period. Prognosis in these young patients

is thought to be poor, with close to 70% of patients presenting with SCD. In the patients who survive, early diagnosis by angiography may lead to successful treatment with angioplasty, stent, or CABG.

DIFFERENTIAL DIAGNOSIS

Myocarditis should be considered in the differential diagnosis, given its ability to mimic AMI. Even after an extensive clinical evaluation looking for a recent febrile illness, pericardial involvement with pleuritic pain, a friction rub, and typical ST elevations, myocarditis can be overlooked. An endomyocardial biopsy is not a reasonable diagnostic test given its invasiveness, low sensitivity, and high risk/benefit ratio. Advances in cardiac imaging using nuclear cardiology and magnetic resonance imaging (MRI) may further enhance diagnostic capabilities and enable differentiation of an MI from inflammatory myocarditis.

MANAGEMENT

Treatment of AMI of normal coronary arteries should be the same as with any AMI. There should be an emphasis on early intervention, limitation of remodeling, and aggressive risk modification.

PROGNOSIS

Most studies report a favorable prognosis with a lower rate of morbidity; however, as with all AMI patients, the ejection fraction is the greatest predictor of prognosis.

CASE RECORD

A 63-year-old female patient underwent a radical hysterectomy for cervical carcinoma. She had a history of diabetes, but no prior history of CAD. During the early postoperative period she became hypotensive, due to possible intra-abdominal hemorrhage requiring urgent exploration, transfusion, and use of IV pressors. Her hemodynamic state remained unstable, and subsequent ECG showed minimal ST segment elevation in V2–V4 along with some elevation of troponins. An echocardiographic examination confirmed a new apical akinetic segment (**300A**), confirming a diagnosis of an acute anterior wall MI. She underwent an urgent cardiac catheterization procedure, which showed no critical stenosis in any of the coronary arteries (**300B, C**), and normal flow in both coronary arteries.

She was postulated to have an acute obstruction of the LCA with spontaneous recanalization. The persistent hypotension, blood products, and the effect of power pressor agents could have led to spasm and thrombosis of the LAD, with subsequent recanalization.

The patient did well and finally was discharged home, with no recurrent angina or heart failure.

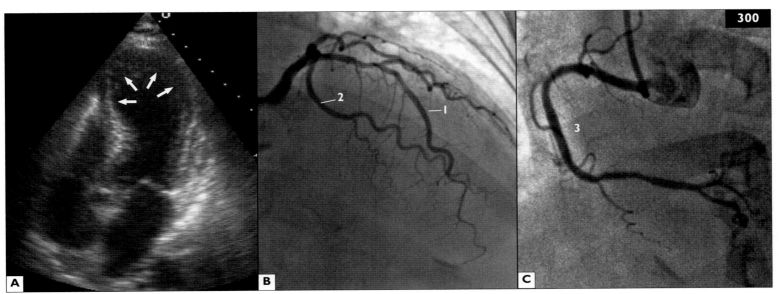

300 Images from a patient with an acute myocardial infarction with normal coronary arteries (Case record). **A**: Echocardiogram in an apical four-chamber view showing large area of apical akinesia (arrows) consistent with an acute myocardial infarction. **B**: Left coronary arteriogram showing no obvious stenosis in the left anterior descending (1) or circumflex (2) arteries. **C**: Right coronary arteriogram showing no stenosis or occlusion in the right coronary artery (3).

Chapter Thirteen

Heart Attack: Management Strategy

PREHOSPITAL

JENS FLENSTED LASSEN, MD, PhD

INTRODUCTION

Acute myocardial infarction (AMI) carries a high mortality and is the commonest single cause of death in developed countries. Its clinical presentation is a heart attack and effective treatment is obviously of paramount importance. The main issue in prehospital management of heart attack is to minimize the time from symptom onset to treatment and in the mean time to stabilize the patient, prevent or treat fatal arrythmias, obtain a working diagnosis for patient triage, initiate the primary medical treatment, and to assure patient transferral to relevant life-saving reperfusion therapy or to further medical treatment and diagnosis as soon as possible.

PATHOGENESIS

Heart attack usually occurs when blood flow in a major coronary artery is compromised by a thrombus rapidly developing at the site of a ruptured plaque, or from endothelial erosion. The result is either a total occlusion of the coronary artery or a state of dynamic closure and reperfusion with peripheral embolization that compromises the microcirculation and leads to acute myocardial ischemia, causing pain and eventually cardiac arrest. Patient survival is determined by a number of factors but the most important is early restoration of adequate flow to the ischemic part of the myocardium.

CLINICAL PRESENTATION

A heart attack often presents with dynamic chest pain and changes in the ST segment in the electrocardiogram (ECG) (**301**). The clinical presentation ranges from a patient with mild chest pain at rest or only on minimal exertion to a person with severe chest pain at rest and eventually cardiogenic shock, lipothymia, or cardiac arrest. The typical patient suffers from chest pain descibed as a pressure, tightness, or heaviness at the chest and with the pain radiating to the left or both arms, shoulders, jaw, neck, or back. Furthermore, persistent shortness of breath, nausea, and vomiting as well as weakness, dizziness, or loss of consciousness can be present. The term acute coronary syndrome (ACS) is used for this acute phase of coronary heart disease (CHD) and comprises the

subgroups: unstable angina pectoris (UAP), non-ST elevation acute myocardial infarction (NSTEMI), ST elevation acute myocardial infarction (STEMI), and sudden coronary death (SCD) (**302**).

TRIAGE OF HEART ATTACK PATIENTS

Patients with symptoms suggesting ACS should have a 12-lead ECG recorded as soon as possible. The ECG can differentiate patients with heart attack into two large groups that require different therapeutic approaches. If ST segment elevation is present, the development of a myocardial infarction (MI) seems likely (STEMI) and immediate reperfusion is usually indicated.

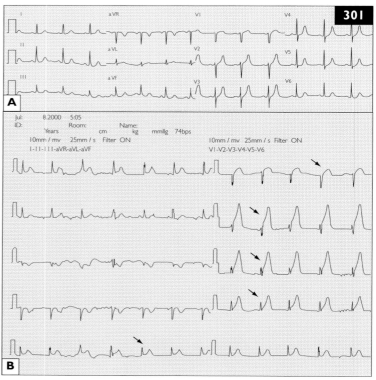

301 Dynamic electrocardiogram (ECG) changes in a 45-year-old male with anterior ST segment elevation myocardial infarction. **A**: Normal ECG recorded in the ambulance. **B**: At arrival at the hospital 17 minutes later a new ECG is recorded with clear signs of anterior myocardial infarction (arrows indicating elevation of the ST segment).

Reperfusion therapy has been a major advance in the treatment of acute STEMI, with a 25% reduction in mortality with thrombolysis and with even better results for primary percutaneous coronary intervention (PCI) as indicated by the most recent meta-analysis. Accordingly, patients with ST segment elevation should be referred without delay to either a cardiac center that offers primary PCI or to a hospital department suitable for delivery of thrombolytic therapy.

In the absence of ST segment elevation, patients can be referred to the nearest hospital to receive antithrombotic treatment and further diagnostic evaluation. Raised biochemical markers of myocardial damage within the first 12–24 hours indicate that these patients must have had NSTEMI. These patients should be offered an early invasive strategy involving cardiac catheterization within 48 hours, which could be accomplished with initial management at a noncatheterization facility and subsequent transfer. Patients without raised concentrations of biomarkers of myocardial damage can be regarded as having UAP.

THE IMPORTANCE OF TIME FROM SYMPTOM ONSET TO TREATMENT

Ventricular fibrillation (VF) is the most common mechanism of death in MI and most cases occur very early in the course of a heart attack before the heart muscle is damaged. Primary VF is almost invariably fatal in the absence of electrical defibrillation, but is highly reversible with rapid defibrillation; many patients make an excellent recovery if treated promptly. Otherwise, the condition is fatal within minutes even when cardiopulmonary resuscitation is provided immediately. After delays of 4–5 minutes the survival rate decreases to 15–40% and after 10 minutes or longer 95% will die. Patients with heart attack who pass through the initial period without VF still have a high risk of death, which increases dramatically with time from symptom onset to

treatment. The gain in saved lives in patients with STEMI receiving reperfusion therapy is large within the first 2 hours of symptom onset, but declines rapidly during the next hours to a stable minimum after approximately 24 hours. Recent large-scale clinical trials indicate that thrombolytic therapy saves 30 lives per 1,000 patients and that the mean time from symptom onset to initiation of therapy has remained unchanged during the last decade, at approximately 2 hours and 45 minutes. However, reducing this delay by 1 hour is likely to increase the number of lives saved per 1,000 patients by a further 25, emphasizing the importance of keeping the delay from symptom onset to relevant treatment to a minimum (**303**).

PREHOSPITAL RESUSCITATION

Large observational studies of outcomes in patients with heart attack indicate that resuscitation is superior to thrombolysis in reducing death. Of 3,972 patients receiving medical care, resuscitation was successful in 257 (6.5%) and fibrinolysis prevented death in 63 (1.6%). About 80% of the lives saved were attributable to resuscitation from cardiac arrest and about 20% from fibrinolytic treatment. Of the patients whose lives were saved by resuscitation, 40% had had their first arrest outside hospital and so owed their lives primarily to bystanders or to the ambulance services.

CARDIAC ARREST

Given that most cardiac arrests cannot be predicted and that there are delays in the response of emergency medical services, the most practical strategy to improve survival is to make defibrillators available in public places and to encourage bystanders to use them. Unfortunately, only a minor proportion of unexpected cardiac arrests occur in public places, making rapid treatment very difficult for most patients. Furthermore, education of the general

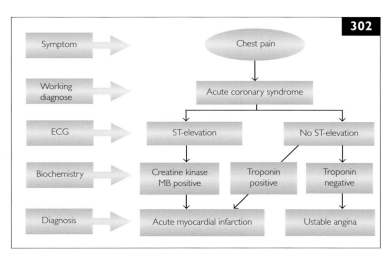

302 Algorithm to show the evaluation of patients with heart attack and the terminology of acute coronary syndromes. ECG: electrocardiogram.

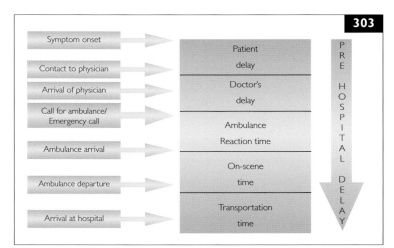

303 Diagram to illustrate sources of prehospital delay in patients with heart attack. The prehospital delay is on average 2.5 hours. Not all steps are mandatory. Some patients access the hospital directly and some make direct emergency calls bypassing the family physician.

population in the initial treatment of cardiac arrest is very important for the success of this strategy.

INITIAL MANAGEMENT

Time is of paramount importance. It still seems to take over 2 hours from symptom onset to the patient coming into the health-care system, indicating the need for public campaigns to encourage patients to use emergency calls in cases of unfamiliar chest pain. Furthermore, health-care professionals should always be aware of reducing prehospital delay as much as possible for patients with a heart attack, and should remember that a patient history indicating ACS is enough for admittance to hospital. The patient should be calmed down as much as possible and kept at rest while waiting for the ambulance service to arrive. Initial medical treatment with nitroglycerin and aspirin should be given prehospital if available, and a 12-lead ECG should be recorded as soon as possible as the essential basis for a further treatment strategy.

FUTURE DEVELOPMENTS

The use of prehospital diagnosis of AMI by 12-lead ECG ST segment monitoring by either physicians or paramedics on site or by use of telemedicine is developing, and should reduce in-hospital delay to treatment by warning the hospital prior to the patient's arrival. Furthermore, the technique facilitates the use of either prehospital thrombolysis or, even better, of direct referral of the patient to a cardiac center that offers primary PCI as the optimal reperfusion strategy. If this can be accomplished in a timely fashion, such an approach clearly will improve outcomes based on current evidence (**304**).

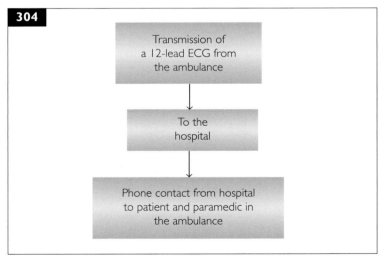

304 Use of telemedicine for diagnosis and in triage of patients with heart attack. Recording of a 12-lead electrocardiogram followed by transmission to a cardiac invasive center. The physician at the invasive center calls back to the ambulance and takes a brief history directly from the patient as a basis for patient triage to either primary percutaneous coronary intervention at the center or further diagnosis and stabilizing treatment at the local hospital.

EMERGENCY DEPARTMENT

KRISTIAN THYGESEN, MD, PhD AND
JOSEPH S. ALPERT, MD

INTRODUCTION

Emergency Departments (EDs) are dedicated to supporting each patient's vital functions while performing rapid diagnostic and triage functions. The time available for the ED personnel to evaluate and initiate therapy varies according to the need for an immediate response in the case of cardiac arrest to a more leisurely but nevertheless expedited diagnostic work-up. Patients with high-risk cardiac conditions, for example ACS, should be transferred to the Coronary Care Unit (CCU) or the catheterization laboratory without delay. Patients with ACS that is intermediate in risk benefit the most from admission to a specialized chest pain unit (**305**).

Epidemiological data suggest that about 20% of all admissions to a medical ED are due to acute chest pain, with 20–25% of these individuals actually having confirmed myocardial ischemia or infarction; however, no cardiac disease is found in 50% of these patients[1].

CLINICAL PRESENTATION

The evaluation of patients presenting with acute chest pain is primarily focused on suspected ACS. However, it is important to remember that other entities such as aortic dissection, pulmonary embolism, and pneumothorax also require immediate diagnostic and therapeutic interventions (**306**).

Ischemic cardiac pain

Chest discomfort or pain is usually localized over a wide area of the anterior chest wall, possibly radiating to the left and/or right arm as well as to the neck and back. Other symptoms, such as dyspnea, syncope, epigastric pain, or sweating, may be the presenting complaint in patients with ACS.

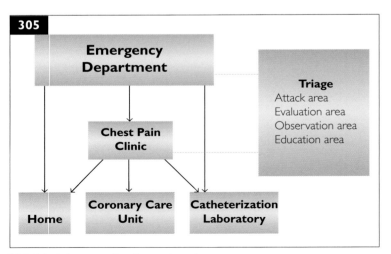

305 Admission route for chest pain patients.

Nonischemic chest pain

Patients with cardiomyopathy or myocarditis may describe pain that is similar to anginal discomfort. However, nonischemic pain will usually not respond to nitrate therapy. Pain that arises from the pericardium typically increases with inspiration and is ameliorated by leaning forward. Musculoskeletal pain is often provoked by postural change as well as by movement. Patients with major pulmonary emboli often complain of severe dyspnea. Chest pain associated with pneumonia is almost always pleuritic in nature. Pneumothorax usually occurs in young men who describe the sudden onset of chest pain and dyspnea.

Esophageal disorders, gastritis, and peptic ulcers may sometimes cause chest discomfort, which is often reported to occur in response to eating or drinking. Patients with anxiety, depression, or panic disorders may describe chest discomfort which closely resembles that of myocardial ischemia. Dissecting aneurysm is often accompanied by severe crushing pain diffusely localized to the chest or back.

DIAGNOSIS

Besides the clinical evaluation, immediate diagnostic testing in patients with acute cardiac conditions includes ECG, blood sampling and, if necessary, a variety of imaging studies.

Electrocardiogram

The ECG is an easily accessible method of identifying patients with myocardial ischemia. The ECG may also reveal arrhythmias, signs of left ventricular hypertrophy (LVH), bundle branch block (BBB), and even acute right ventricular strain in patients with massive pulmonary embolism. However, it must be remembered that the sensitivity and specificity of the ECG are only moderate in the diagnosis of cardiac diseases.

Between 40 and 50% of patients admitted to the ED with acute chest pain have pathologic ECG changes including BBB, paced rhythms, and signs of a previous MI. An additional 15% of patients will demonstrate either ST elevation or ST depression, suggesting an evolving AMI. About one-third of patients admitted with acute chest pain have a normal ECG, but up to 40% of these individuals are subsequently shown to have suffered an AMI[1].

Biochemical markers

Blood samples to assess myocardial damage should be taken if the chest pain is suggestive of myocardial ischemia. These blood tests may be employed to measure creatine kinase (CK) MB activity or mass, troponin I or T, or myoglobin. Troponins and CKMB mass are the most specific markers for cardiac cell damage[2].

The various biomarkers have different abilities to detect myocardial damage following critical narrowing of a coronary artery. Myoglobin is released most rapidly, followed by CKMB and the troponins within 3–6 hours of ischemic myocardial damage. Measurements of troponin T or I have been shown to be the most sensitive and specific marker of MI. Approximately 10–12 hours are needed in order to rule out an MI. An optimal diagnostic strategy should include blood sampling on admission and at 6–9 hours after the onset of symptoms. An optional additional sample is often obtained at 12–24 hours (**307**).

Chest radiography

A chest X-ray is often helpful in patients with chest pain and no obvious myocardial ischemia. Chest roentgenography may reveal pulmonary conditions as well as aortic aneurysm. Dissection of the aorta may, however, cause no overt changes in the standard chest X-ray. Therefore, transesophageal echocardiography (TEE) or computed tomography (CT) should be considered for patients with chest pain radiating to the back, particularly if a new murmur of aortic insufficiency is heard.

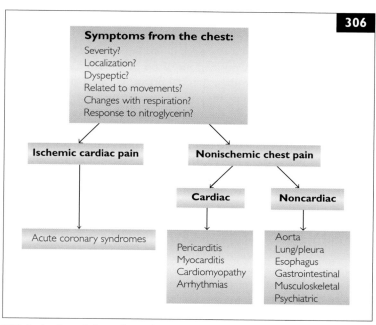

306 Evaluation of chest discomfort.

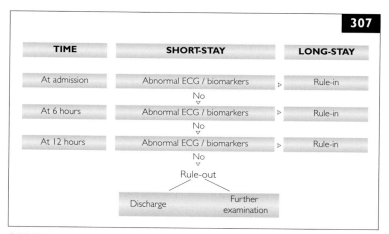

307 Diagnostic strategy for acute chest pain.

Echocardiography

Echocardiography is an essential diagnostic examination employed in the triage of patients with emergent cardiac conditions. Regional wall motion abnormalities develop within seconds following coronary occlusion and well before myocardial necrosis commences. However, wall motion abnormalities are not specific for AMI and may be due to ischemia or a prior infarction. Echocardiography is of particular value for the diagnosis of other causes of chest pain such as acute aortic dissection, pericardial effusion, or massive pulmonary embolism.

Radionuclide imaging

Myocardial perfusion scintigraphy has also been used successfully for triaging patients presenting with acute chest pain. A normal resting technetium-99m myocardial perfusion scintigram effectively excludes major MI. An abnormal scintigram is not diagnostic of acute infarction unless it is known previously to have been normal, but it does indicate the presence of coronary artery disease (CAD) and the need for further evaluation. Perfusion scintigraphy may be more useful than echocardiography in patients with a poor echocardiographic window.

MANAGEMENT OF HIGH-RISK PATIENTS

Once vital signs have been stabilized and hypoxemia corrected, aspirin should be given in the earliest possible phase to patients with suspected ACS. Furthermore, in order to decrease myocardial ischemia, nitrates should be used liberally in addition to intravenous beta blocking drugs. Persistent chest pain should be relieved with morphine[1].

If fibrinolytic therapy has not already been administered in the prehospital phase, it must be started promptly in the ED or in the CCU in patients with ST segment elevation. However, these patients are often transferred directly to the catheterization laboratory for immediate coronary angiography (CAG) and angioplasty[3].

ACS patients with UAP or NSTEMI may benefit from the administration of low-molecular weight heparin, particularly if these patients have an elevated blood troponin level. Furthermore, platelet glycoprotein (GP) IIb/IIIa inhibitors have also been shown to be beneficial in high-risk patients who undergo PCI[4,5].

ROLE OF CHEST PAIN UNITS

Diagnostic work-up, risk assessment, and treatment of chest pain can be problematic. Most chest pain patients can be more efficiently and expeditiously evaluated in a specialized Chest Pain Unit (CPU) than in the ED.

Since hospitals have different ED configurations, CPUs may have different designs; however, such units should be equipped to resuscitate patients, appropriately monitor these individuals for cardiac rhythm disturbances and ischemia, and follow blood pressure and arterial blood oxygenation. Patients usually remain in the CPU for 10–12 hours following the onset of symptoms.

CORONARY CARE UNIT

**KRISTIAN THYGESEN, MD, PhD AND
JOSEPH S. ALPERT, MD**

INTRODUCTION

Patients with acute cardiac conditions, i.e. unstable coronary syndromes, acute pulmonary edema, complex arrhythmias, massive pulmonary emboli, and acute perimyocarditis require continuous monitoring with special medical and nursing care. These patients should be admitted to a CCU or a cardiac intensive care unit adequately designed and equipped, and staffed by specially trained professionals who function under the leadership of a cardiologist knowledgeable in the management of these critically ill patients.

All patients with suspected MI should initially undergo clinical and diagnostic assessment followed by appropriate therapy, including pain relief, antithrombotic and anti-ischemic drugs and, if indicated, reperfusion interventions. Moreover, resuscitation strategies should be employed if required.

NONINVASIVE MONITORING

ECG monitoring for arrhythmias and ischemia should be started immediately in any patient suspected of having sustained an ACS. Monitoring should be continued for at least 24 hours or until an alternative diagnosis has been made. More prolonged monitoring may be appropriate for patients with sustained heart failure, shock, or serious arrhythmias. During the early phases of an ACS, the risk for potentially malignant arrhythmias is high. Monitoring the recovery of ST segment deviations, or the lack thereof, during the first hours following admission in these patients provides important prognostic information and may be helpful for selecting further treatment such as rescue PCI.

INVASIVE MONITORING

All CCUs should have the equipment and personnel with the skills needed to undertake invasive monitoring of systemic arterial and pulmonary arterial pressures. Arterial pressure monitoring should be initiated immediately in patients with cardiogenic shock. Balloon flotation catheters are of value in the assessment and care of some patients with low cardiac output. Pulmonary arterial catheterization permits measurement of right atrium, pulmonary arterial, and pulmonary wedge pressures, as well as cardiac output.

MANAGEMENT OF ACUTE ISCHEMIC SYNDROMES

The initial assessment in patients with chest pain or other symptoms of presumed cardiac ischemic origin should include a careful history and a physical examination. An ECG should also be performed to confirm the preliminary diagnosis and to guide treatment. Laboratory assessment should include biochemical markers of myocardial damage, preferably cardiac troponin T or I, in order to establish or reject the diagnosis according to the European Society of Cardiology (ESC)/American College of Cardiology (ACC) criteria for the diagnosis of AMI (*Table 42*)[1].

Prophylactic therapies in the early phase of an acute coronary syndrome

Convincing evidence for the effectiveness of aspirin in doses of 75–325 mg per day has been shown in both short- and long-term studies. There are few contraindications to the use of aspirin; for example, known hypersensitivity to aspirin, active peptic ulcer, or hemorrhagic diatheses[2,3].

Many trials have shown the benefit of beta blockers in AMI because of the potential of these agents to limit infarct size, reduce the occurrence of fatal arrhythmias, and to relieve pain. The IV route of administration is initially preferred in patients at high risk. Oral therapy should subsequently be instituted to achieve a target heart rate between 50 and 60 beats per minute. Patients with impaired atrioventricular (AV) conduction, a history of asthma, or with acute left ventricular dysfunction should not receive beta blockers.

The use of nitrates is largely based on pathophysiologic considerations and clinical experience. The major therapeutic benefit is probably related to the venodilator effects of these agents, leading to a decrease in myocardial preload and left ventricular end-diastolic volume. In addition, nitrates dilate coronary arteries, increase coronary collateral flow, and inhibit platelet aggregation.

Persistent ST segment elevation or new left bundle branch block

For patients with the clinical presentation of MI and with persistent ST segment elevation or new or presumed new left BBB (LBBB), early mechanical or pharmacologic reperfusion should be performed unless contraindications are present (**308**)[2].

Fibrinolytic treatment

Patients with chest discomfort and ST elevation or new LBBB should receive aspirin and IV fibrinolytic therapy with the minimum of delay. A realistic aim is to initiate fibrinolysis within 90 minutes of the patient calling for medical treatment ('call to needle' time) or within 30 minutes of arrival at the hospital ('door to needle' time). Fibrinolytic therapy should not be given to patients in whom infarction has been ongoing for more than 12 hours, unless there is evidence of active ischemia, together with ECG criteria for fibrinolysis.

Adjunctive antiplatelet and anticoagulant are almost always indicated in conjunction with fibrinolytic therapy. The first dose of aspirin, 150–325 mg, should be chewed, and a lower dose (75–160 mg) given orally daily thereafter. If oral ingestion is not possible, IV aspirin can be given (250 mg). Heparin is usually employed during and after fibrinolysis, especially with tissue plasminogen activator. Heparin does not improve immediate clot lysis but coronary patency appears to be better when IV heparin has been used. Low-molecular weight heparin has a number of advantages over standard heparin due to its greater factor-Xa inhibition, more predictable kinetics, less protein binding, less platelet activation, a lower rate of thrombocytopenia, and avoidance of monitoring activated partial thromboplastin time (aPTT). Thrombolytic therapy is associated with a small but significant excess risk of approximately 3.9 extra strokes per 1,000

Table 42 Definition of myocardial infarction

Criteria for acute, evolving myocardial infarction
Either of the following criteria satisfies the diagnosis for an acute, evolving myocardial infarction:
- Typical rise and fall of biochemical markers of myocardial necrosis with at least one of the following:
  - Ischemic symptoms
  - Development of pathologic Q waves
  - Development of ST segment changes indicative of ischemia
  - Coronary artery intervention, e.g., angioplasty.
- Pathologic findings of an acute myocardial infarction.

Criteria for established myocardial infarction
- Development of new pathologic Q waves on serial ECGs.
  The patient may or may not remember any symptons.
  Biochemical markers of myocardial necrosis may have normalized.
- Pathologic findings of a healed or healing myocardial infarction.

ECG: electrocardiogram.

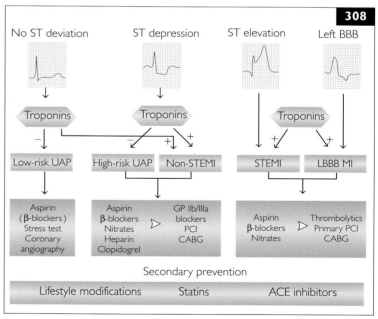

308 Approaches to therapy in acute ischemic syndromes. ACE: angiotensin-converting enzyme; CABG: coronary artery bypass graft; GP: glycoprotein; LBBB: left bundle branch block; PCI: percutaneous coronary intervention; STEMI: ST segment elevation myocardial infarction; UAP: unstable angina pectoris. –/+: negative/positive test result.

patients treated, largely attributable to cerebral hemorrhage. Major noncerebral bleeds can occur in 4–13% of patients treated[2].

Primary percutaneous coronary interventions
PCI is defined as angioplasty and/or stenting without prior or concomitant fibrinolytic therapy. PCI is the preferred therapeutic option for acute STEMI when it can be performed within 90 minutes after the first medical contact. PCI is also indicated when it can be initiated within 3 hours of admission to a community hospital with subsequent transfer to a medical center with catheterization facilities. Primary PCI is the preferred therapy for patients in shock following AMI. Primary PCI is effective in securing and maintaining coronary artery patency and avoids some of the bleeding risks of fibrinolysis[2].

Patients without persistent ST segment elevation

Patients with a presumptive ACS who initially present with ST depression, negative T waves, or a normal ECG usually receive treatment that includes aspirin, heparin, beta blockade, and oral or IV nitrates. Nondihydropyridine calcium antagonists may be selected instead of beta blockers in those patients who cannot tolerate beta blockade. Continuous multi-lead ischemia monitoring is frequently helpful and troponin measurements should be assessed serially. Based on these clinical, ECG and biochemical data, risk assessment can be performed and therapeutic strategies can be selected (**309**)[3,4].

High-risk patients
Patients with recurrent ischemia or chest pain, patients with elevated troponin levels, or patients who develop hemodynamic instability or major arrhythmias usually receive intravenous GP IIb/IIIa receptor blockers followed by CAG and possible PCI or coronary bypass surgery.

Low-risk patients
Low-risk patients include those who have no recurrence of chest pain, patients without elevation of biochemical markers of myocardial necrosis, and patients without ST deviation. In these patients, therapeutic interventions include oral aspirin, beta blockers, and possibly nitrates or calcium antagonists. Furthermore, an exercise or pharmacologic stress test is recommended to confirm or establish a diagnosis of CAD and/or to monitor the results of anti-ischemic therapy. Patients who demonstrate ischemia during the stress test are usually referred for CAG. It should be appreciated that a standard exercise test may be inconclusive. In such patients an additional stress echocardiogram, or stress myocardial perfusion scintigram, may be appropriate.

PUMP FAILURE AND SHOCK

Left ventricular failure during the acute phase of MI is associated with a poor prognosis. The presence of pulmonary congestion can be assessed clinically and by chest X-ray. Echocardiography is also very useful in assessing the extent of myocardial damage, as well as residual left ventricular function and the presence of complications. The severity of heart failure may be categorized clinically by the Killip classification: class 1: no rales or third heart sound; class 2: presence of rales over <50% of the lung fields and/or a third heart sound; class 3: presence of rales over >50% of the lung fields; class 4: shock.

Management of acute heart failure

Oxygen should be administered early by mask or intranasally. Minor degrees of failure often respond promptly to diuretics such as furosemide 20–40 mg given slowly IV, repeated at 1–4 hourly intervals. If the response to diuretics is inadequate, intravenous nitroglycerin should be employed. Consideration should be given to initiating hemodynamic monitoring. Inotropic agents such as dobutamine may be of value if there is evidence of low cardiac output or hypotension.

Cardiogenic shock

Cardiogenic shock is a clinical state of hypoperfusion characterized by systolic blood pressure <90 mmHg (12 kPa) and central filling pressure >20 mmHg (2.7 kPa), or a cardiac index <1.8 l/min/m². The presence of severe left ventricular dysfunction and/or associated mechanical complications should be evaluated by means of echocardiography. Hemodynamic assessment is usually performed with a balloon flotation catheter. Intravenous dopamine should be administered as described above as well as intra-aortic balloon counter pulsation. Emergency PCI or cardiac surgery may be life saving and should be considered at an early stage.

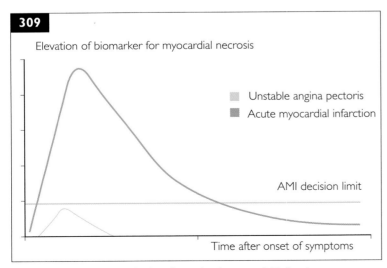

309

Elevation of biomarker for myocardial necrosis

■ Unstable angina pectoris
■ Acute myocardial infarction

AMI decision limit

Time after onset of symptoms

309 Biochemical markers in the diagnosis of myocardial infarction.

ARRHYTHMIAS AND CONDUCTION DISTURBANCES

Arrhythmias and conduction disturbances are extremely common during the early hours after MI. In some cases, for example ventricular tachycardia (VT), VF, and complete AV block, the arrhythmia should be treated immediately. Often, arrhythmias are a manifestation of a serious underlying disorder, such as continuing ischemia, pump failure, altered autonomic tone, hypoxia, or electrolyte or acid–base disturbances that require corrective measures. The necessity for treatment and its urgency depend on the hemodynamic consequences of the rhythm disorder.

LENGTH OF STAY IN THE CORONARY CARE UNIT

The length of stay in the CCU is usually 2–4 days, dictated by the individual clinical presentation. Patients with STEMI without complications usually receive treatment in the intensive care unit for 36–48 hours. Patients with unstable coronary syndromes with dynamic ST segment shifts and elevated troponins must stay in the CCU until they are stable. High-risk ACS patients who undergo angioplasty must stay in the CCU until they are stable.

POSTHOSPITAL

MOGENS LYTKEN LARSEN, MD, DMSC

INTRODUCTION

The hospital stay for ACS has now been shortened to 3–5 days. With shorter stays, however, the opportunity to counsel patients about risk reduction and exercise is minimal. Furthermore, the use of medications, including aspirin, beta blockers, lipid-lowering agents, and angiotensin-converting enzyme (ACE) inhibitors implies close monitoring and follow-up.

Cardiac rehabilitation programs were first developed in the 1960s, and the goal is to ensure the best possible physical, psychological, and social conditions so that patients after a heart attack may, by their own efforts, preserve or resume their proper place in society. This is directed towards maintaining job activities, as well as influencing the underlying atherosclerotic process and the prognosis of the patient with CHD (see Goble and Worchester, 1999; Further Reading). Meta-analyses of 21 randomized, controlled trials performed in the 1980s provided data on the effect of cardiac rehabilitation on long-term mortality from cardiovascular causes, and recent Cochrane analyses showed that cardiac rehabilitation is effective in reducing cardiac mortality.

In 1994, the American Heart Association stated that cardiac rehabilitation programs should consist of a multi-faceted and multi-disciplinary approach to overall cardiovascular risk reduction, and that programs that consist of exercise training alone are not considered cardiac rehabilitation. Today, many centers have broadened the concept of cardiac rehabilitation programs to include secondary prevention programs with the assessment and modification of risk factors.

CARDIAC REHABILITATION/SECONDARY PREVENTION

According to the World Health Organization, three phases after a heart attack can be distinguished (*Table 43*). Phase I is

Table 43 World Health Organization definition of the three phases after a heart attack

Phase I	Phase II	Phase III
Management at CCU	Cardiac rehabilitation/ secondary prevention	Follow-up in co-operation with primary health care
Prevention of relapse	Assessment of risk factors	Specify long-term goals
Smoking cessation	Vocational counseling	
Referral to rehabilitation program	Dietary counseling	
	Smoking cessation	
	Exercise test	
	Aerobic training	
	Adjustments of medication	

management at the CCU until discharge. Phase II is the outpatient program from discharge until return to vocational activities or the ability to manage daily activities. Phase III is the further course after phase II. The interval between in-hospital (phase I) and outpatient program (phase II) should be as short as 1–2 weeks. Early attendance reduces the level of anxiety and depression.

Each patient should undergo a careful medical evaluation and exercise test prior to participating in an outpatient cardiac rehabilitation program, for the purpose of establishing a safe and effective program of comprehensive cardiovascular risk reduction and rehabilitation. The duration of the initial rehabilitation program usually ranges from 4 to 12 weeks. In order to maintain a healthy lifestyle, continuation of the program, i.e. a follow up phase (III), should be aimed for, coordinated with the general practitioner.

NONPHARMACOLOGIC INTERVENTIONS

Nutritional counseling and modifications of dietary habits have an important role in cardiac rehabilitation and secondary prevention. Dietary recommendations usually provide the first-line approach to reducing plasma cholesterol, and randomized dietary intervention trials have led to a significant reduction in total mortality in patients after a heart attack. However, the relationship of diet to CHD is more complex, and many of the mechanisms are still not known. Therefore, all patients with CHD should receive professional advice on modification of the diet, with the emphasis on a low proportion of saturated animal fat, avoidance of trans-unsaturated fats, an adequate supply of mono- and polyunsaturated fats, with a moderate amount of low-fat dairy products, at least two fish meals per week, a high fiber content, and plenty of fruit and vegetables.

Smoking cessation reduces risk and is highly cost-effective. Observational studies have shown that giving up smoking will reduce the risk of further nonfatal heart attacks and cardiovascular mortality rate by up to 50% over a 2-year follow-up period. Patients should be encouraged and supported professionally to stop smoking all forms of tobacco for life. Individual counseling and support of the patient is the most successful approach, and nicotine replacement therapies can be initially helpful for some patients, particularly those who are heavily addicted to nicotine.

Weight management should be considered in patients with excess weight. Whether obesity itself is an independent risk factor has not been proven, but due to the adverse effects of obesity on other risk factors, reduction of weight is important. The goal is not primarily to reach the ideal body weight, but to achieve improvements in obesity-related risk factors, such as dyslipidemia and insulin resistance. To achieve weight loss a combined diet, exercise, and behavioral program is necessary.

Physical-activity counseling and exercise training in rehabilitation programs have been shown to reduce the risk of total mortality, cardiovascular mortality, and fatal reinfarctions. An increased physical activity level and improvement in cardio-respiratory fitness are also associated with better survival. Training programs used in different trials differ greatly, but programs with

regular aerobic exercise for at least 12 weeks have been successful, and it is recommended that patients after a heart attack and with no contraindications should be encouraged to take regular aerobic exercise, e.g. at least three times a week for 20–30 minutes. If possible, however, the physician should tailor the exercise program to the clinical characteristics of the patient. The improved exercise performance is only maintained as long as training is kept up, and patients should be encouraged to continue training after finishing the rehabilitation program.

Psychosocial management during cardiac rehabilitation leads to improved measures of anxiety, emotional stress, lack of self-confidence, depression, social isolation, and patient-reported quality of life. Since depression and social isolation after a heart attack are associated with increased mortality rates, cardiac rehabilitation programs should be able to offer specific psycho-social interventions such as stress management and professional psychiatric help to patients with clinical depression.

PHARMACOLOGIC INTERVENTIONS

Many different pharmaceutical classes have demonstrated benefit in secondary prevention after a heart attack. In recent years, most guidelines have recommended that discharge therapy should be based on the results of secondary prevention trials, together with a more specific treatment of underlying lipid disorders, hypertension, and/or diabetes (*Table 44*).

Discharge therapy recommended as part of a secondary prevention program and aggressive risk management includes aspirin, beta blockers, and ACE inhibitors. Many coronary units also initiate lipid-lowering therapy before discharge. The meta-analyses of antiplatelet trials following a heart attack provide convincing evidence of a significant reduction in all-cause mortality, vascular mortality, nonfatal reinfarctions, and nonfatal stroke. Therefore, continuation of aspirin is recommended, at a dosage of 75–325 mg, for long-term medical therapy after a heart attack. Likewise, firm evidence shows that long-term beta blockade remains an effective and well tolerated treatment that reduces mortality and morbidity in unselected patients after a heart attack. Consequently, most guidelines recommend that beta blockers should be administered to all patients without a contraindication following a heart attack and treatment should be continued indefinitely. Finally, treatment with ACE inhibitors has reduced cardiovascular mortality after a heart attack in patients with congestive heart failure, left ventricular dysfunction, hypertension, or diabetes. Treatment with ACE inhibitors is therefore initiated before discharge in these patient groups. More recent data have indicated a benefit of ACE inhibitors in an even more broad population of patients at risk for cardiovascular events, but there is no formal recommendation given for this expanded population. At discharge most patients will be on low doses of beta blockers and ACE inhibitors, and it is very important that the rehabilitation program includes follow-up on medication to monitor dose adjustments and side-effects.

Lipid management aimed at normalizing blood lipids results in a marked reduction in the rate of clinical coronary events and

Table 44 Evaluation and interventions in relation to different components of a multifactorial rehabilitation program

	Evaluation	Intervention
Patient assessment	Medical history Physical examination	Compose patient care program
Nutritional counseling	Obtain estimate of daily food intake Assess eating habits	Prescribe dietary modifications Individualize eating plan Educate and counsel patient (and family)
Smoking cessation	Document smoking status Determine readiness to change	Provide formal smoking cessation program Update status at each visit
Weight management	Measure weight, height, and circumference Calculate BMI	In patients with BMI>25 establish reasonable short-term and long-term weight goals Develop a combined diet, exercise and behavioral program
Exercise training	Obtain an exercise test	Develop a documented individualized exercise prescription for aerobic resistance training
Psychosocial management	Use interview and/or standardized measurement tools to identify psychosocial distress	Offer individual education and counseling Develop supportive rehabilitation environment to enhance social support Cooperate with appropriate mental health specialist
Discharge therapy	Evaluate relevant long-term therapy with aspirin, beta blockers, and ACE inhibitors	Monitor dose adjustments and side-effects (ECG, kidney function)
Lipid management	Obtain fasting measures of total cholesterol, HDL, LDL and TG Repeat lipid profiles 4–6 weeks after hospitalization and 2 months after changes in therapy	Provide nutritional counseling and add drug treatment until: LDL <100 mg/dl (2.8 mmol/l), HDL >35 mg/dl (1.0 mmol/l), TG <200 mg/dl (2.5 mmol/l)
Hypertension and diabetes management	Measurement of resting BP on at least 2 visits	Continue assessment and optimize treatment until: BP <140/90 mmHg [18.7/12 kPa] or BP <130/85 mmHg [17.3/11.3 kPa] (diabetics)
	Identify diabetic subjects Obtain fasting plasma glucose in all patients and HbA1c in diabetic patients to monitor therapy	Continue monitoring and optimize diet, exercise, and oral hypoglycemic agents or insulin until near normalization of glycemic control with HbA1c <7.0%

ACE: angiotensin-converting enzyme; BMI: body mass index; BP: blood pressure; ECG: electrocardiogram; HbA1c: glycated hemoglobin; HDL: high-density lipoprotein; LDL: low-density lipoprotein; TG: triglyceride. (Modified from Core components of cardiac rehabilitation/secondary prevention programs. A statement for healthcare professionals from the American Heart Association and American Association of Cardiovascular and Pulmonary Rehabilitation [2000]. *Circulation* **102**:1069–1073.)

mortality in patients with CHD, and diet, exercise, and drugs are all indicated to achieve levels of low density lipoprotein (LDL) cholesterol <100 mg/dl (2.8 mmol/l). Therefore, patients with a heart attack should follow the dietary recommendations already given. Moreover, all patients should have their blood lipids measured 4–6 weeks after their heart attack while attending the cardiac rehabilitation program, to characterize their lipid profile and to initiate or optimize proper lipid-lowering drug therapy. The currently available lipid-lowering drugs include inhibitors of HMG CoA reductase (statins), fibrates, bile acid sequestrants (resins), and nicotinic acid and its derivatives. They have all been used in trials, demonstrating benefit to various extents, but the most convincing evidence has been obtained with statins, which are also the most potent of the lipid-lowering drugs with the best safety record. At present, the statins are therefore first-line drugs.

Hypertension and diabetes management plays an important role in cardiac rehabilitation and secondary prevention programs, since approximately two-thirds of the patients have hypertension and one-third have type 2 diabetes. These conditions, however, complicate secondary prevention because of ongoing therapy and the need for frequent dose adjustments. Nonpharmacologic interventions will improve blood pressure and metabolic control, but also imply more frequent monitoring. The goals of hypertension and diabetes management are blood pressure values <140/90 mmHg (18.7/12 kPa) (or <130/85 mmHg [17.3/11.3 kPa] in diabetics) and a glycated hemoglobin level <7.0% in diabetics. Drug therapy should be intensified until these goals are achieved.

FUTURE DEVELOPMENTS

The studies of cardiac rehabilitation on long-term mortality were performed before the widespread use of thrombolytic therapy, coronary stent replacement, and aggressive pharmacologic risk management. Cardiac rehabilitation, however, has been shown to improve functional capacity, emotional well-being, return-to-work rate, and longevity. In the future outcome measures will need to be changed, as current pharmacologic therapies become widespread. In addition, cardiac rehabilitation as it is practiced at different centers needs to be examined. So far implementation of programs is only beginning in many countries, but the combination of cardiac rehabilitation and secondary prevention should be the future posthospital management strategy for patients after a heart attack.

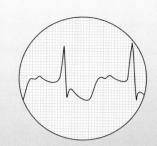

Chapter Fourteen

Silent Myocardial Ischemia

SILENT MYOCARDIAL ISCHEMIA

HANS MICKLEY, MD, DMSC

DEFINITION

Silent myocardial ischemia (SMI) is defined as objective documentation of myocardial ischemia in the absence of angina or anginal equivalents.

EPIDEMIOLOGY

SMI can be detected in patients with stable coronary artery disease (CAD) and in patients with acute coronary syndromes (ACS). Growing insights into the epidemiology of SMI have resulted from the use of ambulatory monitoring. Patients with stable CAD have been most extensively studied, and ischemic episodes can be demonstrated in 41–73%. Around three-quarters of episodes are silent. In patients with unstable angina, episodes of myocardial ischemia can be detected in >50% and approximately 90% are asymptomatic. The prevalence of ischemic episodes in patients with a recent acute myocardial infarction (AMI) ranges from 14% to 42% with 81–100% being silent. The proportion of patients with postinfarction SMI appears to be fairly stable over the following 3-year period (**310**)[1], but considerable variability is found within and between patients. In general, SMI is more prevalent in the elderly and in diabetics[2]. Women remain underrepresented in studies of SMI, but collectively it appears that objective evidence of myocardial ischemia is equally common among male and female patients with stable CAD. Concomitant chest pain, however, is more frequently reported among males, suggesting a higher prevalence of SMI in females[3].

PATHOGENESIS

Experimental invasive studies have shown that when a coronary artery is occluded, a cascade of physiologic abnormalities is initiated. The occurrence of angina is a relatively late finding that is preceded by a sequence of clinically silent changes (**311**)[4]. However, there does exist a relatively small group of patients who

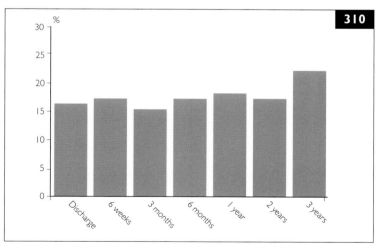

310 Prevalence of transient myocardial ischemia on serial ambulatory monitoring after first acute myocardial infarction. More than 90% are silent. (From Mickley et al. [1998]. Prevalence, variability, and long-term prognostic importance of transient myocardial ischemia. *Cardiology* **90**:160–167. With permission from the publishers, Karger, Basel.)

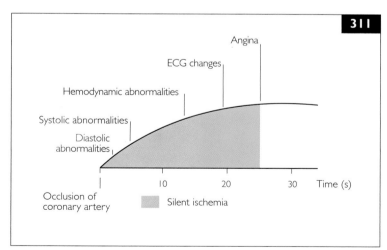

311 Sequential cascade of myocardial ischemia. ECG: electrocardiogram. (From Sigwart et al. [1984]. Ischemic events during coronary artery balloon obstruction. In: *Silent Myocardial Ischemia*. W Rutishauser, H Roskam (eds). Springer-Verlag, Berlin, p. 29. With permission from the publishers, copyright Springer-Verlag, Heidelberg [1984].)

remain totally asymptomatic during myocardial ischemia. Why some patients have chest pain and others are nonsymptomatic has been extensively studied, and several explanations have been proposed: a possible role for endorphins, differences in the pain threshold, a generalized hyposensitivity to pain, and lesser amounts of myocardium being jeopardized during silent than symptomatic ischemia. The results, however, are inconsistent and no definite conclusions can be drawn. From ambulatory monitoring we know that many ischemic episodes occur at low heart rates, lower than the heart rates we associate with demand-related ischemia on stress testing.

CLINICAL PRESENTATION

SMI is not an isolated coronary syndrome and ischemic episodes can be detected in patients with chronic as well as acute CAD. During ambulatory monitoring some patients will only demonstrate SMI, whereas other patients will have both symptomatic and asymptomatic episodes. During exercise testing, however, inducible ischemia will be either symptomatic or asymptomatic. Myocardial ischemia detected by exercise testing often predicts who will have ischemic episodes on ambulatory monitoring. Episodes of ambulatory ischemia will display a

circadian rhythm, with a peak incidence in the morning, a smaller peak in the evening, and a low incidence at night. The circadian pattern is evident in both symptomatic and silent ischemia. The available data suggest that objective evidence of myocardial ischemia, whether symptomatic or silent, is a clinical marker for the presence of significant CAD and perfusion abnormalities.

DIAGNOSIS

Electrocardiographic evidence of myocardial ischemia can be detected by changes in the ST segment on the standard electrocardiogram (ECG), by use of an exercise test or ambulatory monitoring. Exercise testing is commonly used to examine for potentially inducible ischemia, albeit symptomatic or silent. Similarly to the standard ECG, exercise testing reveals information concerning the magnitude and extent of myocardial ischemia. Ambulatory monitoring gives information on the frequency and duration of ischemia occurring spontaneously or during daily activities, with or without symptoms. Significant ischemia on exercise testing (**312**) and ambulatory monitoring (**313**) is defined as the development of horizontal or down-sloping ST segment depression ≥1 mm measured 80 ms after the J point when compared with the baseline ECG. In ambulatory monitoring, one

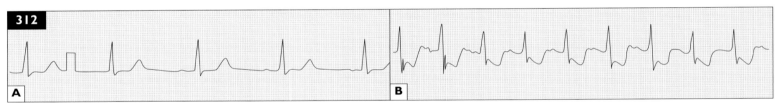

312 Electrocardiograms at rest before exercise testing (heart rate 70 bpm) (**A**) and during exercise testing at maximum work load (heart rate 145 bpm) (**B**). ST segment depression >4 mm of down-sloping nature.

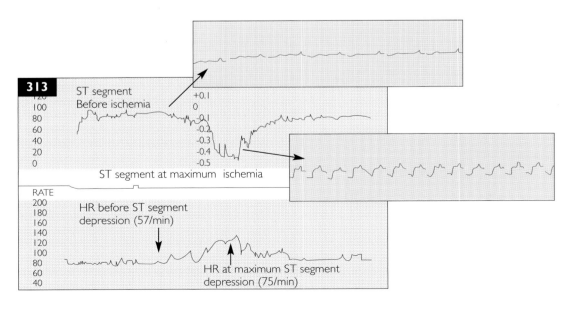

313 Section of trend curves of the ST segment (**upper panel**) with electrocardiographic tracings before and during maximum silent ischemia (4mm ST segment depression of horizontal type) and heart rate (HR) values (**lower panel**).

episode has to last ≥1 minute. More sophisticated methods such as perfusion scintigraphy, stress echocardiography, or positron emission tomography (PET) can also be used to detect myocardial ischemia.

MANAGEMENT

Multiple clinical trials have demonstrated that episodes of symptomatic and SMI can be reduced by anti-anginal drugs including nitrates, calcium antagonists, and beta blockers. The sum of evidence indicates that beta blockers are the most efficacious agents and that coronary revascularization is superior to medical treatment in the suppression of SMI. However, it is important to realize that no medical treatment whether driven by clinical symptoms or ECG evidence of ischemia, or the performance of mechanical revascularization can totally abolish objective evidence of myocardial ischemia. Thus, the 12-week results of the ACIP study have shown that among patients who present with significant ST segment depression, 45–89% continue to have (mainly) SMI during ambulatory monitoring or exercise testing (*Table 45*)[5]. In patients with ACS undergoing one-vessel coronary stenting, one-third exhibited SMI after the procedure[6]. What remains to be resolved is the question of whether a reduction in SMI *per se* directly improves clinical outcome, or whether a reduction in SMI is only a marker of treatment effect.

PROGNOSIS

At present there is substantial evidence that episodes of predominantly SMI provide prognostic information in selected patients with CAD. Studies from 1988 to 1990 addressing high-risk patients with stable angina suggest that ischemic episodes identify subjects at increased risk of future death or nonfatal myocardial infarction (MI)[7]. Larger and more recent long-term follow-up studies of individuals representing the general population of patients with stable CAD have failed to confirm these early observations[8,9]. Available data do not support the hypothesis that repetitive episodes of SMI will result in any clinically measurable damage of left ventricular (LV) function[10]. In patients with unstable angina, the persistence of transient ST segment depression may provide more prognostic information than that obtained by clinical assessment of chest pain. In the general population of patients with AMI, episodes of transient ischemia can be used to identify subjects at increased risk of subsequent combined hard and soft cardiac events. Ambulatory monitoring may supplement predischarge exercise testing in risk stratification, but the validity remains controversial. In patients deemed unable to perform a predischarge exercise test, the demonstration of ambulatory, mainly SMI can identify patients at heightened risk for recurrent MI and cardiac death. Despite some controversy, the bulk of literature suggests that silent exercise-induced postinfarction ischemia is associated with a significantly better outcome than painful ischemia.

SUMMARY

In most cases, the presence of SMI places the patient at additional risk. However, the highest risk is undoubtly found in patients who concurrently have left main or three-vessel disease and reduced LV function. To date, there is no direct evidence that episodes of SMI are associated with future hard cardiac events in a cause-and-effect relationship[11]. Controlled studies comparing the prognostic implications of different treatment regimens in different subgroups of patients with CAD, with and without SMI, are needed in order to elucidate if such episodes are themselves deleterious. Currently, a routine search for ambulatory ischemia cannot be recommended either in unselected patients with stable angina or in survivors of AMI who can perform predischarge exercise test. The presence of transient SMI seems to provide independent prognostic information in selected patients with ACS.

Table 45 12-week results of the ACIP study in patients with significant ST segment depression

	Rates of silent myocardial ischemia		
	Angina driven (n = 204)	Ischemia driven (n = 202)	Coronary revascularization (n = 212)
Ambulatory (%)	61	59	45
Exercise-induced (%)	85	89	70

(From Knatterud et al. [1994]. Effects of treatment strategies to suppress ischemia in patients with coronary artery disease: 12-week results of the aymptomatic cardiac ischemia pilot (ACIP) study. *J. Am. Coll. Cardiol.* **24**:11–20.)

Chapter Fifteen

Chronic Arrhythmias and Conduction Disorders

CHRONIC ARRHYTHMIAS AND CONDUCTION DISORDERS

ANDERS KIRSTEIN PEDERSEN, MD, DMSC

INTRODUCTION

Chronic ischemic heart disease (IHD) is accompanied by an increased risk of both tachyarrhythmias and bradyarrhythmias. Myocardial ischemia leads to changes in impulse conduction velocity and influences the refractory periods. The development of myocardial infarcts (MI) creates zones of nonconducting tissue surrounded by border-zones with changed electrophysiological properties, thus making the settings for re-entry loops.

The development of heart failure by post-MI remodeling additionally enhances the general risk of ventricular tachyarrhythmias, and the increased wall stress in the left atrium (LA) induced by increased filling pressures increases the risk of developing atrial fibrillation (AF). Temporary or permanent ischemia in the nodal tissues or in the specialized conduction system may lead to temporary or permanent impairment of impulse formation or impulse propagation, resulting in manifestations of bradycardia. Ischemic damage to the specialized conduction system in the ventricles may result in bundle branch block (BBB), which impairs the synchronous contraction pattern of the ventricles, resulting in mitral regurgitation and heart failure.

ATRIAL FIBRILLATION

IHD, along with age, arterial hypertension, diabetes, valvular disease and heart failure, is an independent specific risk factor for the development of chronic AF. A fibrillating atrium abolishes the atrial contractile contribution to the cardiac output and abolishes the sinus node regulation of heart rate, leaving the heart rate to be controlled by the atrioventricular-nodal (AVN) conduction properties. The result is a significant (at least 15%) decrease in cardiac output, which might precipitate heart failure, accompanied by a risk of arterial thromboembolism of 3–9% per year, depending on the presence of additional risk factors.

The management of AF in the presence of one or several risk factors should always include anticoagulation, preferably with a coumarin derivative, with a thrombin inhibitor or with an antiplatelet agent if proper anticoagulation is not tolerated. The management of the rhythm disturbance *per se* gives two options: to accept the fibrillation and just regulate the AV conduction to a near-physiological level with drugs, if necessary (rate control), or to convert the fibrillating atrium to sinus rhythm with DC-conversion or drugs (rhythm control). The latter option usually involves chronic anti-arrhythmic drug therapy to avoid relapse into AF, but even with the most aggressive drug regimen a recurrence rate of >50% is common. Several controlled clinical trials have recently failed to demonstrate a clinical benefit of an aggressive rhythm-controlling therapy in terms of morbidity (symptoms, thromboembolic risk) or mortality. Such a strategy often involves the use of drugs with proarrhythmic properties (sotalol, flecainide, chinidine) which should be avoided if decreased ejection fraction (EF) or heart failure is present. Amiodarone in doses of 100–200 mg/day is probably the most effective drug in rhythm control but chronic therapy should be well monitored due to the high incidence of side-effects. Rate control is most effectively exerted with a beta blocker or a calcium antagonist. Amiodarone may be the only drug tolerated if heart failure is present. Digoxin is not very effective in preserving physiologic rate controls due to its vagus-dependent action. Catheter-based AVN ablation with pacemaker-based rate control is an option in drug intolerance.

VENTRICULAR TACHYARRHYTHMIAS AND SUDDEN CARDIAC DEATH

Sudden cardiac death (SCD), defined as unexpected and instantaneous (<1 hour of symptoms) death due to cardiac causes without pre-existing cardiac disease, is a common cause of death in chronic IHD. SCD is clearly related to the development of lethal arrhythmias, in particular ventricular tachycardia and ventricular fibrillation (VF). In monitored SCD cases, 70–80% are due to tachyarrhythmia and 20% due to bradyarrhythmia. SCD is seen with or without MI. In autopsy series, a fresh coronary lesion is a common finding in hearts without previous scarring, but in hearts with significant previous infarcted areas, a larger proportion is without signs of unstable coronary lesions. These deaths are supposedly caused by primary arrhythmia. The relationship of previous damage of the heart in the thrombolysis era (low EF) to the risk of arrhythmic death is shown in *Table 46*.

A number of other risk factors for SCD in IHD have been identified: (1) increased ventricular ectopy, (2) nonsustained ventricular tachycardia, (3) sustained ventricular tachycardia,

(4) inducible ventricular tachycardia by electrophysiological study (see Chapter 8, Electrophysiology), (5) markers of autonomic activity (resting heart rate, heart rate variability, baroreceptor sensitivity), (6) markers of ventricular scarring (late potentials), and (7) markers of repolarization abnormalities (T wave alternans, T wave dispersion). A previous, aborted SCD is also a prominent risk factor. VF during the first 24 hours of an acute MI is not considered a significant risk factor for later SCD.

The management of any arrhythmia in IHD is guided by two principles: (1) a careful evaluation of the symptoms of the particular arrhythmia and the risk of progression into a life-threatening condition, and (2) a careful evaluation of the effect of a therapeutic strategy on both symptoms and risk. Unfortunately, a chosen strategy may at the same time effectively limit symptoms and increase the risk. Consequently, evidence-based strategies are fundamental in the management of arrhythmias.

Increased ventricular ectopy is often seen in acute exacerbations of IHD. It frequently accompanies MI or unstable ischemia. Also in chronic stable conditions, ventricular ectopy or even nonsustained ventricular tachycardia may produce palpitations. Importantly, the risk for SCD associated with these arrhythmias seems to be most prominent when combined with low EF. Suppression of the arrhythmias by drugs is not associated with a risk reduction: on the contrary, some drugs (lidocaine, flecainide, d-sotalol) clearly increase the short-term and long-term mortality. Therefore, symptom suppression should be performed only with drugs with a beneficial or neutral effect on the risk (e.g. beta blockers or amiodarone).

Sustained ventricular tachycardia is a particular manifestation seen in patients with significant myocardial scarring, often produced by remote clinical infarctions. The typical patient has a dilated left ventricle (LV) with large infarct areas or even an aneurysm. The occurrence of tachycardia is most often unrelated to any primary coronary event, and the mechanism of the tachycardia is usually a macrore-entry around a scar area, giving a characteristic monomorphic electrocardiographic (ECG) pattern. The risk of future SCD is greatly enhanced if the tachycardia is associated with hemodynamic collapse, or is accompanied by symptoms such as syncope, angina, or heart failure. Not rarely, a monomorphic ventricular tachycardia, though initially tolerable,

degenerates into VF within a few minutes, and a clinical presentation as primary arrhythmic death with primary VF is not uncommon.

The primary aim of the management of sustained ventricular tachycardia is to terminate the tachycardia, most often with DC-conversion. If the tachycardia is slow and the patient is completely stable, amiodarone infusion (150–300 mg IV followed by 1000 mg/day) might terminate the tachycardia, but extreme surveillance is necessary to observe hemodynamic deterioration which will necessitate DC-conversion.

The secondary aim of the management of any ventricular arrhythmia is to reduce the risk of future SCD. In nonsustained ventricular tachycardia in the absence of acute ischemia and associated with EF <35%, an electrophysiological study is recommended (see Chapter 8, Electrophysiology). If the patient has inducible ventricular tachycardia or fibrillation, implantation of an automatic implantable cardioverter-defibrillator (ICD) is recommended (**314**). If the patient presents with monomorphic ventricular tachycardia or VF in the absence of MI, ICD implantation is additionally recommended. Often, recurrent tachycardia is controlled by antitachycardia pacing by the device or by drug therapy. Another therapeutic option is radiofrequency catheter ablation of the re-entry circuit (**315**) to eliminate recurrence of the tachycardia (but probably not the risk of SCD). Recent trials have evaluated the risk of ICD in patients with low EF and no arrhythmias. It appears that the risk reduction of SCD is of the same magnitude as in patients with presenting arrhythmias.

BRADYARRHYTHMIAS AND BLOCK
Sinus node dysfunction may be caused by chronic coronary disease in the artery related to the sinus node artery branch, usually the right coronary artery (RCA). More commonly it is seen in

Table 46 Rate of death for each mode of mortality at various dichotomy limits of left ventricular ejection fraction

LVEF (%)	Rate (%) per person-year (total events)		
	All cause	Arrhythmic	Cardiac
<20	23.1	9.4	10.6
21–30	17.5	7.7	6.3
31–40	6.8	3.2	2.2

LVEF: left ventricular ejection fraction. (From Priori et al. [2001]. Task Force on sudden cardiac death of the European Society of Cardiology. *Eur. Heart J.* **22**:1374–1450.)

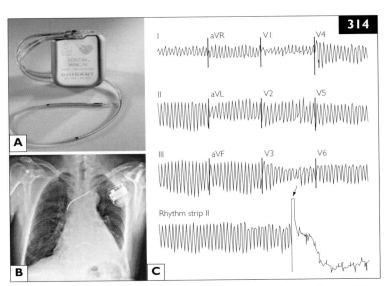

314 An implantable cardioverter-defibrillator (**A**), the position in thorax (**B**) and an electrocardiogram with ventricular fibrillation and automatic defibrillation into DDD paced rhythm (**C**).

conjunction with the use of drugs with depressant action on the sinus node (beta blockers, calcium antagonists, amiodarone, digoxin). If the sinus node dysfunction is symptomatic, and the continuous use of depressant drugs is necessary, implantation of a pacemaker system might be warranted.

Temporary ischemic damage to the AVN is common in acute inferior MI. Since the AVN often receives atrial branches from both the RCA and the left coronary artery (LCA), the AV-block is usually at supra-His level, of a lower degree, and is rarely permanent because of the development of collaterals. On the other hand, anterior infarction associated with complete heart block or right BBB (RBBB) and episodes of second or third degree AV-block have a high risk of recurrence or permanency, since it is caused by damage in the infra-His structures, the specialized conduction bundles. A permanent pacemaker is most often indicated in these cases.

A special situation is the post-MI patient with left BBB (LBBB) or RBBB combined with a left hemiblock. In both situations, the patient has a bifascicular conduction block, but a pacemaker implant is only recommended in the presence of symptoms of bradycardia or if intermitent second degree AV-block is documented. Permanent BBB might induce ventricular dyssynchrony in a dilated LV which may aggravate heart failure and mitral incompetence. For these patients, biventricular pacing with right septal pacing combined with left lateral wall pacing through the coronary veins is a promising therapeutic modality (**316**).

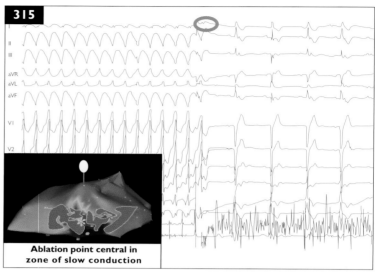

Ablation point central in zone of slow conduction

315 Radiofrequency catheter ablation of stable monomorphic ventricular tachycardia, guided by electroanatomical mapping (**insert**). The onset of energy delivery immediately terminates the tachycardia.

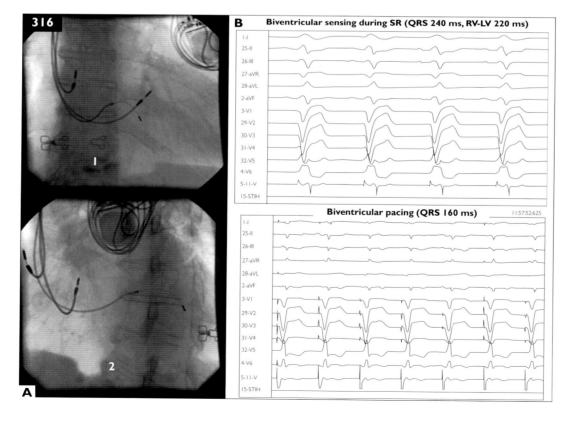

316 Position of electrodes in biventricular pacing (**A**) and the effect of biventricular pacing on QRS width (**B**). 1: anteroposterior projection; 2: left anterior oblique projection.

Chapter Sixteen

Left Ventricular Dysfunction

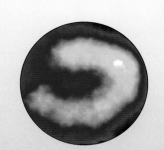

HEART FAILURE

JOHN G.F. CLELAND, MD, FRCP, FESC, NIKOLAY NIKITIN, PhD, DSC, FARQAD ALAMGIR, MBBS, MRCP, AND ANDREW CLARK, MA, MD, FRCP

DEFINITION

There is no universally accepted definition of heart failure. There are two conceptual approaches: (1) primarily subjective: a clinical syndrome characterized by symptoms (especially breathlessness) and signs of fluid retention caused by cardiac dysfunction or (2) primarily objective: cardiac dysfunction leading to activation of compensatory mechanisms and a reduction in exercise capacity. Patients who fulfill the subjective definition should also fulfill the objective criteria but the reverse is often not true (i.e. patients may have severe but asymptomatic cardiac dysfunction). An ejection fraction (EF) <40% is commonly used as a threshold for defining left ventricular systolic dysfunction (LVSD) but there are many other forms of cardiac dysfunction that may lead to symptoms of heart failure or to premature death.

EPIDEMIOLOGY

The epidemiology of heart failure is complex and poorly described, partly due to a lack of a universally accepted objective definition. Heart failure (using primarily subjective criteria) is the commonest single cause of medical admissions. Annually, about 500 admissions/100,0000 population will be due to, or complicated by, heart failure.

The incidence of subjectively defined heart failure rises steeply with age but this may not be true for LVSD. The overall annual incidence of heart failure is about 4/1,000 population but rises to about 1% of people aged 65–74 years and even higher in older age groups. About half of these cases are associated with LVSD. The incidence of suspected heart failure, which reflects the demand for diagnostic services, will be 2–5-fold higher.

About 2% of the population will have LVSD, most of which will be due to ischemic heart disease (IHD) and about half will be accompanied by symptoms and signs of heart failure (**317**). Another 1% will have clinical evidence of heart failure with preserved left ventricular (LV) systolic function, often termed diastolic heart failure, which is commonly associated with hypertension and/or atrial fibrillation (AF). Valvular disease is another common cause of heart failure.

The incidence and prevalence of heart failure appear to be increasing, probably due to improved primary and secondary 'prevention' (more accurately termed procrastination) and treatment of heart failure.

PATHOGENESIS

In simple terms, heart failure may be due to the heart being 'weak' (LVSD), 'stiff' (diastolic heart failure), 'overloaded' (severe hypertension, valve stenosis, or volume overload), 'leaking' (valvular regurgitation), or 'confused' (AF or cardiac dyssynchrony). IHD accounts for >50% of cases of heart failure and possibly >80% in patients aged 50–75 years, but less in younger (dilated cardiomyopathy) and older (hypertension) age groups. IHD is also the commonest cause of LVSD in western society.

Most patients who develop heart failure as a consequence of myocardial infarction (MI) develop symptoms and signs within days of the event, due to the sudden loss of contractile power associated with cardiac myocyte stunning and death. Estimates of the proportion of MIs that exhibit evidence of heart failure within the first week varies widely, from 10% to 50%. Heart failure will often resolve as the heart adapts (by ventricular dilatation and myocardial hypertrophy) and stunning recovers. If ventricular damage is sufficiently severe then progressive ventricular remodeling (ventricular dilatation with stretching of scar and the

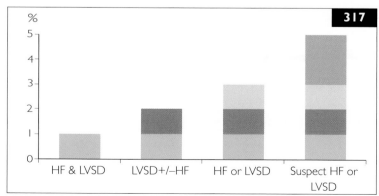

317 Prevalence of heart failure and left ventricular systolic dysfunction. HF: heart failure; LVSD: left ventricular systolic dysfunction. (Adapted from Cleland et al. [2001]. The heart failure epidemic: exactly how big is it? *Eur Heart J* **22**:623–626.

development of hypertrophy and fibrosis in remote, previously undamaged myocardium) will occur, increasing the risk of sudden death or the subsequent development of chronic heart failure.

In about 50% of patients with IHD and LVSD, a substantial volume of myocardium with contractile dysfunction will still be viable, reflecting stunning (without structural changes in cardiac myocytes) or hibernation (with loss of structural elements in cardiac myocytes). Accelerated loss of cardiac myocytes (apoptosis) in hibernating myocardium may lead to irreversible contractile failure. Beta blockers and revascularization may protect and improve function in such segments. The risks and benefits of conservative management versus revascularization are being evaluated in randomized trials.

A substantial proportion of patients with IHD, LVSD, and heart failure have no obvious history of MI. About 25% of MIs are 'silent' and are not recognized acutely. Myocardial stunning and hibernation may occur independently of MI. Regional contractile asynchrony commonly complicates regional contractile failure and is also an important target for therapy. Damage to the valve apparatus may also lead to mitral regurgitation and heart failure.

CLINICAL PRESENTATION

A diagnosis of heart failure will first be made during a hospital admission in 60–80% of patients. The primary reason for such admissions is often an MI, an arrhythmia, or a respiratory infection.

Patients may present with acute breathlessness due to pulmonary edema shortly after an MI or with more subtle evidence of heart failure, including tachycardia, a third heart sound, elevated venous pressure, and pulmonary crepitation. Patients with chronic ventricular dysfunction late after MI may present with a gradual increase in exertional breathlessness or with a sudden worsening of symptoms due to a precipitating factor such as myocardial ischemia, AF, pulmonary embolism, or infection. Severe cardiac dysfunction may be asymptomatic and present as sudden death.

DIAGNOSIS
Diagnosis of heart failure (i.e. is heart failure present?)

Heart failure is a syndrome that cannot be diagnosed by any single test. The diagnosis depends on the presence of symptoms and objective evidence of cardiac dysfunction, usually LVSD for patients with IHD. Many clinicians require evidence of fluid retention as part of the diagnosis, although signs are often absent due to the use of diuretics. Echocardiography, radionuclide studies, and cine-magnetic resonance imaging may all be used to assess ventricular function (**318–322**).

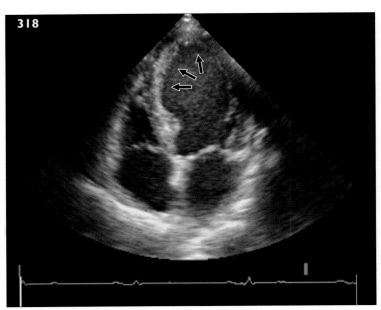

318 Echocardiographic apical four-chamber view showing an apical aneurysm (arrows) in a patient after anterior myocardial infarction. Plasma concentration of N-terminal brain natriuretic peptide prior to echocardiography was 662 pmol/l (normal upper limit = 36 pmol/l).

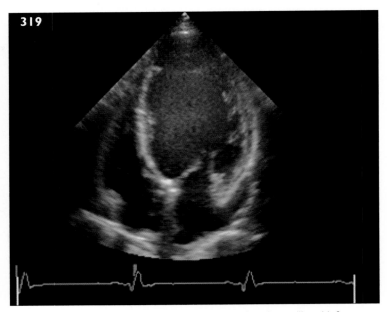

319 Echocardiographic apical four-chamber view showing a dilated left ventricle (end-diastolic volume = 340ml) with severely impaired global function (ejection fraction = 22%) as a result of progressive postinfarction ventricular remodeling. Plasma concentration of N-terminal brain natriuretic peptide prior to echocardiography was 1,515 pmol/l (normal upper limit = 36 pmol/l).

A normal electrocardiogram (ECG) makes a diagnosis of heart failure very unlikely. Measurement of the plasma concentration of natriuretic peptides is an alternative method with which to assess cardiac function and prognosis, but not the cause of cardiac dysfunction, which still requires imaging.

A diagnosis of heart failure requires exclusion of severe anemia, renal failure, or hepatic dysfunction, which may all mimic heart failure. Pulmonary function should be assessed to exclude lung disease as a cause of symptoms or as a factor complicating the management of heart failure.

Diagnosis in heart failure (i.e. what is the cause of heart failure?)

Tests should generally be directed at diagnoses that will alter management. Imaging tests will identify valve regurgitation, ventricular dyssynchrony, and other causes of heart failure such as aortic valve disease, from which patients with IHD are not immune. There is no evidence that the risk outweighs the benefit of revascularization in patients with heart failure, even if myocardial ischemia, hibernation, or stunning is present. Accordingly, coronary arteriography is only required in patients with heart failure if angina is present and uncontrolled by medical therapy, or if it is felt necessary to confirm a suspected diagnosis of dilated cardiomyopathy.

DIFFERENTIAL DIAGNOSIS

The differential diagnosis depends on the signs and symptoms. Where breathlessness predominates, respiratory disease, infection, pulmonary embolism, and anemia should be considered and excluded where appropriate. Where signs of fluid retention predominate, renal failure, hepatic failure, and venous disease should be excluded. The above conditions may coexist with and /or precipitate heart failure.

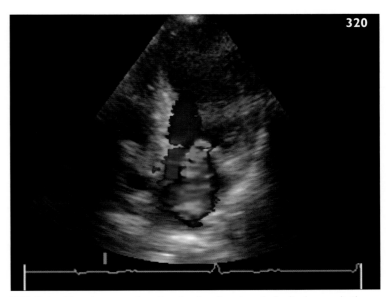

320 Color Doppler recording showing functional central mitral regurgitation. Plasma concentration of N-terminal brain natriuretic peptide prior to echocardiography was 2,369 pmol/l (normal upper limit = 36 pmol/l).

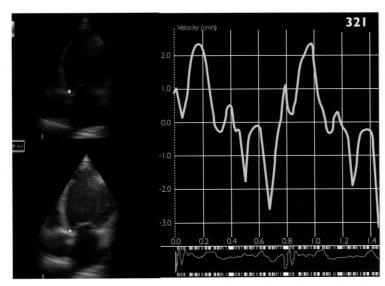

321 Color tissue Doppler imaging showing a decreased systolic mitral annular velocity (2.4 cm/second) at the septal end of the mitral annulus, as a result of impaired longitudinal ventricular function.

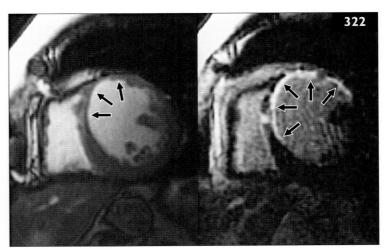

322 Cardiovascular magnetic resonance images obtained in a patient with heart failure due to ischemic heart disease. An end-diastolic short-axis image (**left**) shows an area of myocardial thinning and contractile dysfunction (arrows). The second image (**right**), taken 15 minutes after contrast injection, shows a bright area of hyperenhancement (arrows) confirming the presence of irreversible myocardial injury (infarcted region).

MANAGEMENT

Conceptually, treatment for heart failure due to IHD could be targeted at the coronary arteries or at ventricular function (**323**).

There is no evidence that aspirin, lipid-lowering therapy, and revascularization are safe or effective in patients with heart failure. Each of these interventions is now the subject of a major outcome trial. Those concerned about polypharmacy in heart failure should consider stopping the above treatments until their safety and efficacy are established.

In patients with IHD and LVSD, angiotensin-converting enzyme (ACE) inhibitors and beta blockers have been shown to improve symptoms or delay their progression, reduce the rate of hospitalization (all-cause and for heart failure), reduce the risk of recurrent MI, and delay death. The effects are large compared to those of most other interventions for cardiovascular conditions (e.g. revascularization for triple vessel disease). Beta blockers appear to be effective pharmacologic therapy for myocardial hibernation.

All patients with IHD and LVSD should receive ACE inhibitors and beta blockers unless contraindications exist, such as hypotension, renal dysfunction and, for beta blockers, reversible obstructive airways disease and bradycardia. Patients with relative contraindications should only receive these agents on expert advice. Care and experience are required for safe and efficient titration to optimal maintenance doses. Symptoms,

weight, heart rate, blood pressure, and renal function should be monitored.

The clinical benefits and adverse effects of angiotensin receptor blockers (ARBs) and ACE inhibitors are similar, but ARBs are not associated with cough and rarely with angio-oedema. Accordingly, ARBs may be used as an alternative to ACE inhibitors in appropriate patients. ARBs may also be given in addition to ACE inhibitors to improve symptoms, if these are poorly controlled, and reduce the rate of hospitalization for heart failure. Whether they can also reduce mortality is controversial.

Aldosterone receptor antagonists (ARAs) have been shown to reduce hospitalizations and mortality in patients with postinfarction LVSD and in patients with severe heart failure. It can be assumed, therefore, that they are also effective in patients with mild chronic heart failure due to LVSD, although guidelines hesitate on this issue. Feminizing side-effects, especially gynecomastia, are common with spironolactone and may be avoided by using a selective agent such as eplerenone.

Most patients with failure and LVSD should now be on triple therapy with an ACE inhibitor, beta blocker, and either an ARB or ARA, but possibly not both. In older patients and those with renal dysfunction, there is a risk of serious hyperkalemia with either agent but especially ARAs. There is little evidence to support the use of digoxin in addition to beta blockers and ACE inhibitors except in patients with AF. Nitrates may be used for angina but there is no good evidence of benefit in heart failure. Calcium channel antagonists, with perhaps the exception of amlodipine, and class-I antiarrhythmic agents should be avoided. Amiodarone suppresses arrhythmias and is relatively safe but there is no good evidence that it improves prognosis.

Patients who remain symptomatic despite standard pharmacologic treatment who have evidence of cardiac dyssynchrony (LV ejection fraction ≤35%, QRS >120 msec and echocardiographic interventricular mechanical delay) on the surface ECG should routinely be considered for biventricular pacing to provide resynchronization leading to improved symptoms, reduced hospitalization, and prolonged life. These devices are relatively inexpensive. It is controversial whether devices that provide both resynchronization and a defibrillator function will increase longevity but they are more costly and carry the risk of inappropriate shocks. Implantable defibrillators reduce sudden death and this has a small but definite overall survival benefit. These devices do not improve heart failure symptoms and may make them worse (especially if they provide back-up right ventricular pacing) and are relatively expensive. Improved targeting of defibrillators would reduce the associated morbidity and costs but runs the risk of missing some patients who might benefit.

Out-of-hospital telemonitoring devices, both invasive and noninvasive, could revolutionize the management of heart failure with drugs or devices.

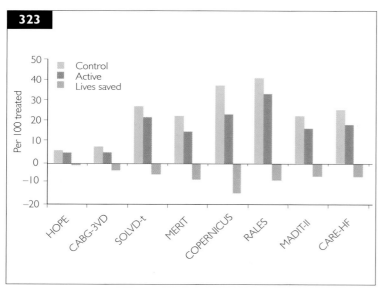

323 Two-year mortality and benefits of therapy in studies of heart failure. (Adapted from Cleland *et al.* [2003]. Update of clinical trials from the American College of Cardiology. EPHESUS, SPORTIF-III, ASCOT, COMPANION, UK-PACE, and T-wave Alternans. *Eur. J. Heart Fail.* **5**:389–394; Cleland and Clark [2003]. Delivering the cumulative benefits of triple therapy for heart failure. Too many cooks will spoil the broth. *J. Am. Coll. Cardiol.* **42**:1226–1233).

Agents such as levosimendan or nitrates/nesiritide (in that order of evidence) should be used for the management of acute excacerbations of heart failure and IHD, in addition to morphine and, if hypoxemia exists, high-flow oxygen. Inotropic agents should be avoided unless the patient has severe hypotension and developing shock.

PROGNOSIS

The prognosis of new-onset heart failure is poor, both in terms of morbidity and mortality. About 25% of patients will be readmitted within 3 months of a hospital discharge for heart failure, making it the commonest reason for early readmission (**324**). About one-third of patients will die within 6 months of first diagnosis (**325**). Amongst patients who have survived the first 6 months, the subsequent annual mortality is about 15%. LVSD and IHD both indicate a worse prognosis. About half of patients with heart failure will die out of hospital, usually suddenly, due to arrhythmias or recurrent MI. The rest will die during a hospital readmission either as a direct consequence of another vascular event (MI or stroke), infection (respiratory), or malignant arrhythmia. A minority of patients will die in intractable heart failure.

ORGANIZATION OF A HEART FAILURE SERVICE

Although heart failure is one of the very few conditions for which there is randomized controlled trial evidence to prove that organization of services makes a difference to patient outcome, few hospitals have developed specialized services. Reorganization of services for the management of heart failure should be a major health priority (**326**).

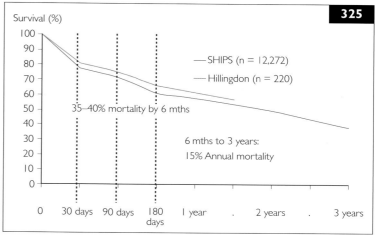

325 Prognosis of incident (acute) heart failure. (Adapted from Cleland et al. [1999]. Is the prognosis of heart failure improving? *Eur. J. Heart Fail.* **1**:229–241; Cowie et al. [2000]. Prognosis of heart failure: a population-based study of the outcome in incident cases *Heart* **83**:505–510.)

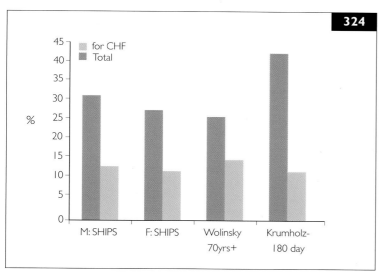

324 Rate of early (90 days) readmission for heart failure. CHF: chronic heart failure. (Adapted from Cleland et al. [1999.] Is the prognosis of heart failure improving? *Eur. J. Heart Fail.* **1**:229–241; Krumholz et al. [1997]. Readmission after hospitalization for congestive heart failure among Medicare beneficiaries. *Arch. Intern. Med.* **157**: 99–104; Wolinsky et al. [1997]. The sequelae of hospitalization for congestive heart failure among older adults. *J. Am. Geriatr. Soc.* **45**:558–563.)

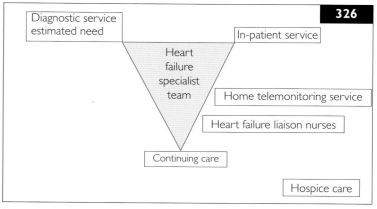

326 Elements for the organization of a Heart Failure Service.

ISCHEMIC CARDIOMYOPATHY, HIBERNATION, AND VIABILITY

AREND F.L. SCHINKEL, MD, PhD, JEROEN J. BAX, MD, PhD AND DON POLDERMANS, MD, PhD

DEFINITION

Ischemic cardiomyopathy refers to a state of severe LV dysfunction caused by chronic coronary artery disease (CAD). The extent of LV wall motion abnormalities may vary from circumscript dysfunctional regions to global impairment of function of the LV; the severity of dysfunction can vary from mild hypokinesia to akinesia and eventually dyskinesia. Frequently, a varying degree of wall motion abnormalities is present and LV EF is impaired (<35%).

EPIDEMIOLOGY

Chronic CAD is the most important cause of LV dysfunction leading to heart failure. In nearly 70% of the patients in 13 major heart failure trials, CAD was the underlying cause of heart failure[1]. The incidence and prevalence of ischemic cardiomyopathy have increased rapidly over the last decades. It has become clear that patients with ischemic cardiomyopathy represent a high-risk group. In the studies of LV dysfunction (SOLVD) registry, the 1-year mortality of patients with ischemic cardiomyopathy was 18%[2]. Although survival after the onset of heart failure has improved over the past 50 years, heart failure remains highly fatal. Among patients with heart failure in the 1990s, >50% were dead at 5 years[3]. Moreover, the extent of CAD and the severity of LV dysfunction are related to clinical outcome[1].

PATHOPHYSIOLOGY

The pathophysiology of ischemic cardiomyopathy is complex. For many years, LV dysfunction in patients with chronic CAD was considered irreversible, since LV dysfunction most often results from scar formation as a consequence of MI. However, it was recognized that the contractility in dysfunctional myocardium distal to a coronary stenosis can be improved following coronary revascularization[4,5]. The concept of hibernating myocardium was introduced to describe this state of hypoperfusion with persistently impaired LV function that can be partially or completely restored by revascularization[6,7]. Over the years, much knowledge has been acquired on hibernating myocardium and many studies have shown that segments with dysfunctional but hibernating (viable) myocardium improved in function after revascularization[8]. Pooled data from 105 viability studies with 3,003 patients, included 15,045 dysfunctional segments, with 7,941 (53%) improving in function after revascularization[8]. The time course of functional recovery of hibernating myocardium may vary. The recovery time may depend on multiple factors including duration and severity of ischemia, the time and completeness of myocardial revascularization, and the ultrastructural changes within the dysfunctional

myocardium[9,10]. The authors have demonstrated that 25% of dysfunctional but viable segments improved within 3 months of revascularization, whereas an additional 18% exhibited (additional) improvement at 14 months after revascularization (**327**). Indeed, the more severely damaged myocardium needed longer to recover in function after revascularization[9].

CLINICAL PRESENTATION

Patients with ischemic cardiomyopathy typically present with clinical symptoms of heart failure, although angina may be present. These patients should be evaluated extensively, including 2D echocardiography to evaluate regional and global LV function and (mitral) valvular functions, some form of stress imaging to assess ischemia, and coronary angiography (CAG) to evaluate suitability for potential revascularization[11]. Next, some form of viability assessment (see below) should be included. Based on the findings, therapy can be tailored to the individual patient.

MANAGEMENT

The options for treatment include medical therapy, myocardial revascularization (with mitral valve repair and LV remodeling if indicated), cardiac resynchronization (biventricular pacing), and heart transplantation. Newer treatment modalities include laser treatment, advanced surgery, assist devices, artificial hearts, and

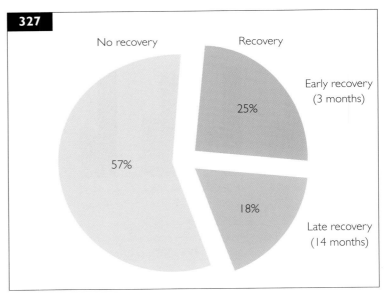

327 Early (3 months) and late (14 months) recovery after myocardial revascularization in dysfunctional segments in patients with ischemic cardiomyopathy. (Data based on Bax et al. [2001]. Time course of functional recovery of stunned and hibernating segments after surgical revascularization. *Circulation* **104**:1314–318.)

transplantation of different (progenitor) cells. These options should currently be considered experimental. Heart transplantation is associated with favorable survival but the availability of donor hearts is limited. Significant improvement in survival has been achieved with ACE inhibitors, beta blockers, and spironolactone. Despite all these new drugs, mortality of patients with severe heart failure remains high; Cowie *et al.*[12] showed that the 12-month mortality was 38%, and extrapolation of these results demonstrated 5-year mortality >70%.

Myocardial revascularization can be an effective alternative therapy in the subgroup of patients with a substantial amount of dysfunctional but viable myocardium. In these patients, revascularization may improve, and even normalize LV EF, heart failure symptoms, and survival[13]. Because revascularization in patients with ischemic cardiomyopathy is associated with an increased periprocedural morbidity and mortality[14], candidates for revascularization should be carefully selected. The extent of improvement in LV function is related to the extent of dysfunctional viable tissue[15]. Hence, a substantial amount of viable tissue has to be present, otherwise improvement of global LV function is not likely to occur. On the basis of the presence of dysfunctional but viable myocardium, >50% of patients with ischemic cardiomyopathy may be considered for revascularization. Schinkel and coworkers recently determined the prevalence of myocardial viability in a large group of patients with ischemic cardiomyopathy[16]. Dobutamine stress echocardiography demonstrated viability in 35% of the dysfunctional segments (**328**). When the cut-off value of ≥4 dysfunctional but viable segments was applied to classify a patient as viable, 57% of the patients had substantial viability. In these patients coronary revascularization may be considered as therapy.

VIABILITY TECHNIQUES
Several techniques have emerged to delineate dysfunctional scarred from dysfunctional but viable myocardium[17]. These techniques rely on the identification of different characteristics of viable myocardium (*Table 47*).

Thallium-201 stress-redistribution-reinjection and thallium-201 rest-redistribution single photon emission computed tomography (SPECT), are commonly used and accepted nuclear techniques to assess myocardial perfusion and cell membrane integrity[18]. Technetium-99m sestamibi or technetium-99m tetrofosmin can be used to assess perfusion and intact mitochondria.

Perfusion and metabolism can be evaluated with positron emission tomography (PET) or SPECT using dedicated (511 keV) collimators. Glucose utilization can be evaluated with ^{18}F-fluorodeoxyglucose (FDG). The introduction of SPECT imaging has contributed to a more widespread use of metabolic imaging.

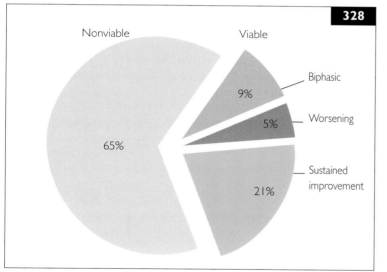

328 The prevalence of viable and nonviable tissue in patients with ischemic cardiomyopathy; 35% of dysfunctional myocardium was viable, whereas 65% was nonviable. Twenty-one percent of dysfunctional myocardium showed sustained improvement, 5% worsening, and 9% a biphasic wall motion pattern during low-high-dose dobutamine stress echocardiography. (Data based on Schinkel et al. [2001]. How many patients with ischemic cardiomyopathy exhibit viable myocardium? *Am. J. Cardiol.* **88**:561–564.)

Table 47 Characteristics of dysfunctional but viable myocardium

Characteristic	Viability technique	Markers of viability
Perfusion/intact cell membrane	Thallium-201 SPECT	Tracer activity >50%; redistribution >10%
Perfusion/intact mitochondria	Technetium-99m TF/MIBI SPECT	Tracer activity >50%; improved tracer uptake after nitrates
Glucose metabolism	FDG imaging (PET or SPECT)	Tracer activity >50%; preserved perfusion/ FDG uptake; perfusion–metabolism mismatch
Contractile reserve	Dobutamine echo cardiography	Improved contraction during infusion of low-dose dobutamine

Generally, cardiac FDG uptake is compared with regional perfusion. A normal perfusion/FDG uptake, or reduced perfusion with enhanced FDG uptake, indicates viable myocardium (**329**).

Viability on dobutamine echocardiography is indicated by improvement of wall motion during the infusion of low-dose dobutamine (5–10 µg/kg/minute)[19] (**330**). Recent studies have employed a high-dose protocol (with dosages up to

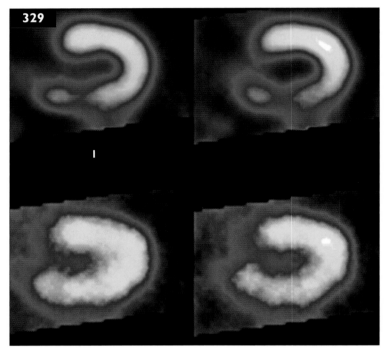

329 Prefusion defect (top) with preserved FDG uptake (bottom). Dual isotope simultaneous acquisition single photon emission computerized tomography scan (horizontal long-axis slices) showing a substantial perfusion–metabolism mismatch in the inferior wall (I), indicating viable myocardium. FDG: fluorodeoxyglucose.

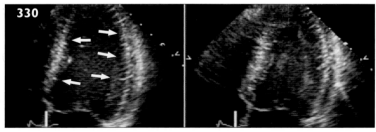

330 2D echocardiography recorded in the apical four-chamber view (end-systolic) at rest (**left panel**) and during infusion of low-dose dobutamine (**right panel**) in a patient with ischemic cardiomyopathy and severe hypokinesia of the interventricular septum and the lateral wall of the left ventricle (arrows). During low-dose dobutamine, improved contraction of the dysfunctional segments (inward motion and thickening of the myocardium) indicated myocardial viability.

40 µg/kg/minute, with the addition of atropine). This protocol allows assessment of both viability and stress-induced ischemia.

All these techniques are accurate and accepted for the assessment of myocardial viability. However, the predictive accuracies vary among various studies. In general, the nuclear imaging techniques appear to have a higher sensitivity for the prediction of functional recovery whereas stress echocardiography appears to be more specific[17]. A comparison of pooled data[17] demonstrated that the sensitivity and specificity of low-dose dobutamine echocardiography were, respectively, 84% and 81%, of thallium-201 reinjection 86% and 47%, thallium-201 rest-redistribution 90% and 54%, technetium-99m sestamibi 83% and 69%, and FDG PET 88% and 73%. Hence, all modalities had a high sensitivity, whereas low-dose dobutamine echocardiography had the highest specificity ($p < 0.01$). Both thallium-201 methods were less specific than low-dose dobutamine echocardiography ($p < 0.01$), technetium-99m sestamibi ($p < 0.05$), and FDG PET ($p < 0.01$). The discrepancy between nuclear imaging and dobutamine echocardiography for the prediction of functional outcome after revascularization may be related to different levels of ultrastructural cell damage in dysfunctional myocardium[9,10]. The inotropic response during dobutamine stimulation may be lost while more basal characteristics such as cell membrane integrity and glucose utilization are still intact. Nevertheless, all these techniques, SPECT, PET and stress echocardiography, accurately identify high-risk patients who may benefit from revascularization.

Recently, magnetic resonance imaging (MRI) combined with gadolinium-based contrast agents was proposed to evaluate myocardial viability; hyperenhancement of dysfunctional myocardium indicates scar tissue[20]. Importantly, the transmural extent of viable/nonviable myocardium can be determined because of the high spatial resolution of MRI. This may have important clinical implications since the extent of transmural injury is related to functional improvement after revascularization.

Electromechanical assessment of myocardial viability has also been developed using the NOGA system, a catheter-based, nonfluoroscopic, 3D endocardial mapping system[21] (see Chapter 8, Electromechanical Mapping). This new technique shows good concordance with nuclear imaging and stress echocardiography[21]. This is an invasive method for assessing viability, as compared to the previously described noninvasive techniques. Still, the NOGA technique is of interest, since it may serve as a platform for other procedures, such as laser revascularization, myoblast injection, or coronary angioplasty.

SUMMARY

Ischemic cardiomyopathy is an increasing clinical problem in terms of the number of affected patients. Myocardial revascularization may substantially improve heart failure symptoms, global LV function, and prognosis in patients with a substantial amount of dysfunctional but viable myocardium. Therefore, patients with heart failure symptoms secondary to chronic CAD should undergo noninvasive assessment of myocardial viability.

Chapter Seventeen

Percutaneous Coronary Intervention

INDICATIONS, PROCEDURE, AND TECHNIQUE

LEIF THUESEN, MD, PhD

INDICATIONS

Revascularization by percutaneous coronary intervention (PCI) or coronary artery bypass graft operation (CABG) is indicated when coronary angiography (CAG) has shown one or multiple coronary artery stenoses of diameter >50% in a patient with stable angina pectoris, unstable angina pectoris (UAP), acute myocardial infarction (AMI), positive test for myocardial ischemia, ischemic-induced arrhythmia, or left ventricular stunning/hibernation.

PCI can be performed when the following criteria are fulfilled:
- The treatment can be carried out successfully without significant complications.
- The treatment will result in symptomatic relief or reduced risk of complications to ischemic heart disease.
- The treatment will have a long-lasting positive effect.
- The treatment is equivalent to, or better than, CABG.

RISK FACTORS

Risk factors for PCI are related to the patient and to the coronary artery lesion. Patient-related risk factors:
- Age >65 years.
- Complicating diseases (diabetes, renal failure, peripheral atherosclerosis, and cerebrovascular disease).
- Acute coronary syndrome (ACS).
- Reduced left ventricular function.
- Cardiogenic shock.

Lesion-related risk factors:
- Ostial location.
- Bifurcate lesion.
- Tortuous vessel proximal to the lesion.
- Angled lesion.
- Long lesion (>20 mm).
- Diffuse coronary artery disease.
- Calcified lesion.
- Intracoronary thrombus.
- Degenerated saphenous vein graft.

- Multi-vessel PCI.
- PCI of left main coronary artery.

Improved PCI technique, primarily implantation of intracoronary stents, and treatment with glycoprotein (GP) IIb/IIIa inhibitors have reduced the risk of the acute procedure-related complications, death, MI, and acute bypass operation. Therefore, the acute procedure-related risk is primarily related to the possibility of successful stent implantation in the lesion. Stent implantation may be difficult in tortuous arteries, calcified arteries, and in small vessels.

PERCUTANEOUS CORONARY INTERVENTION VERSUS CORONARY ARTERY BYPASS GRAFT OPERATION

In a suitable coronary anatomy, PCI treatment with and without implantation of intracoronary stents is equivalent to CABG; this is also the case in patients with multi-vessel disease. However, in diabetic patients with multi-vessel disease, CABG may be preferred, especially if the left anterior descending coronary artery (LAD) is affected.

In chronic total occlusions, long lesions, very tortuous lesions, ostial lesions, bifurcate lesions, and in saphenous vein grafts, PCI may be difficult, impossible, or be associated with poor long-term results and thus be inferior to CABG.

PROCEDURE AND TECHNIQUE

PCI is performed through the femoral, the brachial, or the radial artery. A guiding catheter is placed in the ostium of the diseased coronary artery, a 0.014 inch guide wire is advanced through the lesion, and a balloon catheter is introduced over the guide wire and placed in the stenosis. Usually the balloon is inflated for 15–30 seconds by 6 atmospheres.

STENTS

After the balloon dilatation (**331**), a balloon premounted coronary stent is placed in the stenosis, and the stent balloon inflated to a pressure of ≥10 atmospheres for 15–30 seconds (**332**). The use of intracoronary stents has reduced the acute complication rate in PCI to <1%. Furthermore, stent implantation has reduced the risk of restenosis to 10–30%, depending on vessel diameter, lesion length, and the technique of implantation. Therefore, most centers implant stents in all lesions where it is technically possible.

In selected lesions, the stent can be implanted directly without balloon predilatation.

DRUG-ELUTING STENTS

In-stent restenosis is primarily caused by proliferation of myointimal cells. It is likely that new stent technology will reduce the problem of in-stent restenosis close to zero. The drug-eluting stent is a conventional stainless steel stent coated with an antiproliferative drug or with a polymer containing an antiproliferative drug. Sirolimus and taxol are such antiproliferative drugs, which have a clinically documented long-lasting anti-restenotic effect.

ROTATIONAL ATHERECTOMY

Rotational atherectomy uses a high-speed rotablator bur to enlarge the coronary artery lumen by plaque pulverization and embolization, rather than tissue removal (**333**). The indication has been fibrotic, calcified vessels and ostial lesions. Other indications are failure to insert a balloon through a lesion or failure to dilate a lesion with a balloon. Some interventionalists claim that rotational atherectomy softens the internal vessel wall and facilitates treatment with conventional balloons and stents.

DIRECTIONAL ATHERECTOMY

Directional atherectomy was developed for the purpose of excising obstructing atheroma tissue. The technique is advocated by a few dedicated centers for the treatment of a heavy plaque burden in larger vessels. The procedure is usually finalized by balloon dilatation or stent implantation.

BRACHYTHERAPY

Vascular brachytherapy is effective in the treatment of in-stent restenosis and is the first choice treatment of diffuse in-stent restenosis and relapsing focal in-stent restenosis. Both gamma and beta sources can be used. Brachytherapy of in-stent restenosis is preceded by dilatation with a conventional balloon or a so-called cutting balloon. It is likely that intravascular brachytherapy may be substituted by treatment with drug-eluting stents in the near future.

ADJUNCTIVE MEDICAL THERAPY

All PCI patients should be treated with aspirin in a dose between 75 and 325 mg per day. In combination with aspirin, the platelet inhibitor clopidogrel reduces the risk of acute stent thrombosis following PCI with stent from 2.5% to <1%. Clopidogrel should be given to all PCI patients prior to PCI treatment and for at least 1 month after the treatment. Unfractionated heparin is used for PCI procedures in a dose of 70–100 U/kg. It may be safe to use low-molecular weight heparin instead of unfractionated heparin.

GP IIb/IIIa receptor antagonists reduce the risk of procedure-related reinfarction and death in patients with diabetes, unstable coronary syndromes, and in patients treated with a stent. Abciximab has the best documented effect, but integrelin and tirofiban also seem to be effective. Ideally, the GP IIb/IIIa inhibitor should be given before the intervention.

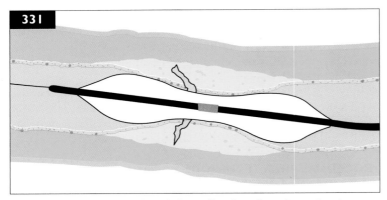

331 Schematic diagram to show balloon dilatation of an atherosclerotic plaque.

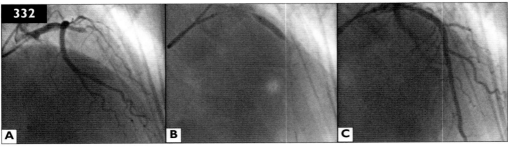

332 Coronary angiography showing a suboccluded left anterior descending coronary artery (**A**). The stenosis is dilated with a balloon mounted drug-eluting stent (**B**), and angiography after stenting confirms that the stenosis has been successfully eliminated (**C**).

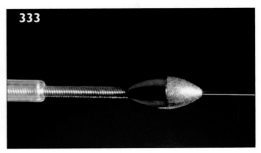

333 Rotablator diamond-coated bur.

RESULTS AND COMPLICATIONS

SJOERD H. HOFMA, MD, PhD AND PIM J. DE FEYTER MD, PhD

PERCUTANEOUS CORONARY INTERVENTION IN ANGINA PECTORIS

Twenty-five years have elapsed since the introduction of PCI. Starting with balloon angioplasty for discrete single vessel, single lesion coronary artery stenosis, the field has evolved into treating triple vessel disease, total occlusions, bifurcations, main stem stenosis, and AMI with stenting, combined with adjunctive antithrombotic medical therapies including thienopyridines and GP IIb/IIIa inhibitors.

The major complications of balloon angioplasty were procedural (sub)occlusive dissections (**334**) and late restenosis, predominantly due to early elastic recoil and late negative vessel remodeling, as well as some neointimal proliferation.

In the beginning of the 1990s, stents where introduced in the clinical arena (after some first attempts since 1986). The initial stent trials in 1994 proved superior in single lesions in normal sized coronary arteries[1,2]. Stents prevent early elastic recoil and late negative remodeling by 'scaffolding' the artery. Suboptimal balloon angioplasty results and acute dissections were also effectively treated with stents. The new problem of (sub)acute stent thrombosis was virtually solved with the introduction of thienopyridines as standard cotreatment for at least the first month after stenting, and is now approximately <1%.

The major challenge of the late 1990s was the problem of in-stent restenosis. The late lumen loss is almost entirely caused by neointimal hyperplasia inside the stented coronary segment. This is mainly due to vessel wall injury as well as inflammatory response and delayed endothelial healing of the stented segment[3,4]. Many stent coatings have been investigated, both to reduce initial thrombus formation (seen as a nidus for stimulation of neointima proliferative factors), and to limit the proliferative response itself.

The introduction of drug-eluting stents has provided major progress in the fight against in-stent restenosis. The most successful so far are sirolimus- (an antiproliferative cell cycle inhibitor) and paclitaxel- (a microtubule inhibitor) eluting stents (*Table 48*). In noncomplex lesions, restenosis has been virtually abolished. Currently, the performance of the sirolimus-eluting stent for a variety of indications, such as long lesions, small vessels, total occlusions, main stem, and AMI is under investigation.

Percutaneous stent treatment has also been shown to be effective in multi-vessel disease. With continuing catheter-based improvements, the surgical treatment of multi-vessel disease will gradually be replaced by stent treatment. The ARTS study has already shown similar protection against death, stroke, and MI in patients with multi-vessel disease treated with CABG or bare stent-based percutaneous intervention[5]. However, stenting was associated with a greater need for repeat revascularization. Drug-eluting stents will significantly decrease the need for repeat revascularization and thus will become more competitive to surgery. This will be investigated in the ARTS-II trial.

The risk of (sub)acute complications of PCI in the stent era is shown in *Table 49*.

CORONARY INTERVENTION IN MYOCARDIAL INFARCTION

Opening the thrombotic occlusion of the infarct-related coronary artery in AMI is effective in reducing the infarct size and thus in preserving of the left ventricular function (**335**).

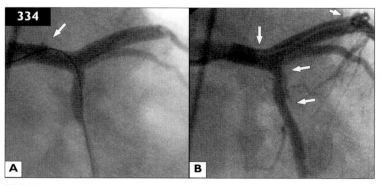

334 Major complication in percutaneous coronary intervention (PCI). **A:** Guiding catheter poking into the vessel wall of the left main coronary artery (arrow) during PCI of a lesion in the left circumflex coronary artery (LCx). **B:** Main stem dissection with tear visible into the left anterior descending coronary artery as well as into the LCx (arrows; several minutes later than panel A).

Table 48 Results of percutaneous coronary intervention with balloon, bare stents, and drug-eluting stents

Trial	Intervention	MACE* (% at 6 mths)	MACE* (% at 1 year)	Restenosis (% at 6 mths)
EPISTENT[13]	Balloon + abciximab	-	25.3	-
	vs.			
	Stent + abciximab	-	20.1	-
BENESTENT II[14]	Balloon	19.3	22.4 (p=0.01)	31 (p<0.001)
	vs.			
	Heparin-coated stent	12.8	15.7	16
RAVEL[12]	Bare stent	27.1(7 mths) (p<0.001)	28.8 (p<0.001)	26.6 (p<0.001)
	vs.			
	Sirolimus-eluting	3.3	5.8	0
SIRIUS**	Bare stent	18.9(9 mths) (p<0.001)		35.4 (in-stent) (p<0.001)
	vs.			
	Sirolimus-eluting	7.1		3.2
TAXUS II moderate release**	Bare stent	20.0 (p=0.0064)		20.2 (in-stent) (p=0.0002)
	vs.			
	Paclitaxel-eluting	7.8		4.7

*MACE: death/nonfatal myocardial infarction/target vessel revascularization; ** SIRIUS and TAXUS data presented at TCT meeting Washington, September 2002.

Angiographic studies show only 60% normal coronary flow at 90 minutes in patients treated with thrombolysis. Newer thrombolytic agents are faster and easier to administer to the patient, but fail to increase normal flow significantly. As early as 1993 pioneers such as Zijlstra *et al.* and Grines *et al.* demonstrated the benefit of primary percutaneous transluminal coronary angioplasty (PTCA) in AMI[6,7]. In 1997 Weaver *at al.* showed a 32% mortality reduction in primary PTCA compared to fibrinolysis in a meta-analysis of 2606 infarct patients[8]. The CADILLAC trial[9] demonstrated additional benefit of stenting versus balloon angioplasty in AMI. The benefit was entirely due to less target vessel revascularization in the stent group. Mortality was only 2% at 30 days! The sustained effect of primary PCI was reported by Zijlstra *et al.* at 5 ± 2 years follow-up of their patients[10].

The benefit of additional use of GP IIb/IIIa inhibitors in primary PCI is not clear yet, as the CADILLAC and ADMIRAL studies[9,11] showed conflicting results.

Recent data also show the benefit of transportation of patients acutely from noninterventional hospitals to interventional centers. The PRAGUE-2 study compared on-site streptokinase with transport to an interventional center with subsequent PCI. Treatment delay was 32 minutes in the PCI group. Despite this delay, 30-day death, reinfarction, or stroke was significantly reduced (*Table 50*). The Danish DANAMI-2 trial using recombinant tissue plasminogen activator (tPA) versus transport and PCI demonstrated the same benefit in twice as many patients and with a treatment delay of 60 minutes.

To decrease the transport delay in the authors' region, the ambulance personnel (without a physician) estimate the infarct size and location, with the help of an electrocardiogram (ECG) computer program. In cases with a large infarction, the patient is transferred immediately to the interventional center for PCI. After PCI, patients are relocated to neighboring community hospitals for further treatment. This approach may significantly reduce the time to first balloon inflation and further decrease the mortality rate.

Table 49 Complications of percutaneous coronary intervention in the stent era

Complication	%
Death	0.3–0.6
Q-wave MI	1–2
(Sub)acute stent thrombosis	1
Emergency CABG[15,16]	0.3–0.6
• Cause:	
Extensive dissection	38–50
Acute closure	25
Perforation	8–24
Aortic dissection	0–4
• Surgical mortality	11–21
• Death/MI	19–25
Femoral access complications[17]	
Pseudoaneurysm	3
Arteriovenous fistula	0.4
Retroperitoneal bleeding	0.1–0.4

CABG: coronary artery bypass graft; MI: myocardial infarction.

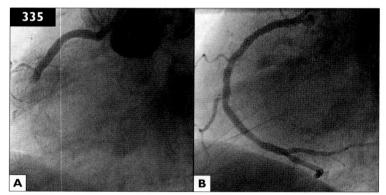

335 Percutaneous coronary intervention in acute myocardial infarction. **A:** Total occlusion of the right coronary artery (RCA). **B:** Patent RCA after recanalization and stenting.

Table 50 Recent results of primary percutaneous coronary intervention in acute myocardial infarction patients

Trial	Design	No. of patients	Mortality, % (p value)	Composite, % (p-value)
Zwolle et al.[10]	SK vs. Angioplasty	395	5±2y FU 23.9 vs. 13.4 (p < 0.01)	
ADMIRAL[12]	PCI vs. PCI+GP IIb/IIIa	300	6 month FU 7.4 vs. 3.4 (p < 0.13)	6 month FU* 33.8 vs. 22.8 (p < 0.03)
CADILLAC[10]	Balloon vs. Stent	2082	4.5 vs. 3.0 (n.s)	20.0 vs. 11.5 (p < 0.001)
PRAGUE-2[†]	SK vs. Transport+PCI	850	30 day FU 10.0 vs. 6.8 (p < 0.13)	30 day FU** 15.2 vs. 8.4 (p < 0.003)
DANAMI-2[†]	tPA vs. Transport+PCI	1572	7.6 vs. 6.6 (p < 0.35)	13.7 vs. 8.0 (p < 0.0003)

MI: myocardial infarction; SK: streptokinase; tPA: recombinant tissue plasminogen activator;* Composite endpoint at 6 months: death, re-MI, stroke, target vessel revascularization;** Composite endpoint at 30 days: death, re-MI, stroke;[†] PRAGUE and DANAMI data presented at ESC Berlin, August 2002.

LATE RESTENOSIS

BENNO J. RENSING, MD

DEFINITION

Restenosis is defined as the renarrowing of the vessel after an initially successful PCI. It has been the Achilles' heel of PCI since the inception of the technique and still severely hampers its long-term efficacy. Restenosis typically occurs 1–4 months after successful angioplasty[1,2] (**336**) and often manifests itself by a recurrence of anginal complaints and/or recurrence of ischemia at functional tests. Angiographic restenosis is now generally accepted to have occurred if a >50% lumen diameter reduction is present at the treated segment at follow-up angiography. Binary angiographic restenosis rates after balloon angioplasty are 25–60%, depending on several lesion and patient risk factors. Until recently the only method to reduce the chance for restenosis was implantation of a coronary stent[3]. This has led to a proliferative use of stents and these devices are now used in >70% of PCI cases in most centers. Although restenosis is less common after stenting, it still occurs quite frequently but is harder to treat. Reported re-restenosis rates after PCI for in-stent restenosis are between 20% and 85%.

MECHANISM OF RESTENOSIS

From serial intravascular ultrasound (IVUS) studies it became clear that restenosis after balloon angioplasty is caused by a combination of early elastic vessel recoil, negative remodeling (shrinkage) of the vessel wall, and neointima formation. The neointima is created by smooth muscle cell migration and proliferation from the media towards the intima and excessive extracellular matrix formation (**337A**). The contribution of neointima formation to late lumen loss is only 20–30%, while negative remodeling accounts for 70–80% of late loss[4,5]. On the other hand, the scaffolding properties of a stent effectively prevent recoil and negative remodeling and therefore in-stent restenosis is almost exclusively caused by neointima formation, (**337B, 338**)[6].

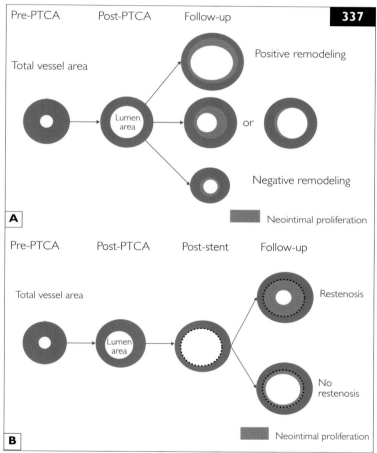

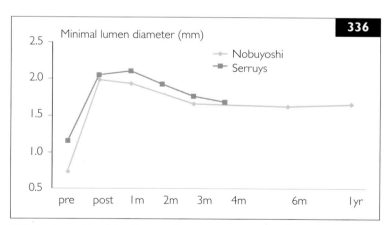

336 Angiographic minimal lumen diameter at several time intervals after coronary balloon angioplasty. Lumen diameter reduction typically occurs 1–4 months after the intervention. pre: preangioplasty; post: immediately postangioplasty; m: month; yr: year. (As reported by Serruys et al. [1988]. Incidence of restenosis after successful coronary angioplasty: a time related phenomenon. A quantitative angiographic study in 342 consecutive patients at 1, 2, 3, and 4 months. *Circulation* **77**:361–367; Nobuyoshi et al. [1988]. Restenosis after successful percutaneous transluminal coronary angioplasty: serial angiographic follow-up of 299 patients. *J. Am. Coll. Cardiol.* **12**:616–623.)

337A: Restenosis after balloon dilatation. Cross sections at the dilatation site. Because of the balloon angioplasty both the total vessel cross sectional area and the lumen area are increased. Several follow-up scenarios are now possible. **Upper course:** The total vessel area can increase (positive remodeling). Even with moderate neointimal formation no restenosis will develop. **Middle course:** No remodeling, total vessel area is unchanged and restenosis will be dependent on the amount of neointima formation. **Lower course:** Negative remodeling, total vessel area decreases and restenosis occurs almost independently of the amount of neointima formation. **B**: Restenosis after stent implantation. After stent implantation both total vessel area and lumen area are further increased. Because recoil and remodeling are effectively prevented by the radial forces exerted on the vessel wall, the occurrence of restenosis is solely dependent on the amount of neointima formation. PTCA: percutaneous transluminal coronary angioplasty.

PREDICTORS OF RESTENOSIS

In animal models, a good correlation exists between the amount of injury inflicted on the vessel wall as assessed histologically, and the subsequent amount of neointima formation. Unfortunately there is currently no imaging technique that can accurately visualize *in vivo* the severity of vascular damage after balloon angioplasty or stenting.

Several patient-related, procedural-related, and lesion-related variables predictive of restenosis have been identified. The most important patient-related predictor is diabetes; both insulin-dependent and noninsulin-dependent diabetics are known to have a higher restenosis risk. Patients with a skin allergy to the stainless steel components nickel or molybdenum are also more prone to restenosis after stent implantation, probably because most stents are made of stainless steel. Lesion-related variables include totally occluded arteries, lesions in vein grafts, ostial lesions, long lesions, lesions in small vessels, or lesions at a coronary bifurcation.

Procedural variables are stent implantation (less restenosis), number of stents implanted, length of stented segment, and type of stent implanted; certain coil type stents, stents with thicker struts, and gold coated stents elicit a stronger neointimal response and are therefore attended with a higher restenosis rate. Finally, a high percent diameter stenosis or low minimal lumen cross sectional area postprocedure are also powerful predictors of restenosis after balloon angioplasty and stenting. Using quantitative angiographic and quantitative IVUS measurements of vessel size, percent diameter stenosis postprocedure, stent length, and postprocedural minimal lumen cross sectional area, de Feyter and Serruys were able to construct reliable reference charts from which the expected restenosis rate after stent implantation can be read[7,8] (*Table 51, Table 52*).

Mehran and coworkers[9] recognized four patterns of in-stent restenosis with different long-term outcomes after repeat PCI: type I: focal (<10 mm long); type II: diffuse (>10 mm in stent); type III: proliferative (>10 mm, extending outside stent margins); type IV: occlusive restenosis (**339**). Target lesion revascularization 6 months after successful repeat PCI was 19% in type I in-stent restenosis, 35% for type II, 50% for type III, and 83% for type IV.

PREVENTION OF RESTENOSIS

In the balloon angioplasty era, a myriad drugs with potential to reduce restenosis have been tested in clinical trials, but almost all failed. Most of these drugs were aimed at inhibiting neointima formation, which is now known to account for only 20–30% of late lumen loss after balloon angioplasty. Probucol is the only drug

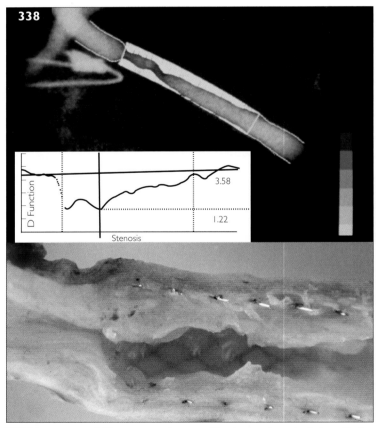

338 Upper panel: Coronary angiogram of in-stent restenosis. Automatically detected vessel edges and quantitative measurements have been superimposed on the angiographic image. The minimal lumen diameter is 1.22 mm, the reference vessel size is 3.58 mm. **Lower panel**: Gross anatomic specimen of the same vessel segment. The longitudinally cut artery clearly shows the stent and the in-stent neointimal tissue. The neointima extends proximally into the nonstented part of the vessel wall.

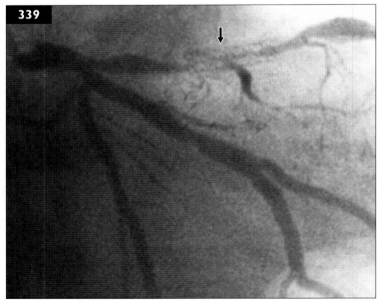

339 Example of a Type III in-stent restenosis 4 months after stent implantation in the proximal left anterior descending artery. The contours of the metallic stent can clearly be seen (arrow). The restenotic process extends proximally and distally from the stent.

Table 51 Restenosis rates calculated from in-stent area and stent length

Stent Length mm	Minimum in-stent area, mm²									
	3.0–3.9	3.9–4.8	4.8–5.7	5.7–6.6	6.6–7.5	7.5–8.4	8.4–9.3	9.3–10.2	10.2–11.1	11.1–12.0
10–15	0.30 (0.22–0.40)	0.25 (0.19–0.32)	0.21 (0.16–0.26)	0.17 (0.13–0.21)	0.13 (0.11–0.17)	0.11 (0.08–0.14)	0.08 (0.06–0.12)	0.07 (0.04–0.10)	0.05 (0.03–0.09)	0.04 (0.02–0.08)
15–20	0.33 (0.25–0.42)	0.28 (0.22–0.34)	0.23 (0.19–0.28)	0.19 (0.16–0.22)	0.15 (0.12–0.18)	0.12 (0.09–0.16)	0.10 (0.07–0.13)	0.08 (0.05–0.12)	0.06 (0.04–0.10)	0.05 (0.02–0.09)
20–25	0.36 (0.28–0.46)	0.31 (0.25–0.37)	0.25 (0.21–0.30)	0.21 (0.18–0.24)	0.17 (0.14–0.20)	0.14 (0.11–0.17)	0.11 (0.09–0.15)	0.09 (0.06–0.13)	0.07 (0.04–0.11)	0.05* (0.03–0.10)
25–30	0.40 (0.31–0.49)	0.34 (0.27–0.41)	0.28 (0.24–0.33)	0.23 (0.20–0.27)	0.19 (0.16–0.23)	0.15 (0.12–0.20)	0.12 (0.09–0.17)	0.10 (0.06–0.15)	0.08 (0.05–0.13)	0.06 (0.03–0.11)
30–35	0.43 (0.34–0.53)	0.37 (0.30–0.44)	0.31 (0.26–0.38)	0.26 (0.22–0.31)	0.21 (0.17–0.26)	0.17 (0.13–0.22)	0.14 (0.10–0.19)	0.11 (0.07–0.17)	0.09* (0.05–0.15)	0.07* (0.04–0.13)
35–40	0.46 (0.36–0.57)	0.40 (0.32–0.49)	0.34 (0.28–0.41)	0.29 (0.23–0.35)	0.24 (0.19–0.29)	0.19 (0.14–0.25)	0.16 (0.11–0.22)	0.13 (0.08–0.19)	0.10* (0.06–0.17)	0.08* (0.04–0.15)
40–45	0.50 (0.39–0.61)	0.43* (0.34–0.53)	0.37 (0.29–0.46)	0.31 (0.25–0.39)	0.26 (0.20–0.34)	0.22* (0.15–0.29)	0.18 (0.12–0.25)	0.14* (0.09–0.22)	0.11 (0.06–0.19)	0.09* (0.05–0.17)
45–50	0.53* (0.41–0.65)	0.48 (0.36–0.58)	0.40 (0.31–0.50)	0.34 (0.26–0.44)	0.29 (0.21–0.38)	0.24 (0.17–0.33)	0.20 (0.13–0.29)	0.16* (0.09–0.25)	0.13 (0.07–0.22)	0.10* (0.05–0.19)
50–55	0.57* (0.43–0.69)	0.50 (0.38–0.62)	0.44 (0.33–0.55)	0.38 (0.28–0.49)	0.32* (0.22–0.49)	0.27* (0.18–0.38)	0.22* (0.14–0.33)	0.18* (0.10–0.29)	0.14* (0.08–0.26)	0.11* (0.05–0.22)
55–60	0.60* (0.45–0.73)	0.54* (0.40–0.67)	0.47* (0.34–0.60)	0.41* (0.29–0.54)	0.35 (0.24–0.48)	0.29* (0.19–0.42)	0.24 (0.15–0.38)	0.20* (0.10–0.29)	0.16* (0.08–0.29)	0.13* (0.06–0.26)

From IVUS-determined post–stent-implantation minimum in-stent area and stent length, one can extrapolate the expected 6-month QCA restenosis rate. The range of the 2 variables is divided into 10 groups each. The expected restenosis rate for the median of each range was calculated along with the 95% CI for this particular value (indicated in parentheses).
*There were no actual observations in this range; figures presented are calculated by extrapolation from the model.
Adapted from de Feyter et al. ([1999][7].)

Table 52 Restenosis rates calculated from stenosis diameter and vessel size

Vessel Size mm	Percent diameter stenosis after procedure									
	1.5–5.9	5.9–10.3	10.3–14.7	14.7–19.1	19.1–23.5	23.5–27.9	27.9–32.3	32.3–36.7	36.7–41.1	41.1–45.5
1.83–2.14	0.24* 0.15–0.36	0.28 0.19–0.40	0.33 0.23–0.45	0.38 0.28–0.50	0.44 0.32–0.56	0.49 0.37–0.62	0.55 0.41–0.69	0.61 0.44–0.75	0.66* 0.48–0.80	0.71* 0.51–0.85
2.14–2.45	0.17 0.11–0.26	0.21 0.14–0.28	0.25 0.18–0.32	0.29 0.22–0.37	0.34 0.26–0.42	0.39 0.30–0.49	0.45 0.34–0.57	0.50 0.37–0.64	0.56 0.40–0.71	0.62* 0.43–0.78
2.45–2.76	0.12 0.08–0.18	0.15 0.11–0.20	0.18 0.14–0.22	0.21 0.17–0.26	0.25 0.21–0.30	0.30 0.24–0.37	0.35 0.27–0.44	0.40 0.29–0.52	0.46 0.32–0.61	0.51* 0.35–0.68
2.76–3.07	0.08 0.05–0.12	0.10 0.07–0.14	0.12 0.10–0.16	0.15 0.13–0.18	0.18 0.15–0.22	0.22 0.18–0.27	0.26 0.20–0.33	0.31 0.22–0.41	0.36 0.24–0.49	0.41 0.26–0.58
3.07–3.38	0.06 0.03–0.09	0.07 0.05–0.10	0.09 0.06–0.11	0.11 0.08–0.13	0.13 0.10–0.16	0.16 0.12–0.20	0.19 0.14–0.25	0.23 0.15–0.32	0.27 0.17–0.39	0.32 0.19–0.48
3.38–3.69	0.04 0.02–0.07	0.05 0.03–0.07	0.06 0.04–0.09	0.07 0.05–0.10	0.09 0.06–0.12	0.11 0.08–0.15	0.13 0.09–0.19	0.16 0.10–0.25	0.20 0.12–0.31	0.23 0.13–0.38
3.69–4.00	0.03 0.01–0.05	0.03 0.02–0.06	0.04 0.02–0.07	0.05 0.03–0.08	0.06 0.04–0.10	0.07 0.05–0.12	0.09 0.05–0.15	0.11 0.06–0.19	0.14 0.07–0.24	0.17 0.08–0.30
4.00–4.31	0.02* 0.01–0.04	0.02 0.01–0.04	0.03 0.01–0.05	0.03 0.02–0.06	0.04 0.02–0.08	0.05 0.03–0.09	0.06 0.03–0.12	0.08 0.04–0.15	0.10* 0.05–0.19	0.12* 0.05–0.24
4.31–4.62	0.01* 0.00–0.03	0.01* 0.01–0.03	0.02* 0.01–0.04	0.02* 0.01–0.05	0.03 0.01–0.06	0.03 0.02–0.07	0.04 0.02–0.09	0.05* 0.02–0.12	0.07* 0.03–0.15	0.08* 0.03–019
4.62–4.93	0.01* 0.00–0.02	0.01* 0.00–0.03	0.01* 0.00–0.03	0.01* 0.01–0.04	0.02 0.01–0.05	0.02* 0.01–0.06	0.03* 0.01–0.07	0.04* 0.01–0.09	0.04* 0.02–0.11	0.05* 0.20–0.15

The cells marked with numbers in italics and an asterisk indicate the range without actual observations in the data set. Cells with bold numbers indicate the range with actual observations.
Adapted from de Serruys et al. ([1999][8].)

that was effective in balloon angioplasty trials. It had a positive remodeling effect on the vessel wall without a reduction in neointimal hyperplasia, the result of which was a lesser restenosis rate. Because of side-effects it is, however, not approved in the USA. In a mixed population of balloon angioplasty and stent implantation patients, homocysteine reduction therapy with folic acid, pyridoxine and vitamin B12 reduced 6-month restenosis rates. The effect was more pronounced in the balloon angioplasty group than in the stented group.

Pharmacologic restenosis prevention trials after stent implantation have so far been disappointing. No systemically administered drug has shown efficacy. Local drug delivery at the stent implantation site is more promising. With this technique higher dosages can be delivered to the target site while avoiding systemic side-effects. In a small study enoxaparin, locally delivered through a micro porous balloon, indeed reduced restenosis after stenting.

The breakthrough in restenosis prevention now seems to be drug-eluting stents. Here a special drug-containing coating is applied to the metallic struts of the stent. Depending on the physico-chemical characteristics of the coating, the drug elutes in a predicable manner from the stent and can act specifically on the underlying vessel wall. Using the stent as a delivery vehicle has the further advantage of drug administration during a longer time period, which allows a more effective inhibition of smooth muscle cell migration and proliferation. Two drug-eluting stents are currently available for routine use. Both use a polymer coating for elution of either sirolimus (Rapamycin) or paclitaxel.

Sirolimus inhibits cell division between the G1 and S phases and effectively inhibits smooth muscle cell proliferation. Recently published trial results are spectacular[10,11]. The RAVEL study[10] showed absence of angiographic restenosis at 6 months and a 1-year survival free of MI or revascularization of 94% (**340**). The SIRIUS trial[11] included patients at higher risk of restenosis but nevertheless showed a 6-month angiographic restenosis rate of only 8.9% and a 270-day event free survival of 91.5% in the sirolimus stent group.

The drug paclitaxel inhibits cellular division, motility, and signal transduction and therefore also effectively inhibits smooth muscle cell proliferation. The large randomized TAXUS IV trial[12] showed similar results to the SIRIUS trial, a 6-month angiographic restenosis rate of 7.9% and a 9-month event free survival of 92.4% in the paclitaxel eluting stent group. However, the long-term influence of sirolimus, paclitaxel, and the polymer on the vessel wall is unknown and concerns have been raised that these stents will only delay and not prevent neointimal proliferation.

MANAGEMENT OF RESTENOSIS

Treatment of restenosis after balloon angioplasty is relatively straightforward. Stent implantation reduces the repeat restenosis rate by 50% and is the method of choice. Repeat restenosis rate is in the order of 20% after stenting versus 40% after reballoon angioplasty. Treatment of in-stent restenosis on the other hand is a far more vexing problem. Repeat balloon angioplasty is

associated with repeat restenosis rates of 20–85%, depending on the type of restenosis used. Additional stenting, rotational atherectomy, directional atherectomy, and laser angioplasty have all been tried but with long-term results similar to balloon angioplasty. Acute lumen enlargement is therefore not enough and additional measures have to be taken to inhibit neointima formation. Currently the only proven therapy for the inhibition of repeat in-stent neointima formation is intracoronary radiation therapy with β and γ sources. Several studies have shown that repeat in-stent restenosis is reduced from 60% to 30% after intracoronary brachytherapy. Concerns with radiation therapy are delayed re-endothelialization with late thrombotic problems, and the possibility that radiation therapy merely delays and does not prevent restenosis. Furthermore, the long-term influence and risk of radiation therapy on cardiac and extracardiac tissues remain unclear. Whether additional stenting with a drug-eluting stent can prevent repeat restenosis is currently being investigated. Preliminary results with a sirolimus-eluting stent are promising.

CONCLUSION

Late vascular narrowing or restenosis is still the major shortcoming of every PCI technique. Following balloon angioplasty it is primarily caused by negative remodeling or shrinkage of the vessel, and to a lesser extent by neointima formation. Stenting prevents negative remodeling and in-stent restenosis is thus entirely caused by intimal hyperplasia. Restenosis rates are lower after stenting; however, in-stent restenosis is traditionally very difficult to treat. The final step in the development of an effective preventive therapy for restenosis seems to be implantation of a stent loaded with a drug that locally inhibits the neointimal hyperplastic response.

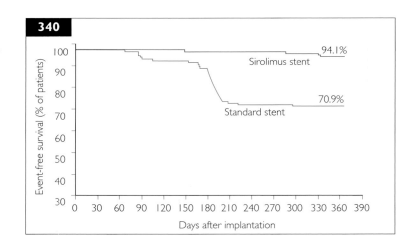

340 Kaplan–Meier curve for survival free of myocardial infarction and repeat revascularization. Event-free survival was significantly better in the sirolimus stent group (*P*<0.001 log rank test). (Adapted with permission from Morice *et al.* [2002]. A randomized comparison of a sirolimus-eluting stent with a standard stent for coronary revascularization. *N. Engl. J. Med.* **346**:1778–1780. Copyright 2002 Massachusetts Medical Society. All rights reserved.)

Chapter Eighteen

Coronary Artery Bypass Graft Surgery

PROCEDURES AND INDICATIONS

MATTHEW J. PRICE, MD

INTRODUCTION

The purpose of coronary artery bypass grafting (CABG) is to supply blood to the distal coronary circulation beyond significant coronary stenoses, using venous or arterial conduits. Favaloro and colleagues popularized CABG using aorto-coronary saphenous vein conduits in the late 1960s, and since then CABG has become one of the most common surgical procedures. Four major forces have influenced the development of CABG surgery: (1) the introduction of cardiopulmonary bypass; (2) the use of arterial conduits; (3) off-pump coronary artery bypass (OP-CAB); and (4) improvements in percutaneous cardiovascular intervention.

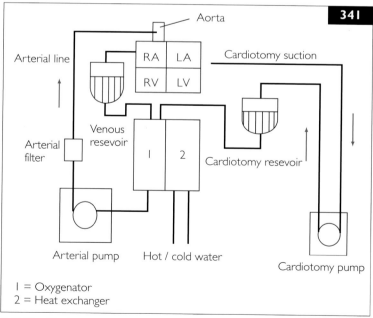

341 Simplified schematic diagram of the cardiopulmonary bypass machine. LA: left atrium; LV: left ventricle; RA: right atrium; RV: right ventricle.

PROCEDURES

Cardiopulmonary bypass

Gibbons first introduced the cardiopulmonary bypass (CPB) machine in 1953 (**341**). The central function of the CPB machine is oxygenation and circulation of blood independent of the heart and lungs. A secondary function is cooling and warming of the blood to regulate the patient's body temperature. In the standard technique, a circuit is created between the venous and arterial systems by cannulating the right atrium (or the vena cava) and the ascending aorta. Deoxygenated blood is removed from the venous system and passed through a chamber within which the red blood cells, exposed to oxygen, undergo gas exchange. The blood is propelled through the circuit and into the arterial system by a pumping device and passed through a heat exchanger to be cooled. Blood that is removed by suction catheters from within the operating field can also be filtered and introduced into this circuit to be returned to the patient's circulation. Heparin is used to prevent thrombus formation within the CPB tubing. Once the patient is cooled, the proximal aorta can then be cross-clamped to stop blood flow through the heart. Myocardial preservation is accomplished through general hypothermia, the administration of cardioplegia solution which contains a high potassium concentration to stop the electrical activity of the heart, and often through direct application of ice slush to the heart's surface.

Venous and arterial conduits

Saphenous veins are the most commonly used conduits. They are usually harvested from the lower extremities, either through open incisions or endoscopically, and anastomosed to the proximal aorta and to the coronary circulation. Grafts may supply a single coronary artery or may feed multiple arteries through 'jump' grafts that take advantage of side-to-side anastomoses. Since venous grafts suffer a high rate of late closure (see below), arterial conduits are used whenever possible. The left internal mammary artery (LIMA) is the most commonly used arterial conduit. The LIMA is dissected from behind the left anterior chest wall and anastomosed to the distal left anterior descending artery (LAD) or diagonal artery. The right internal mammary artery, radial artery, right gastroepiploic artery, and inferior epigastric artery may also be used as conduits. Given the high long-term patency rate and demonstrated survival benefit of the LIMA in comparison to venous grafts, a LIMA should be used to bypass the LAD whenever possible, and venous grafts or radial arteries used to supply the left circumflex artery (LCx) and right coronary artery (RCA) (**342**).

Contraindications to the use of a LIMA include significant subclavian stenosis, significant LIMA atherosclerosis (which is very uncommon), mediastinal fibrosis, or technical difficulties. Bilateral IMA grafting is relatively contraindicated in diabetics due to marked reduction of blood flow to the sternum and the risk of wound infection. Although the LIMA is relatively immune to atherosclerosis, it is not uncommon for the radial artery to have significant atherosclerosis, which prevents its use.

Off-pump coronary artery bypass
Recent technical advances in operative techniques have enabled surgeons to perform coronary anastomoses successfully on the beating heart, thus eliminating the need for cardiac arrest and CPB. Given the numerous complications of CPB (see below), there is great potential for OP-CAB to decrease significantly the morbidity associated with CABG. OP-CAB has been associated with decreased bleeding complications, fewer blood transfusions, shorter ventilatory support times, decreased systemic inflammatory response, shorter hospital length of stay, and possibly decreased neurological, renal, and pulmonary complications. However, OP-CAB is technically demanding and some vessels may not be accessible without CPB. The benefits of OP-CAB in comparison to CABG with CPB need to be confirmed by large, randomized, controlled clinical trials.

INDICATIONS FOR CORONARY ARTERY BYPASS GRAFT
Most patients undergo CABG surgery for symptoms of chronic angina. The presumed benefits of CABG in comparison to medical therapy or percutaneous revascularization are largely based on clinical trials that have limited application in the current era of cardiovascular management. Patients in these trials did not receive statins, and angiotensin-converting enzyme (ACE) inhibitors and

beta blockers were not routinely used. The trials were performed prior to significant technical advances in percutaneous intervention, such as intracoronary stents. Most studies comparing percutaneous transluminal coronary angioplasty (PTCA) with CABG have potential selection bias, short follow-up, and limited statistical power to determine mortality differences. With these caveats, mortality benefits were seen for CABG compared to medical therapy for left main disease (>50%) or left main-equivalent disease (proximal LAD and circumflex disease), three-vessel disease (especially with left ventricular dysfunction), and severe proximal LAD disease (especially with left ventricular dysfunction). Diabetics may have improved survival with CABG compared to PTCA.

The major difference in outcome between CABG and PTCA groups is the increased need for repeat revascularization in the PTCA group because of the high rates of restenosis. The decision whether to pursue percutaneous or surgical revascularization will become even more complicated with the advent of drug-eluting stents that limit in-stent restenosis, and as technology continues to improve allowing the interventional cardiologist to approach successfully even the highest-risk lesions relatively safely. Hybrid techniques which involve percutaneous intervention of the LCx and/or RCA in combination with minimally-invasive or endoscopic LIMA-to-LAD bypass grafting, may represent an alternative approach in the future. With this background, the generally accepted indications for CABG in patients with stable, chronic angina are:

- Left main artery stenosis >50%, or >70% stenoses in both the proximal LAD (before the first septal) and LCx arteries.
- Three-vessel disease, especially in diabetics and patients with left ventricular dysfunction.
- Two-vessel disease that includes a severe proximal LAD stenosis (before the first septal).
- One- or two-vessel disease without significant LAD disease, but with high-risk features on stress testing or a large amount of jeopardized myocardium.

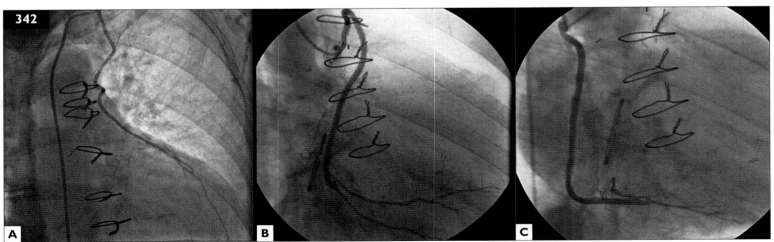

342 A: Left internal mammary (LIMA) arteriography demonstrating LIMA grafted to the left anterior descending artery. **B**: Angiogram of a saphenous vein graft to the distal left circumflex artery. **C**: Angiogram of a saphenous vein graft to the posterior descending artery arising from the right coronary artery.

COMPLICATIONS AND OUTCOMES

MATTHEW J. PRICE, MD AND STEVEN S. KHAN, MD

INTRODUCTION
Indications for CABG and the associated procedures are described in the previous section.

COMPLICATIONS OF CORONARY ARTERY BYPASS GRAFT

Sequelae of cardiopulmonary bypass
The use of CPB triggers a systemic inflammatory response manifested by the development of platelet dysfunction, accelerated fibrinolysis, a consumptive coagulopathy, and elevation of a variety of inflammatory mediators. As a result, the postoperative course may be complicated by bleeding and capillary leak. Transfusion with packed red blood cells, platelets, and coagulation factors may be needed, as well as the administration of desmopressin (ddAVP) to enhance platelet function and protamine to reverse the effects of heparin. Cannulation and cross-clamping of the aorta during initiation of CPB may dislodge atheroma or particulate matter, leading to atheroemboli of the central nervous system and kidneys. Proximal aortic atherosclerosis, previous stroke, and older age are predictors of major stroke perioperatively. CPB is also associated with subtle, nonfocal neurological abnormalities, identified by extensive neuropsychological testing. Intraoperative hypotension or loss of pulsatile flow during CPB can lead to neurological, renal, and splanchnic impairment. Patients with significant preoperative renal dysfunction (creatinine >2.5 mg/dl [221 μmol/l]) are at increased risk of requiring postoperative hemodialysis.

Postoperative atrial fibrillation
New onset of atrial fibrillation (AF) occurs in approximately 30% of patients undergoing CABG, and occurs more frequently in patients undergoing concomitant valve repair or replacement. The highest incidence is on postoperative days 2 and 3. Predictors of postoperative AF include older age, male gender, chronic obstructive pulmonary disease or other respiratory compromise, hypertension, previous AF, longer aortic cross-clamp times, and hypokalemia. Patients with postoperative AF have a two- to threefold increased risk of stroke as well as increased hospital stay and greater hospital costs. Moreover, these patients have a significantly higher 30-day and 6-month mortality rate, possibly because they represent a more critically ill set of patients. Prophylactic treatment with beta blockers, amiodarone, sotalol, and possibly biatrial pacing significantly reduces the incidence of postoperative AF.

Early and late graft closure
Bypass graft attrition is a major cause of morbidity after CABG. Early occlusion within the first month after surgery is predominantly secondary to thrombosis, and occurs in 3–12% of saphenous vein grafts (**343**). Thrombosis is caused by a combination of endothelial disruption, technical factors that reduce graft flow (such as anastomotic stricture or significant distal vessel disease), and the systemic prothrombotic state that follows bypass surgery. During the first postoperative year, 15% of venous grafts occlude, and by 10 years, 40% are no longer patent. As a result, additional revascularization is required in approximately one-third of patients within 12 years of saphenous vein graft (SVG). This attrition in venous graft patency is secondary to intimal hyperplasia that develops over the first year followed by the development of progressive atherosclerosis, leading to significant luminal obstruction. Venous graft atherosclerosis is more diffuse, concentric, less calcified, and more rapidly progressive compared with native vessel atherosclerosis. With advanced plaque formation, late thrombotic occlusion of venous grafts frequently occurs.

Hypercholesterolemia, smoking, diabetes mellitus, and the age of the graft are predisposing factors for venous graft disease. Aspirin (begun 6 hours after surgery), smoking cessation, and statin therapy are important preventive therapies.

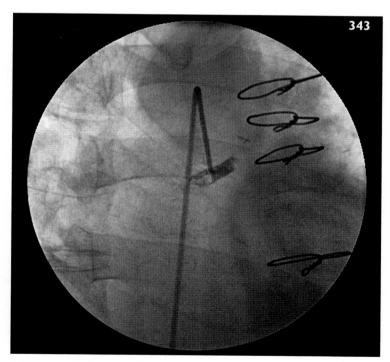

343 Early graft closure. A 63-year-old male presented with left arm pain, congestive heart failure, and elevated cardiac enzymes 10 days after four-vessel coronary artery bypass graft. Cardiac catheterization revealed thrombotic occlusion of the saphenous vein graft to the ramus intermedius. Due to the heavy thrombus burden, percutaneous intervention was unsuccessful.

In contrast to venous grafts, arterial conduits have a much higher long-term patency rate. The 10-year patency rate of internal mammary conduits is 90%, compared with 60% for saphenous vein conduits. LIMA graft failure is commonly due to technical errors and/or stenosis at the anastomotic site, significant native disease distal to the graft insertion or, rarely, unligated intercostal branches (**344**). Internal mammary artery grafts are relatively resistant to the development of atherosclerosis.

OUTCOMES AFTER CORONARY ARTERY BYPASS GRAFT

Approximate survival rates after CABG are 90–95% at 5 years, 80–90% at 10 years, and 65–75% at 15 years. Major predictors of increased in-hospital mortality after CABG include urgent (rather than elective) operation, older age, previous heart surgery, increased number of major coronary arteries with significant obstruction, female sex, and left ventricular dysfunction. Of these, nonelective surgery, older age, and repeat CABG surgery are associated with the greatest increase in early risk. Major predictors of long-term outcome include advanced age, diabetes mellitus, female gender, left ventricular dysfunction, and the number of diseased coronary vessels. Angina is the most common cardiac event in follow-up, and is most commonly due to SVG occlusion. Internal mammary artery graft use is associated with lower rates of recurrent angina and improved survival. As with all patients with cardiovascular disease, optimum medical therapy with aspirin, beta blockers, ACE inhibitors, and statins combined with smoking cessation, diet, and exercise are crucial in preventing cardiac events.

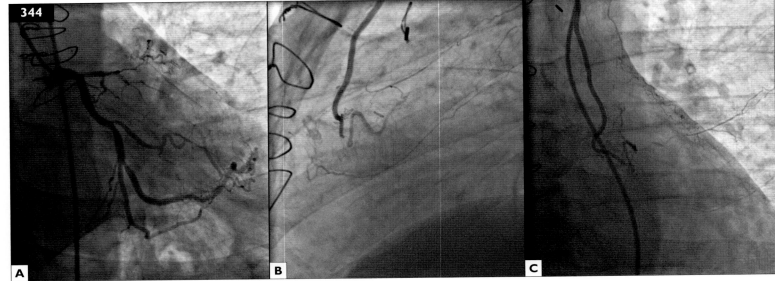

344 Left internal mammary artery (LIMA) graft failure. A 74-year-old male presented with recurrent angina 4 months after three-vessel coronary artery bypass graft (CABG), which included a LIMA conduit to the left anterior descending artery (LAD). Stress myocardial perfusion imaging revealed a large reversible defect in the anterior, septal, and apical distribution. Cardiac catheterization was performed. Left coronary angiography in the RAO projection (**A**) reveals a proximally occluded LAD. No competitive flow was seen distally. Selective LIMA arteriography in the lateral (**B**) and AP (**C**) projections reveals compromise of the LIMA graft due to critical narrowing at the anastomotic site with the LAD. LIMA graft compromise early after CABG is primarily due to technical failure. AP: anteroposterior; RAO: right anterior oblique.

Chapter Nineteen

Ischemic Heart Disease: Special Problems

WOMEN AND HORMONES

STEVE LEE, MD AND STEVEN KHAN, MD

INTRODUCTION

Heart disease is the number one cause of death in American women and a significant cause of morbidity. In 1999 in the USA alone, over 260,000 women died from heart attacks and other coronary events, whereas over 41,000 women died from breast cancer and 63,000 died from lung cancer. As with men, the incidence of coronary heart disease (CHD) in women rises with age, though women typically develop symptoms of heart disease around 10–15 years later than men. Men typically experience their first heart attack around age 50 years, while women are usually aged 60–70 years. In addition, heart disease is unusual in premenopausal women, and women who have had their ovaries surgically removed are more likely to have a heart attack and to suffer a heart attack at an earlier age. These observations suggest that hormones may play a role in the delayed development of heart disease in women, and that hormones may potentially have a protective effect.

HORMONE REPLACEMENT THERAPY

Traditionally, hormone replacement therapy (HRT) in post-menopausal women with an intact uterus consisted of estrogen and progestin replacement. Estrogen is produced predominantly from a woman's ovaries, and its levels decline during menopause. Estrogen is felt to have a number of potentially beneficial cardiovascular effects, including modulation of vasomotor tone, reductions in low-density lipoprotein (LDL) and high-density lipoprotein (HDL) cholesterol, and helping to prevent weight gain. Because the use of estrogen alone increases the risk of uterine (endometrial) cancer, progestin is usually added to reduce this risk in women who have an intact uterus.

HRT is commonly used to alleviate the symptoms of menopause such as hot flashes, night sweats, mood swings, and vaginal dryness, along with slowing the progression of osteoporosis. However, the use of HRT in the prevention of heart disease has been a much more controversial topic. While it has long been accepted that HRT can have adverse effects such as an increased incidence of thromboembolism and gallbladder disease, there were no randomized prospective trials investigating the cardiovascular benefits of HRT until recently. Previous population studies have

suggested that HRT may indeed reduce the incidence of cardiac events. However, the recent results of the Heart and Estrogen–progestin Replacement Study (HERS), HERS II, and Women's Health Initiative have provided compelling evidence against the use of HRT for the purpose of cardiac protection.

HERS, HERS II, AND WOMEN'S HEALTH INITIATIVE

HERS was the first large-scale, randomized trial to study the effects of HRT in postmenopausal women with known coronary artery disease (CAD). A total of 2,763 postmenopausal women with a history of previous heart attack, angioplasty, bypass surgery, or >50% occlusion of a major coronary artery, were randomly assigned to either placebo or HRT with estrogen and progestin. The primary end-points of the trial were nonfatal heart attack and cardiac death, and patients were monitored for over 4 years. The results showed that during the first year of treatment, there was an increase in cardiac events in the patients on HRT (**345**), primarily due to an

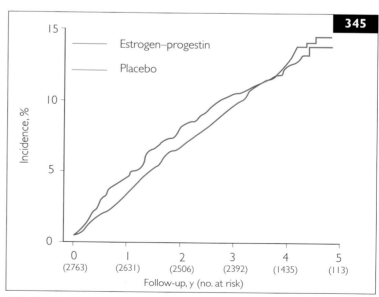

345 Graph of primary endpoint from the Heart and Estrogen–progestin Replacement Study (HERS): nonfatal myocardial infarction (MI) and coronary heart disease (CHD) death. y: years. (Modified from Hulley et al. [1998]. Randomized trial of estrogen plus progestin for secondary prevention of coronary heart disease in postmenopausal women. Heart and Estrogen/progestin Replacement Study (HERS) Research Group. *JAMA* **280**:605–613.)

increase in nonfatal myocardial infarction (MI) in the first year (**346**). However, at the end of the study at 4–5 years, there appeared to be fewer nonfatal heart attacks in women on HRT. Overall, the HRT and placebo groups showed no significant differences for any cardiovascular endpoints. The conclusion from HERS was that there was no evidence to support starting HRT in postmenopausal women with known coronary disease. However, if women with coronary disease had already been on HRT for more than 1 year, it could be continued due to its possible late protective effects.

There were several criticisms of HERS, including the need for longer-term follow-up and the selection of only women with previous cardiac disease as study patients. HERS II addressed the former criticism by providing an additional 3 years of follow-up on 2,321 of the original HERS patients. In this follow-up study, the patients were informed whether they were receiving placebo or HRT, and were encouraged to continue the same treatment. The additional years of follow-up from HERS II showed that there was in reality no late benefit from HRT in reducing the risk of nonfatal MI or overall cardiac events (**347**). However, as in the original HERS, there was an increase in the incidence of thromboembolic events and gallbladder disease. The overall conclusion from HERS and HERS II was that HRT should not be used in postmenopausal women with known coronary disease for the purpose of decreasing the risk of a cardiac event.

The reported results from the Women's Health Initiative have extended these findings to women without any previous cardiac history (i.e. for primary prevention). The Women's Health Initiative was a randomized, controlled trial which involved 16,608 women aged 50–79 years with an intact uterus and no previous heart disease or symptoms of heart disease. The women were randomized to either placebo or HRT with estrogen and progestin. Although originally intended to run 8.5 years, the trial was halted after 5.2 years because of an increased risk of invasive breast cancer in the patients assigned to HRT. In addition, it was found that there was a significantly higher incidence of cardiac events (both nonfatal heart attacks and cardiac deaths) and of strokes in the patients randomized to HRT. Based on these results, women without a previous cardiac history should not be advised to start HRT for a potential cardiovascular benefit.

SUMMARY

The results of the HERS, HERS II, and the Women's Health Initiative trials therefore do not support the use of HRT in women for either primary or secondary prevention of cardiac events. While it remains true that women generally experience heart disease later in life than men, it does not appear that the administration of combined estrogen and progestin protects against cardiovascular disease. Further research is needed to investigate the reasons why women seem to be protected in the premenopausal years, and whether estrogen treatment without progestin or selective estrogen receptor modulators have a role in the primary or secondary prevention of heart disease.

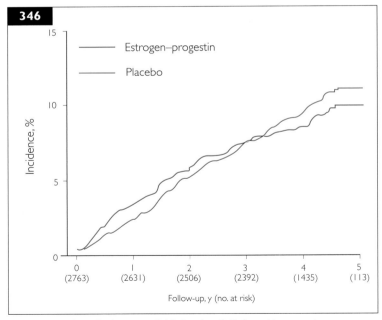

346 Graph of nonfatal myocardial infarction (MI) from Heart and Estrogen/progestin Replacement Study (HERS). y: years. (Modified from Hulley *et al.* [1998]. Randomized trial of estrogen plus progestin for secondary prevention of coronary heart disease in postmenopausal women. Heart and Estrogen/progestin Replacement Study (HERS) Research Group. *JAMA* **280**:605–613.)

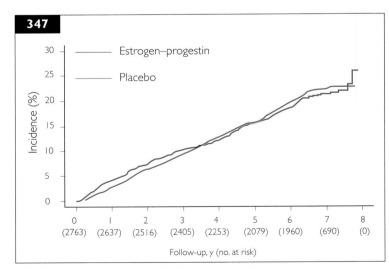

347 Coronary heart disease (CHD) events from Heart and Estrogen/progestin Replacement Study II (HERS II). y: years. (Modified from Grady *et al.* [2002]. Cardiovascular disease outcomes during 6.8 years of hormone therapy: Heart and Estrogen/progestin Replacement Study follow-up (HERS II). *JAMA* **288**:49–57.)

DIABETIC ATHEROGENIC DYSLIPIDEMIAS

ALLAN D. SNIDERMAN, MD, FRCP(C)

INTRODUCTION

Diabetes is not just dysglycemia. Diabetes, particularly type 2 diabetes, is also dyslipidemia. This extension from glucose to lipids, which is, arguably, the most important change in our understanding of diabetes since the discovery of insulin, is the consequence of three major clinical observations. First, whereas the incidence of microvascular disease is very much the same in different ethnic groups across the world, the incidence of macrovascular disease differs substantially amongst them. This suggests that some other factor, such as the differences in lipids which are present amongst these groups, might be responsible for the differences in the frequency of macrovascular disease that are observed. Second, the United Kingdom Diabetes Prevention Study documented that better control of blood sugar did reduce the frequency of microvascular disease but did not significantly affect the frequency of macrovascular disease. Third, statin therapy substantially reduces major coronary event rates in patients with type 2 diabetes. This beneficial effect was observed in smaller diabetic subgroups in a number of the major statin clinical trials, and has now been definitively demonstrated in the Heart Protection Study and the CARDS Study.

DYSLIPIDEMIA IN DIABETES

Given these findings, there can be no doubt that dyslipidemia matters in type 2 diabetes and, given that LDL lowering is the principal beneficial effect of statin therapy, that LDL matters in diabetes. Appreciation of the lipid abnormalities in diabetes has changed with time. Classically, LDL has not mattered in diabetes. The characteristic triad of abnormalities was elevated triglycerides (Tg), normal LDL cholesterol (LDL C), and low HDL C. By this formulation, very low-density lipoproteins (VLDLs) and HDLs are abnormal, whereas LDL is not. However, some time ago it was established that LDL particles differ in composition, some being larger because they contain more cholesterol ester in their core, others being smaller because they contain less. Each LDL particle contains one molecule of a large protein, apoB100 (apoB), which encapsulates the particle and one region of which binds to the LDL receptor in the liver to allow the LDL particle to be removed from the plasma. Because lipids are less dense than proteins, smaller LDL particles contain relatively less lipid and more protein and are, therefore, denser than larger LDL particles.

There is now overwhelming evidence from *in vitro* and *in vivo* pathophysiologic studies and from cross-sectional and prospective epidemiologic studies that smaller, denser cholesterol-depleted LDL particles are more atherogenic than larger, more buoyant, cholesterol-replete LDL particles. In diabetes, given the frequency of hypertriglyceridemia, small dense LDLs are common and this feature is now generally included in the definition, although LDL

size cannot be measured clinically. Even worse, it is still not widely appreciated that not only is LDL composition altered in patients with type 2 diabetes, but LDL particle number is frequently increased as well, the combination resulting in hyperTg hyperapoB, one of the commonest, most atherogenic dyslipoproteinemias. The objective in this brief chapter is to illustrate hyperTg hyperapoB in terms of particle number and composition and to distinguish it from normal and simple hypertriglyceridemia (hyperTg normoapoB).

NORMAL

The relative number and composition of VLDL and LDL particles in a normal individual are illustrated in **348**. VLDLs are the triglyceride-enriched particles secreted by the liver, which, after hydrolysis of their triglyceride at the endothelial surfaces of adipose tissue and muscle, are transformed into cholesterol-enriched LDL particles. Note there are nine times more LDL particles than VLDL particles. This relation follows from the difference in their half-lives, with each LDL particle, on average, persisting in the circulation nine times longer than each VLDL particle. Note also that VLDL particles are substantially larger than LDL particles. The differences in their number and size explain why LDL is so much more atherogenic than VLDL. LDL is much more numerous and much smaller than VLDL and therefore much more likely to encounter and penetrate the arterial vascular wall.

Tg is the major core lipid in VLDL, whereas cholesterol ester is the major core lipid in LDL. Each VLDL and LDL particle contains one molecule of apoB and therefore plasma apoB is an exact measure of VLDL and LDL particle numbers. Given the ratio of LDL to VLDL particles, plasma apoB is a clinically accurate measure of LDL particle number. Note also that most of

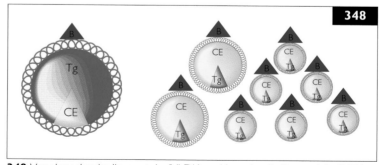

348 Very low-density lipoprotein (VLDL) and low-density lipoprotein (LDL) particle number and composition in a normal individual. Note there are nine times more LDL than VLDL particles. Note also that LDL particles differ in composition, with most being smaller and cholesterol enriched. B: apoB 100 protein; CE: cholesterol ester; Tg: triglyceride.

the LDL particles in a normal individual are the larger, cholesterol-replete variety.

HYPERTG NORMOAPOB

The characteristic profile of hyperTg normoapoB is illustrated in **349**. The VLDL particles secreted by the liver are larger than normal because they contain more Tg than normal. These illustrations, necessarily of course, show differences in area. In real life, however, the differences are in volume and are therefore much larger. In the syndrome of hyperTg normoapoB, although the VLDL particles are much larger than normal, thus accounting for the hypertriglyceridemia, they are secreted by the liver at a normal rate. Because they are secreted at a normal rate, LDL particle number is normal. (In fact, fewer than normal VLDL particles are converted to LDL, and therefore particle number tends to be average or even lower than average.) However, in contrast to normal, most of the LDL particles are smaller and denser than normal. HyperTg normoapoB is common, but is not associated with a substantially increased risk of vascular disease.

PRODUCTION OF SMALL, DENSE, LOW-DENSITY LIPOPROTEIN

The generally accepted mechanism by which small dense LDLs are created is illustrated in **350**. It is a two-step process. Step 1 involves the exchange of core lipids between VLDL and LDL. This occurs via the action of a protein in plasma, cholesterol ester transfer protein (CETP). CETP promotes the exchange of a Tg molecule from VLDL to LDL for a cholesterol ester molecule, which is transferred from LDL to VLDL. The consequence is that the VLDL particle is enriched in cholesterol ester, whereas the LDL particle is enriched in Tg. Neither changes in size. Step 2 involves hydrolysis of the Tg in the LDL particle, either by hepatic lipase or phospholipase A2. Hydrolysis of Tg does reduce the volume of core lipids and so the product is a smaller, denser LDL particle. It also seems likely that the composition of precursor particles plays an important role in determining the composition of the product

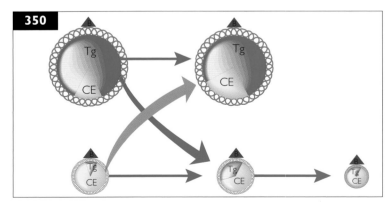

350 The process of generation of a small dense low-density lipoprotein (LDL) particle is illustrated. There are two steps. The first alters LDL composition but not its size. The second results in a smaller LDL particle being produced. B: apoB 100 protein; CE: cholesterol ester; Tg: triglyceride.

particles, Tg-enriched VLDL producing principally small, dense LDL, cholesterol-enriched VLDL producing principally large, buoyant LDL.

HYPERTG HYPERAPOB

This is the commonest atherogenic dyslipoproteinemia in patients with vascular disease and is also the commonest atherogenic dyslipoproteinemia in type 2 diabetes. Its major features are illustrated in **351**. VLDL secretion rate is increased and, therefore, compared to normals or to patients with hyperTg normoapoB, VLDL particle number is increased. However, in contrast to hyperTg normoapoB, the VLDL particles contain normal amounts of Tg. Because the VLDL secretion rate is increased, the generation of LDL particles is increased proportionately. Because VLDL particle number is increased,

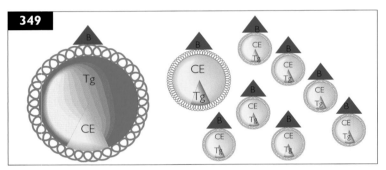

349 Very low-density lipoprotein (VLDL) and low-density lipoprotein (LDL) number and composition in a patient with hyperTg normoapoB. Note that neither VLDL nor LDL particle number is increased. The VLDL particle is triglyceride enriched whereas most LDL particles are cholesterol depleted. B: apoB 100 protein; CE: cholesterol ester; Tg: triglyceride.

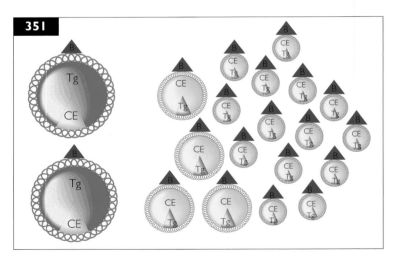

351 Very low-density lipoprotein (VLDL) and low-density lipoprotein (LDL) particle number and composition in a patient with hyperTg hyperapoB. Note that both are increased in number, with the proportion maintained between those that are VLDL and those that are LDL. Note also that most of the LDL particles are smaller and cholesterol depleted. B: apoB 100 protein; CE: cholesterol ester; Tg: triglyceride.

hypertriglyceridemia is present and small, dense LDL are the rule.

Hypertriglyceridemia is defined as a plasma Tg ≥ 1.5 mmol/l (133 mg/dl) because above this level, small, dense LDL are common, whereas below it they are not. An elevated apoB is defined as a value ≥120 mg/dl, a value that represents approximately the 75th percentile of the North American population. This cut-off was chosen to correspond to the cut-off for LDL C, for which a level of approximately 4 mmol/l (155 mg/dl) represents the 75th percentile of the population.

It is critical to appreciate that the risk of vascular disease with hyperTg hyperapoB is higher than with uncomplicated hypercholesterolemia, and that the reduction in risk with statins exceeds that achieved by treatment of simple hypercholesterolemia.

DYSLIPIDEMIAS IN TYPE 2 DIABETES MELLITUS

352 contrasts the results obtained in patients with type 2 diabetes using two different lipid classifications. The first is based on Tgs and LDL C, the second on Tgs and apoB. With the conventional Tg/LDL C approach, 23% have elevated LDL, with half of these also having increased Tgs. The largest group (41.3%) had hypertriglyceridemia with normal LDL C. These results contrast with those obtained using Tg/apoB. Now, almost 40% have elevated apoB and therefore increased LDL particle number, virtually double the number using Tg/LDL C. Thirty percent have hyperTg hyperapoB, the most atherogenic of the dyslipoproteinemias. Only 26.5% have hyperTg normoapoB; thus the less dangerous dyslipidemia has been reduced in number and the more dangerous increased by using apoB rather than LDL C. In both methods, just over one-third are normal. Unquestionably, the most common atherogenic dyslipoproteinemia in type 2 diabetes is hyperTg hyperapoB.

APOB-GUIDED STATIN THERAPY

Not only is apoB a better index than LDL C to predict risk, it is also a more accurate guide to the adequacy of statin therapy. This conclusion is based on the results of AFCAPS/TexCAPS, 4S, the Leiden Heart Study, the THROMBO Study, and LIPID. Given that risk of disease relates in the first instance more closely to the number of atherogenic particles than to LDL C, so also should the residual risk of disease.

SUMMARY

Contrary to conventional wisdom, LDL remains the main atherogenic lipoprotein in type 2 diabetes. However, this can only be appreciated if apoB is measured as well as lipoprotein lipids. It is also important to note that the measurement of apoB is standardized, automated, inexpensive, and can be done on fasting plasma, whereas there are serious errors in the calculation of LDL C with values of Tg ≥2.0 mmol/l (177 mg/dl).

The most important conclusion is that marked reduction of apoB, that is to say, marked reduction of atherogenic particles, will substantially reduce vascular mortality and morbidity in patients with type 2 diabetes.

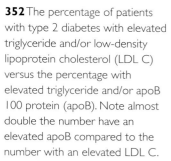

352 The percentage of patients with type 2 diabetes with elevated triglyceride and/or low-density lipoprotein cholesterol (LDL C) versus the percentage with elevated triglyceride and/or apoB 100 protein (apoB). Note almost double the number have an elevated apoB compared to the number with an elevated LDL C.

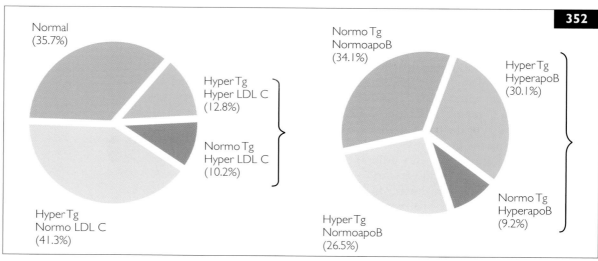

REVASCULARIZATION: PERCUTANEOUS CORONARY INTERVENTION VERSUS CORONARY ARTERY BYPASS GRAFTING

DAVID TÜLLER, MD AND BERNHARD MEIER, MD

INTRODUCTION

The goals of medical therapy, percutaneous coronary intervention (PCI) and coronary artery bypass surgery (CABG) in patients with CAD are to reduce cardiovascular mortality, decrease cardiac morbidity, and to alleviate symptoms. Both PCI and CABG have been proven to be valuable treatment options in selected patients with stable and unstable CAD. The choice of the appropriate management strategy is influenced by patient age, severity of symptoms, extent of CAD, lesion characteristics, comorbidity, left ventricular function, and the presentation of CAD as stable or unstable.

PERCUTANEOUS CORONARY INTERVENTION VERSUS CORONARY ARTERY BYPASS SURGERY IN PATIENTS WITH STABLE ANGINA PECTORIS

Several observational and randomized trials have been performed to give guidance for the optimal revascularization strategy[1-7]. The results of these trials have been quite consistent:

- Over a period of 1–5 years there was no significant difference with respect to mortality and nonfatal MI between PCI and CABG, except for diabetic patients in the BARI-Trial, where patients treated with CABG had significantly better survival rates after 5 years (80.6% vs. 65.5%, p <0.003)[5].

- Patients treated initially with angioplasty are in greater need of subsequent revascularization, especially in the first year, mainly due to restenosis. About 20–42% of patients initially treated with angioplasty require an additional revascularization procedure (CABG or PCI) within the first year. The availability of coronary stents markedly reduced these rates. In the recently published ARTS Trial, which randomly compared CABG with coronary stenting in multi-vessel disease in 1205 patients, only 17% of patients in the stenting group required additional revascularization within the first year[7].

- The prevalence of angina is higher in the patients treated with angioplasty than with CABG. This difference diminishes over 3 years[8]. In a report from the BARI Investigators, the functional status of the patients after CABG was significantly superior during the first 3 years of follow-up to that of those undergoing angioplasty. This difference, however, was no longer significant after 4 and 5 years[9].

- The mean cost of the initial procedure of angioplasty is lower than that of CABG ($21,113 versus $32,347, p <0.001 in the BARI Trial), but after 5 years the total medical cost of angioplasty was increased to 95% of that of surgery ($56,225 versus $58,889)[9]. The 5-year cost of angioplasty was significantly lower for patients with two-vessel disease but not three-vessel

disease[9]. The newer ARTS Trial, where coronary stents were used in all PCI patients, showed reduced cost in the stenting group after 1 year of follow-up (difference of $2,973 in favor of stenting)[7].

In summary, PCI or CABG are both clinically feasible treatment options for many patients with stable angina pectoris. The optimal management strategy depends mainly on the number of coronary vessels involved, the ability to achieve complete revascularization, left ventricular function, and patient preference. An ACC/AHA Task Force has published guidelines for the use of CABG and PCI in various clinical settings[10]. The choice of procedure must be individualized for a particular patient but certain recommendations can be made as described below.

Single-vessel disease

Most patients with single-vessel CAD can be managed by the less invasive percutaneous treatment. Single vessel disease remains the main indication for PCI with over 80% of procedures performed in Europe and over 90% in the USA being limited to a single vessel. In the RITA Trial, 45% of 1011 randomized patients had single-vessel disease. After 6.5 years of follow-up there was no significant difference in risk of death or nonfatal MI between the patients treated with angioplasty or surgery. The results were similar for patients with single or multi-vessel disease[3]. Some data from the New York State Cardiac Procedure Registry suggest that patients with isolated obstruction of the proximal left anterior descending artery (LAD) have better survival rates with CABG than with PCI[2]. However, the results from the Lausanne and SIMA Trials[11,12], two prospective randomized trials which compared balloon angioplasty (Lausanne Trial) or stenting (SIMA Trial) versus surgery for isolated proximal LAD stenosis, reveal that PCI and CABG are equally effective treatment options for isolated proximal LAD stenosis in patients with left ventricular ejection fraction (EF) >45% (**353, 354**). In patients with proximal LAD disease and diminished left ventricular function, surgery may be the prefered treatment.

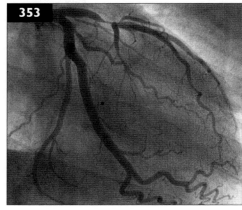

353 A 30-year-old patient with stable angina pectoris CCS II. The left coronary angiogram shows a subtotal proximal left anterior descending artery (LAD) stenosis. The right coronary artery (not shown) was normal. This patient successfully underwent coronary artery bypass surgery with an isolated left mammary artery graft to the distal LAD.

Multi-vessel disease

The lack of difference in late mortality and nonfatal MI in the randomized trials of PCI versus CABG mentioned above, suggests that PCI may be a reasonable initial strategy for patients with normal ventricular function who accept the possible need for repeat revascularization. Patients with focal triple-vessel disease may fare well with PCI (**355**). Complete revascularization is a major goal in patients with left ventricular dysfunction and multi-vessel disease. Because of the greater chance of complete revascularization with CABG than with PCI, the majority of patients with three-vessel disease, left main disease, multiple chronic total occlusions, or left ventricular dysfunction should be referred for surgery. In many patients either method of revascularization is suitable and both can be offered to the patients (*Table 53*).

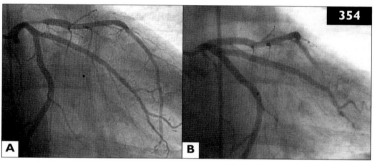

354 A 49-year-old patient with stable angina pectoris CCS II and normal left ventricular function. **A**: coronary angiogram of the left coronary artery with a subtotal ostial left anterior descending artery stenosis. This patient underwent successful balloon angioplasty with subsequent stenting of this lesion. **B**: Postprocedural result.

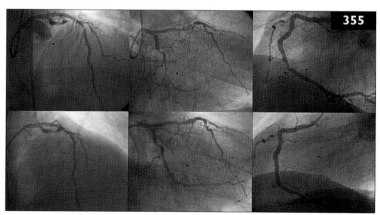

355 A 43-year-old patient with focal triple-vessel disease. Coronary angiography shows significant stenoses of the left anterior descending artery (LAD), the left circumflex coronary artery, and the right coronary artery (upper panel, from left to right). The patient was successfully treated with primary stenting of the LAD, balloon angioplasty and stenting of the left circumflex artery, and primary stenting of the right coronary artery in one session (lower panel from left to right).

PERCUTANEOUS CORONARY INTERVENTION VERSUS CORONARY ARTERY BYPASS SURGERY IN PATIENTS WITH ACUTE CORONARY SYNDROMES

An early invasive strategy is increasingly used in patients with acute coronary syndromes (ACS), especially in those with high-risk indicators, such as elevated troponin I or T, recurrent chest pain despite aggressive treatment, or dynamic ST changes in the electrocardiogram (ECG). Angioplasty can be performed with a success rate of >95% in patients with ACS[13]. Periprocedural MI occurs in 2.7%, and emergency CABG is required in 1.4% of patients.

The choice between CABG and PCI in ACS involves similar considerations as in patients with stable angina pectoris. Patients with single-vessel disease are usually treated with PCI. Because of the risk of acute vessel closure or acute stent thrombosis, CABG is usually preferred if a large amount of myocardium is at risk, as in left main disease, two-vessel disease involving the proximal LAD, or severe three-vessel disease and impaired left ventricular function. In a subset of patients with multi-vessel disease and an ACS, angioplasty of the 'culprit lesion' can initially be performed to stabilize the patient, followed by full revascularization in a second session. PCI may be the preferred management strategy in patients with high surgical risk. The AWSOME trial compared CABG to PCI in 454 patients with unstable angina and an increased risk for surgery (prior CABG, age >70 years, left ventricular ejection fraction <35%, MI within 7 days, or intra-aortic balloon pump required). There was no difference in short-term (30 days) or long-term (3 years) mortality in patients treated with CABG and PCI, suggesting that PCI is an alternative to CABG in patients with a high operative risk[14].

Table 53 Factors that may influence the decision of percutaneous coronary intervention (PCI) versus coronary artery bypass graft (CABG) in patients with multi-vessel disease

PCI preferred	CABG preferred
Patients with focal coronary disease and preserved left ventricular function.	Diabetic patients with three-vessel disease.
Younger patients (<50 years), who may need CABG in the future, in order to delay surgery to avoid later reoperation.	Patients with angina and left ventricular dysfunction, in whom complete revascularization cannot be achieved by PCI.
Older patients and patients with significant comorbidity who have high surgical risk or short life expectancy.	Patients with large amount of myocardium at risk (two-vessel disease with proximal left anterior descending artery, left main disease, diffuse three-vessel disease).
Patient's preference.	Patient's preference.

ALLOGRAFT CORONARY ARTERY DISEASE

HENRIK EGEBLAD, MD, DMSC

INTRODUCTION

Five years after heart transplantation 25–50% of all recipients have developed allograft arteriopathy visible on a coronary angiogram (see chapter 5, Transplant Vasculopathy). It is a serious condition and a major limitation to long-term survival in heart transplant patients. The vasculopathy presents as diffuse concentric thickening of the intima, with lengthy, more or less irregular, narrowing of the lumen. The condition includes endothelial dysfunction and decreased flow reserve. Progression leads to severe obstruction and obliteration of minor intramyocardial coronary artery branches and of the major epicardial arteries. Eventually the process commonly results in myocardial failure, acute MI (AMI), or sudden death (**356–360**). Signs of mild vasculopathy by coronary arteriography worsen to severe vasculopathy in 40–50% of cases per year, and in patients with severe vasculopathy the mortality is about 40% per year.

The reason for this type of arteriopathy is unclear but some risk factors and protective measures retarding the process have been identified. Vasculopathy may sometimes appear shortly after transplantation even in younger recipients, and there is a relationship to the degree of human leukocyte antigen (HLA) mismatch and an association between the number of allograft rejection episodes and vasculopathy. Thus, first of all allograft vasculopathy is believed to be the result of an immunologic process and chronic rejection is another commonly used term for the arteriopathy. Infection with cytomegalovirus, a common opportunistic infection in transplant patients, also plays a role as well as elements of the immunosuppressive treatment (cyclosporine and prednisone). Pre-existent atherosclerosis in the recipient and known risk factors such as dyslipidemia, smoking, overweight, and hypertension are also supposed to predispose to post-transplant CAD.

SYMPTOMS, SIGNS, AND DIAGNOSIS

Re-innervation occurs to a certain extent in many donor hearts but angina pectoris caused by post-transplant arteriopathy is a rare symptom. More commonly, dyspnea or vague chest discomfort on exercise develops. Arrhythmias may also occur. ECG changes in terms of ST-T changes and signs of AMI are late phenomena.

Stress echocardiography or myocardial scintigraphy is used as screening in some centers, but the sensitivity for myocardial dysfunction induced by vasculopathy is <80–90% in many series. Yet in experienced hands a normal stress echocardiogram seems to warrant a very small incidence of ischemic myocardial events over the next year. Tissue Doppler imaging may also have potential (**358, 359**). In many centers, even asymptomatic patients are offered coronary arteriography at regular intervals, often on a yearly basis or every second year. In symptomatic patients, it is not feasible clinically or by echocardiography to distinguish between myocardial failure caused by rejection or vasculopathy. Clinical suspicion of heart failure should prompt an endomyocardial biopsy and a coronary arteriogram, particularly when symptoms occur a few years after the transplantation. Intravascular ultrasound (IVUS) is much more sensitive for revealing incipient vasculopathy than is the

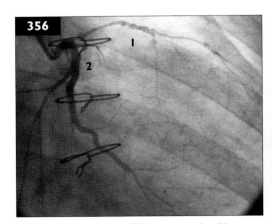

356 Angiogram from a 27-year-old male with severe allograft coronary artery disease. The left anterior descending branch (1) of the left coronary artery is obliterated. The secondary branches of the circumflex branch (2) are poor, apart from one major obtuse marginal artery ending with branches somewhat like a pollarded tree. Only four years after heart transplantation the patient had been admitted with chest pain and an electrocardiogram showed anterior acute myocardial infarction. Heart failure developed and the patient underwent successful retransplantation.

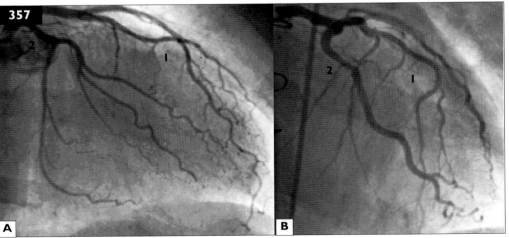

357 Coronary angiograms of the left coronary artery. **A**: A 48-year-old male who underwent heart transplantation 5 years earlier because of dilated cardiomyopathy. **B**: A 61-year-old male who was transplanted 6 years earlier also because of dilated cardiomyopathy. In both patients the peripheral part of the left anterior descending artery (1) is relatively thin and poor, a common finding after heart transplantation. In **B** the circumflex branch (2) shows mild wall changes and the minor branches are not so clearly seen as in **A** but the difference is not dramatic. **A** was asymptomatic while **B** had developed increasing dyspnea on exercise with a simultaneous 3 kg gain in weight over a couple of months. Endomyocardial biopsy showed no signs of rejection. See also **358, 359**.

conventional contrast angiogram. IVUS and Doppler determination of the coronary flow reserve (CFR) are usually performed to test the value of a new potentially preventive protocol.

PREVENTION AND TREATMENT

Heart transplant recipients are advised to follow a lifestyle known to minimize the risk of regular atherosclerosis. Aspirin is administered to reduce the risk of coronary artery thrombosis. In randomized studies, pravastatin and diltiazem have been shown to yield some protection against the development of vasculopathy. Another measure is the administration of ganciclovir as prophylaxis against infection with cytomegalovirus. Administration of vitamins C and E appear to delay the development of early post-transplant CAD. Recently, it has also been shown that novel immuno–suppressive agents (proliferation signal inhibitors) may offer some protection against the development of vasculopathy.

Once severe arteriopathy has developed with symptoms and visible changes in the major epicardial artery branches on a conventional angiogram, the prognosis is very poor and retransplantation is the only treatment possibility to consider (**356**). However, PCI may be successful in selected patients with more focal coronary artery stenoses (**360**).

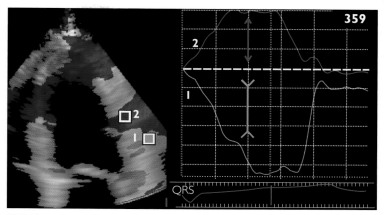

359 Abnormal myocardial strain in allograft vasculopathy. Strain is the relative deformation within a myocardial region. Negative strain means contraction while positive strain indicates passive stretching of the fibers. The left panel is identical to **358B**. As indicated by the small green (1) and red (2) squares, the basic region and the region in the middle of the lateral wall are interrogated for regional myocardial strain. The strain curves from the two regions are depicted in the right panel where the systole is delineated by the two blue dotted lines. The green graph (1) from the base of the lateral wall shows negative strain in systole, i.e. contraction, while the red graph (2) from the mid part of the lateral wall indicates that this region is being stretched by the adjacent active myocardium. Thus, in support of the diagnosis of coronary artery vasculopathy, the red graph indicates that there is ischemia or infarction in the mid part of the lateral wall of patient **B** of **357**, **358**.

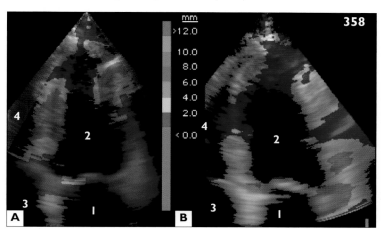

358 Tissue Doppler four-chamber views in a modality named tissue tracking. By means of a color coded scale, tissue tracking displays the systolic motion amplitude towards the apex in each myocardial segment. Thus tissue tracking focuses on the systolic shortening of the subendocardial and subepicardial myocardial fibers, their course being predominantly longitudinal from basis to apex. **A** and **B** are from the same patients as in **357**. **A** exhibits almost normal overall motion with a maximum systolic shortening of >12 mm close to the mitral annulus. As in a normal heart, the motion amplitude decreases in colored bands of almost equal size throughout the interventricular septum. In the lateral wall, there is repetition of the color band sequence close to the apex indicating a minor contraction abnormality here. In **B** the overall systolic motion amplitude is severely decreased (4–6 mm close to the mitral annulus) and in the middle of the lateral wall the motion amplitude decreases to 2 mm indicating that this area may not contract. The conventional 2D and M-mode echocardiograms of patient **B** showed only ambiguous reduction of the left ventricular function. A diagnosis of small vessel vasculopathy was supposed on the basis of an endomyocardial biopsy showing no rejection, angiographic suspicion of coronary arteriopathy (**357**), and severe depression of the systolic function of the longitudinal myocardial fibers. See also **359**. 1: left atrium; 2: left ventricle; 3: right atrium; 4: right ventricle.

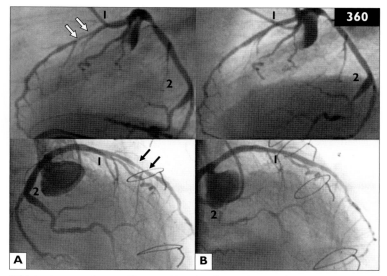

360 Angiograms from a 62-year-old male who underwent heart transplantation 8 years earlier because of ischemic heart disease. **A**: Two different views recorded because of recently developed dyspnea on exertion with accompanying chest discomfort. A rather severe lengthy focal stenosis is seen in the left anterior descending branch (1) of the left coronary artery (arrows). The patient underwent successful percutaneous coronary intervention (PCI) with stent insertion. However, symptom relief lasted only a couple of weeks. A control angiogram (**B**) confirmed a satisfactory result of PCI but verified other signs of advanced epicardial allograft vasculopathy now clearly visible in the branches of the circumflex branch of the left coronary artery (2).

CHRONIC REFRACTORY ANGINA

MICHAEL C. KIM, MD, FACC AND SAMIN K. SHARMA, MD, FACC

INTRODUCTION

Angina pectoris, the symptom that most often brings patients with ischemic heart disease to medical attention, represents an imbalance between myocardial oxygen supply and demand. Conventional therapies used to combat this condition have included a combination of medical therapies and mechanical revascularization techniques, mostly coronary artery bypass graft surgery (CABG) and PCI. As the survival of patients with primary coronary events continues to improve, however, the number of patients with coronary artery disease (CAD) unresponsive to conventional therapies has also risen. This increasingly important group of patients have chronic refractory angina pectoris and represent a growing population desperate for new or alternative treatment modalities.

Two criteria must be met before a patient is labeled with chronic refractory angina. First, there must be objective evidence of severe symptomatic ischemia. Second, all known conventional therapies must be exhausted. Most studies on this population have required Canadian Cardiovascular Society function class (CCSC) III or IV symptoms. Importantly, the coronary anatomy causing these symptoms must be deemed unamenable to either PCI or CABG by a consensus of different interventional cardiologists and cardiac surgeons.

ALTERNATIVE MEDICAL THERAPIES

When traditional anti-anginal agents have been tried and are inadequate in controlling symptoms, the addition of more recent antiplatelet and anticoagulant medications may be helpful.

Adenosine diphosphate receptor inhibitors

Clopidogrel is a thienopyridine derivative that blocks adenosine diphosphate- (ADP) mediated platelet aggregation. Combination therapy with aspirin has shown promising benefits in cerebrovascular diseases and, more recently, in the management of non-ST elevation myocardial infarction (NSTEMI) from the CURE trial. It is not known, however, if clopidogrel actually improves symptoms on a daily basis.

Low-molecular weight heparin

Compared to unfractionated heparin, low-molecular weight heparins (LMWH) reduce the generation of thrombin due to an increased ratio of antifactor Xa:antifactor II activity. Two randomized, placebo-controlled trials have studied the potential efficacy of LMWH in patients with stable angina. Although the number of subjects was small, the patients receiving LMWH in addition to their current medical regimen did have decreased symptoms and decreased ischemia on the treadmill.

Thrombolytic agents

While thrombolytic agents have not been shown to be beneficial in patients with NSTEMI, it has been postulated that low-dose thrombolytic therapy may improve both microcirculatory and macrocirculatory coronary flow by decreasing blood viscosity. Two randomized nonplacebo-controlled studies have been conducted demonstrating decreased fibrinogen levels, red cell aggregation, and plasma viscosity. Exercise capacity and anginal episodes were decreased with the addition of low-dose urokinase therapy. However, a placebo effect cannot be ruled out.

Partial fatty acid oxidation inhibitors

Ranolazine is the first in a new class of compounds called partial fatty acid oxidation inhibitors, which represent the first new anti-anginal drug class in more than 20 years. Preliminary studies have shown an increase in exercise duration and a decrease in anginal events compared to placebo.

NEUROSTIMULATION

Transcutaneous electrical nerve stimulation (TENS) and spinal cord stimulation (SCS) have been proposed to decrease sympathetic output and potentially attenuate pain sensation in chronic angina. SCS currently is the more promising of the two techniques and has been studied in two large scale studies. Results have demonstrated its safety and a decrease in the frequency of anginal events and an increase in exercise tolerance. Again, a placebo effect cannot be ruled out. Skin irritation and paresthesias are the main side-effects.

ENHANCED EXTERNAL COUNTERPULSATION

Enhanced external counterpulsation (EECP) increases venous return and diastolic coronary perfusion pressure using timed, sequential cuff inflations from the calves to the upper thighs. Two recent randomized, placebo-controlled studies have evaluated this emerging technique in patients with refractory angina and have shown promising results, with a decrease in anginal episodes and an increase in exercise tolerance. Reversible thallium perfusion defects also decreased after EECP therapy in one study. The exact mechanism by which EECP may improve symptoms is not clear. It has been postulated that collateral circulation may be increased in addition to improved diastolic coronary flow.

SURGICAL AND PERCUTANEOUS LASER REVASCULARIZATION

Laser revascularization by surgical or percutaneous means has been extensively studied for patients with refractory angina (**361**). The laser creates a network of channels by which the majority of the heart's blood supply is delivered directly to the myocardium. It has been further postulated that these laser channels may create new blood vessels via angiogenesis and may produce an anesthetic effect by attenuating nerve sensation. *Table 54* summarizes the major surgical and percutaneous trials involving laser revascularization. Most have shown short-term improvements in anginal class, quality-of-life perception, and exercise duration. However, a recent placebo-controlled percutaneous study demonstrated the marked placebo effect of this modality, with no difference between the laser and placebo groups. This has cast a shadow of doubt over the entire area of laser revascularization in this very desperate patient population.

EXPERIMENTAL ANGIOGENESIS

Perhaps the most provocative and promising emerging therapy for refractory angina is cardiovascular gene therapy in the hope of promoting angiogenesis. Angiogenesis is the process of forming new vessels which lack tunica media. An example of this is the formation of capillaries along the border zone of an MI. Since Isner's seminal study using a plasmid to introduce vascular endothelial growth factor (VEGF) into a patient with an ischemic limb, multiple studies have been performed introducing VEGF or fibroblast growth factor (FGF). *Table 55* gives a summary of the major experimental angiogenic trials. Using a variety of markers (magnetic resonance imaging, single photon emission computerized tomography imaging, electromechanical mapping) to document ischemia, these trials have documented decreased objective ischemia and improvements in symptoms. Unlike the other modalities discussed to treat refractory angina, large placebo-controlled studies have also shown statistically significant improvements in exercise tolerance over placebo. Furthermore, all trials to date have demonstrated a good safety profile when given these genes or gene products.

EMERGING REVASCULARIZATION TECHNIQUES

Percutaneous *in situ* coronary venous arterialization (PICVA) and percutaneous *in situ* coronary artery bypass (PICAB) are two new revascularization techniques being investigated for patients with chronic refractory angina. PICVA uses the corresponding venous

system adjacent to the stenosed or occluded coronary artery to perfuse the ischemic myocardium via retroperfusion (**362**). PICAB actually bypasses the blocked coronary artery again by accessing the adjacent coronary vein but then reconnecting to the artery distal to the obstruction and perfusing the ischemic territory in an antegrade fashion. These techniques are currently in their infancy but may prove to be a viable alternative to traditional means of revascularization.

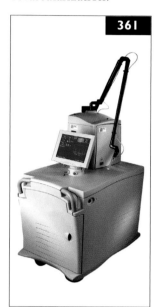 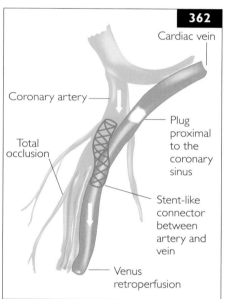

361 CO_2 transmyocardial revascularization laser. With permission from Edwards.

362 Diagram to show percutaneous *in situ* coronary venous arterialization.

Table 54 Major surgical and percutaneous trials involving laser revascularization

First author	Year	Number of patients	Follow-up (months)	Laser type	Angina 2 class improvement (vs. placebo)	1-year survival (laser vs. placebo)
Frazier	1999	192	12	CO_2	72% vs. 13% (p <0.01)	85% vs. 79%
Allen	1999	275	12	H Yag	76% vs. 32% (p <0.01)	84% vs. 89%
Burkhoff	1999	182	12	H Yag	48% vs. 14% (p <0.01)	95% vs. 90%
Schofield	1999	188	12	CO_2	24% vs. 4% (p <0.01)	89% vs. 96%
Oesterle (PTMR)	2000	221	12	H Yag	34% vs. 14% (p <0.01)	93% vs. 97%
Leon	2000	298	6	H Yag	34% vs. 42% (p <0.01)	98% vs.97%
Whitlow (PTMR)	2001	330	12	H Yag	32% vs. 10% (p <0.01)	92% vs. 93%

(From: Frazier *et al.* [1999]. Transmyocardial revascularization with a carbondioxide laser in patients with end-stage coronary artery disease. *N. Engl. J. Med.* **34**:1021–1028; Allen *et al.* [1999]. Comparison of transmyocardial revascularization with medical therapy in patients with refractory angina. *N. Engl. J. Med.* **341**:1029–1036; Burkhoff *et al.* [1999]. Transmyocardial laser revascularization compared with continued medical therapy for treatment of refractory angina pectoris: a prospective randomized trial. ATLANTIC Investigators. *Lancet* **354**:885–890; Schofield *et al.* [1999]. Transmyocardial laser revascularization in patients with refractory angina: a randomized controlled trial. *Lancet* **353**:519–524; Oesterle *et al.* [2000]. Percutaneous transmyocardial laser revascularization for severe angina: the PACIFIC randomized trial. *Lancet* **356**:1705–1710: Leon [2000]. TCT Meetings, Washington; Whitlow [2001]). TCT Meetings, Washington.

CARDIAC TRANSPLANTATION

When every attempt to treat significant angina has failed, cardiac transplantation remains as a last resort for patients with refractory angina. Because of the severe shortage of donor transplants and the expected mortality from receiving a transplanted heart (20% at 1 year and 60% at 10 years), this decision must be made by both physician and patient with great care.

CHELATION THERAPY

There is no convincing evidence showing any benefits to chelation therapy using the calcium chelating agent ethylene diamine tetra acetic acid (EDTA). On the contrary, there may be fatal side-effects to such treatment, including severe renal damage and lethal hypocalcemia.

Table 55 Major experimental angiogenic trials

First author	Agent used	Number of patients/target	Results
Baumgartner	Plasmid VEGF	9/limb ischemia	VEGF levels increased, ABI, MRA improved, 4/7 ulcers improved
Losordo	Plasmid VEGF	5/intramyocardial	Dobutamine SPECT and collaterals improved in all 5 patients
Rosengart	Adenoviral VEGF	21/intramyocardial	Angiography and stress sestamibi scan assessment of wall motion improved in most patients
Laham	BFGF via microcapsules	24/intramyocardial	High-dose group showed significant improvement on stress nuclear imaging after 3 months
Udelson	Recombinant FGF	59/IV and intracoronary	Improvement in both stress and rest SPECT imaging after 180 days

ABI: ankle brachial index; (B)FGF: (basic) fibroblast growth factor; MRA: magnetic resonance angiography; SPECT: single photon emission computerized tomography; VEGF: vascular endothelial growth factor.
(Baumgartner et al. [1998]. Constitutive expression of phVEGF 16s after intramuscular gene transfer promotes collateral vessel development in patients with critical limb ischemia. *Cirulation* **97**:1114–1123; Losordo et al. [2002]. Phase 1/2 placebo-controlled, double-blind dose escalating trial myocardial vascular endothelial growth factor 2 gene transfer to catheter delivery in patients with chronic myocardial ischemia. *Circulation* **105**:2012–2018; Rosengart et al. [1999]. Angiogenesis gene therapy: Phase I assessment of direct intramyocardial administration of an adenovirus vector expressing VEGF 121 cDNA to individuals with significant coronary artery disease. *Circulation* **100**:468–474; Laham et al. [2000]. Intracoronary basic fibroblast growth factor (FGF-2) in patients with severe ischemic heart diease: results of a phase I open-label dose escalation study. *J. Am. Coll. Cardiol.* **36**:2132–2139; Udelson (see Laham ref).

ETHNICITY AND CARDIOVASCULAR DISEASE

STEPHANIE OUNPUU, PhD AND SALIM YUSUF, FRCP, DPhil

INTRODUCTION

The concept of risk factors associated with cardiovascular disease (CVD) was derived from prospective epidemiologic studies conducted mainly in Western populations. Therefore, while globally, nonwhite populations constitute the majority of the world's population, the most influential risk factors for CVD in these populations have largely been unexplored. The burden of CVD varies substantially between geographic regions, with the majority of CVD occurring in developing countries (see chapter 1, Burden of Ischemic Heart Disease). CVD mortality is projected to double between 1990 and 2020, with the developing countries experiencing approximately 80% of the increase. Ethnic variations in disease rates are closely tied to geographic patterns of disease.

DIVERSITY

Ethnicity is a construct that encompasses both genetic and cultural (e.g. language, religion, dietary) differences. Individuals of different ethnic backgrounds tend to live in distinct regions and societies; therefore, variations in disease rates by ethnicity are intertwined with geographic differences. However, lifestyle patterns adopted by a given ethnic group may vary substantially in differing regions. Consequently, a study of variations in disease by ethnic group is intertwined with additional variations in lifestyle, geography, socio-economic status, and so on.

PATHOGENETIC DIFFERENCES

Initial observations about ethnic variations in disease burden are provided by data on differences in risk factors and disease rates between countries. In the Seven Countries Study, low rates of coronary heart disease (CHD) were observed in Japan and the Mediterranean countries, with high CHD rates in Finland and the USA. These differences were largely explained by differences in diet, serum cholesterol, and blood pressure. Data published by the World Health Organization demonstrate a greater than 10-fold difference in age standardized CHD mortality rates among men and women in different countries (**363**).

Several factors are likely to contribute to the interpopulation differences in CHD, as descibed below.

Stage of epidemiological transition

The stage of epidemiological transition varies by country and even by regions within a country. The stages of the transition are characterized by variations in life expectancy and demographic profiles, and differing contributions from competing causes of death. Both the total burden of CVD and the composition of the CVD spectrum will vary with the dynamics of health transition. For example, the prominent CVDs in the earliest stage of the epidemiological transition are rheumatic heart disease and nutritional cardiomyopathies. By the fourth stage of the transition, stroke and ischemic heart disease are the predominant CVDs.

Prevalence of environmental risk factors

The prevalence of environmental risk factors varies widely across populations, which is probably related to both culture and stage of industrialization. Tobacco use is expected to increase in most transitional countries compared to decreases observed in most industrialized nations. For example, cigarette smoking is highly prevalent among Chinese males (>60%) and this rate is increasing. Physical inactivity, which predisposes to obesity, hypertension, glucose intolerance, hypertriglyceridemia, and low HDL is an example of adverse lifestyle changes that accompany urbanization.

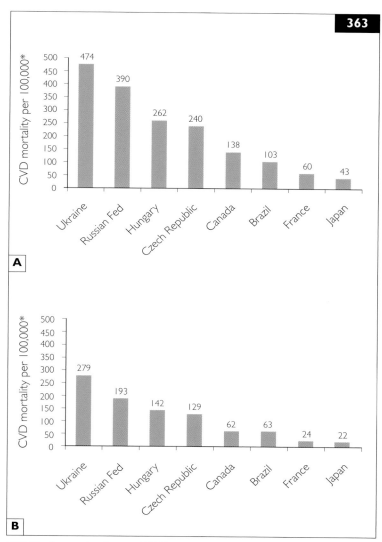

363 Cardiovascular disease (CVD) mortality in selected countries demonstrating marked international variations. *: rates adjusted to World Health Organization standard population. **A**: men; **B**: women.

Preliminary data from a population-based study in south India (The Prospective Urban and Rural Epidemiologic [PURE] Study) indicate that over half of the urban sample have sedentary lifestyles compared with only 15% of the rural sample. The globalization of food production and marketing has resulted in increased availability of vegetable oils and fats and increased consumption of energy-dense foods, a shift from plant to animal protein, and towards refined carbohydrates. These shifts in dietary patterns have been observed in both Africa and Asia, are occurring in countries and groups with a relatively low level of income, and are accelerated by urbanization.

Genetic factors

Genetic factors explain variation in the risk of incident CVD within populations by providing the basis for differences in individual susceptibility in shared and relatively homogeneous populations. They also contribute to interpopulation differences, due to variable frequencies of one or more genetic determinants in different ethnic groups. Lp(a), for example, is a genetically determined plasminogen-like apolipoprotein that may be related to both atherogenesis and thrombogenesis, and has been demonstrated to be a powerful independent risk factor for premature atherosclerosis. Preliminary cross-sectional data indicate that Lp(a) may vary significantly between ethnic groups. A recent migration study confirmed that urban Indians in Britain, when compared to their siblings in rural India, had similarly elevated levels of Lp(a), despite differences in their glucose and lipid profiles. When compared to Malays and Chinese living in Singapore, Indians have higher levels of Lp(a). Genetic contributions to lipid disorders, obesity, salt sensitivity, insulin resistance, coagulation derangements, and endothelial dysfunction are being explored.

Programming effect

The programming effect of factors promoting selective survival may also determine individual responses to environmental challenges and, thereby, contribute to the population differences in CVD. The thrifty gene hypothesis describes a process of selective survival, where a population was occasionally exposed to adverse environmental conditions and associated famine. For example, selection of a gene that increases the efficiency of fat storage through an oversecretion of insulin in response to a meal, would favor survival in a period of famine. However, a high level of energy intake (because of the relatively easy access to 'rich' foods) with urbanization may lead to a less desirable response that includes obesity, hyperinsulinemia, diabetes, and atherosclerosis. Such gene–environmental interactions may relate to higher blood pressure levels (e.g. salt retention or sensitivity genes), or higher homocysteine levels (due to higher consumption of meats and lower consumption of vegetables interacting with various genes that affect homocysteine synthesis or break down).

Other programming factors

Other programming factors which may underlie population differences in CHD include the state of intrauterine, infant, and early childhood nutrition. An adverse intrauterine growth environment due to poor maternal nutrition may confer a selective survival advantage to the fetus who has been programmed for reduced insulin sensitivity. However, as the child is exposed to overnutrition in later childhood and early adulthood, such programming could lead to high blood pressure, glucose intolerance, and dyslipidemia. It has been suggested that the susceptibility of south Asians to diabetes may be modified by improving intrauterine growth.

NATURAL EXPERIMENT

Therefore, differences in demographic profiles, environmental factors, and early childhood programming influences as well as differences in gene frequency or expression can all contribute to variations in CVD between different populations. Studies in migrant groups provide a natural experiment, where environmental changes due to altered lifestyles are superimposed over genetic influences. For example, the Ni-Hon-San study of Japanese migrants revealed that blood cholesterol levels and CHD rates rose from relatively low levels among those in Japan, to intermediate levels in Honolulu, and to high levels in San Francisco. Comparison of Afro-Caribbeans, south Asians, and Europeans in the UK indicate marked differences in central obesity, glucose intolerance, hyperinsulinemia, and related dyslipidemia, despite similar blood pressure, body mass index, and total plasma cholesterol. In Canada, there are marked differences between different ethnic groups in the prevalence and death rates from CHD, with the highest rates being among those of European and south Asian origin, but lowest among those of Chinese origin. There was a greater rate of clinical events among south Asians compared with the other two ethnic groups for similar degrees of atherosclerosis, suggesting that the propensity to plaque rupture may vary in different ethnic groups. Thus, where the environment is common but gene pools differ, the nonconventional risk factors may be explanatory of risk variance; whereas, when the same gene pool is confronted with different environments, the conventional risk factors play a major role. The challenge of preventing CVDs lies in identifying and addressing the components most relevant to each community at their present and projected levels of the epidemiologic transition.

CARDIOVASCULAR DISEASE IN CHRONIC KIDNEY DISEASE

DANIEL E. WEINER, MD AND MARK J. SARNAK, MD

INTRODUCTION

CVD is the primary cause of morbidity and mortality in chronic kidney disease (CKD). In the current chapter, a brief overview of recent developments in the classification of CKD is provided and the epidemiology of CVD in CKD is described, focusing on the prevalence of CVD and risk factors for CVD. Potential methods to reduce the tremendous burden of CVD in CKD are discussed.

CLASSIFICATION OF CHRONIC KIDNEY DISEASE

The National Kidney Foundation (NKF) Kidney Disease Outcomes Quality Initiative (KDOQI) has recently developed a new classification of CKD (*Table 56*)[1]. Individuals in stages 1–4 CKD have either reduced glomerular filtration rate (GFR) below 60 ml/minute/1.73 m^2, or structural kidney damage as manifest by proteinuria, albuminuria, or abnormalities on imaging studies. Kidney transplant recipients are included in stages 1–4. Dialysis patients have GFR values below 15 ml/minute/1.73 m^2 and are considered stage 5 CKD.

There are approximately 20 million individuals in the USA with stages 1–4 CKD and 300,000 dialysis patients classified as stage 5. Additionally, there are approximately 100,000 kidney transplant recipients in the USA, making CKD a significant public health problem.

Table 56 Stages of chronic kidney disease

Stage	Description	GFR (ml/minute/ 1.73 m^2)	US prevalence (×10^3)
1	Kidney damage with normal or ↑GFR	90	5,900
2	Kidney damage with mild ↓GFR	60–89	5,300
3	Moderate ↓GFR	30–59	7,600
4	Severe ↓GFR	15–29	400
5	Kidney failure	<15 or dialysis	300

GFR: glomerular filtration rate. (Reproduced and modified with permission from the National Kidney Foundation [2002]. K/DOQI Clinical practice guidelines on hypertension and antihypertensive agents in chronic kidney disease. *Am. J. Kidney. Dis.* **39**(Suppl.1, s1–s266[1].)

SPECTRUM OF CARDIOVASCULAR DISEASE IN CHRONIC KIDNEY DISEASE

CKD patients may have any combination of cardiomyopathy, ischemic heart disease, and large vessel arteriosclerosis. Cardiomyopathy is usually a consequence of either ischemic heart disease (volume overload secondary to anemia, retention of salt and water, and potentially the presence of an arteriovenous fistula) or pressure overload secondary to hypertension, arteriosclerosis, and aortic stenosis if present. Ischemic heart disease is primarily due to large vessel coronary disease, but may also be nonatherosclerotic in nature, particularly in the setting of underlying left ventricular hypertrophy (LVH) and small vessel disease. Large vessel arteriosclerosis is characterized by diffuse dilatation and hypertrophy of large arteries with loss of arterial elasticity, and occurs in response to both atherogenic factors causing direct vascular injury as well as changes in systemic hemodynamic burden.

EPIDEMIOLOGY OF CARDIOVASCULAR DISEASE IN CHRONIC KIDNEY DISEASE

Stages 1–4

Reduced GFR and the presence of albuminuria are both associated with a higher likelihood of CVD in cross-sectional analyses, and are independent risk factors for CVD outcomes in longitudinal studies[2]. In the Heart Outcomes and Prevention Evaluation (HOPE) study, a creatinine level ≥1.4 mg/dl (124 μmol/l) at baseline was independently associated with a 40% increased risk for the primary outcome of CVD death, MI, or stroke[3]. Similarly, the presence of albuminuria was independently associated with an 83% increased risk for the same primary outcome[4].

The prevalence of LVH is also directly associated with the severity of kidney disease: approximately 27% of CKD subjects with creatinine clearance >50 ml/minute, 31% with a creatinine clearance between 25 and 50 ml/minute, and over 45% with creatinine clearance <25 ml/minute have LVH by echocardiographic criteria[5]. Similarly, elevated urine albumin levels have been associated with LVH in multiple studies.

Stage 5

CVD mortality rates are ~10–30-fold higher in dialysis patients than in the general population, even after stratification for age, gender, and race (**364**)[6]. Furthermore, CVD accounts for approximately half of all deaths and contributes to an annual mortality rate of ~20% among dialysis patients.

There are two reasons for the high CVD mortality rate in dialysis patients. First, there is a high prevalence of CVD, with 40% of patients having a history of heart failure, 40% with ischemic heart disease, and as many as 75% with LVH by echocardiographic criteria[6]. Second, dialysis patients with CVD have a high case fatality rate. For example, dialysis patients who have suffered an MI have a 59% mortality rate at 1 year and 90% mortality at 5 years (**365**)[7].

Because of the tremendous burden of CVD in CKD, several recent guidelines have classified all patients with CKD into the 'highest-risk' status for future CVD events[8]. This implies that

when guidelines and treatment targets from the general population are extrapolated to subjects with CKD, recommendations that apply to the 'highest-risk' group should be used.

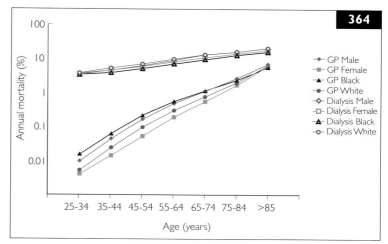

364 Cardiovascular mortality defined by death due to arrhythmias, cardiomyopathy, cardiac arrest, myocardial infarction, atherosclerotic heart disease, and pulmonary edema in the general population (GP) (NCHS multiple cause of mortality data files ICD 9 codes 402, 404, 410–414, and 425–429, 1993) compared to ESRD treated by dialysis (USRDS special data request HCFA form 2746 #'s 23, 26–29 and 31, 1994–96). Data are stratified by age, race, and gender. (Reproduced with permission from Foley et al. [1998]. Epidemiology of cardiovascular disease in chronic renal disease. *Am. J. Kidney Dis.* **32**(Suppl. 3):S112–S119.)

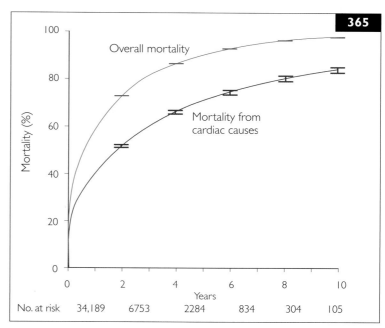

365 Estimated cumulative mortality after acute myocardial infarction among patients on dialysis. (Reproduced with permission from Herzog et al. [1998]. Poor long-term survival after myocardial infarction among patients on long-term hemodialysis. *N. Engl. J. Med.* **339**:799–805.)

CARDIOVASCULAR RISK FACTORS

In subjects with CKD, cardiac risk factors can be classified as traditional and nontraditional (*Table 57*). Traditional risk factors have been defined primarily in the Framingham Heart Study. Nontraditional risk factors are those factors that increase in prevalence or severity as kidney function declines. These may include factors that are recognized as risk factors in the general population but have a higher prevalence in CKD, such as hyperhomocysteinemia, or factors that are unique to subjects with CKD, such as anemia and abnormal calcium × phosphate concentration product.

Traditional risk factors

Traditional CVD risk factors such as age, diabetes mellitus, systolic hypertension, LVH, reduced physical activity, low HDL cholesterol, and elevated Tgs are highly prevalent in subjects with CKD. The relationship between traditional risk factors and CVD outcomes in CKD is for the most part consistent with the relationships described in the general population, but some differences have been noted. For example, 'U'-shaped relationships exist between all-cause mortality and both blood pressure and cholesterol levels in dialysis patients. Interestingly, the troughs (lowest risk) occur at higher levels of blood pressure and cholesterol than seen in the general population, perhaps reflecting confounding from underlying cardiomyopathy in subjects with lower blood pressure and malnutrition in subjects with lower cholesterol.

Table 57 Traditional and nontraditional cardiovascular risk factors in chronic kidney disease

Traditional	Nontraditional
Older age	Albuminuria
Male gender	Hyperhomcysteinemia
Hypertension	Anemia
Higher LDL C	Abnormal calcium/phosphate metabolism
Lower HDL C	Extracellular fluid volume overload
	Electrolyte imbalance
Diabetes	Oxidative stress
Smoking	Inflammation
Physical inactivity	Malnutrition
Menopause	Thrombogenic factors
Family history of cardiovascular disease	Altered nitric oxide/endothelin balance
Left ventricular hypertrophy	Sleep disturbances

HDL C: high-density lipoprotein cholesterol; LDL C: low-density lipoprotein cholesterol. (Reproduced and modified with permission from Sarnak et al. [2000]. Cardiovascular disease and chronic renal disease: a new paradigm. Am. J. Kidney Dis. **35**(Suppl. 1):S117–S131.)

Nontraditional risk factors

Homocysteine

Levels of homocysteine are inversely correlated with the level of GFR; thus 85% of dialysis patients have hyperhomocysteinemia defined by levels >95th percentile in the general population. There are no studies which have shown that treatment of hyperhomocysteinemia reduces CVD outcomes in CKD. Furthermore, hyperhomocysteinemia in dialysis patients is relatively refractory to folate supplementation, making treatment challenging.

C-reactive protein

C-reactive protein (CRP) is a circulating marker of inflammation that is often elevated in dialysis patients. Several studies have demonstrated independent associations between levels of CRP and CVD outcomes, suggesting that inflammation may play an important role in promoting atherosclerosis in CKD.

Oxidant stress

Oxidant stress is also more prevalent and oxidant defenses less available in CKD. This may result in inhibition of normal endothelial function, predisposing to atherosclerosis. Two small, randomized controlled trials in dialysis patients have demonstrated reductions in CVD outcomes with the antioxidants vitamin E and N-acetyl cysteine[9,10].

Abnormal calcium and phosphorus metabolism

Patients with CKD often have elevated phosphorus levels, elevated calcium × phosphorus concentration products, and increased parathyroid hormone levels. These abnormalities result in extremely high electron-beam computed tomography (EBCT) coronary calcium scores and widespread tissue calcification. The latter may lead to diminished large vessel compliance and increased CVD events.

Anemia

With loss of kidney function, endogenous erythropoietin production decreases leading to chronic anemia. Chronic anemia in turn is a risk factor for LVH and both *de novo* and recurrent heart failure, as well as all-cause mortality in dialysis patients. Recombinant human erythropoietin is used to treat anemia in CKD, with a target hemoglobin of 11–12 g/dl. There are, however, no randomized controlled trials that have shown that correction of anemia results in decreased CVD events or all-cause mortality.

SUMMARY

Methods to decrease the burden of CVD in CKD involve earlier recognition of kidney disease, with a goal of both reducing kidney disease progression and preventing CVD. Subjects with CKD are in the highest risk group for CVD outcomes, and aggressive treatment of both traditional as well as nontraditional CVD risk factors is therefore recommended.

Chapter Twenty

Primary Prevention

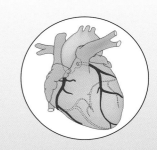

PRIMARY PREVENTION

STEVE LEE, MD AND NOEL BAIREY MERZ, MD

INTRODUCTION

Primary prevention of cardiovascular disease (CVD) refers to preventing the onset of disease in patients who have no previous history of cardiovascular disease. This involves both preventing the development of risk factors before they occur, and modifying any cardiovascular risk factors that may already be present. Population studies have identified a number of risk factors that are associated with the development of CVD:

- Age (men ≥45 years, women ≥55 years or postmenopausal).
- Family history of coronary artery disease (CAD) in first degree relatives (male <55 years, female <65 years).
- Smoking.
- Hypertension (blood pressure ≥140/90 mmHg [18.7/12 kPa]).
- Diabetes mellitus.
- Low-density lipoprotein (LDL) cholesterol ≥160 mg/dl (4.1mmol/l).
- High-density lipoprotein (HDL) cholesterol <40 mg/dl (1mmol/l) in men, <50 mg/dl (1.3 mmol/l) in women; if HDL cholesterol ≥ 60 mg/dl (1.55 mmol/l), subtract 1 risk factor.

While age and family history are risk factors that cannot be modified, smoking, hypertension, diabetes, and cholesterol levels are factors that can potentially be prevented or, if already present, optimized (*Table 58*).

SMOKING

Cigarette smoking is considered the single most modifiable risk factor for the development of CVD. According to the Centers for Disease Control, up to 30% of all coronary heart disease deaths in the USA can be attributed to cigarette smoking, with the risk being strongly dose-related. Moreover, numerous studies have shown a decrease in cardiac deaths when smoking is stopped, with the increased cardiovascular risk for smokers returning to that of a nonsmoker approximately 5 years after cessation. Cigar and pipe smoking also carry an increased risk.

Table 58 Categories of risk factors

Causative risk factors:
- Cigarette smoking.
- Elevated blood pressure.
- Elevated serum cholesterol (or LDL C) or elevated apolipoprotein B.
- Low HDL C.
- Diabetes mellitus.

Coronary plaque burden as a risk factor:
- Age.
- Nonspecific ST segment changes on resting ECG.

Conditional risk factors:
- Triglycerides*.
- Small LDL particles*.
- Lp(a)*.
- Homocysteine*.
- Coagulation factors*:
  Plasminogen activating factor inhibitor-1.
  Fibrinogen.
- C-reactive protein.

Predisposing risk factors:
- Overweight and obesity (especially abdominal obesity)[†].
- Physical inactivity[†].
- Male sex.
- Family history of premature CAD.
- Socioeconomic factors.
- Behavioral factors (e.g. mental depression).
- Insulin resistance.

Susceptibility risk factor:
- Left ventricular hypertrophy.

*These factors are considered conditional risk factors when serum levels are abnormally high. [†]Obesity and physical inactivity are counted as major risk factors by the American Heart Association. CAD: coronary artery disease; ECG: electrocardiogram; HDL C: high-density lipoprotein cholesterol; LDL: low-density lipoprotein cholesterol; Lp(a): lipoprotein a. (Modified from Smith *et al.* [2000]. AHA Conference Proceedings. Prevention conference V: Beyond secondary prevention: Identifying the high-risk patient for primary prevention: executive summary. American Heart Association. *Circulation* **101**:111–116.)

The goal for smokers is complete cessation. It is recommended to ask about smoking status as part of every routine evaluation, to reinforce nonsmoking status when possible, and to encourage patients and family members strongly to stop smoking and to avoid secondhand smoke. When required, it may be necessary to provide counseling, formal cessation programs, and nicotine replacement.

CHOLESTEROL

Elevated blood total and LDL cholesterol, elevated triglycerides (Tgs), and low HDL cholesterol are associated with a higher risk for the development of CVD. Conversely, a high HDL cholesterol (≥60 mg/dl [1.55 mmol/l]) is considered to have a protective effect and is therefore considered a negative cardiovascular risk factor. Numerous studies have shown that controlling cholesterol levels reduces the incidence of cardiac events.

Although specific recommendations for cholesterol screening vary, it is generally accepted that cholesterol levels should be checked routinely in individuals at high risk for CVD (e.g. multiple other risk factors) as well as in young healthy adults in whom cholesterol awareness may lead to lifestyle modifications. The American Heart Association (AHA) recommends that total and HDL cholesterol levels be measured in all adults over 20 years of age, and positive and negative risk factors for heart disease be evaluated at least every 5 years. If total cholesterol is >200 mg/dl (5.2 mmol/l) or if HDL is <40 mg/dl (1 mmol/l) in men or <50 mg/dl (1.3 mmol/l) in women, then the LDL cholesterol should be measured.

The AHA recommends the following goals for primary prevention:

Primary goals:
- LDL <160 mg/dl (4.1 mmol/l) if 0–1 risk factors are present.
- LDL <130 mg/dl (3.4 mmol/l) if 2 risk factors are present.
- LDL <100 mg/dl (2.6 mmol/l) if diabetic.

Secondary goals:
- HDL ≥40 mg/dl (1 mmol/l) for men, or ≥50 mg/dl (1.3 mmol/l) for women.
- Tgs <150 mg/dl (1.7 mmol/l).

Options for controlling cholesterol levels include diet modification, weight control, exercise, and drug therapy (e.g. statins, fibrates, niacin) (**366, 367**).

BLOOD PRESSURE

Hypertension is an independent risk factor for CVD. Numerous studies have shown that elevations in both systolic and diastolic blood pressure are consistently and proportionally associated with increased cardiovascular morbidity and mortality. Moreover, blood pressure control has been shown to reduce the incidence of cardiovascular events.

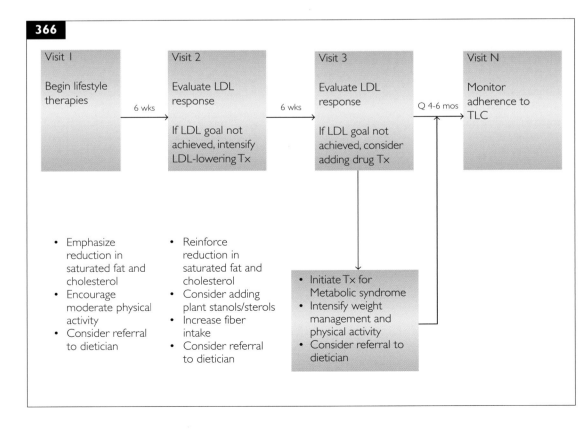

366

Visit I	Visit 2	Visit 3	Visit N
Begin lifestyle therapies	→ 6 wks → Evaluate LDL response	→ 6 wks → Evaluate LDL response	→ Q 4-6 mos → Monitor adherence to TLC
	If LDL goal not achieved, intensify LDL-lowering Tx	If LDL goal not achieved, consider adding drug Tx	

- Emphasize reduction in saturated fat and cholesterol
- Encourage moderate physical activity
- Consider referral to dietician

- Reinforce reduction in saturated fat and cholesterol
- Consider adding plant stanols/sterols
- Increase fiber intake
- Consider referral to dietician

- Initiate Tx for Metabolic syndrome
- Intensify weight management and physical activity
- Consider referral to dietician

366 Low-density lipoprotein lowering: lifestyle changes. LDL: low-density lipoprotein; TLC: therapeutic lifestyle changes; Tx: treatment. (Modified from Grundy *et al.* [2002]. Third Report of the National Cholesterol Education Program (NCEP) Expert Panel on Detection, Evaluation, and Treatment of High Blood Cholesterol in Adults (Adult Treatment Panel III): Final Report. NIH Publication No. 02-5215; reprinted in *Circulation* **106**:3143–3421.)

The AHA recommends checking blood pressure in all adults at least every 2–2.5 years, and to maintain a goal blood pressure of <140/90 mmHg (18.7/12 kPa) (<130/80 mmHg [17.3/10.7 kPa] in patients with heart failure, diabetes, or renal insufficiency). Options for controlling blood pressure include diet modification (including moderation in alcohol consumption, sodium restriction, and an eating plan that is low in saturated fat, 5–9 daily combined servings of fruits and vegetables, and three daily servings of nonfat dairy product [DASH diet]), weight control, exercise, and drug therapy (*Table 59*).

DIABETES MELLITUS

Diabetes is an independent risk factor for the development of CVD. Up to 80% of deaths in diabetic patients are from complications of CVD, with the majority of these deaths from CAD. In addition, people with diabetes but no history of CAD are considered to have the same risk for coronary events as people with established CAD. However, the United Kingdom Prospective Diabetes Survey (UKPDS) showed that improved blood glucose control reduces the incidence of heart attacks and heart failure. Therefore, diabetes and blood glucose should be controlled as aggressively as possible with diet, exercise, weight control, and appropriate hypoglycemic therapy.

DIET, OBESITY, AND PHYSICAL INACTIVITY

In addition to the risk factors listed above, studies have shown that diet, obesity, and physical inactivity are associated with CVD. These factors are of course also strongly linked to elevated cholesterol, hypertension, and diabetes/glucose intolerance. Eating a healthy diet (*Table 59*), controlling weight, and exercising regularly will therefore potentially carry manifold benefits.

HORMONE REPLACEMENT THERAPY

Hormone replacement therapy (HRT) with estrogen and progestin has traditionally been considered an option for primary prevention of heart disease in postmenopausal women. Recent findings from the Women's Health Initiative, however, have provided compelling evidence that HRT does not reduce a woman's risk of developing heart disease, but rather is associated with an increased risk of CVD and thrombotic events (see chapter 19, Women and Hormones).

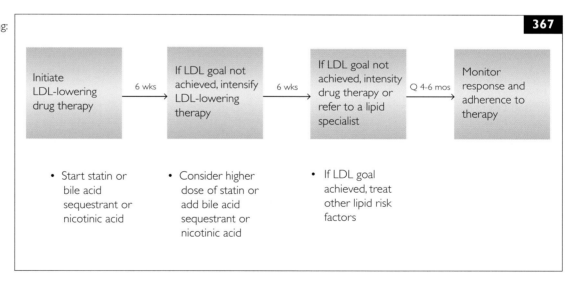

367 Low-density lipoprotein (LDL) lowering: drug therapy. (Modified from: Grundy *et al.* [2002]. Third Report of the National Cholesterol Education Program (NCEP) Expert Panel on Detection, Evaluation, and Treatment of High Blood Cholesterol in Adults (Adult Treatment Panel III): Final Report. NIH Publication No. 02-5215; reprinted in *Circulation* **106**:3143–3421.)

367

Initiate LDL-lowering drug therapy

→ 6 wks →

If LDL goal not achieved, intensify LDL-lowering therapy

→ 6 wks →

If LDL goal not achieved, intensity drug therapy or refer to a lipid specialist

→ Q 4-6 mos →

Monitor response and adherence to therapy

- Start statin or bile acid sequestrant or nicotinic acid

- Consider higher dose of statin or add bile acid sequestrant or nicotinic acid

- If LDL goal achieved, treat other lipid risk factors

Table 59 The DASH diet

Following the DASH Eating Plan

The DASH eating plan shown below is based on 2,000 calories a day. The number of daily servings in a food group may vary from those listed, depending on your caloric needs. Use this chart to help you plan your menus or take it with you when you go to the store.

Food group	Daily servings (except as noted)	Serving sizes	Examples and notes	Significance of each food group to the DASH eating plan
Grains and grain products	7–8	1 slice bread 1 oz dry cereal* 1/2 cup cooked rice, pasta, or cereal	Whole wheat bread, English muffin, pita bread, bagel, cereals, grits, oatmeal, crackers, unsalted pretzels and popcorn	Major sources of energy and fiber
Vegetables	4–5	1 cup raw leafy vegetable 1/2 cup cooked vegetable 6 oz vegetable juice	Tomatoes, potatoes, carrots, green peas, squash, broccoli, turnip greens, collards, kale, spinach, artichokes, green beans, lima beans, sweet potatoes	Rich sources of potassium, magnesium, and fiber
Fruits	4–5	6 oz fruit juice 1 medium fruit 1/4 cup dried fruit 1/2 cup fresh, frozen, or canned fruit	Apricots, bananas, dates, grapes, oranges, orange juice, grapefruit, grapefruit juice, mangoes, melons, peaches, pineapples, prunes, raisins, strawberries, tangerines	Important sources of potassium, magnesium, and fiber
Lowfat or fat free dairy foods	2–3	8 oz milk 1 cup yogurt 1 1/2 oz cheese	Fat free (skim) or lowfat (1%) milk, fat free or lowfat buttermilk, fat free or lowfat regular or frozen yogurt, lowfat and fat free cheese	Major sources of calcium and protein
Meats, poultry, and fish	2 or less	3 oz cooked meats, poultry, or fish	Select only lean; trim away visible fats; broil, roast, or boil, instead of frying; remove skin from poultry	Rich sources of protein and magnesium
Nuts, seeds, and dry beans	4–5 per week	1/3 cup or 1 1/2 oz nuts 2 Tbsp or 1/2 oz seeds 1/2 cup cooked dry beans	Almonds, filberts, mixed nuts, peanuts, walnuts, sunflower seeds, kidney beans, lentils, peas	Rich sources of energy, magnesium, potassium, protein, and fiber
Fats and oils†	2–3	1 tsp soft margarine 1 Tbsp lowfat mayonnaise 2 Tbsp light salad dressing 1 tsp vegetable oil	Soft margarine, lowfat mayonnaise, light salad dressing, vegetable oil (such as olive, corn, canola, or safflower)	DASH has 27 percent of calories as fat, including fat in or added to foods
Sweets	5 per week	1 Tbsp sugar 1 Tbsp jelly or jam 1/2 oz jelly beans 8 oz lemonade	Maple syrup, sugar, jelly, jam, fruit-flavored gelatin, jelly beans, hard candy, fruit punch, sorbet, ices	Sweets should be low in fat

*Equals 1/2 – 1 1/4 cups, depending on cereal type. Check the product's Nutrition Facts Label.
†Fat content changes serving counts for fats and oils: For example, 1 Tbsp of regular salad dressing equals 1 serving; 1 Tbsp of a lowfat dressing equals 1/2 serving; 1 Tbsp of a fat free dressing equals 0 servings.

(Modified from The DASH (Dietary Approaches to Stop Hypertension) Study (2001). NIH Publication No. 01-4082.)

Chapter Twenty-One

Genetics of Ischemic Heart Disease

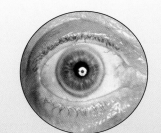

GENETICS OF ISCHEMIC HEART DISEASE

ANNE TYBJÆRG-HANSEN, MD, PhD

INTRODUCTION

Genetic variation affecting the risk of ischemic heart disease (IHD) is mainly due to mutations in genes encoding apolipoproteins, lipid metabolizing enzymes, and lipoprotein receptors influencing lipid and lipoprotein metabolism. The most common of these mutations affect the regulation of low density lipoprotein (LDL) cholesterol in plasma, leading to severe monogenic hyper-cholesterolemia. Elevated plasma LDL cholesterol levels are causally related to IHD[1,2], and a reduction in these levels reduces the incidence of IHD[3–5] and the associated mortality rate[3,4]. Elevated LDL cholesterol levels may be caused by decreased removal of LDL from plasma, as a result of either mutations in the LDL receptor (LDLR) gene (*LDLR*), as in classic familial hypercholesterolemia (FH)[6], or mutations in the ligand domain of the apolipoprotein B gene (*APOB*), affecting binding of LDL to the LDLR. Apolipoprotein B (apoB) is the chief protein component of LDL and serves as the ligand for the removal of LDL from the circulation by the LDLR. Familial ligand-defective apolipoprotein B (FLDB) results from mutations affecting the structure and function of the ligand binding domain of apoB[7–10], while FH results from numerous different mutations affecting the structure and function of the LDLR itself[6].

EPIDEMIOLOGY

Both types of disorder are characterized biochemically by an elevation in the concentration of LDL-bound cholesterol in plasma, pathologically by premature IHD and, in some patients, by cholesterol deposits that form tendon xanthomas, and genetically by autosomal dominant inheritance. In populations of European descent, FLDB with hypercholesterolemia is mainly due to a single mutation in *APOB* (CGG>CAG; Arg3500Gln) with a heterozygote frequency of 1 in 500 to 1 in 1000[11–13]. The mutation is rare among individuals of non-European origin. Haplotype analysis in several populations suggests a strong founder gene effect[14]. By contrast, FH is caused by more than 500 different mutations all together, with a heterozygote frequency of about 1 in 500[6]. A remarkably high prevalence of FH has been noted in certain areas of the world[6]. As expected, homozygotes, who inherit two mutant genes at the FLDB locus, the LDL receptor locus, or one at each locus, are very rare (2 in 1,000,000), and are more severely affected than the corresponding heterozygotes.

PATHOGENESIS

In humans, most plasma cholesterol is transported in LDL. This lipoprotein consists of a central core composed of apolar lipids (triglycerides and cholesteryl esters) and an outer shell of phospholipids, unesterified cholesterol, and a single apoB molecule as its protein component. Cholesterol in plasma is used for the synthesis of steroid hormones and cell membranes. Excess cholesterol is removed by the liver mainly via receptor-mediated endocytosis by the LDL-receptor and is either used for resynthesis of lipoproteins or excreted. Thus, defects in the LDLR or in the receptor-binding region of apoB due to mutations in the *LDLR* or in the putative binding domain of *APOB* will result in increased LDL cholesterol levels in plasma, and an increased risk of atherosclerosis and premature IHD (**368**). Heterozygous FLDB is generally associated

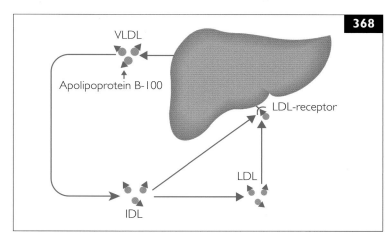

368 Uptake of low-density lipoprotein (LDL) via the LDL receptor (LDLR) and apolipoprotein B (apoB). Very low-density lipoprotein (VLDL) is produced in the liver and most VLDL triglycerides are hydrolyzed in extrahepatic tissues by lipoprotein lipase to yield intermediate-density lipoprotein (IDL) or remnant particles. LDLRs on hepatocytes recognize apolipoprotein E on VLDL and mediate the endocytosis of some of these particles. A substantial fraction, however, are further processed by hepatic lipase to yield LDL. LDL is taken up by LDLRs, which recognize a binding domain on apoB. When mutations are present in the *LDLR* or *APOB* genes this uptake of LDL may be dysfunctional and result in accumulation of LDL particles in plasma and thus in hypercholesterolemia.

with lower mean LDL cholesterol levels than heterozygous FH and, perhaps, with less coronary atherosclerosis[6,13].

CLINICAL PRESENTATION

For heterozygotes, the earliest manifestation is hypercholesterolemia, which is present already in childhood in many affected subjects, and remains the only clinical finding throughout the second to third decade. Tendon xanthomas – especially in the Achilles tendons, in the extensor tendons of the hand, and in the patellar tendons – may appear at the end of the third decade in those with the highest cholesterol levels (**369**). Clinical symptoms of IHD appear from the fourth decade onwards, generally about 10 years earlier in men than in women [6,15]. Although both FH and FLDB may be associated with a wide range of expression of LDL cholesterol levels, the average increase in cholesterol levels for FLDB heterozygotes is about 2.0 mmol/l (77 mg/dl) (**370**) while it is about 3–5 mmol/l (116–193 mg/dl) for FH heterozygotes[6,13]. The average increase in risk of IHD is 7–20-fold (**370**), dependent mainly on the magnitude of the increase in cholesterol levels[6,13]. While homozygotes for FLDB seem to have cholesterol levels similar to those of the more severely affected FH heterozygotes, FH homozygotes have very severe hypercholesterolemia (16–25 mmol/l [618–968 mg/dl]). Cutaneous xanthomas appear within the first years of life and death from IHD is most often before 20 years of age[6].

GENETIC ASPECTS

A tentative clinical diagnosis can be made if the hypercholesterolemic patient has tendon xanthomas (**369**) or a pedigree in which one of the parents and about one-half of the first degree relatives have hypercholesterolemia in association with tendon xanthomas, and/or

premature IHD. However, many heterozygotes, especially those with FLDB, lack tendon xanthomas. The ultimate diagnosis of FLDB or FH relies on the detection of Arg3500Gln or Arg3500Trp in *APOB*, or a mutation in the *LDLR* in genomic deoxyribonucleic acid (DNA) from the patient. DNA can be extracted from fresh or frozen whole blood, from blood spots on filter paper, or from buccal swabs. Mutations are generally detected by polymerase chain reaction (PCR) amplification of relevant parts of the gene (*APOB*) or the whole gene (*LDLR*), followed by determination of the base sequence of the PCR products, often preceded by a prescreening method (dHPLC, SSCP, DGGE). Deletions, insertions, or major rearrangements may be detected by Southern blot analysis or other methods. Once the specific family mutation has been identified in the patient, all the first degree relatives regardless of disease status should be screened for this mutation. The value of these predictive screenings above measuring plasma cholesterol once a year in all relatives for the rest of their life is the same as for all other predictive genetic screening: only individuals who test positive for the mutation (about one-half of all first degree relatives) enter the surveillance program, and the diagnosis in these individuals can be made at a very early stage before complications arise.

TREATMENT

Treatment of FLDB and FH is aimed at reducing levels of LDL cholesterol in order to retard the progression of atherosclerotic lesions and decrease the risk of IHD. Statins are efficient drugs in lowering LDL cholesterol both in FLDB and in most FH heterozygotes, and may be tried in the rare FLDB homozygotes[6,15]. Patients with homozygous FH respond poorly to any kind of drug therapy. The current preferred treatment of homozygous FH is selective removal of apoB-containing lipoproteins by LDL apheresis[16].

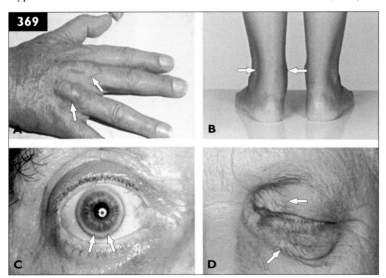

369 Cholesterol deposits outside the vascular wall. Tendon xanthomas in the extensor tendons of the hand (**A**) and in the Achilles tendons (**B**); arcus corneae (**C**); xanthelasmas around the eyes (**D**). While tendon xanthomas are characteristic of very high cholesterol levels caused by *LDLR* mutations or mutations in the binding domain of *APOB*, arcus corneae and xanthelasmas are also found with lower cholesterol levels and in some cases are familial. Tendon xanthomas or xanthelasmas regress or disappear when plasma cholesterol levels are reduced.

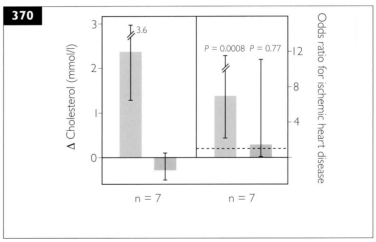

370 Average increase in plasma cholesterol (left) and odds ratio for ischemic heart disease (right) in heterozygotes for two different ligand defective mutations in apolipoprotein B: Arg3500Gln (pink bars) and Arg3531Cys (green bars). Only the Arg3500Gln mutation is associated with a significant increase in cholesterol levels and an increased odds ratio for ischemic heart disease. The broken line corresponds to an odds ratio = 1. From Tybjaerg-Hansen et al. [1998]. Association of mutations in the apolipoprotein B gene with hypercholesterolemia and the risk of ischemic heart disease. *N. Engl. J. Med.* **338**:1577–84.)

Chapter Twenty-Two

Stem Cell Therapy in Acute Myocardial Infarction

STEM CELL THERAPY IN ACUTE MYOCARDIAL INFARCTION

JENS KASTRUP, MD, DMSC

INTRODUCTION

The prognosis after an acute ST elevation myocardial infarction (STEMI) has improved considerably after the introduction of acute treatment regimes with aspirin, thrombolysis, and primary percutaneous coronary intervention (primary PCI). However, many people still suffer from severe congestive heart failure symptoms after a STEMI, caused by necrosis and remodeling of the left ventricular myocardium. In an attempt to find and introduce new treatment regimes, stem cell therapy is currently under investigation, to see whether it could improve the myocardial perfusion and function of the left ventricle after STEMI.

STEM CELLS FOR VASCULOGENESIS OR MYOGENESIS, OR BOTH?

Human bone marrow contains adult mesenchymal stem cells, which, by stimulation, can differentiate into different cell lines, including endothelial, osteal, chondral, and muscle cell types[1]. Within cardiology, the focus has been on initiating vasculogenesis and myogenesis in ischemic myocardium from stem cells[2]. By stimulating the cells with a variety of growth factors, it has been possible to differentiate several different mesenchymal stem cell lines into endothelial cells and also some to myoblasts[1,2]. In animal studies, stem cells delivered systemically have been demonstrated to incorporate into newly developed blood vessels after STEMI, but not all have been found to differentiate into myocytes. In human stem cell studies, therefore, the aim has been to initiate the development of new blood vessels in ischemic myocardium from stem cells.

Whether the myocardium after a STEMI by itself produces the factors such as stromal-derived factor 1 (SDF-1) to attract circulating stem cells, or the growth factors to induce differentiation of stem cells is, at present, uncertain[3].

WHICH CELLS TO USE IN CLINICAL TRIALS?

It is possible to obtain adult stem cells from bone marrow aspirations or circulating blood. The cells used in most clinical trials have been mononucleated cells (MNCs) obtained by Ficoll density separation (**371A**)[4-7]. However, this cell suspension only contains 1–3% CD34+/CD45+ stem cells, the majority of the cells being leucocytes, lymphocytes, monocytes, and megacaryocytes[8]. A further separation can increase the CD133+ stem cells to 3–8% (**371B**)[9]. In one center, circulating progenitor cells were harvested from venous blood and cultivated for 3 days before use for injection therapy, and >90% of these cells demonstrated endothelial markers (**371C**)[5-7]. In addition, purified stem cells can be expanded in cultivation (**371C**). Whether there are any differences in clinical treatment effects between the different cell lines used is unknown. In addition, several stem cell lines with other surface markers have demonstrated the capacity to differentiate into endothelial cells and form blood vessels[1]. The stem cell CD34-/CD45- can differentiate into endothelial cells using vascular endothelial growth factor (VEGF) stimulation (**372**). The MNC solution content of leucocytes and monocytes produces a variety of growth factors, which themselves may effect treatment or may be of benefit for the differentiation of the stem cell solution produced.

HOW TO DELIVER THE STEM CELLS?

The main problem immediately after a primary PCI-treated STEMI is the amount of necrotic myocardium and number of poorly perfused coronary vessels (no reflow), due to distal microembolization and/or microvascular spasm in combination with impaired perfusion in necrotic myocardium (as described in Chapter 12, Downstream (Micro)Embolization, Slow Flow, and No Reflow). How the stem cells should be delivered to the target region is therefore under discussion. Acutely after a STEMI, the stem cells cannot be injected directly into or around the necrotic myocardium with a percutaneous approach as performed in gene or stem cell therapy studies in chronic myocardial ischemia[9,10]. In one study, stem cells were injected directly into the infarct border zone during bypass surgery 10–90 days after STEMI[8]. The most frequently used method has been the direct intracoronary delivery method[4,5]. Approximately 5 days after primary PCI treatment with a stent, a perfusion balloon was placed within the stent in the infarct related artery (**373**). During a 3-minute balloon inflation, 2–3 ml cell suspension was infused into the artery. After a short reperfusion period, the process was repeated until the final volume of 6–9 ml had been delivered. However, it is debatable how many of the cells

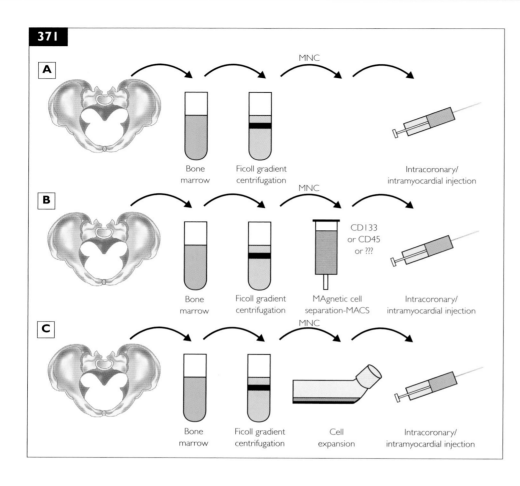

371 Methods of preparing stem cells for clinical trials. **A**: Mononuclear cells (MNC) are prepared from a bone marrow aspirate by Ficoll gradient centrifugation, and after washing are used for injection therapy. **B**: After the Ficoll gradient separation, the MNC can be divided into subgroup stem cell populations characterized by surface markers as CD133 or CD45 by magnetic cell sorting (MACS), and are used for injection therapy. **C**: Stem cells from bone marrow or blood can be expanded from the MNC population by cultivation. The cells attached to the dishes are considered to be mesenchymal stem cells.

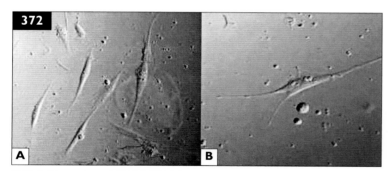

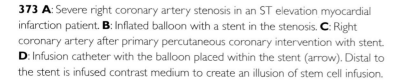

372 A: Mesenchymal CD34-/CD45- stem cells expanded by cultivation for 2 weeks. **B**: Endothelial cell differentiated from a CD34-/CD45- stem cell by stimulation with vascular endothelial growth factor.

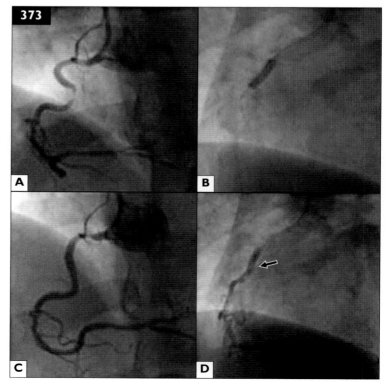

373 A: Severe right coronary artery stenosis in an ST elevation myocardial infarction patient. **B**: Inflated balloon with a stent in the stenosis. **C**: Right coronary artery after primary percutaneous coronary intervention with stent. **D**: Infusion catheter with the balloon placed within the stent (arrow). Distal to the stent is infused contrast medium to create an illusion of stem cell infusion.

actually reached the target tissue area due to no reflow, and whether the injected cells were attracted to and had time to cross the capillary wall into the tissue, or whether the majority of cells were simply transferred through the myocardium. It can also be speculated whether the intracoronary delivery method involves too short a cell stimulation period to induce vasculogenesis. A more rational and less invasive treatment protocol could be a prolonged stimulation period by mobilization of stem cells from the bone marrow into the circulation for several days immediately after the STEMI by subcutaneous injection of the stem cell mobilization factor, granulocyte colony-stimulating factor (G-CSF). An ongoing double-blind placebo-controlled trial is currently investigating this treatment regime.

CLINICAL TRIALS

Based on the encouraging results in animal studies, three small clinical safety and efficacy trials in STEMI patients from three centers have been published[5–8]. A total of 56 patients were treated with different cell types and application methods, and in two of the studies a nonrandomized, nonplacebo-treated control group was included. None of the studies reported any serious side-effects of the treatments. They all demonstrated a beneficial effect on left ventricular function, geometry, and contractility within the cell-treated group but not within the control group, using echocardiography, single photon emission computerized tomography (SPECT), magnetic resonance imaging (MRI), positron emission tomography (PET), and ventriculography. However, there seemed to be no significant difference between the cell-treated group and the control group for these parameters, maybe due to the small number of patients included. It has been suggested that a beneficial effect of stem cell treatment in STEMI patients is due to stimulation of neoangiogenesis, which limits myocyte apoptosis, reduces collagen deposition and scar formation, and thereby influences late remodeling.

CONCLUSION

Stem cell therapy in STEMI patients treated with primary PCI is still an experimental but promising treatment. The results of larger randomized double-blind placebo-controlled studies are awaited before it can be decided whether stem cell therapy should be added to the existing treatment regimes.

Chapter Twenty-Three

Guidelines and Recommendations

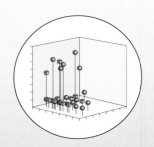

GUIDELINES AND RECOMMENDATIONS

STEEN E. HUSTED, MD, DSCI AND BIRGITTE K. ZIEGLER, MD

INTRODUCTION

The main reasons for developing clinical guidelines are the desire of health care professionals to offer, and patients to receive, the best care possible. Since not every individual patient fits into a box in a clinical guideline, the latter alone is not enough; guideline information must be combined with the clinical experience of the doctor in order to decide whether the evidence applies to the individual patient and how it should be integrated into clinical practice. This combination creates a dynamic state of learning and teaching, which may help to improve health care and cost-effectiveness.

GUIDELINES MUST BE REGULARLY UPDATED

A guideline is a distillation of the available evidence within a certain area, and in an area such as ischemic heart disease with continuous research and an increasing number of trials and amount of evidence, the guidelines must be reviewed on a regular basis in order to keep them up to date in relation to current science.

HOW TO IMPLEMENT GUIDELINES

The results from a randomized controlled trial (RCT) are obtained with optimized diagnostic and treatment regimens, and often in selected groups of patients fulfilling strict inclusion and exclusion criteria. In order to achieve the same effect in daily clinical practice and thereby improve morbidity and mortality in patients, it is important that the guidelines are implemented with the correct dose in comparable groups of patients with thorough control of treatment effect. Moreover, it has been documented that guideline-concordant treatment is associated with improved outcome[1].

BARRIERS FOR IMPLEMENTATION

Barriers for implementing a guideline are numerous. Examples are:
- Distance (both geographic and professional) between the authors of the guideline and the treating physicians.
- Increasing health care costs, with the newest drugs/interventions being more expensive than the older ones.
- Different sets of guidelines from various organizations makes it difficult for clinicians to follow one universal set of recommendations.
- Lack of time for most doctors to spend time on literature search and reading.
- Unawareness of the guideline; lack of motivation.
- Lack of patient compliance due to polypharmacy.

CONTINUOUS SURVEILLANCE

Control of any impact due to implementation of a guideline is very important, since it can identify both over- and undertreatment[2]. An international survey such as the EUROASPIRE or a national database can form a continuous, dynamic surveillance with the possibility of providing up-to-date information on which treatment is actually given for specific populations of patients, and whether it influences prognosis. Another reason for the need for control is that most trials are restricted in some way, i.e. in patient population, concomitant treatment, treatment procedures, and others. In clinical practice, deviations from this are unavoidable and may reveal some so far unknown side-effects or interactions. As an example, national databases have shown that the median age of the patient population treated in daily practice with thrombolysis in acute myocardial infarction (AMI) is >10 years older than the median age of patients in the major RCTs. This is important since older patients have a significantly higher risk of bleeding complications. In the future, a web-based approach that integrates computerized guidelines and electronic medical records may be a solution to some of these problems.

NATIONAL GUIDELINES

There are different definitions of levels of evidence and grades of recommendation. The most commonly used evidence levels are A, B, and C and recommendation grades 1 and 2 (*Table 60*). The recommendation to use or not to use a specific treatment or diagnostic test is a trade-off between benefits and risk/cost. When benefits and risk/cost are balanced, conflicts between different guidelines and recommendations may be seen, and in this situation the characteristics of the specific patient become important in the decision of whether or how to treat. Guidelines should aim to minimize those variations in service delivery that are presumed to be due to inappropriate care. The variations can be observed both locally, nationally, and internationally.

It is not realistic to expect all nations to implement all parts of a large international guideline. The national scientific societies should aim to adjust the guidelines according to national needs and options. These adaptations may have a strong impact on the implementation of a guideline. For general physicians and for doctors who are not working only in cardiology, surveys have shown that summaries of information reinforced by recommendations by local respected specialists/authorities have a much higher chance of affecting the behavior of the physicians than international guidelines.

Table 61 shows examples of existing international recommendations for the USA and Europe and a national Danish

Table 60 Levels of evidence and grades of recommendation

Grade	Clarity of benefit/risk	Methodological strength of underlying evidence	Implications
1A	Clear	Meta-analysis; randomized trials without important limitations and with consistent results	Strong recommendation; can apply to most patients in most circumstances. Useful and effective
1B	Clear	Randomized trials with limitations (small numbers of patients, inconsistent results, methodological problems). Careful analyzed nonrandomized/observational studies	Strong recommendations, likely to apply to most patients
1C	Clear	Observational studies, expert opinion	Intermediate strength recommendations; may change when stronger evidence becomes available
2A	Unclear	Randomized trials without important limitations	Recommendations in favor of usefulness and efficacy
2B	Unclear	Randomized trials with limitations (small number of patients, inconsistent results, methodological problems)	Recommendations weaker in favor of usefulness and efficacy
2C	Unclear	Observational studies, expert opinion	Very weak recommendations; other alternatives may be equally reasonable

Table 61 Example of levels of recommendations for selected treatment modalities in patients with unstable angina pectoris or non-ST segment elevation myocardial infarction in the USA, Europe, and Denmark

Treatment	USA (March 2002)	Europe (Sept. 2000)	Denmark (April 2002)
Acetylsalicylic acid	1A	A	1A
Clopidogrel alone (acetylsalicylic acid allergy/ intolerance)	1A	C	1A
Clopidogrel + acetylsalicylic acid	1B	-	1B
Beta blocker acutely	1B	B	1B
Beta blocker long-term	1A	A	1A
GP IIb/IIIa for planned PCI	1A	A	1A
GP IIb/IIIa for high-risk patients and no PCI	1A	-	-
Statin, LDL >130 mg/dl (3.4 mmol/l)	1A	-	1B
LMWH	1A	A	1A
Early intervention with ST depression and/ or raised markers	1A	B	1A
Exercise test in low/intermediate-risk patients	1C	-	-

GP IIb/IIIa: glycoprotein IIb/IIIa receptor antagonist; LDL: low-density lipoprotein; LMWH: low-molecular weight heparin; PCI: percutaneous coronary intervention.

recommendation, covering treatment of unstable angina pectoris (UAP) and non-ST segment elevation myocardial infarction (NSTEMI). The differences are probably caused by variations in the interpretation of existing data and by adjustment to local options, and are additionally influenced by the fact that two of the guidelines were updated in 2002 while the European recommendation is from 2000.

LEGAL BINDING OF GUIDELINES

It is worth noting that guidelines from, for instance, the European Society of Cardiology, have no specific authority and are not legally binding[3]. They may, though, have potential legal significance as state-of-the-art and expert evidence. On the contrary, in the USA, guidelines can be legally binding and serve as an important evidence document in a possible trial. However, recommendations and guidelines should not be seen as dictates, but as an important tool in daily clinical decision making. They cannot take into account the compelling individual circumstances of the single patient.

HOMEPAGES

The guidelines and updates from the large international societies of cardiology (American and European) can be downloaded from their homepage. On these homepages, there are links to most national societies of cardiology, where national guidelines can be found if available on-line:

- European Society of Cardiology[4]: www.escardio.org
- American Heart Association[5]: www.americanheart.org
- American College of Cardiology[6]: www.acc.org

FUTURE NEEDS

Very few of the guidelines contain data on cost-effectiveness. The gap between treatment possibilities and actual treatment availability is growing, mostly due to an escalation in the treatment possibilities; implantation of cardioverter defibrillators (ICD) is a good example. Rising health care costs is an increasing problem throughout the world, and future research should incorporate this issue. A possibility could be for future guidelines to indicate a 'minimum standard of care' and thereby prevent unrealistic expectations[3]. It would be an optimal goal if the currently available resources were used to assure implementation of treatment modalities which are known to improve mortality and morbidity of patients.

References

REFERENCES

CHAPTER 1 Burden of Ischemic Heart Disease
References

1 International Cardiovascular Disease Statistics, American Heart Association. Available at: http://www.americanheart.org/downloadable/heart/1077185395308FS06INT4(ebook).pdf

2 American Heart Association. Heart Disease and Stroke Statistics, 2004 Update. Dallas, Tex., AHA 2003. Available at: http://www.americanheart.org/downloadable/heart/1079736729696HDSStats2004UpdateREV3-19-04.pdf

3 Death Rates by State, American Heart Association. Available at: http://www.americanheart.org/downloadable/heart/1077873552170FS20DR4(ebook).pdf

4 Kuller LH (2004). Ethnic differences in atherosclerosis, cardiovascular disease, and lipid metabolism. *Curr. Opin. Lipidol.* **15**:109–113.

5 The World Health Report 2002, World Health Organization. Available at: http://www.who.int/whr/2002/en

6 Tunstall-Pedoe H, Kuulasmaa K, Mähönen M, Tolonen H, Ruokokoski E, Amouyel P (1999). Contribution of trends in survival and coronary event rates to changes in coronary heart disease mortality: 10-year results from 37 WHO MONICA Project populations. *Lancet* **353**:1547–1557.

7 Morbidity and Mortality: 2002 Chart Book on Cardiovascular, Lung, and Blood Diseases, National Institutes of Health. Available at: http://www.nhlbi.nih.gov/resources/docs/02_chtbk.pdf

8 Murray CJ, Lopez AD (1997). Mortality by cause for eight regions of the world: Global Burden of Disease Study. *Lancet* **349**:1269–1276.

9 Murray CJ, Lopez AD (1997). Alternative projections of mortality and disability by cause 1990–2020: Global Burden of Disease Study. *Lancet* **349**:1498–1504.

10 Yusuf S, Reddy S, Ounpuu S, Anand S (2001). Global burden of cardiovascular diseases: Part II: variations in cardiovascular disease by specific ethnic groups and geographic regions and prevention strategies. *Circulation* **104**:2855–2864.

11 A Race Against Time: The Challenge of Cardiovascular Disease in Developing Economies. Columbia University, New York, 2004. Available at: http://www.earth.columbia.edu/news/2004/images/raceagainsttime_FINAL_0410404.pdf

CHAPTER 2 Anatomy of the Heart
Coronary arteries
References

1 Manabe H, Yutani C (1997). *Atlas of Ischemic Heart Disease.* Churchill Livingstone, New York.

2 Davies MJ (1998). *Atlas of Coronary Artery Disease.* Lippincott-Raven, Philadelphia.

3 Alderman EL, Stadius M (1992). The angiographic definitions of the Bypass Angioplasty Revascularization Investigation. *Coron. Artery Dis.* **3**:1189–1207.

4 Scanlon PJ, Faxon DP, Audet AM, *et al.* (1999). ACC/AHA guidelines for coronary angiography. A report of the American College of Cardiology/American Heart Association Task Force on practice guidelines (Committee on Coronary Angiography). Developed in collaboration with the Society for Cardiac Angiography and Interventions. *J. Am. Coll. Cardiol.* **33**:1756–1824.

Myocardium
Further reading

Brette F, Orchard C (2003). T-tubule function in mammalian cardiac myocytes. *Circ. Res.* **92**:1182–1192.

Coghlan HC, Coghlan L (2001). Cardiac architecture: Gothic versus Romanesque. A cardiologist's view. *Semin. Thorac. Cardiovasc. Surg.* **13**:417–430.

de Tombe PP (2003). Cardiac myofilaments: mechanics and regulation. *J. Biomech.* **36**:721–730.

Jongsma HJ, Wilders R (2000). Gap junctions in cardiovascular disease. *Circ. Res.* **86**:1193–1197.

Severs NJ (2000). The cardiac muscle cell. *Bioessays* **22**:188–199.

Torrent-Guasp F, Buckberg GD, Clemente C, Cox JL, Coghlan HC, Gharib M (2001). The structure and function of the helical heart and its buttress wrapping. I. The normal macroscopic structure of the heart. *Semin. Thorac. Cardiovasc. Surg.* **13**:301–319.

Walker CA, Spinale FG (1999). The structure and function of the cardiac myocyte: a review of fundamental concepts. *J. Thorac. Cardiovasc. Surg.* **118**:375–382.

Conduction system
Further reading

Katz AM (2001). Structure of heart, myocardial cells, and biological membranes. In: *Physiology of the Heart*, 3rd edn. AM Katz (ed). Lippincott Williams and Wilkins, Philadelphia, pp. 1–38.

Oosthoek PW, Viragh S, Mayen AE, van Kempen MJ, Lamers WH, Moorman AF (1993). Immunohistochemical delineation of the conduction system. I: The sinoatrial node. *Circ. Res.* **73**(3):473–481.

Oosthoek PW, Viragh S, Lamers WH, Moorman AF (1993). Immunohistochemical delineation of the conduction system. II: The atrioventricular node and Purkinje fibers. *Circ. Res.* **73**(3):482–491.

Rupart M, Zipes DP (2001). Genesis of cardiac arrhythmias. Electrophysiologic considerations. In: *Braunwald's Heart Disease. A Textbook of Cardiovascular Medicine*, 6th edn. E Braunwald, DP Zipes, P Libby (eds). WB Saunders, Philadelphia, pp. 659–699.

Scheinman M (1997). Arrhythmias. In: *Essential Atlas of Heart Diseases*. E Braunwald (ed), Current Medicine, Philadelphia, pp. 6.1–6.34.

CHAPTER 3 Physiology of the Heart
Coronary circulation
Further reading

Bache RJ, Duncker DJ (1994). Coronary steal. *A.C.C. Curr. J. Rev.* Mar/Apr:9–12.

Duncker DJ, Bache RJ (2000). Regulation of coronary vasomotor tone under normal conditions and during acute myocardial hypoperfusion. *Pharmacol. Ther.* **86**:87–110.

Duncker DJ, Merkus D (2005). Acute adaptations of the coronary circulation to exercise. *Cell Biochem. Biophys.* **43**:17–35.

Feigl EO (1983). Coronary Physiology. *Physiol. Rev.* **63**:1–205.

Hoffman JIE, Spaan JA (1990). Pressure-flow relations in coronary circulation. *Physiol. Rev.* **70**:331–390.

Kajiya F, Goto M (1999). Integrative physiology of coronary microcirculation. *Jpn. J. Physiol.* **49**:229–241.

Laughlin MH, Korthuis R, Duncker DJ, Bache RJ (1996). Regulation of blood flow to cardiac and skeletal muscle during exercise. In: *Handbook of Physiology*, Section 12. LB Rowell, JT Shepherd (eds). *Exercise: Regulation and Integration of Multiple Systems*. Oxford University Press, New York. Chapter 16, 705–769.

Merkus D, Chilian WM, Stepp DW (1999). Functional characteristics of the coronary microcirculation. *Herz* **24**:496–508.

Myocardium and determinants of oxygen demand
References

1 Gould K(1999). Physiology of the coronary circulation and endothelium. In: *Coronary Artery Stenosis and Reversing Atherosclerosis*, 2nd edn. Arnold/Oxford University Press, New York.

2 Klein LJ, Visser FC, Knaapen P, Peters JH, Teule GJ, Visser CA, Lammertsma AA (2001). Carbon-11 acetate as a tracer of myocardial oxygen consumption. *Eur. J. Nucl. Med.* **28**(5):651–668.

3 Depre C, Vanoverschelde JL, Taegtmeyer H (1999). Glucose for the heart. *Circulation* **99**(4):578–588.

4 Kass DA, Maughan WL (1988). From 'Emax' to pressure-volume relations: a broader view. *Circulation* **77**(6):1203–1212.

5 Ganz P, Braunwald EB (1998). Coronary blood flow and myocardial ischemia. In: *Heart Disease: A Textbook of Cardiovascular Medicine*, 5th edn. EB Braunwald (ed). WB Saunders, Philadelphia.

6 Bassingthwaighte JB, King RB, Roger SA (1989). Fractal nature of regional myocardial blood flow heterogeneity. *Circ. Res.* **65**(3):578–590.

7 Decking UK, Schrader J (1998). Spatial heterogeneity of myocardial perfusion and metabolism. *Basic Res. Cardiol.* **93**(6):439–445.

8 Huggins GS, Pasternak RC, Alpert NM, Fischman AJ, Gewirtz H (1998). Effects of short-term treatment of hyperlipidemia on coronary vasodilator function and myocardial perfusion in regions having substantial impairment of baseline dilator reverse [see comments]. *Circulation* **98**(13):1291–1296.

9 Losordo DW, Vale PR, Symes JF, *et al.* (1998). Gene therapy for myocardial angiogenesis: initial clinical results with direct myocardial injection of phVEGF165 as sole therapy for myocardial ischemia. *Circulation* **98**(25):2800–2804.

10 Apstein CS, Taegtmeyer H (1997). Glucose–insulin–potassium in acute myocardial infarction: the time has come for a large, prospective trial. *Circulation* **96**(4):1074–1077.

Conduction system
References

1 Bharati S, Lev M (1995). Anatomy of the normal conduction system, disease related changes, and their relationship to arrhythmogenesis. In: *Cardiac Arrhythmia: Mechanisms, Diagnosis, and Management*. PJ Podrid, PR Kowey (eds). Williams & Wilkins, Baltimore, pp.1–15.

2 West TC (1955). Ultramicroelectrode recording from the cardiac pacemaker. *J. Pharmacol. Exp. Ther.* **115**:283–290.

3 Michaels DC, Matyas EP, Jalife J (1990). Experimental and mathematical observations on pacemaker interactions as a mechanism of synchronization in the sinoatrial node. In: *Cardiac Electrophysiology: From Cell to Bedside.* DP Zipes, J Jalife (eds). WB Saunders, Philadelphia, pp. 182–192.

4 Meijler FL, Janse MJ (1988). Morphology and electrophysiology of the mammalian atrioventricular node. *Physiol. Rev.* **68**:608–647.

5 Munk AA, Adjemian RA, Zhao J, Ogbaghebriel A, Shrier A (1996). Electrophysiological properties of morphologically distinct cells isolated from the rabbit atrioventricular node. *J. Physiol.* **493**(3):801–818.

6 Denes P, Wu D, Dhingra R, *et al.* (1975). Dual atrioventricular nodal pathways: a common electrophysiological response. *Br. Heart J.* **37**:1069–1076.

7 Myerburg RJ, Gelband H, Hoffman BF (1971). Functional characteristics of the gating mechanism in the canine AV conducting system. *Circ. Res.* **28**:136–147.

8 Gorgels AP, Al Fadley F, Zaman L, Kantoch MJ, Al Halees Z (1998). The long QT syndrome with impaired atrioventricular conduction: a malignant variant in infants. *J. Cardiovasc. Electrophysiol.* **9**:1225–1232.

9 Scheinman MM, Peters RW, Sauve MJ, *et al.* (1982). Value of the H-Q interval in patients with bundle branch block and the role of permanent pacing. *Am. J. Cardiol.* **50**:1316.

10 Shaw DB, Linker NJ, Heaver PA, Evans R (1987). Chronic sinoatrial disorder (sick sinus syndrome): a possible result of cardiac ischaemia. *Br. Heart J.* **58**:598–607.

11 Alboni P, Baggioni GF, Scarfo S, *et al.* (1991). Role of sinus node artery disease in sick sinus syndrome in inferior wall acute myocardial infarction. *Am. J. Cardiol.* **67**:1180–1184.

12 Kyriakidis M, Trikas A, Triposkiadis F, *et al.* (1997). Sinus node dysfunction in acute inferior myocardial infarction. Role of sinus node artery and clinical course in patients with one-vessel coronary artery disease. *Cardiology* **88**:166–169.

13 Mark AL (1983). The Bezold–Jarisch reflex revisited: clinical implications of inhibitory reflexes originating in the heart. *J. Am. Coll. Cardiol.* **1**:90–102.

14 Feigl D, Ashkenazy J, Kishon Y (1984). Early and late atrioventricular block in acute inferior myocardial infarction. *J. Am. Coll. Cardiol.* **4**:35–38.

15 Topol EJ, Van de Werf FJ (2002). Acute myocardial infarction: early diagnosis and management. In: *Textbook of Cardiovascular Medicine.* EJ Topol (ed). Lippincott Williams & Wilkins, Philadelphia, pp. 385–419.

**CHAPTER 4 Pathophysiology of Myocardial Ischemia
Coronary artery anomalies**
References

1 Baltaxe HA, Wixson D (1977). The incidence of congenital anomalies of the coronary arteries in the adult population. *Radiology* **122**:47–52.

2 Topaz O, DeMarchena EJ, Perin E, Sommer LS, Mallon SM, Chahine RA (1992). Anomalous coronary arteries: angiographic findings in 80 patients [see comments]. *Int. J. Cardiol.* **34**:129–138.

3 Yamanaka O, Hobbs RE (1990). Coronary artery anomalies in 126,595 patients undergoing coronary arteriography. *Cathet. Cardiovasc. Diagn.* **21**:28–40.

4 Alexander RW, Griffith GC (1956). Anomalies of the coronary arteries and their clinical significance. *Circulation* **14**:800–805.

5 Taylor AJ, Rogan KM, Virmani R (1992). Sudden cardiac death associated with isolated congenital coronary artery anomalies. *J. Am. Coll. Cardiol.* **20**:640–647.

6 Kragel AH, Roberts WC (1988). Anomalous origin of either the right or left main coronary artery from the aorta with subsequent coursing between aorta and pulmonary trunk: analysis of 32 necropsy cases. *Am. J. Cardiol.* **62**:771–777.

7 Maron BJ, Poliac LC, Roberts WO (1996). Risk for sudden cardiac death associated with marathon running [see comments]. *J. Am. Coll. Cardiol.* **28**:428–431.

8 Taylor AJ, Byers JP, Cheitlin MD, Virmani R (1997). Anomalous right or left coronary artery from the contralateral coronary sinus: 'high-risk' abnormalities in the initial coronary artery course and heterogeneous clinical outcomes. *Am. Heart J.* **133**:428–435.

9 Roberts WC (1986). Major anomalies of coronary arterial origin seen in adulthood. *Am. Heart J.* **111**:941–963.

10 Johnsrude CL, Perry JC, Cecchin F, *et al.* (1995). Differentiating anomalous left main coronary artery originating from the pulmonary artery in infants from myocarditis and dilated cardiomyopathy by electrocardiogram. *Am. J. Cardiol.* **75**:71–74.

11 Ohmoto Y, Hara K, Kuroda Y, Fukuda S, Tamura T (1997). Stent placement in surgically reimplanted left main coronary artery in patient with anomalous origin of left main coronary artery from pulmonary artery. *Cathet. Cardiovasc. Diagn.* **42**:48–50.

12 Saito T, Fuse K, Kato M, Hasegawa N, Oki S (1996). Anomalous left main coronary artery arising from the pulmonary artery in an adult: treatment by direct reimplantation. *Surg. Today* **26**:453–456.

13 Letcher JR, McCormick D, Tendler S, Ross JJ, Chandrasekaran K, Brockman S (1991). Left main coronary artery arising from the pulmonary trunk in a 56-year-old patient presenting with acute myocardial infarction. *Am. J. Cardiol.* **68**:1257–1258.

14 Bagger JP, Vesterlund T, Nielsen TT (1985). Cardiac metabolism and coronary hemodynamics before and after bypass surgery for anomalous origin of the left main coronary artery from the pulmonary trunk. *Am. J. Cardiol.* **55**:864–865.

15 Koike K, Musewe NN, Smallhorn JF, Freedom RM (1989). Distinguishing between anomalous origin of the left

coronary artery from the pulmonary trunk and dilated cardiomyopathy: role of echocardiographic measurement of the right coronary artery diameter. *Br. Heart J.* **61**:192–197.

16 Vaksmann G, Mauran P, Rey C, Francart C, Dupuis C (1988). Visualization of anomalous origin of the left main coronary artery from the pulmonary trunk by pulsed and color Doppler echocardiography. *Am. Heart J.* **116**:181–182.

17 King DH, Danford DA, Huhta JC, Gutgesell HP (1985). Noninvasive detection of anomalous origin of the left main coronary artery from the pulmonary trunk by pulsed Doppler echocardiography. *Am. J. Cardiol.* **55**:608–609.

18 Backer CL, Stout MJ, Zales VR, *et al.* (1992). Anomalous origin of the left coronary artery. A twenty-year review of surgical management. *J. Thorac. Cardiovasc. Surg.* **103**:1049–1057.

19 Ogden JA, Goodyer AV (1970). Patterns of distribution of the single coronary artery. *Yale J. Biol. Med.* **43**:11–21.

20 Barth CW, Roberts WC (1986). Left main coronary artery originating from the right sinus of Valsalva and coursing between the aorta and pulmonary trunk. *J. Am. Coll. Cardiol.* **7**:366–373.

21 Liberthson RR, Dinsmore RE, Fallon JT (1979). Aberrant coronary artery origin from the aorta. Report of 18 patients, review of literature, and delineation of natural history and management. *Circulation* **59**:748–754.

22 Rinaldi RG, Carballido J, Giles R, Del Toro E, Porro R (1994). Right coronary artery with anomalous origin and slit ostium. *Ann. Thorac. Surg.* **58**:829–832.

23 Fernandes ED, Kadivar H, Hallman GL, Reul GJ, Ott DA, Cooley DA (1992). Congenital malformations of the coronary arteries: the Texas Heart Institute experience. *Ann. Thorac. Surg.* **54**:732–740.

24 Taylor AJ, Farb A, Ferguson M, Virmani R (1997). Myocardial infarction associated with physical exertion in a young man [clinical conference]. *Circulation* **96**:3201–3204.

Anerobic myocardial metabolism
References

1 Opie LH (1991). *The Heart: Physiology and Metabolism.* Raven Press, New York.

2 Bax JJ, Knapp FF, Visser FC (1998). Single photon imaging of myocardial metabolism: the role of iodine 123 fatty acids and fluorine-18 deoxyglucose. In: *Nuclear Medicine in Clinical Diagnosis and Treatment.* IPC Murray, PJ Ell (eds). Churchill Livingstone, London.

3 Visser FC (2001). Imaging of cardiac metabolism using radiolabelled glucose, fatty acids, and acetate. *Coron. Artery Dis.* **12**(Suppl 1):S12–S18.

4 Rupp H, Zarain-Herzberg A, Maisch B (2002). The use of partial fatty acid oxidation inhibitors for metabolic therapy of angina pectoris and heart failure. *Herz.* **27**(7):621–636.

Collateral development
Further reading

Burkhoff D, Weisfeldt M (2000). Cardiac function and circulatory control. In: *Cecil Textbook of Medicine*, 21st edn. L Goldman, JC Bennett (eds). WB Saunders, Philadelphia, p. 176.

Ganz P, Ganz W (2001). Coronary blood flow and myocardial ischemia. In: *Heart Disease: A Textbook of Cardiovascular Medicine*, 6th edn. E Braunwald, DP Zipes, P Libby (eds). WB Saunders, Philadelphia, p. 1087.

Tabibiazar R, Rockson SG (2001). Angiogenesis and the ischaemic heart. *Eur. Heart J.* **22**:903–918.

Van Royen N, Piek JJ, Schaper W, Bode C, Buschmann I (2001). Arteriogenesis: mechanisms and modulation of collateral artery development. *J. Nucl. Cardiol.* **8**:687–693.

Preconditioning, stunning, and hibernation
Further reading

Bonow RO (1996). Identification of viable myocardium. *Circulation* **94**:2674–2680.

Braunwald E, Kloner RA (1982). The stunned myocardium: prolonged, postischemic ventricular dysfunction. *Circulation* **66**:1146–1149.

Charlat ML, O'Neill PG, Hartley CJ, Roberts R, Bolli R (1989). Prolonged abnormalities of left ventricular diastolic wall thinning in the 'stunned' myocardium in conscious dogs: time course and relation to systolic function. *J. Am. Coll. Cardiol.* **13**:185–194.

Heyndrickx GR, Millard RW, McRitchie RJ, Maroko PR, Vatner SF (1975). Regional myocardial functional and electrophysiologic alterations after brief coronary artery occlusion in conscious dogs. *J. Clin. Invest.* **56**:978–985.

Kloner RA, Bolli R, Marban E, Reinlib L, Braunwald E (1998). Medical and cellular implications of stunning, hibernation, and preconditioning: An NHLBI workshop. *Circulation* **97**:1848–1867.

Kloner RA, Yellon D (1994). Does ischemic preconditioning occur in patients? *J. Am. Coll. Cardiol.* **24**:1133–1142.

Mahaffey KW, Puma JA, Barbagelata NA, *et al.* (1999). Adenosine as an adjunct to thrombolytic therapy for acute myocardial infarction: results of a multi-center, randomized, placebo-controlled trial: the Acute Myocardial Infarction STudy of ADenosine (AMISTAD) trial. *J. Am. Coll. Cardiol.* **34**(6):1711–1720.

Murry CE, Jennings RB, Reimer KA (1986). Preconditioning with ischemia: a delay of lethal cell injury in ischemic myocardium. *Circulation* **74**:1124–1136.

Rahimtoola SH (1989). The hibernating myocardium. *Am. Heart J.* **117**:211–221.

CHAPTER 5 Myocardial Ischemia: Compromised Supply Atherothrombosis
References

1 Lusis AJ (2000). Atherosclerosis. *Nature* **407**:233–241.

2 Libby P (2002). Inflammation in atherosclerosis. *Nature* **420**:868–874.

3 Steinberg D (2002). Atherogenesis in perspective: hypercholesterolemia and inflammation as partners in crime. *Nat. Med.* **8**:1211–1217.

4 Fuster V, Fayad ZA, Badimon JJ (1999). Acute coronary syndromes: biology. *Lancet* **353**(Suppl 2):SII5–SII9.

5 Falk E (1999). Stable versus unstable atherosclerosis: clinical aspects. *Am. Heart J.* **138**(5 Pt 2):S421–S425.

6 Davies MJ (2000). The pathophysiology of acute coronary syndromes. *Heart* **83**:361–366.

7 Shah PK, Kaul S, Nilsson J, Cercek B (2001). Exploiting the vascular protective effects of high-density lipoprotein and its apolipoproteins: an idea whose time for testing is coming. Part I and II. *Circulation* **104**:2376–2383, 2498–2502.

8 Bøttcher M, Falk E (1999). Pathology of coronary arteries in smokers and nonsmokers. *J. Cardiovasc. Risk* **6**:299–302.

9 Verma S, Anderson TJ (2002). Fundamentals of endothelial function for the clinical cardiologist. *Circulation* **105**:546–549.

10 Ruggeri ZM (2002). Platelets in atherothrombosis. *Nat. Med.* **8**:1227–1234.

11 Falk E, Shah PK, Fuster V (1995). Coronary plaque disruption. *Circulation* **92**:657–671.

12 Sambola A, Osende J, Hathcock J, *et al.* (2003). Role of risk factors in the modulation of tissue factor activity and blood thrombogenicity. *Circulation* **107**:973–977.

13 Topol EJ, Yadav JS (2000). Recognition of the importance of embolization in atherosclerotic vascular disease. *Circulation* **101**:570–580.

14 Libby P, Ridker PM, Maseri A (2002). Inflammation and atherosclerosis. *Circulation* **105**:1135–1143.

15 Goldstein JA (2002). Angiographic plaque complexity: the tip of the unstable plaque iceberg. *J. Am. Coll. Cardiol.* **39**:1464–1467.

16 Rioufol G, Finet G, Ginon I, *et al.* (2002). Multiple atherosclerotic plaque rupture in acute coronary syndrome: a three-vessel intravascular ultrasound study. *Circulation* **106**:804–808.

17 Schoenhagen P, Tuzcu EM, Ellis SG (2002). Plaque vulnerability, plaque rupture, and acute coronary syndromes: (multi)-focal manifestation of a systemic disease process. *Circulation* **106**:760–762.

18 Buffon A, Biasucci LM, Liuzzo G, D'Onofrio G, Crea F, Maseri A (2002). Widespread coronary inflammation in unstable angina. *N. Engl. J. Med.* **347**:5–12.

19 Servoss SJ, Januzzi JL, Muller JE (2002). Triggers of acute coronary syndromes. *Prog. Cardiovasc. Dis.* **44**:369–380.

Coronary vasoconstriction and spasm
References

1 Maseri A, Mimmo R, Chierchia S, *et al.* (1975). Coronary spasm as a cause of acute myocardial ischemia in man. *Chest* **68**:625–633.

2 Beltrame JF, Sasayama S, Maseri A (1999). Racial heterogeneity in coronary artery vasomotor reactivity: differences between Japanese and Caucasian patients. *J. Am. Coll. Cardiol.* **33**:1442–1452.

3 Maseri A, Davies G, Hackett D, *et al.* (1990). Coronary artery spasm and vasoconstriction. The case for a distinction. *Circulation* **81**:1983–1991.

4 Maseri A, Lanza GA, Manolfi M, *et al.* (1996). Lo spasmo coronarico 20 anni dopo. *Cardiologia* **41**:351–356.

5 Kaski JC, Maseri A, Vejar M, *et al.* (1989). Spontaneous coronary artery spasm in variant angina results from a local hyperreactivity to a generalized constrictor stimulus. *J. Am. Coll. Cardiol.* **14**:1456–1463.

6 Masumoto A, Mohri M, Shimokawa H, *et al.* (2002). Suppression of coronary artery spasm by the rho-kinase inhibitor fasudil in patients with vasospastic angina. *Circulation* **105**:1545–1547.

7 Lanza GA, Pedrotti P, Pasceri V, *et al.* (1996). Autonomic changes associated with spontaneous coronary spasm in patients with variant angina. *J. Am. Coll. Cardiol.* **28**:1249–1256.

8 Lanza GA, Patti G, Pasceri V, *et al.* (1999). Circadian distribution of ischemic attacks and ischemia-related ventricular arrhythmias in patients with variant angina. *Cardiologia* **44**:913–920.

9 Gaspardone A, Tomai F, Versaci F, *et al.* (1999). Coronary artery stent placement in patients with variant angina refractory to medical treatment. *Am. J. Cardiol.* **84**:96–98.

10 Myerburg RJ, Kessler KM, Mallon SM, *et al.* (1992). Life-threatening ventricular arrhythmias in patients with silent myocardial ischemia due to coronary artery spasm. *N. Engl. J. Med.* **326**:1451–1455.

Nonatherothrombotic coronary artery disease
Further reading

Ball GV, Bridges SL (2002). *Vasculitis.* Oxford University Press, Oxford.

Lanzer P, Topol EJ (2002). *Panvascular Medicine.* Springer-Verlag, Berlin.

Stehbens WE, Lie JT (1995). *Vascular Pathology.* Chapman & Hall, London.

Voung PN, Berry C (2002). *The Pathology of Vessels.* Springer-Verlag, Paris.

Microvascular disease
Further reading

Strauer BE (1990). The significance of coronary reserve in clinical heart disease. *J. Am. Coll. Cardiol.* **15**:775–783.

Bøtker HE (2001). Microvascular angina and syndrome X. In: *International Textbook of Cardiology in Color.* MH Crawford, JP DiMarco (eds). Mosby, London.

Systemic causes
Further reading

Hutchinson SJ, Chandraratna AN (2001). Hematologic diseases. In: *Cardiology*. MC Crawford *et al.* (eds). Mosby, London, 8.8:1–2.

James TN (2000). Homage to James B. Herrick: a contemporary look at myocardial infarction and at sickle cell heart disease: the 32nd Annual Herrick Lecture of the Council on Clinical Cardiology of the American Heart Association. *Circulation.* **101**(15):1874–1887.

Saltzberg MT, Soble JS, Parrillo JE (2001). Acute heart failure and shock. In: *Cardiology*. MC Crawford *et al.* (eds). London, Mosby, 5.3:1–12.

Transplant vasculopathy
References

1 Kapadia SR, Nissen SE, Tuzcu EM (1999). Impact of intravascular ultrasound in understanding transplant coronary artery disease. *Curr. Opin. Cardiol.* **14**:140–150.

2 Johnson DE, Gao SZ, Schroeder JS, DeCampli WM, Billingham ME (1989). The spectrum of coronary artery pathologic findings in human cardiac allografts. *J. Heart Transplant.* **8**:349–359.

3 Kapadia SR, Nissen SE, Ziada KM, *et al.* (1998). Development of transplantation vasculopathy and progression of donor-transmitted atherosclerosis: comparison by serial intravascular ultrasound imaging. *Circulation* **98**:2672–2678.

4 Tuzcu EM, Kapadia SR, Tutar E, *et al.* (2001). High prevalence of coronary atherosclerosis in asymptomatic teenagers and young adults: evidence from intravascular ultrasound. *Circulation* **103**:2705–2710.

5 Glagov S, Weisenberg E, Zarins CK, Stankunavicius R, Kolettis GJ (1987). Compensatory enlargement of human atherosclerotic coronary arteries. *N. Engl. J. Med.* **316**:1371–1375.

6 Tuzcu EM, Hobbs RE, Rincon G, *et al.* (1995). Occult and frequent transmission of atherosclerotic coronary disease with cardiac transplantation. Insights from intravascular ultrasound. *Circulation* **91**:1706–1713.

7 Costanzo MR, Eisen HJ, Brown RN, *et al.* (2001). Are there specific risk factors for fatal allograft vasculopathy? An analysis of over 7,000 cardiac transplant patients. *J. Heart Lung Transplant.* **20**:152.

8 Kobashigawa J (2000). What is the optimal prophylaxis for treatment of cardiac allograft vasculopathy? *Curr. Control Trials Cardiovasc. Med.* **1**:166–171.

9 Tsutsui H, Ziada KM, Schoenhagen P, *et al.* (2001). Lumen loss in transplant coronary artery disease is a biphasic process involving early intimal thickening and late constrictive remodeling: results from a 5-year serial intravascular ultrasound study. *Circulation* **104**:653–657.

10 Massy ZA (2001). Hyperlipidemia and cardiovascular disease after organ transplantation. *Transplantation* **72**:S13–S15.

11 Stoica SC, Goddard M, Large SR (2002). The endothelium in clinical cardiac transplantation. *Ann. Thorac. Surg.* **73**:1002–1008.

12 Young JB (2000). Perspectives on cardiac allograft vasculopathy. *Curr. Atheroscler. Rep.* **2**:259–271.

13 Drinkwater DC, Laks H, Blitz A, *et al.* (1996). Outcomes of patients undergoing transplantation with older donor hearts. *J. Heart Lung Transplant.* **15**:684–691.

14 Schroeder JS, Hunt SA (1991). Chest pain in heart-transplant recipients [editorial; comment]. *N. Engl. J. Med.* **324**:1805–1807.

15 Young JB (1992). Cardiac allograft arteriopathy: an ischemic burden of a different sort. *Am. J. Cardiol.* **70**:9F–13F.

16 Aranda JM Jr, Hill J (2000). Cardiac transplant vasculopathy. *Chest* **118**:1792–1800.

17 Kapadia SR, Nissen SE, Tuzcu EM (1999). Impact of intravascular ultrasound in understanding transplant coronary artery disease. *Curr. Opin. Cardiol.* **14**:140–150.

18 Konig A, Theisen K, Klauss V (2000). Intravascular ultrasound for assessment of coronary allograft vasculopathy. *Z. Kardiol.* **89**:IX/45–49.

19 Tuzcu EM, Kapadia SR, Sachar R, *et al.* (2005). Intravascular ultrasound evidence of angiographically silent progression in coronary atherosclerosis predicts long-term morbidity and mortality after cardiac transplantation. *J. Am. Coll. Cardiol.* **45**:1538–1542.

20 Kobashigawa JA, Tobis JM, Starling RC, *et al.* (2005). Multicenter intravascular ultrasound validation study among heart transplant recipients: outcomes after 5 years. *J. Am. Coll. Cardiol.* **45**:1532–1537.

21 Schroeder JS, Gao SZ, Alderman EL, *et al.* (1993). A preliminary study of diltiazem in the prevention of coronary artery disease in heart-transplant recipients [see comments]. *N. Engl. J. Med.* **328**:164–170.

22 Kobashigawa JA, Katznelson S, Laks H, *et al.* (1995). Effect of pravastatin on outcomes after cardiac transplantation [see comments]. *N. Engl. J. Med.* **333**:621–627.

23 Halle AA 3rd, Wilson RF, Massin EK, *et al.* (1992). Coronary angioplasty in cardiac transplant patients. Results of a multi-center study. *Circulation* **86**:458–462.

24 Halle AA 3rd, DiSciascio G, Massin EK, *et al.* (1995). Coronary angioplasty, atherectomy and bypass surgery in cardiac transplant recipients. *J. Am. Coll. Cardiol.* **26**:120–128.

Traumatic coronary artery disease
References

1 Buckman RF Jr, Badellino MM, Mauro LH, *et al.* (1993). Penetrating cardiac wounds: a prospective study of factors influencing initial resuscitation. *J. Trauma* **34**:717–725.

2 Asensio JA, Murray J, Demetriades D, *et al.* (1998). Penetrating cardiac injuries: a prospective study of variables predicting outcomes. *J. Am. Coll. Surg.* **186**:24–34.

3 Asensio JA, Berne JD, Demetriades D, *et al.* (1998). One hundred and five penetrating cardiac injuries: a 2-year prospective evaluation. *J. Trauma* **44**:1073–1082.

4 Rea WJ, Sugg WL, Wilson LC, *et al.* (1969). Coronary artery lacerations. *Ann. Thorac. Surg.* 7:518–528.

5 Espada R, Whisennand HH, Mattox KL, Beall AC (1975). Surgical management of penetrating injuries to the coronary arteries. *Surgery* **78**:755–760.

6 Wall MJ, Mattox KL, Chen CD, Baldwin JC (1997). Acute management of complex cardiac injuries. *J. Trauma* **42**:905–912.

7 DeBakey ME, Simeone FA (1946). Battle injuries of the arteries in World War II: an analysis of 2471 cases. *Ann. Surg.* **123**:534.

8 Hughes CW (1958). Arterial repair during the Korean war. *Ann. Surg.* **147**:555–561.

9 Rich NM, Baugh JH, Hughes CW (1970). Acute arterial injuries in Vietnam: 1000 cases. *J. Trauma* **10**:359–369.

10 Seipelt RG, Vazquez-Jimenez JF, Messmer BJ (2000). Missiles in the heart causing coronary artery disease 44 years after injury. *Ann. Thorac. Surg.* **70**:979–980.

11 Salmi A, Blank M, Slomski C (1996). Left anterior descending occlusion after blunt chest trauma. *J. Trauma* **40**:832–834.

12 Westaby S, Drossos G, Giannopoulos N (1995). Posttraumatic coronary artery aneurysm. *Ann. Thorac. Surg.* **60**:712–713.

13 Reissman P, Rivkind A, Jurim O, Simon D (1992). Case Report: the management of penetrating cardiac trauma with major coronary artery injury: is cardiopulmonary bypass essential? *J. Trauma* **33**:773–775.

14 Ginzburg E, Dygert J, Parra-Davila E, *et al.* (1998). Coronary artery stenting for occlusive dissection after blunt chest trauma. *J. Trauma* **45**:157–161.

15 Cherng WJ, Bullard MJ, Chang HJ, Lin FC (1995). Diagnosis of coronary artery dissection following blunt chest trauma by transesophageal echocardiography. *J. Trauma* **39**:772–774.

16 Friesen CH, Howlet JG, Ross DB (2000). Traumatic coronary fistula management. *Ann. Thorac. Surg.* **69**:1973–1983.

CHAPTER 6 Myocardial Ischemia: Morbid Demand
Cardiac hypertrophy
References

1 Frey N, Olson EN (2003). Cardiac hypertrophy: the good, the bad, and the ugly. *Ann. Rev. Physiol.* **65**: 21.1–21.35.

2 Schirmer H, Lunde P, Rasmussen K (1999). Prevalence of left ventricular hypertrophy in the general population. The Tromso Study. *Euro. Heart J.* **20**:429–438.

3 Opie LH (2001). Mechanism of cardiac contraction and relaxation. In: *Heart disease – A Textbook of Cardiovascular Medicine*, 6th edn. E Braunwald, PZ Douglas, P Libby (eds). WB Saunders, Philadelphia, pp. 464–466.

4 Lorell BH, Carabello BA (2000). Left ventricular hypertrophy: pathogenesis, detection, and prognosis. *Circulation* **102**: 470–479.

5 Ardehali A, Ports TA (1990). Myocardial oxygen supply and demand. *Chest* **98**:703.

6 Linzbach AJ (1960). Heart failure from the point of view of quantitative anatomy. *Am. J. Cardiol.* **5**:370–382.

7 Bove KE (1974). Myocardial hypertrophy and enlargement . In: *The Heart – International Academy of Pathology Monograph*. JE Edwards, M Lev, MR Abell (eds). Williams & Wilkins, Baltimore, Monograph No.15 pp. 31–55.

8 Weber KT, Clark WA, Janicki JS, *et al.* (1987). Physiologic versus pathologic hypertrophy and the pressure-overloaded myocardium. *J. Cardiovasc. Pharm.* **10**(Suppl.6):S37–S49.

9 Neyses L, Pelzer T (1995). The biological cascade leading to cardiac hypertrophy. *Eur. Heart J.* **16**(Suppl N):8–11.

10 Opie LH (1997). Overload hypertrophy and its molecular biology. In: *The Heart: Physiology, from Cell to Circulation*, 3rd edn. LH Opie (ed). Lippincott-Raven, Philadelphia, pp. 391–418.

11 Meerson FZ (1983). Adaptation and deadaptation. In: *The Failing Heart*. AM Kats (ed). Raven Press, New York.

Systemic causes
Further reading

Chobanian AV, Bakris GL, Black HR, *et al.*; National Heart, Lung, and Blood Institute Joint National Committee on Prevention, Detection, Evaluation, and Treatment of High Blood Pressure; National High Blood Pressure Education Program Coordinating Committee (2003). The seventh report of the Joint National Committee on prevention, detection, evaluation, and treatment of high blood pressure: the JNC 7 report. *JAMA* **289**:2560–2572.

Conlon C, Perry IJ (2001). Epidemiology of hypertension. In: *Cardiology*. MC Crawford, *et al.* (eds). Mosby, London, pp. 3.2.1–3.2.10.

Jamrozik K (2001). Epidemiology of atherosclerotic disease. In: *Cardiology*. MC Crawford, *et al.* (eds). Mosby, London, 1.2.1–1.2.14.

Kaplan NM (2001). Systemic hypertension: mechanisms and diagnosis. In: *Heart Disease: A Textbook of Cardiovascular Medicine*, 6th edn. E Braunwald, PZ Douglas, P Libby (eds). WB Saunders, Philadelphia, pp. 921–950.

Klein I, Ojamaa K (1998). Thyrotoxicosis and the heart. *Endocrinol. Metabol. Clin. N. Am.* 27(1):51–62.

Ridker PM, Genest J, Libby P (2001). Risk factors for atherosclerotic disease. In: *Heart Disease: A Textbook of Cardiovascular Medicine*, 6th edn. E Braunwald, PZ Douglas, P Libby (eds). WB Saunders, Philadelphia, p. 1023.

Roffi M, Cattaneo F, Topol EJ (2003). Thyrotoxicosis and the cardiovascular system: subtle but serious effects. *Cleve. Clinic. J. Med.* **70**(1):57–63.

Toft AD, Boon NA (2000). Thyroid disease and the heart. *Heart* **84**:455–460.

Vela BS (2001). Endocrinology and the heart. In: *Cardiology*. MC Crawford, *et al.* Mosby, London, pp. 8.4.2–8.4.4.

CHAPTER 7 Detection of Coronary Artery Disease
Diagnostic coronary angiography
References

1 Scanlon PJ, Faxon DP, Audet AM, *et al.* (1999). ACC/AHA guidelines for coronary angiography: executive summary and recommendations: a report of the American College of Cardiology/American Heart Association Task Force on Practice Guidelines (Committee on Coronary Angiography). Developed in collaboration with the Society for Cardiac Angiography and Interventions. *Circulation* **99**:2345–2357.

2 Davis K, Kennedy JW, Kemp HG Jr, *et al.* (1979). Complications of coronary arteriography from the Collaborative Study of Coronary Artery Surgery (CASS). *Circulation* **59**:1105–1112.

3 Krone RJ, Johnson L, Noto T (1996). Five year trends in cardiac catheterization: a report from the Registry of the Society for Cardiac Angiography and Interventions. *Cathet. Cardiovasc. Diagn.* **39**:31–35.

Quantitative coronary arteriography
References

1 Lespérance J, Bilodeau L, Reiber JHC, Koning G, Hudon G, Bourassa M (1998). Issues in the performance of quantitative coronary angiography in clinical research trials. In: *What's New in Cardiovascular Imaging?* JHC Reiber, EE van der Wall (eds). Kluwer Academic Publishers, Dordrecht, pp. 31–46.

2 Janssen JP, Koning G, de Koning PJH, Tuinenburg JC, Reiber JHC (2002). A novel approach for the detection of pathlines in X-ray angiograms: the wavefront propagation algorithm. *Int. J. Cardiovasc. Im.* **18**:235–248.

3 van der Zwet PM, Reiber JHC (1994). A new approach for the quantification of complex lesion morphology: the gradient field transform; basic principles and validation results. *J. Am. Coll. Cardiol.* **24**(1):216–224.

4 Koning G, Tuinenburg JC, Hekking E, *et al.* (2002). A novel measurement technique to assess the effects of coronary brachytherapy in clinical trials. In: *Image Analysis in Drug Discovery and Clinical Trials. IEEE Transactions on Medical Imaging (TMI)*. M Sonka, M Grunkin (eds). Vol. 21(10) pp. 1254–1263.

5 Reiber JHC, Jukema JW, Koning G, Bruschke AVG (1996). Quality control in quantitative coronary arteriography. In: *Lipid Lowering Therapy and Progression of Coronary Atherosclerosis*. AVG Bruschke, JHC Reiber,

KI Lie, HJJ Wellens (eds). Kluwer Academic Publishers, Dordrecht, pp. 45–63.

Magnetic resonance coronary angiography
References

1 Li D, Paschal CB, Haacke EM, Adler LP (1993). Coronary arteries: three-dimensional MR imaging with fat saturation and magnetization transfer contrast. *Radiology* **187**(2):401–406.

2 Wang Y, Riederer SJ, Ehman RL (1995). Respiratory motion of the heart: kinematics and the implications for the spatial resolution in coronary imaging. *Magn. Reson. Med.* **33**(5):713–719.

3 van Geuns RJM, Wielopolski PA, Wardeh AJ, de Bruin HG, Oudkerk M, de Feyter PJ (2001). VCATS: volume coronary angiography using targeted scans: a new strategy in MR coronary angiography. *Int. J. Cardiol. Imag.* **17**(5):405–410.

4 White RD, Caputo GR, Mark AS, Modin GW, Higgins CB (1987). Coronary artery bypass graft patency: noninvasive evaluation with MR imaging. *Radiology* **164**(3):681–686.

5 Post JC, van Rossum AC, Bronzwaer JG, *et al.* (1995). Magnetic resonance angiography of anomolous coronary arteries. A new gold standard for delineating proximal course? *Circulation* **92**(11):3163–3171.

6 Manning WJ, Li W, Edelman RR (1993). A preliminary report comparing magnetic resonance coronary angiography with conventional angiography. *N. Engl. J. Med.* **328**(12):828–832.

7 Pennell DJ, Bogren HG, Keegan J, Firmin DN, Underwood SR (1996). Assessment of coronary artery stenosis by magnetic resonance imaging. *Heart* **75**(2):127–133.

8 Duerinckx AJ, Urman MK (1994). Two-dimensional coronary MR angiography: analysis of initial clinical results. *Radiology* **193**(3):731–738.

9 Post JC, van Rossum AC, Hofman MB, de Cock CC, Valk J, Visser CA (1997). Clinical utility of two-dimensional magnetic resonance angiography in detecting coronary artery disease. *Eur. Heart J.* **18**(3):426–433.

10 Kim WY, Danias PG, Stuber M, *et al.* (2001). Coronary magnetic resonance angiography for the detection of coronary stenoses. *N. Engl. J. Med.* **345**:1863–1869.

11 Rubinstein RI, Askenase AD, Thickman D, Feldman MS, Agarwal JB, Helfant RH (1987). Magnetic resonance imaging to evaluate patency of aortocoronary bypass grafts. *Circulation* **76**:786–791.

12 Jenkins JP, Love HG, Foster CJ, Isherwood I, Rowlands DJ (1988). Detection of coronary artery bypass graft patency as assessed by magnetic resonance imaging. *Br. J. Radiol.* **61**:2–4.

13 Frija G, Schouman-Claeys E, Lacombe P, Bismuth V, Ollivier JP (1989). A study of coronary artery bypass graft patency using MR imaging. *J. Comput. Assist. Tomogr.* **13**:226–232.

14 Galjee MA, van Rossum AC, Doesburg T, van Eenige MJ, Visser CA (1996). Value of magnetic resonance imaging in assessing patency and function of coronary artery bypass grafts. An angiographically controlled study. *Circulation* **93**:660–666.

15 White RD, Pflugfelder PW, Lipton MJ, Higgins CB (1988). Coronary artery bypass grafts: evaluation of patency with cine MR imaging. *Am. J. Roentgenol.* **150**:1271–1274.

16 Aurigemma GP, Reichek N, Axel L, Schiebler M, Harris C, Kressel HY (1989). Noninvasive determination of coronary artery bypass graft patency by cine magnetic resonance imaging. *Circulation* **80**:1595–1602.

17 Kalden P, Kreitner KF, Wittlinger T, *et al.* (1999). Assessment of coronary artery bypass grafts: value of different breath-hold MR imaging techniques. *Am. J. Roentgenol.* **172**:1359–1364.

18 Vrachliotis TG, Bis KG, Aliabadi D, Shetty AN, Safian R, Simonetti O (1997). Contrast-enhanced breath-hold MR angiography for evaluating patency of coronary artery bypass grafts. *Am. J. Roentgenol.* **168**:1073–1080.

19 Wintersperger BJ, Engelmann MG, von Smekal A, *et al.* (1998). Patency of coronary bypass grafts: assessment with breath-hold contrast-enhanced MR angiography: value of a nonelectrocardiographically triggered technique. *Radiology* **208**:345–351.

20 Langerak SE, Vliegen HW, de Roos A, *et al.* (2002). Detection of vein graft disease using high-resolution magnetic resonance angiography. *Circulation* **105**:328–333.

21 Yoshino H, Nitatori T, Kachi E, *et al.* (1997). Directed proximal magnetic resonance coronary angiography compared with conventional contrast coronary angiography. *Am. J. Cardiol.* **80**:514–518.

22 Post JC, van Rossum AC, Hofman MB, Valk J, Visser CA (1996). Three-dimensional respiratory-gated MR angiography of coronary arteries: comparison with conventional coronary angiography. *Am. J. Roentgenol.* **166**:1399–1404.

23 Müller MF, Fleisch M, Kroeker R, Chatterjee T, Meier B, Vock P (1997). Proximal coronary artery stenosis: three-dimensional MRI with fat saturation and navigator echo. *J. Magn. Reson. Imaging.* **7**:644–651.

24 Kessler W, Achenbach S, Moshage W, *et al.* (1997). Usefulness of respiratory gated magnetic resonance coronary angiography in assessing narrowings 50% in diameter in native coronary arteries and in aortocoronary bypass conduits. *Am. J. Cardiol.* **80**:989–993.

25 Sandstede JJ, Pabst T, Beer M, *et al.* (1999). Three-dimensional MR coronary angiography using the navigator technique compared with conventional coronary angiography. *Am. J. Roentgenol.* **172**:135–139.

26 Huber A, Nikolaou K, Gonschior P, Knez A, Stehling M, Reiser M (1999). Navigator echo-based respiratory gating for three-dimensional MR coronary angiography: results from healthy volunteers and patients with proximal coronary artery stenoses. *Am. J. Roentgenol.* **173**:95–101.

27 van Geuns RJ, de Bruin HG, Rensing BJ, *et al.* (1999). Magnetic resonance imaging of the coronary arteries: clinical results from three dimensional evaluation of a respiratory gated technique. *Heart* **82**:515–519.

28 Sardanelli F, Molinari G, Zandrino F, Balbi M (2000). Three-dimensional, navigator-echo MR coronary angiography in detecting stenoses of the major epicardial vessels, with conventional coronary angiography as the standard of reference. *Radiology* **214**:808–814.

29 Nikolaou K, Huber A, Knez A, Becker C, Bruening R, Reiser M (2002). Intraindividual comparison of contrast-enhanced electron-beam computed tomography and navigator-echo-based magnetic resonance imaging for noninvasive coronary artery angiography. *Eur. Radiol.* **12**:1663–1671.

30 Regenfus M, Ropers D, Achenbach S, *et al.* (2002). Comparison of contrast-enhanced breath-hold and free-breathing respiratory-gated imaging in three-dimensional magnetic resonance coronary angiography. *Am. J. Cardiol.* **90**:725–730.

31 Wittlinger T, Voigtlander T, Rohr M, *et al.* (2002). Magnetic resonance imaging of coronary artery occlusions in the navigator technique. *Int. J. Cardiovasc. Imaging* **18**:203–211; discussion 213–215.

32 Lethimonnier F, Furber A, Morel O, *et al.* (1999). Three-dimensional coronary artery MR imaging using prospective real-time respiratory navigator and linear phase shift processing: comparison with conventional coronary angiography. *Magn. Reson. Imaging* **17**:1111–1120.

33 Weber C, Steiner P, Sinkus R, Dill T, Bornert P, Adam G (2002). Correlation of 3D MR coronary angiography with selective coronary angiography: feasibility of the motion-adapted gating technique. *Eur. Radiol.* **12**:718–726.

34 Plein S, Jones TR, Ridgway JP, Sivananthan MU (2003). Three-dimensional coronary MR angiography performed with subject-specific cardiac acquisition windows and motion-adapted respiratory gating. *Am. J. Roentgenol.* **180**:505–512.

35 van Geuns RJM, Wielopolski PA, de Bruin HG, *et al.* (2000). MR coronary angiography with breath-hold targeted volumes: preliminary clinical results. *Radiology* **217**:270–277.

36 Regenfus M, Ropers D, Achenbach S, *et al.* (2000). Noninvasive detection of coronary artery stenosis using contrast-enhanced three-dimensional breath-hold magnetic resonance coronary angiography. *J. Am. Coll. Cardiol.* **36**:44–50.

37 Bunce NH, Lorenz CH, John AS, Lesser JR, Mohiaddin RH, Penell DJ (2003). Coronary artery bypass graft patency: assessment with true ast imaging with steady-state precession versus gadolinium-enhanced MR angiography. *Radiology* **227**: 440–446.

38 Bogaert J, Kuzo R, Dymarkowski S, Beckers R, Piessens J, Rademakers FE (2003). Coronary artery imaging with

real-time Navigator three-dimensional turbo-field echo MR coronary angiography: initial experience. *Radiology* **226**:707–716.

39 Jahnke C, Paetsch I, Schnackenburg B, *et al.* (2004). Coronary MR angiography with steady state free precession: individually adapted breath-hold technique versus free breathing technique. *Radiology* **232**:669–676.

40 Gerber BL, Coche E, Pasquet A, *et al.* (2005). Coronary artery stenosis: direct comparison of four section multidetector row CT and 3D Navigator MR imaging for detection: initial results. *Radiology* **234**:98–108.

41 Sakuma H, Ichikawa Y, Suzawa N, *et al.* (2005). Assessment of coronary arteries with total study time of less than 30 minutes using whole heart coronary MR angiography. *Radiology* **237**:316–321.

42 Jahnke C, Paetsch I, Nehrke K, *et al.* (2005). Rapid and complete coronary artery tree visualization with magnetic resonance imaging: feasibility and diagnostic performance. *Eur. Heart J.* **26**:2313–2319.

43 Jahnke C, Paetsch I, Schnackenburg B, *et al.* (2004). Coronary MR angiography with steady state free precession: individually adapted breath-hold technique versus free breathing technique. *Radiology* **232**:669–676.

44 Herborn CU, Schmidt M, Bruder O, Nagel E, Shamsi K, Barkhausen J (2004). MR coronary angiography with SH L 643 A: initial experience in patients with coronary artery disease. *Radiology* **233**:567–563.

45 Yang PC, Meyer CH, Terashima M, *et al.* (2003). Spiral magnetic resonance coronary angiography with rapid real-time localization. *J. Am. Coll. Cardiol.* **41**(7):1134–1141.

Further reading

Cai JM, Hatsukami TS, Ferguson MS, Small R, Polissar NL, Yuan C (2002). Classification of human carotid atherosclerotic lesions with *in vivo* multi-contrast magnetic resonance imaging. *Circulation* **106**:1368–1373.

Edelman RR, Manning WJ, Burstein D, Paulin S (1991). Coronary arteries: breath-hold MR angiography. *Radiology* **181**:641–643.

Fayad ZA, Fuster V, Fallon JT, *et al.* (2000). Noninvasive *in vivo* human coronary artery lumen and wall imaging using black-blood magnetic resonance imaging. *Circulation* **102**:506–510.

Li D, Kaushikkar S, Haacke EM, *et al.* (1996). Coronary arteries: three-dimensional MR imaging with retrospective respiratory gating. *Radiology* **201**:857–863.

Stuber M, Botnar RM, Danias PG, *et al.* (1999). Double-oblique free-breathing high resolution three-dimensional coronary magnetic resonance angiography. *J. Am. Coll. Cardiol.* **34**:524–531.

Wielopolski PA, van Geuns RJ, de Feyter PJ, Oudkerk M (2000). Coronary arteries. *Eur. Radiol.* **10**:12–35.

Noninvasive multi-slice spiral computed tomography References

1 Ohnesorge B, Flohr T, Becker C, *et al.* (2001). Technical aspects and applications of fast multi-slice cardiac CT. In: *Medical radiology – Diagnostic Imaging and Radiation Oncology.* MF Reiser, M Takahashi, M Modic, R Bruening (eds). Springer, Berlin, pp. 121–130.

2 Nieman K, Oudkerk M, Rensing BJ, *et al.* (2001). Coronary angiography with multi-slice computed tomography. *Lancet* **357**:599–603.

3 Achenbach S, Giesler T, Ropers D, *et al.* (2001). Detection of coronary artery stenoses by contrast-enhanced, retrospectively electrocardiographically-gated, multi-slice spiral computed tomography. *Circulation* **103**:2535–2538.

4 Knez A, Becker CR, Leber A, *et al.* (2001). Usefulness of multi-slice spiral computed tomography angiography for determination of coronary artery stenoses. *Am. J. Cardiol.* **88**:1191–1194.

5 Vogl TJ, Abolmaali ND, Diebold T, *et al.* (2002). Techniques for the detection of coronary atherosclerosis: multi-detector row CT coronary angiography. *Radiology* **223**:212–220.

6 Engelmann MG, von Smekal A, Knez A, *et al.* (1997). Accuracy of spiral computed tomography for identifying arterial and venous coronary graft patency. *Am. J. Cardiol.* **80**:569–574.

7 Tello R, Costello P, Ecker C, *et al.* (1993). Spiral CT evaluation of coronary artery bypass graft patency. *J. Comput. Assist. Tomogr.* **17**:253–259.

8 Stanford W, Brundage BH, MacMillan R, *et al.* (1988). Sensitivity and specificity of assessing coronary bypass graft patency with ultrafast computed tomography: results of a multi-center study. *J. Am. Coll. Cardiol.* **12**:1–7.

9 Bateman TM, Gray RJ, Whiting JS, *et al.* (1986). Cine computed tomographic evaluation of aortocoronary bypass graft patency. *J. Am. Coll. Cardiol.* **8**:693–698.

10 Bateman TM, Gray RJ, Whiting JS, *et al.* (1987). Prospective evaluation of ultrafast cardiac computed tomography for determination of coronary bypass graft patency. *Circulation* **75**:1018–1024.

11 Achenbach S, Moshage W, Ropers D, *et al.* (1997). Non-invasive, three-dimensional visualization of coronary artery bypass grafts by electron beam tomography. *Am. J. Cardiol.* **79**:856–861.

12 Ha JW, Cho SY, Shim WH, *et al.* (1999). Noninvasive evaluation of coronary artery bypass graft patency using three-dimensional angiography obtained with contrast-enhanced electron beam CT. *Am. J. Roentgenol.* **172**:1055–1059.

13 Ropers D, Ulzheimer S, Wenkel E, *et al.* (2001). Investigation of aortocoronary artery bypass grafts by multi-slice computed tomography with electrocardiographic-gated image reconstruction. *Am. J. Cardiol.* **88**:792–795.

14 Detrano RC, Wong ND, Doherty TM, *et al.* (1999). Coronary calcium does not accurately predict near-term

future coronary events in high-risk adults. *Circulation* **99**:2633–2638.

15 Raggi P, Cooil B, Callister TQ (2001). Use of electron beam tomography data to develop models for prediction of hard coronary events. *Am. Heart J.* **141**:375–382.

16 Arad Y, Spadaro LA, Goodman K, *et al.* (2000). Prediction of coronary events with electron beam computed tomography. *J. Am. Coll. Cardiol.* **36**:1253–1260.

17 McLaughlin VV, Balogh T, Rich S (1999). Utility of electron beam computed tomography to stratify patients presenting to the emergency room with chest pain. *Am. J. Cardiol.* **84**:327–328.

18 Schroeder S, Kopp AF, Baumbach A, *et al.* (2001). Noninvasive detection and evaluation of atherosclerotic coronary plaques with multi-slice computed tomography. *J. Am. Coll. Cardiol.* **37**:1430–1435.

19 Nikolaou K, Becker CR, Babaryka G, *et al.* (2001). High-resolution magnetic resonance and multi-slice CT imaging of coronary artery plaques in human *ex vivo* coronary arteries. *Radiology* **221**(Suppl.):503.

Intracoronary ultrasound
References

1 Mintz GS, Painter JA, Pichard AD, *et al.* (1995). Atherosclerosis in angiographically 'normal' coronary artery reference segments: an intravascular ultrasound study with clinical correlations. *J. Am. Coll. Cardiol.* **25**:1479–1485.

2 Nissen SE, Yock P (2001). Intravascular ultrasound: novel pathophysiological insights and current clinical applications. *Circulation* **103**:604–616.

3 Fitzgerald PJ, St. Goar FG, Connolly AJ, *et al.* (1992). Intravascular ultrasound imaging of coronary arteries. Is three layers the norm? *Circulation* **86**:154–158.

4 von Birgelen C, de Feyter PJ, de Vrey EA, *et al.* (1997). Simpson's rule for the volumetric ultrasound assessment of atherosclerotic coronary arteries: a study with ECG-gated three-dimensional intravascular ultrasound. *Coron. Artery Dis.* **8**:363–369.

5 Hamers R, Bruining N, Knook M, Sabate M, Roelandt JRTC (2001). A novel approach to quantitative analysis of intravascular ultrasound images. In: *Computers In Cardiology*. IEEE Computer Society Press, Rotterdam, pp. 589–592.

6 Dijkstra J, Koning G, Reiber JH (1999). Quantitative measurements in IVUS images. *Int. J. Cardiol. Imag.* **15**:513–522.

7 Prati F, Arbustini E, Labellarte A, *et al.* (2001). Correlation between high frequency intravascular ultrasound and histomorphology in human coronary arteries. *Heart* **85**:567–570.

8 Bruining N, von Birgelen C, de Feyter PJ, *et al.* (1998). ECG-gated versus nongated three-dimensional intracoronary ultrasound analysis: implications for volumetric measurements. *Cathet. Cardiovasc. Diagn.* **43**:254–260.

9 Li W, von Birgelen C, Di Mario C, *et al.* (1994). Semi-automated contour detection for volumetric quantification of intracoronary ultrasound. In: *Computers in Cardiology*. IEEE Computer Society Press, Washington, pp. 277–280.

10 Gorge G, Ge J, Haude M, Baumgart D, Buck T, Erbel R (1995). Initial experience with a steerable intravascular ultrasound catheter in the aorta and pulmonary artery. *Am. J. Cardiol. Imag.* **9**:180–184.

11 Hausmann D, Erbel R, Alibelli-Chemarin MJ, *et al.* (1995). The safety of intracoronary ultrasound. A multi-center survey of 2207 examinations. *Circulation* **91**:623–630.

12 Bruining N, von Birgelen C, de Feyter PJ, Roelandt JR, Serruys PW (1998). Ultrasound appearances of coronary stents as obtained by three-dimensional intracoronary ultrasound imaging *in vitro*. *J. Invasive Cardiol.* **10**:332–338.

13 Bruining N, von Birgelen C, de Feyter PJ, Ligthart J, Serruys PW, Roelandt JR (1998). Dynamic imaging of coronary stent structures: an ECG-gated three-dimensional intracoronary ultrasound study in humans. *Ultrasound Med. Biol.* **24**:631–637.

Coronary angioscopy
References

1 Uchida Y, Tomaru T, Nakamura F, Furuse A, Fujimori Y (1987). Percutaneous coronary angioscopy in patients with ischemic heart disease. *Am. Heart J.* **114**:1216–1222.

2 Ishikawa H, Uchida Y (1991). Angioscopic features of coronary artery in Kawasaki disease. *Proceedings of 4th International Kawasaki Disease Conference*, pp. 20–22.

3 Silva JA, Escobar A, Collins TJ, Ramee SR, White CJ (1995). Unstable angina. A comparison of angioscopic findings between diabetic and nondiabetic patients. *Circulation* **92**:1731–1736.

4 Uchida Y (1989). Percutaneous cardiovascular angioscopy. In: *Lasers in Cardiovascular Medicine and Surgery*. G Abela (ed). Kurwer Academic Publishers, Boston, pp. 399–410.

5 Uchida Y (1999). Angioscopic detection of vulnerable plaques and prediction of acute coronary syndromes. In: *The Vulnerable Atherosclerotic Plaque: Understanding, Identification and Modification*. V Fuster (ed). Futura Publishing Co, Armonk, pp. 111–129.

6 Uchida Y (2000). *Coronary Angioscopy*. Futura Publishing Co, Armonk.

7 Uchida Y, Fujimori Y, Ohsawa H, Kanai M, Sakurai T, Yoshinaga K (2000). Angioscopic evaluation of stabilizing effects of bezafibrate on coronary plaques in patients with coronary artery disease: an angioscopic multi-center study. *Therap. Endoscopy* **7**:30–39.

8 Uchida Y, Tomaru T, Sugimoto T (1984). [Angioscopic observation of coronary luminal changes induced by PTCA.] *Proc. Jpn. Coll. Angiol.* **16**:50 (Abstract in Japanese.)

9 Uchida Y, Hasegawa K, Kawamura K, Shibuya I (1989). Angioscopic observation of coronary luminal changes induced by percutaneous coronary angioplasty. *Am. Heart J.* **117**:769–776.

10 Nakamura F, Kvasnicka J, Uchida Y, Geschwind HJ (1992). Percutaneous angioscopic evaluation of luminal changes induced by excimer laser angioplasty. *Am. Heart J.* **124**:1464–1472.

11 Sassower MA, Abela G, Koch JM, Manzo KM, Friedl PG, Nesto RW (1993). Angioscopic evaluation of periprocedural abrupt closure after percutaneous coronary angioplasty. *Am. Heart J.* **126**:444–450.

12 Swatpm TA (1987). Intraoperative angioscopy of saphenous vein and coronary arteries. *J. Thorac. Cardiovasc. Surg.* **9**:339.

13 Uchida Y, Nakamura F, Tomaru T, *et al.* (1995). Prediction of acute coronary syndromes by percutaneous coronary angioscopy in patients with stable angina. *Am. Heart J.* **130**:195–203.

14 Terasawa K, Fujimori Y, Morio H, Uchida Y (2000). [Evaluation of coronary endothelial cell damage caused by PTCA guide wire *in vivo* dye staining angioscopy.] *J. Jpn. Coll. Angiol.* **40**:159–164 (in Japanese).

15 Uchida Y, Ohsawa H, Takeuchi K (1999). Fluorescent image coronary angioscopy. *Jpn. Circulat. J.* **63**(Suppl): 310 (in Japanese).

16 Uchida Y (1989). Percutaneous coronary angioscopy by means of a fiberscope with steerable guide wire. *Am. Heart J.* **117**:1153–1155.

17 Uchida Y, Hirose J, Fujimori Y, Ohshima T (1992). Percutaneous coronary angioscopy. *Jpn. Heart J.* **33**:271–294.

18 Uchida Y, Kanai M, Takeuchi K, Kameda N, Hiruta K, Uchida H (1999). Angioscopic characteristics of vulnerable coronary plaques and their pathological correlations. *Coronary* **16**:302–313 (in Japanese).

19 den Heijer P, Foley DP, Hillege HL, *et al.* (1994). The 'Ermenonville' classification of observations at coronary angioscopy: evaluation of intra- and inter-observer agreement. European Working Group on Coronary Angioscopy. *Eur. Heart J.* **15**:815–822.

Intracoronary Doppler flow
References

1 Berman DS, Kang XP, Van Train KF, *et al.* (1998). Comparative prognostic value of automatic quantitative analysis versus semiquantitative visual analysis of exercise myocardial perfusion single-photon emission computed tomography. *J. Am. Coll. Cardiol.* **32**:1987–1995.

2 Topol EJ, Nissen SE (1995). Our preoccupation with coronary luminology. The dissociation between clinical and angiographic findings in ischemic heart disease. *Circulation* **92**:2333–2342.

3 Kern MJ (2000). Coronary physiology revisited: practical insights from the cardiac catheterization laboratory. *Circulation* **101**:1344–1351.

4 Doucette JW, Corl PD, Payne HM, *et al.* (1992). Validation of a Doppler guide wire for intravascular measurement of coronary artery flow velocity. *Circulation* **85**:1899–1911.

5 Miller DD, Donohue TJ, Younis LT, *et al.* (1994). Correlation of pharmacological 99mTc-sestamibi myocardial perfusion imaging with poststenotic coronary flow reserve in patients with angiographically intermediate coronary artery stenoses. *Circulation* **89**:2150–2160.

6 Joye JD, Schulman DS, Lasorda D, Farah T, Donohue BC, Reichek N (1994). Intracoronary Doppler guide wire versus stress single-photon emission computed tomographic thallium-201 imaging in assessment of intermediate coronary stenoses. *J. Am. Coll. Cardiol.* **24**:940–947.

7 Deychak YA, Segal J, Reiner JS, *et al.* (1995). Doppler guide wire flow-velocity indexes measured distal to coronary stenoses associated with reversible thallium perfusion defects. *Am. Heart J.* **129**:219–227.

8 Tron C, Donohue TJ, Bach RG, *et al.* (1995). Comparison of pressure-derived fractional flow reserve with poststenotic coronary flow velocity reserve for prediction of stress myocardial perfusion imaging results. *Am. Heart J.* **130**:723–733.

9 Heller LI, Cates C, Popma J, *et al.* (1997). Intracoronary Doppler assessment of moderate coronary artery disease: comparison with 201Tl imaging and coronary angiography. FACTS Study Group. *Circulation* **96**:484–490.

10 Danzi GB, Pirelli S, Mauri L, *et al.* (1998). Which variable of stenosis severity best describes the significance of an isolated left anterior descending coronary artery lesion? Correlation between quantitative coronary angiography, intracoronary Doppler measurements and high dose dipyridamole echocardiography. *J. Am. Coll. Cardiol.* **31**:526–533.

11 Verberne HJ, Piek JJ, van Liebergen RAM, Koch KT, Schroeder-Tanka JM, van Royen EA (1999). Functional assessment of coronary artery stenosis by Doppler derived absolute and relative coronary blood flow velocity reserve in comparison with Tc-99m MIBI SPECT. *Heart* **82**:509–514.

12 Piek JJ, Boersma E, di Mario C, *et al.* (2000). Angiographical and Doppler flow-derived parameters for assessment of coronary lesion severity and its relation to the result of exercise electrocardiography. DEBATE study group. Doppler Endpoints Balloon Angioplasty Trial Europe. *Eur. Heart J.* **21**:466–474.

13 Chamuleau SAJ, Meuwissen M, Van Eck-Smit BLF, *et al.* (2001). Fractional flow reserve, absolute and relative coronary blood flow velocity reserve in relation to the results of technetium-99m sestamibi single-photon emission computed tomography in patients with two-vessel coronary artery disease. *J. Am. Coll. Cardiol.* **37**:1316–1322.

14 Meuwissen M, Siebes M, Chamuleau SAJ, *et al.* (2002). Hyperemic stenosis resistance index for evaluation of functional coronary lesion severity. *Circulation* **106**(4):441–446.

15 Duffy SJ, Gelman JS, Peverill RE, Greentree MA, Harper RW, Meredith IT (2001). Agreement between coronary flow velocity reserve and stress echocardiography in intermediate-severity coronary stenoses. *Catheter Cardiovasc. Interv.* **53**:29–38.

16 El-Shafei A, Chiravuri R, Stikovac M, *et al.* (2001). Comparison of relative coronary Doppler flow velocity reserve to stress myocardial perfusion imaging in patients with coronary artery disease. *Catheter Cardiovasc. Interv.* **53**:193–201.

17 Chamuleau SA, Tio RA, de Cock CC, *et al.* (2002). Prognostic value of coronary blood flow velocity and myocardial perfusion in intermediate coronary narrowings and multi-vessel disease. *J. Am. Coll. Cardiol.* **39**:852–858.

18 Ferrari M, Schnell B, Werner GS, Figulla HR (1999). Safety of deferring angioplasty in patients with normal coronary flow velocity reserve. *J. Am. Coll. Cardiol.* **33**:82–87.

19 Kern MJ, Donohue TJ, Aguirre FV, *et al.* (1995). Clinical outcome of deferring angioplasty in patients with normal translesional pressure-flow velocity measurements. *J. Am. Coll. Cardiol.* **25**:178–187.

20 Serruys PW, di Mario C, Piek J, *et al.* (1997). Prognostic value of intracoronary flow velocity and diameter stenosis in assessing the short- and long-term outcomes of coronary balloon angioplasty: the DEBATE Study (Doppler Endpoints Balloon Angioplasty Trial Europe). *Circulation* **96**:3369–3377.

21 Di Mario C, Moses JW, Anderson TJ, *et al.* (2000). Randomized comparison of elective stent implantation and coronary balloon angioplasty guided by online quantitative angiography and intracoronary Doppler. *Circulation* **102**:2938–2944.

22 Lafont A, Dubois-Rande JL, Steg PG, *et al.* (2000). The French randomized optimal stenting trial: a prospective evaluation of provisional stenting guided by coronary velocity reserve and quantitative coronary angiography. FROST Study Group. *J. Am. Coll. Cardiol.* **36**:404–409.

23 Serruys PW, de Bruyne B, Carlier S, *et al.* (2000). Randomized comparison of primary stenting and provisional balloon angioplasty guided by flow velocity measurement. *Circulation* **102**:2930–2937.

24 Kern MJ, Puri S, Bach RG, *et al.* (1999). Abnormal coronary flow velocity reserve after coronary artery stenting in patients. Role of relative coronary reserve to assess potential mechanisms. *Circulation* **100**:2491–2498.

25 Voskuil M, van Liebergen RA, Albertal M, *et al.* (2002). Coronary hemodynamics of stent implantation after suboptimal and optimal balloon angioplasty. *J. Am. Coll. Cardiol.* **39**:1513–1517.

26 Haude M, Baumgart D, Verna E, *et al.* (2001). Intracoronary Doppler- and quantitative coronary angiography-derived predictors of major adverse cardiac events after stent implantation. *Circulation* **103**:1212–1217.

27 Voskuil M, Boersma E, Tijssen JPG, Serruys PW, Piek JJ (2002). Optimized stent implantation according to intracoronary Doppler derived parameters. *Am. J. Cardiol.* **90**(10):1139–1142.

28 Sousa JE, Costa MA, Abizaid AC, *et al.* (2001). Sustained suppression of neointimal proliferation by sirolimus-eluting stents: one-year angiographic and intravascular ultrasound follow-up. *Circulation* **104**:2007–2011.

29 Piek JJ, Kern MJ (2001). Interpretation of trials on provisional stent implantation. *Circulation* **104**:E43.

Endothelial dysfunction
Further reading
Benjamin N, Calver A, Collier J, *et al.* (1995). Measuring forearm blood flow and interpreting the responses to drugs and mediators. *Hypertension* **25**:918–923.

Bøttcher M, Bøtker HE, Sonne HS, Nielsen TT, Czernin J (1999). Endothelium-dependent and -independent perfusion reserve and the effect of L-arginine on myocardial perfusion in patients with syndrome X. *Circulation* **99**:1795–1801.

Celermajer DS (1997). Endothelial dysfunction: does it matter? Is it reversible? *J. Am. Coll. Cardiol.* **30**:325–333.

Celermajer DS, Sorensen K, Gooch V, *et al.* (1992). Noninvasive detection of early endothelial dysfunction in children and adults at risk of atherosclerosis. *Lancet* **340**:111–116.

Corretti MC, Anderson TJ, Benjamin EJ, *et al.* (2002). Guidelines for the ultrasound assessment of endothelial-dependent flow-mediated vasodilation of the brachial artery. *J. Am. Coll. Cardiol.* **39**:257–265.

Electron-beam computed tomography: coronary calcium
References
1 Rumberger JA, Simons DB, Fitzpatrick LA, Sheedy PF, Schwartz RS (1995). Coronary artery calcium area by electron-beam computed tomography and coronary atherosclerotic plaque area. A histopathologic correlative study. *Circulation* **92**:2157–2162.

2 Schmermund A, Erbel R (2001). Current Perspective: unstable coronary plaque and its relation to coronary calcium. *Circulation* **104**:1682–1687.

3 Burke AP, Kolodgie FD, Farb A, *et al.* (2002). Morphological predictors of arterial remodeling in coronary atherosclerosis. *Circulation* **105**:297–303.

4 De Backer G, Ambrosioni E, Borch-Johnsen K, *et al.* (2003). Executive Summary. European guidelines on cardiovascular disease prevention in clinical practice. Third Joint Task Force of European and other Societies on cardiovascular disease prevention in clinical practice. *Eur. Heart J.* **24**:1601–1610.

5 Third Report of the National Cholesterol Education Program (NCEP) Expert Panel on detection, evaluation, and treatment of high blood cholesterol in adults (Adult Treatment Panel III) final report. *Circulation* **106**:3143–3421.

6 Vliegenthart R, Oudkerk M, Hofman A, *et al.* (2005). Coronary calcification improves cardiovascular risk prediction in the elderly. *Circulation* **112**:572–577.

7 O'Rourke RA, Brundage BH, Froelicher VF, *et al.* (2000). American College of Cardiology/American Heart Association expert consensus document on electron-beam computed tomography for the diagnosis and prognosis of coronary artery disease. *J. Am. Coll. Cardiol.* **36**:326–340.

8 Georgiou D, Budoff MJ, Kaufer E, *et al.* (2001). Screening patients with chest pain in the emergency department using EBT: a follow-up study. *J. Am. Coll. Cardiol.* **38**:105–110.

9 Schmermund A, Möhlenkamp S, Berenbein S, Pump H, *et al.* (2006). Population-based assessment of subclinical coronary atherosclerosis using electron beam computed tomography. *Atherosclerosis* **185**:177–182.

10 Hunold P, Vogt FM, Schmermund A, *et al.* (2003). Radiation exposure during cardiac computed tomography: effective doses of multi-detector row computed tomography and electron-beam tomography. *Radiology* **226**:145–152.

Vulnerable atherosclerotic plaques
Further reading
Burke AP, Virmani R, Galis Z, Haudenschild CC, Muller JE (2003). 34th Bethesda Conference: Task force #2. What is the pathologic basis for new atherosclerosis imaging techniques? *J. Am. Coll. Cardiol.* **41**:1874–1886.

Casscells W, Hassan K, Vaseghi MF, *et al.* (2003). Plaque blush, branch location, and calcification are angiographic predictors of progression of mild to moderate coronary stenoses. *Am. Heart J.* **145**:813–820.

Casscells W, Naghavi M, Willerson JT (2003). Vulnerable atherosclerotic plaque: a multi-focal disease. *Circulation* **107**:2072–2075.

Fayad ZA, Choudhury RP, Fuster V (2003). Magnetic resonance imaging of coronary atherosclerosis. *Curr. Atheroscler. Rep.* **5**:411–417.

MacNeill BD, Lowe HC, Takano M, Fuster V, Jang IK (2003). Intravascular modalities for detection of vulnerable plaque: current status. *Arterioscler. Thromb. Vasc. Biol.* **23**:1333–1342.

Naghavi M, Libby P, Falk E, *et al.* (2003). From vulnerable plaque to vulnerable patient: a call for new definitions and risk assessment strategies (Parts I and II). *Circulation* **108**:1664–1672, 1772–1778.

Sarikaya I, Larson SM, Freiman A, Strauss HW (2003). What nuclear cardiology can learn from nuclear oncology. *J. Nucl. Cardiol.* **10**:324–328.

Schaar JA, De Korte CL, Mastik F, *et al.* (2003). Characterizing vulnerable plaque features with intravascular elastography. *Circulation* **108**:2636–2641.

CHAPTER 8 Detection of Myocardial Ischemia and Infarction
Electrocardiography
Further reading
Channer K, Morris F (2002). ABC of clinical electrocardiography: Myocardial ischaemia. *BMJ* **324**:1023–1026.
Zimetbaum PJ, Josephson ME (2003). Use of the electrocardiogram in acute myocardial infarction. *N. Engl. J. Med.* **348**:933–940.

Exercise testing
Further reading
Froelicher VF, Myers JN (2000). *Exercise and the Heart*, 4th edn. WB Saunders, Philadelphia.
Hill J, Timmis A (2002). Exercise tolerance testing. *BMJ* **324**:1084–1087.
Pitt B (1995). Evaluation of the postinfarct patient. *Circulation* **91**:1855–1860.

Continuous vectorcardiographic monitoring
Further reading
Bjorklund E, Lindahl B, Johanson P, *et al.* (2004). Admission troponin T and measurement of ST segment resolution at 60 minutes improve early risk stratification in ST-elevation myocardial infarction. *Eur. Heart J.* **25**(2):113–120.
Dellborg M, Malmberg K, Ryden L, *et al.* (1995). Dynamic online vectorcardiography improves and simplifies inhospital ischemia monitoring of patients with unstable angina. *J. Am. Coll. Cardiol.* **26**(6):1501–1507.
Johanson P, Wagner GS, Dellborg M, *et al.* (2003). ST-segment monitoring in patients with acute coronary syndromes. *Curr. Cardiol. Rep.* **5**(4):278–283. Review.
Nørgaard BL, Thygesen K, Gill S, *et al.* (2000). A technical approach for optimizing surveillance of patients with unstable coronary syndromes: continuous vectorcardiography ischemic monitoring. *Cardiology* **94**:131–138. Review.

Electrophysiology
Further reading
Tracy CM, Akhtar M, DiMarco JP, *et al.* (2000). American College of Cardiology/American Heart Association Clinical Competence Statement on invasive electrophysiology studies, catheter ablation, and cardioversion: a report of the American College of Cardiology/American Heart Association/American College of Physicians-American Society of Internal Medicine Task Force on Clinical Competence. *Circulation* **102**:2309–2320.

Echocardiography
Further reading
Isaaz K (2002). Tissue Doppler imaging for the assessment of left ventricular systolic and diastolic functions. *Curr. Opin. Cardiol.* **17**:431–442.

Kaul S (2001). Myocardial contrast echocardiography: basic principles. *Progr. Cardiovasc. Dis.* **44**:1–11.

Marwick TH (2003). Stress echocardiography. *Heart* **89**:113–118.

Mazur W, Nagueh SF (2001). Myocardial viability: recent developments in detection and clinical significance. *Curr. Opin. Cardiol.* **16**:277–281.

Nijland F, Kamp O, Verhorst PM, de Voogt WG, Visser CA (2002). Early prediction of improvement in ejection fraction after acute myocardial infarction using low dose dobutamine echocardiography. *Heart* **88**:592–596.

Ward RP, Lang RM (2002). Myocardial contrast echocardiography in acute coronary syndromes. *Curr. Opin. Cardiol.* **17**:455–463.

Myocardial scintigraphy
References

1 Hachamovitch R, Berman DS, Kiat H, Cohen I, Friedman JD, Shaw LJ (2002). Value of stress myocardial perfusion single photon emission computed tomography in patients with normal resting electrocardiograms: an evaluation of incremental prognostic value and cost-effectiveness. *Circulation* **105**(7):823–829.

2 Hachamovitch R, Hayes S, Friedman JD, *et al.* (2003). Determinants of risk and its temporal variation in patients with normal stress myocardial perfusion scans: what is the warranty period of a normal scan? *J. Am. Coll. Cardiol.* **41**(8):1329–1340.

Further reading

Berman DS, Kang X, Hayes SW, *et al.* (2003). Adenosine myocardial perfusion single-photon emission computed tomography in women compared with men. Impact of diabetes mellitus on incremental prognostic value and effect on patient management. *J. Am. Coll. Cardiol.* **41**(7):1125–1133.

Udelson JE, Beshansky JR, Ballin DS, *et al.* (2002). Myocardial perfusion imaging for evaluation and triage of patients with suspected acute cardiac ischemia: a randomized controlled trial. *JAMA* **288**(21):2693–2700.

Wackers FJ, Brown KA, Heller GV, *et al.* (2002). American Society of Nuclear Cardiology position statement on radionuclide imaging in patients with suspected acute ischemic syndromes in the emergency department or chest pain center. *J. Nucl. Cardiol.* **9**(2):246–250.

Positron emission tomography
Further reading

Di Carli MF, Asgarzadie F, Schelbert HR, *et al.* (1995). Quantitative relation between myocardial viability and improvement in heart failure symptoms after revascularization in patients with ischemic cardiomyopathy. *Circulation* **92**(12):3436–3444.

Di Carli MF, Hachamovitch R, Berman DS (2002). The art and science of predicting postrevascularization improvement in

left ventricular (LV) function in patients with severely depressed LV function. *J. Am. Coll. Cardiol.* **40**(10):1744–1747.

Haas F, Augustin N, Holper K, *et al.* (2000). Time course and extent of improvement of dysfunctioning myocardium in patients with coronary artery disease and severely depressed left ventricular function after revascularization: correlation with positron emission tomographic findings. *J. Am. Coll. Cardiol.* **36**(6):1927–1934.

Knuuti MJ, Saraste M, Nuutila P, *et al.* (1994). Myocardial viability: fluorine-18-deoxyglucose positron emission tomography in prediction of wall motion recovery after revascularization. *Am. Heart J.* **127**:785–796.

Schelbert HR (1991). Positron emission tomography for the assessment of myocardial viability. *Circulation* **84**:I122–I131.

Wiggers H, Nielsen TT, Bottcher M, Egeblad H, Botker HE (2000). Positron emission tomography and low-dose dobutamine echocardiography in the prediction of postrevascularization improvement in left ventricular function and exercise parameters. *Am. Heart J.* **140**(6):928–936.

Magnetic resonance imaging
References

1 Nagel E, Lehmkuhl HB, Bocksch W, *et al.* (1999). Noninvasive diagnosis of ischemia-induced wall motion abnormalities with the use of high-dose dobutamine stress MRI: comparison with dobutamine stress echocardiography. *Circulation* **99**:763–770.

2 Hundley WG, Hamilton CA, Thomas MS, *et al.* (1999). Utility of fast cine magnetic resonance imaging and display for the detection of myocardial ischemia in patients not well suited for second harmonic stress echocardiography. *Circulation* **100**:1697–1702.

3 Al-Saadi N, Nagel E, Gross M, *et al.* (2000). Noninvasive detection of myocardial ischemia from perfusion reserve based on cardiovascular magnetic resonance. *Circulation* **101**:1379–1383.

4 Schwitter J, Nanz D, Kneifel S, *et al.* (2001). Assessment of myocardial perfusion in coronary artery disease by magnetic resonance: a comparison with positron emission tomography and coronary angiography. *Circulation* **103**:2230–2235.

5 Kim RJ, Wu E, Rafael A, *et al.* (2000). The use of contrast-enhanced magnetic resonance imaging to identify reversible myocardial dysfunction. *N. Engl. J. Med.* **343**:1445–1453.

Further reading

American Heart Association Writing Group on myocardial segmentation and registration for cardiac imaging: Cerqueira MD, Weissman NJ, Dilsizian V, *et al.* (2002). Standardized myocardial segmentation and nomenclature for tomographic imaging of the heart. A statement for healthcare professionals from the cardiac imaging committee of the council on clinical cardiology of the American Heart Association. *Circulation* **105**:539–542.

Nagel E, Klein C, Paetsch I, *et al.* (2003). Magnetic resonance perfusion measurements for the noninvasive detection of coronary artery disease. *Circulation* **108**:432–437.

Nagel E, Lorenz C, Baer F, *et al.* (2001). Stress cardiovascular magnetic resonance: consensus panel report. *J. Cardiovasc. Magn. Reson.* **3**:267–281.

Wagner A, Mahrholdt H, Holly TA, *et al.* (2003). Contrast-enhanced MRI and routine single photon emission computed tomography (SPECT) perfusion imaging for detection of subendocardial myocardial infarcts: an imaging study. *Lancet* **361**:374–379.

Computed tomography
References

1　Budoff MJ, Gillespie R, Georgiou D, *et al.* (1998). Comparison of ultrafast computed tomography and sestamibi in the evaluation of coronary artery disease. *Am. J. Cardiol.* **81**:682–687.

2　Sangiorgi G, Rumberger JA, Severson A, *et al.* (1998). Arterial calcification and not lumen stenosis is highly correlated with atherosclerotic plaque burden in humans: a histologic study of 723 coronary artery segments using nondecalcifying methodology. *J. Am. Coll. Cardiol.* **31**:126–133.

3　Haberl R, Becker A, Leber A, *et al.* (2001). Correlation of coronary calcification and angiographically documented stenoses in patients with suspected coronary artery disease: results of 1, 764 patients. *J. Am. Coll. Cardiol.* **37**:451–457.

4　Schmermund A, Erbel R (2001). Unstable coronary plaque and its relation to coronary calcium. *Circulation* **104**:1682–1687.

5　Shavelle DM, Budoff MJ, Lamont DH, *et al.* (2000). Exercise testing and electron-beam computed tomography in the evaluation of coronary artery disease. *J. Am. Coll. Cardiol.* **36**(1):32–38.

6　Georgiou D, Budoff MJ, Kaufer E, Kennedy JM, Lu B, Brundage BH (2001). Screening patients with chest pain in the emergency department using electron beam tomography: a follow-up study. *J. Am. Coll. Cardiol.* **38**(1):105–110.

7　McLaughlin VV, Balogh T, Rich S (1999). Utility of electron beam computed tomography to stratify patients presenting to the emergency room with chest pain. *Am. J. Cardiol.* **84**:327–328.

8　O'Malley PG, Taylor AJ, Jackson JL, Doherty TM, Detrano RC (2000). Prognostic value of coronary electron-beam computed tomography for coronary heart disease events in asymptomatic populations. *Am. J. Cardiol.* **85**(8):945–948.

9　Rumberger JA, Bell MR, Feiring JA, *et al.* (1991). Measurement of myocardial perfusion using fast computed tomography. In: *Cardiac Imaging*. ML Marcus, HR Schelbert, DJ Skorton, GL Wolf (eds). WB Saunders, Philadelphia, pp. 688–702.

10　Budoff MJ, Oudiz RJ, Zalace CP, *et al.* (1999). Intravenous three-dimensional coronary angiography using contrast enhanced electron beam computed tomography. *Am. J. Cardiol.* **83**:840–845.

11　Achenbach S, Moshage W, Ropers D, Nossen J, Daniel WG (1998). Value of electron-beam computed tomography for the noninvasive detection of high-grade coronary artery stenoses and occlusions. *N. Engl. J. Med.* **339**:1964–1971.

12　Schmermund A, Haude M, Baumgart D, *et al.* (1996). Noninvasive assessment of coronary Palmaz–Schatz stents by contrast enhanced electron beam computed tomography. *Europ. Heart J.* **17**: 1546–1553.

13　Ha JW, Cho SY, Shim WH, *et al.* (1999). Noninvasive evaluation of coronary artery bypass graft patency using three-dimensional angiography obtained with contrast-enhanced electron-beam CT. *Am. J. Roentgenol.* **172**:1055–1059.

14　Goldin JG, Yoon HC, Greaser LE 3rd, *et al.* (2001). Spiral versus electron-beam CT for coronary artery calcium scoring. *Radiology* **221**(1):213–221.

15　Hidajat N, Wolf M, Rademaker J, Knowllmann FD, Oestmann JW, Felix R (2000). Radiation dose in CT of the heart for coronary heart disease and CT of the lung for pulmonary embolism: comparisons between single-slice detector CT, multi-slice detector CT and EBT. *Radiology* **217**:374.

Electromechanical Mapping
Further reading

Bøtker HE, Lassen JF, Hermansen F, *et al.* (2001). Electromechanical mapping for detection of myocardial viability in patients with ischemic cardiomyopathy. *Circulation* **103**:1631–1637.

Wiggers H, Bøtker HE, Søgaard P, *et al.* (2003). Electromechanical mapping versus positron emission tomography and single photon emission computed tomography for the detection of myocardial viability in patients with ischemic cardiomyopathy. *J. Am. Coll. Cardiol.* **41**:843–848.

Invasive hemodynamic monitoring
References

1　Mark JB (1991). Central venous pressure monitoring: clinical insights beyond the number. *J. Cardiothorac. Vasc. Anesth.* **5**(2):163–173.

2　Mangano DT (1980). Monitoring pulmonary pressure in coronary artery disease. *Anesthesiology* **53**(5):364–370.

3　Hall RI, O'Regan N, Gardner M (1995). Detection of intraoperative myocardial ischemia: a comparison among electrographic, myocardial metabolic, and hemodynamic measurements in patients with reduced ventricular function. *Can. J. Anesth.* **42**(6):487–497.

4　Kaplan JA, Wells PH (1981). Early diagnosis of myocardial ischemia using the pulmonary artery catheter. *Anesth. Analg.* **60**:789–793.

5　Pulmonary artery catheter consensus conference: consensus statement (1997). *Crit. Care Med.* **25**(6):909–925.

6 Iberti TJ, Fischer EP, Leibowitz AB, *et al.* (1990). A multi-center study of physicians' knowledge of the pulmonary artery catheter. *JAMA* **264**:2928–2932.

7 Tuman KJ, Caroll GC, Ivankovich AD (1989). Pitfalls in interpretation of pulmonary artery catheter data. *J. Cardiothorac. Anesth.* **3**(5):625–641.

8 Urban MK, Gordon MA, Harris SN, O'Connor T, Barash PG (1993). Intraoperative hemodynamic changes are not good indicators of myocardial ischemia. *Anesth. Analg.* **78**:380–393.

9 Practice guidelines for pulmonary artery catheterization (1993). A report by the American Society of Anesthesiologists' Task Force on pulmonary artery catheterization. *Anesthesiology* **78**:380–393.

10 Shah KB, Rao TKL, Laughlin S, El-Etr AA (1984). A review of pulmonary artery catheterization in 6245 patients. *Anesthesiology* **61**:271–275.

Biochemical markers
Further reading

Apple FS, Wu AHB, Jaffe AS (2002). European Society of Cardiology and American College of Cardiology guidelines for redefinition of myocardial infarction: how to use existing assays clinically and for clinical trials. *Am. Heart J.* **144**:981–986.

Danne O, Möckel M, Lueders C, *et al.* (2003). Prognostic implications of whole blood choline levels in acute coronary syndrome. *Am. J. Cardiol.* **91**:1060–1067.

Heeschen C, Dimmeler S, Hamm CW, *et al.*; CAPTURE Study Investigators (2003). Soluble CD40 ligand in acute coronary syndromes. *N. Engl. J. Med.* **348**:1104–1111.

Jaffe AS, Ravkilde J, Roberts R, *et al.* (2000). It's time for a change to a troponin standard. *Circulation* **102**:1216–1220.

Morrow DA, Braunwald E (2003). Future of biomarkers in acute coronary syndromes: moving toward a multi-marker strategy. *Circulation* **108**:250–252.

Myocardial infarction redefined: a consensus document of The Joint European Society of Cardiology/American College of Cardiology Committee for the redefinition of myocardial infarction (2000). *Eur. Heart J.* **21**:1502–1513.

Olatidoye AG, Wu ABH, Feng Y-J, Waters D (1998). Prognostic role of troponin T versus troponin I in unstable angina pectoris for cardiac events with meta-analysis comparing published studies. *Am. J. Cardiol.* **81**:1405–1410.

Panteghini M, Apple FS, Christenson RH, Dati F, Mair J, Wu AH (1999). Proposals from IFCC Committee on standardization of markers of cardiac damage (C-SMCD): recommendations on use of biochemical markers of cardiac damage in acute coronary syndromes. *Scand. J. Clin. Lab. Invest.* **230**:103–112.

Panteghini M, Pagani F, Yeo K-T J, *et al.* (2004). Evaluation of the imprecision at low-range concentrations of the assays for cardiac troponin determination. *Clin. Chem.* **50**:327–332.

Sabatine MS, Morrow DA, de Lemos JA, *et al.* (2002). Multi-marker approach to risk stratification in non-ST elevation acute coronary syndromes: simultaneous assessment of troponin I, C-reactive protein, and B-type natriuretic peptide. *Circulation* **105**:1760–1763.

CHAPTER 9 Stable Ischemic Syndromes
Stable angina pectoris
Further reading

Blumenthal RS, Cohn G, Schulman SP (2000). Medical therapy versus coronary angioplasty in stable coronary artery disease: a critical review of the literature. *J. Am. Coll. Cardiol.* **36**:668–673.

IONA Study Group. Effect of nicorandil on coronary events in patients with stable angina: the impact of nicorandil in angina (IONA) randomized trial (2002). *Lancet* **359**:1269–1275.

Fox KM, European trial on Reduction of cardiac events with Perindopril in stable Coronary Artery disease Investigators (2003). Efficacy of perindopril in reduction of cardiovascular events among patients with stable coronary artery disease: randomized, double-blind, placebo-controlled, multicenter trial (the EUROPA study). *Lancet* **362**:782–788.

Gibbons RJ, Abrams J, Chatterjee K, *et al.* (2003). ACC/AHA 2002 guideline update for the management of patients with chronic stable angina: summary article: a report of the American College of Cardiology/American Heart Association Task Force on practice guidelines (Committee on the management of patients with chronic stable angina). *J. Am. Coll. Cardiol.* **41**:159–168.

Heidenreich PA, McDonald KM, Hastie T, *et al.* (1999). Meta-analysis of trials comparing beta blockers, calcium antagonists, and nitrates for stable angina. *JAMA* **281**:1927–1936.

Management of stable angina pectoris. Recommendations of the Task Force of the European Society of Cardiology (1997). *Eur. Heart J.* **18**:394–413.

Heart Protection Study Colla Corative Group (2002). MRC/BHF heart protection study of cholesterol lowering with simvastatin in 20,536 high-risk individuals: a randomized placebo-controlled trial. *Lancet* **360**:7–22.

Yusuf S, Sleight P, Poque J, Bosch J, Davies R, Dagenais G (2000). Effects of an angiotensin-converting-enzyme inhibitor, ramipril, on cardiovascular events in high-risk patients. The heart outcomes prevention evaluation study investigators. *N. Engl. J. Med.* **342**:145–153.

The PEACE Trial Investigators (2004). Angiotensin-converting enzyme inhibition in stable coronary artery disease. *N. Engl. J. Med.* **351**:2058–2068.

Prinzmetal's variant angina
Further reading

Hong MK, Park SW, Lee CW, *et al.* (2000). Intravascular ultrasound findings of negative arterial remodeling at sites of focal coronary spasm in patients with vasospastic angina. *Am. Heart J.* **140**(3):395–401.

Kaski JC (2001). Variant angina pectoris: In: *Cardiology*. MH
  Crawford, JP DiMarco, WJ Paulus (eds). Mosby, London.
Ito K, Akita H, Kanazawa K, *et al.* (1999). Systemic endothelial
  function is preserved in men with both active and inactive
  variant angina pectoris. *Am. J. Cardiol.* **84**:1347–1349.
Miki T, Suzuki M, Shibasaki T, *et al.* (2002). Mouse model of
  Prinzmetal angina by disruption of the inward rectifier
  Kir6.1. *Nature Medicine* **8**:466–472.
Pepine CJ, El-Tamimi H, Lambert CR (1992). Prinzmetal's
  angina (variant angina). *Heart Dis. Stroke* **1**:281–286.
Prinzmetal M, Kennamer R, Merliss R, Wade T, Bor N (1959).
  Angina pectoris. I: a variant form of angina pectoris.
  Preliminary report. *Am. J. Med.* **27**:375–388.

Cardiac syndrome X
Further reading
Bøtker HE (2001). Vascular and metabolic abnormalitities in
  patients with angina pectoris and normal coronary
  angiograms. *Dan. Med. Bull.* **48**:1–18.
Cannon RO 3rd, Camici PG, Epstein SE (1992). Pathophysiological dilemma of syndrome X. *Circulation* **85**: 883–892.
Kaski JC (2002). Overview of gender aspects of cardiac
  syndrome X. *Cardiovasc. Res.* **53**:620–626.

CHAPTER 10 Acute Coronary Syndromes
Non-ST elevation acute coronary syndromes
Further reading
Bertrand ME, Simoons ML, Fox KA, *et al.* (2000).
  Management of acute coronary syndromes: acute coronary
  syndromes without persistent ST segment elevation.
  Recommendations of the Task Force of the
  European Society of Cardiology. *Eur. Heart J.*
  21(17):1406–1432.
Braunwald E, Antman EM, Beasley JW, *et al.* (2000).
  ACC/AHA guidelines for the management of patients with
  unstable angina and non-ST segment elevation myocardial
  infarction. A report of the American College of
  Cardiology/American Heart Association Task Force on
  practice guidelines (Committee on the management of
  patients with unstable angina) [In Process Citation].
  J. Am. Coll. Cardiol. **36**(3):970–1062.
Ross R (1999). Atherosclerosis: an inflammatory disease.
  N. Engl. J. Med. **340**:115–126.
Steg P, Goldberg R, Gore J, *et al.* (2002). Baseline
  characteristics, management practices, and in-hospital
  outcomes of patients hospitalized with acute coronary
  syndromes in the Global Registry of Acute Coronary Events
  (GRACE). *Am. J. Cardiol.* **90**(4):358.
Yusuf S, Zhao F, Mehta SR, Chrolavicius S, Tognoni G, Fox KK
  (2001). Effects of clopidogrel in addition to aspirin in
  patients with acute coronary syndromes without ST segment
  elevation. *N. Engl. J. Med.* **345**:494–502.

Acute myocardial infarction with ST segment elevation
References
1 The Joint European Society of Cardiology/American
   College of Cardiology Committee (2000). Myocardial
   infarction redefined: a consensus document of the Joint
   European Society of Cardiology/American College of
   Cardiology Committee for the redefinition of
   myocardial infarction. *J. Am.Coll. Cardiol.*
   36:959–969.
2 White HD, Van de Werf FJJ (1998). Thrombolysis for acute
   myocardial infarction. *Circulation* **97**:1632–1646.
3 Fibrinolytic Therapy Trialists' (FTT) Collaborative Group
   (1994). Indications for fibrinolytic therapy in suspected
   acute myocardial infarction: collaborative overview of early
   mortality and major morbidity results from all randomized
   trials of more than 1000 patients. *Lancet* **343**:311–322.
4 Andrews J, Straznicky IT, French JK, *et al.*, for the HERO-1
   Investigators (2000). ST segment recovery adds to the
   assessment of TIMI 2 and 3 flow in predicting infarct wall
   motion after thrombolytic therapy. *Circulation*
   101:2138–2143.
5 Remmen JJ, Verheugt FWA (2001). The hotline sessions of
   the 23rd European Congress of Cardiology. *Europ. Heart J.*
   22:2033–2037.
6 French JK, Williams BF, Hart HH, *et al.* (1996).
   Prospective evaluation of eligibility for thrombolytic therapy
   in acute myocardial infarction. *BMJ* **312**:1637–1641.
7 Williams ES, Miller JM (2002). Results from late-breaking
   clinical trial sessions at the American College of Cardiology
   51st Annual Scientific Session. *J. Am. Coll. Cardiol.*
   40:1–18.
8 Ryan TJ, Antman EM, Brooks NH, *et al.* (1999). 1999
   update: ACC/AHA guidelines for the management of
   patients with acute myocardial infarction: a report of the
   American College of Cardiology/American Heart
   Association Task Force on practice guidelines (Committee
   on management of acute myocardial infarction). *J. Am. Coll.
   Cardiol.* **34**:890–911.
9 Ohman EM, Harrington RA, Cannon CP, Agnelli G, Cairns
   JA, Kennedy JW (2001). Intravenous thrombolysis in acute
   myocardial infarction. *Chest* **119**(Suppl 1):253S–277S.
10 Antman EM, Morrow DA, McCabe CH, Murphy SA, Ruda
   M, Sadowski Z *et al.* (2006). Enoxaparin versus
   unfractionated heparin with fibrinolysis for ST-elevation
   myocardial infarction. *N Eng J Med* 354: 1477-1488.

Out-of-hospital cardiac arrest and sudden cardiac death
References
1 American Heart Association (2005). AHA guidelines for
   cardiopulmonary resuscitation and emergency cardiovascular
   care. *Circulation* 112 (24 Suppl.):IV1–203.
2 Handley AJ, Koster R, Monsieurs K, Perkins GD, Davies S,
   Bossaert L (2005). European Resuscitation Council

guidelines for resuscitation 2005. Section 2. Adult basic life support and use of automated external defibrillators. *Resuscitation* 67(Suppl. 1):S7–S23.

Further reading

Priori SG, Aliot E, Blomstrom-Lundqvist C, *et al.*, European Society of Cardiology (2003). Update of the guidelines on sudden cardiac death of the European Society of Cardiology. *Eur. Heart J.* 24:13–15.

Corrado D, Pelliccia A, Bjornstad HH, *et al.*, Study Group of Sport Cardiology of the Working Group of Cardiac Rehabilitation and Exercise Physiology and the Working Group of Myocardial and Pericardial Diseases of the European Society of Cardiology (2005). Cardiovascular pre-participation screening of young competitive athletes for prevention of sudden death: proposal for a common European protocol. Consensus Statement of the Study Group of Sport Cardiology of the Working Group of Cardiac Rehabilitation and Exercise Physiology and the Working Group of Myocardial and Pericardial Diseases of the European Society of Cardiology. *Eur. Heart J.* 26:516–524.

Maron BJ (2003). Sudden death in young athletes. *N. Engl. J. Med.* 349:1064–1075.

Hazinski MF, Idris AH, Kerber RE, *et al.* (2005). Lay rescuer automated external defibrillator ('public access defibrillation') programs: lessons learned from an international multicenter trial: advisory statement from the American Heart Association Emergency Cardiovascular Committee; the Council on Cardiopulmonary, Perioperative, and Critical Care; and the Council on Clinical Cardiology. *Circulation* 111:3336–3340.

Priori SG, Bossaert LL, Chamberlain DA, *et al.* (2004). ESC-ERC recommendations for the use of automated external defibrillators (AEDs) in Europe. *Eur. Heart J.* 25:437–445.

Sterk B, van Alem AP, Tukkie R, Simmers TA, Koster RW (2004). ICD-implantation guidelines versus clinical practice: a prospective study of out-of-hospital cardiac arrest survivors. *Europace* 6:179–183.

Buxton AE (2005). Sudden death after myocardial infarction: who needs prophylaxis, and when? *N. Engl. J. Med.* 352:2638–2640.

Lane RE, Cowie MR, Chow AW (2005). Prediction and prevention of sudden cardiac death in heart failure. *Heart* 91:674–680.

Waalewijn RA, de Vos R, Tijssen JG, Koster RW (2001). Survival models for out-of-hospital cardiopulmonary resuscitation from the perspectives of the bystander, the first responder, and the paramedic.*Resuscitation* 51:113–122.

Myerburg RJ, Kessler KM, Castellanos A (1993). Sudden cardiac death: epidemiology, transient risk, and intervention assessment. *Ann. Intern. Med.* 119:1187–1197.

Triggering of acute coronary syndromes
References

1 Kristensen SD, Andersen HR, Falk E (1999). What an interventional cardiologist should know about the pathophysiology of acute myocardial infarction. *Sem. Int. Cardiol.* 4:11–26.

2 Burke AP, Farb A, Virmani R (2001). Coronary thrombosis: what's new. *Pathol. Case Rev.* 6:244–252.

3 Kullo IJ, Edwards WD, Schwartz RS (1998). Vulnerable plaque: pathobiology and clinical implications. *Ann. Int. Med.* 129:1050–1060.

4 Shah PK (1997). Plaque disruption and coronary thrombosis: new insight into pathogenesis and prevention. *Clin. Cardiol.* 20:38–44.

5 Müller JE, Abela GS, Nesto RW, Tofler GH (1994). Triggers, acute risk factors and vulnerable plaques: the lexicon of a new frontier. *J. Am. Coll. Cardiol.* 23:809–813.

6 Tofler GH, Muller JE, Stone PH (1992). Modifiers of timing and possible triggers of acute myocardial infarction in the TIMI II population. *J. Am. Coll. Cardiol.* 20:1049–1055.

7 Gnecchi-Ruscone T, Piccaluga E, Guzzetti S, Contini M, Montano N, Nicolis E (1994). Morning and Monday: critical periods for the onset of acute myocardial infarction. *Eur. Heart J.* 15:882–887.

8 Tofler GH, Gebara OCE, Mittleman MA, *et al.* (1995). Morning peak in ventricular tachyarrhythmias detected by time of implantable cardioverter/defibrillator therapy. *Circulation* 92:1203–1208.

9 Deedwania PC. Hemodynamic changes as triggers of cardiovascular events. Cardiology Clinics 14:229–238, 1996

10 White A, William B (2001). Cardiovascular risk and therapeutic intervention for the early morning surge in blood pressure and heart rate. *Blood Press. Mon.* 6:63–72.

11 Woodhouse PR, Khaw KT, Plummer M, Foley A, Meade TW (1994). Seasonal variation of plasma fibrinogen and factor VII activity in the elderly: Winter infections and death from cardiovascular disease. *Lancet* 343:435–439.

12 Mittleman MA, Maclure M, Tofler GH, Sherwood JB, Goldberg RJ, Muller JE (1993). Triggering of acute myocardial infarction by heavy physical exertion. Protection against triggering by regular exertion. Determinants of myocardial infarction onset study investigators. *N. Engl. J. Med.* 329:1677–1683.

13 Siscovick DS, Weiss NS, Fletcher RH, Lasky T (1984). The incidence of primary cardiac arrest during vigorous exercise. *N. Engl. J. Med.* 311:874–877.

14 Moller J, Hallqvist J, Diderichsen F, Theorell T, Reuterwall C, Ahlbom A (1999). Do episodes of anger trigger myocardial infarction? A case-crossover analysis in the Stockholm Heart Epidemiology Program (SHEEP). *Psychosom. Med.* 61:842–849.

15 Krantz DS, Quigley JF, O'Callahan M (2001). Mental stress as a trigger of acute cadiac events: the role of laboratory studies. *Italian Heart J.* 2:895–899.

16 Phillips DP, Liu GC, Kwok K, Jarvinen JR, Zhang W, Abranson IS (2001). The Hounds of the Baskervilles effect: natural experiment on the influence of psychological stress on timing of death. *Br. Med. J.* **323**:1443–1446.

17 Young M, Benjamin B, Wallis C (1963). The mortality of widowers. *Lancet* **2**:454–456.

18 Berkman LF, Leo-Summers L, Horwitz RI (1992). Emotional support and survival after myocardial infarction: a prospective, population-based study of the elderly. *Ann. Int. Med.* **117**:1003–1009.

19 Blumenthal JA, Babyakk M, Wei J, *et al.* (2002). Usefulness of psychological treatment of mental stress-induced myocardial ischemia in men. *Am. J. Cardiol.* **89**:164–168.

20 Dusseldorp E, van Elderen T, Maes S, Meulman J, Kraaij V (1999). A meta-analysis of psychoeducational programs for coronary heart disease patients. *Health Psychol.* **18**:506–519.

21 Muller JE, Mittleman MA, Maclure M, Sherwood JB, Tofler GH (1996). Triggering myocardial infarction by sexual activity: Low absolute risk and prevention by regular physical exertion. *JAMA* **275**:1405–1409.

22 Mittleman MA, Mintzer D, Maclure M, Tofler GH, Sherwood JB, Muller JE (1999). Triggering of myocardial infarction by cocaine. *Circulation* **99**:2737–2741.

23 Gendreau MA, DeJohn C (2002). Responding to medical events during commercial airline flights. *N. Engl. J. Med.* **346**:1067–1073.

CHAPTER 11 Acute Myocardial Infarction: Complications
Cardiogenic shock
Further reading

Goldberg RJ, Samad NA, Yarzebski J, *et al.* (1999). Temporal trends in cardiogenic shock complicating acute myocardial infarction. *N. Engl. J. Med.* **340**:1162–1168.

Hochman JS, Sleeper LA, Webb JG, *et al.* (1999). Early revascularization in acute myocardial infarction complicated by cardiogenic shock. *N. Engl. J. Med.* **341**:625–634.

Holmes DR Jr, Califf RM, Van de Werf F, *et al.* (1997). Difference in countries' use of resources and clinical outcome for patients with cardiogenic shock after myocardial infarction. Results from the GUSTO trial. *Lancet* **349**:75–78.

Lindholm MG, Køber L, Boesgaard S, *et al.* (2003). Cardiogenic shock complicating acute myocardial infarction: Prognostic impact of early and late shock development. *Eur. Heart J.* **24**:258–265.

Mechanical complications
Further reading

ACC/AHA Guidelines for the management of patients with acute myocardial infarction.
http://www.americanheart.org/presenter.jhtml?identifier=2865.

Birnbaum Y, Fishbein MC, Blanche C, Siegel RJ (2002). Ventricular septal rupture after acute myocardial infarction. *N. Engl. J. Med.* **347**:1426–1432.

Birnbaum Y, Chamoun AJ, Conti VR, Uretsky BF (2002). Mitral regurgitation following acute myocardial infarction. *Coron. Artery Dis.* **13**:337–344.

Birnbaum Y, Chamoun AJ, Anzuini A, Lick SD, Ahmad M, Uretsky BF (2003). Ventricular free wall rupture following acute myocardial infarction. *Coron. Artery Dis.* **14**:463–470.

Van de Werf F, Ardissino D, Betriu A, *et al.* (2003). Management of acute myocardial infarction in patients presenting with ST segment elevation. The Task Force on the Management of Acute Myocardial Infarction of the European Society of Cardiology. *Eur. Heart J.* **24**:28–66.

Arrhythmias complicating acute myocardial infarction
Further reading

Antman EM, Braunwald E (2001). Acute myocardial infarction. In: *Braunwald's Heart Disease. A Textbook of Cardiovascular Medicine*, 6th edn. E Braunwald, DP Zipes, P Libby (eds). WB Saunders, Philadelphia, pp. 1114–1219.

Cheema AN, Sheu K, Parker M, Kadish AH, Goldberger JJ (1998). Nonsustained ventricular tachycardia in the setting of acute myocardial infarction: tachycardia characteristics and their prognostic implications. *Circulation* **98**:2030–2036.

Lloyd MA (2000). Arrhythmias complicating acute myocardial infarction. In: *Mayo Clinic Cardiology Review*, 2nd edn. JG Murphy (ed). Lippincott Williams and Wilkins, Philadelphia, pp. 225–230.

Newby KH, Thompson T, Stebbins A, Topol EJ, Califf RM, Natale A (1998). Sustained ventricular arrhythmias in patients receiving thrombolytic therapy: incidence and outcomes. The GUSTO Investigators. *Circulation* **98**:2567–2573.

Scheinman M (1997). Arrhythmias. In: *Essential Atlas of Heart Diseases*. E Braunwald (ed). Current Medicine, Philadelphia, pp. 6.1–6.34.

Other complications
Further reading

Geerts WH, Heit JA, Clagett GP, *et al.* (2001). Prevention of venous thromboembolism. *Chest* **119**(Suppl.1):132S–175S.

Joint European Society of Cardiology/American College of Cardiology Committee (2000). Myocardial infarction redefined – a consensus document of the Joint European Society of Cardiology/American College of Cardiology Committee for the redefinition of myocardial infarction. *J. Am. Coll. Cardiol.* **36**:959–969.

Meizlish JL, Berger HJ, Plankey M, *et al.* (1984). Functional left ventricular aneurysm formation after acute anterior transmural myocardial infarction: incidence, natural history, and prognostic implications. *N. Engl. J. Med.* **311**:1001–1006.

Northcote RJ, Hutchinson SJ, McGuinness JB (1984). Evidence for the continued existence of the postmyocardial infarction (Dressler's syndrome). *Am. J. Cardiol.* **53**:1201.

Oliva PB, Hammill SC, Talano JV (1994). Effect of definition on incidence of postinfarction pericarditis: is it time to redefine postinfarction pericarditis? *Circulation* **90**:1537–1541.

CHAPTER 12 Acute Myocardial Infarction: Special Problems
Right ventricular acute myocardial infarction
Further reading

Andersen HR, Falk E, Nielsen D (1998). Right ventricular infarction: frequency, size, and topography in coronary heart disease: a prospective study comprising 107 consecutive autopsies from a coronary care unit. *J. Am. Coll. Cardiol.* **10**:1223–1232.

Bowers TR, O'Neill WW, Grines C, Pica MC, Safian RD, Goldstein JA (1998). Effect of reperfusion on biventricular function and survival after right ventricular infarction. *N. Engl. J. Med.* **338**:933–940.

Mehta SR, Eikelboom JW, Natarajan MK, *et al.* (2001). Impact of right ventricular involvement on mortality and morbidity in patients with inferior myocardial infarction. *J. Am. Coll. Cardiol.* **37**:37–43.

Thrombolysis or primary angioplasty?
References

1 Keeley EC, Boura JA, Grines CL (2003). Primary angioplasty versus intravenous thrombolytic therapy for acute myocardial infarction: a quantitative review of 23 randomized trials. *Lancet* **361**:13–20.
2 Aversano T, Aversano LT, Passamani E, *et al.* (2002). Thrombolytic therapy versus primary percutaneous coronary intervention for myocardial infarction in patients presenting to hospitals without on-site cardiac surgery: a randomized controlled trial. *JAMA* **287**:1943–1951.
3 Zijlstra F (2003). Angioplasty versus thrombolysis for acute myocardial infarction: a quantitative overview of the effects of interhospital transportation. *Eur. Heart J.* **24**:21–23.

Reperfusion injury
Further reading

Bolli R (1997). Does lethal myocardial reperfusion injury exist? A controversy that is unlikely to be settled in our lifetime. *J. Thromb. Thrombolysis* **4**:109–110.

Falk E, Thuesen L (2003). Pathology of coronary microembolization and no-reflow. *Heart* **89**:983–985.

Ganz W, Watanabe I, Kanamasa K, Yano J, Han D-S, Fishbein MC (1990). Does reperfusion extend necrosis? A study in a single territory of myocardial ischemia: half reperfused and half not reperfused. *Circulation* **82**:1020–1033.

Rezkalla SH, Kloner RA (2002). No-reflow phenomenon. *Circulation* **105**:656–662.

Wang QD, Pernow J, Sjoquist PO, Ryden L (2002). Pharmacological possibilities for protection against myocardial reperfusion injury. *Cardiovasc. Res.* **55**:25–37.

Downstream (micro)embolization, slow flow, and no reflow
References

1 Topol EJ, Yadav JS (2000). Recognition of the importance of embolization in atherosclerotic vascular disease. *Circulation* **101**:570–580.
2 Falk E, Thuesen L (2003). Pathology of coronary microembolization and no reflow. *Heart* **89**:983–985.
3 Mehran R, Dangas G, Mintz GS, *et al.* (2000). Atherosclerotic plaque burden and CK-MB enzyme elevation after coronary interventions: intravascular ultrasound study of 2256 patients. *Circulation* **101**:604–610.
4 Motwani JG, Topol EJ (1998). Aortocoronary saphenous vein graft disease: pathogenesis, predisposition, and prevention. *Circulation* **97**:916–931.
5 Baim DS, Wahr D, George B, *et al.* for the Saphenous Vein Graft Angioplasty Free of Emboli Randomized (SAFER) Trial Investigators (2002). Randomized trial of a distal embolic protection device during percutaneous intervention of saphenous vein aorto-coronary bypass grafts. *Circulation* **105**:1285–1290.
6 Stone GW, Rogers C, Hermiller J, *et al.* for the FilterWire EX Randomized Evaluation Investigators (2003). Randomized comparison of distal protection with a filter-based catheter and a balloon occlusion and aspiration system during percutaneous intervention of diseased saphenous vein aorto-coronary bypass grafts. *Circulation* **108**:548–553.
7 Stone GW, Cox DA, Babb J, *et al.* (2003). Prospective, randomized evaluation of thrombectomy prior to percutaneous intervention in diseased saphenous vein grafts and thrombus-containing coronary arteries. *J. Am. Coll. Cardiol.* **42**:2007–2013.
8 Schachinger V, Hamm CW, Munzel T, *et al.* for the STENTS (STents IN Grafts) Investigators (2003). A randomized trial of polytetrafluoroethylene-membrane-covered stents compared with conventional stents in aortocoronary saphenous vein grafts. *J. Am. Coll. Cardiol.* **42**:1360–1369.
9 Stankovic G, Colombo A, Presbitero P, *et al.* for the Randomized Evaluation of Polytetrafluoroethylene COVERed Stent in Saphenous Vein Grafts Investigators (2003). Randomized evaluation of polytetrafluoroethylene-covered stent in saphenous vein grafts: the randomized evaluation of polytetrafluoroethylene COVERed stents in saphenous vein grafts (RECOVERS) trial. *Circulation* **108**:37–42.
10 Roffi M, Mukherjee D, Chew DP, *et al.* (2002). Lack of benefit from intravenous platelet glycoprotein IIb/IIIa receptor inhibition as adjunctive treatment for percutaneous interventions of aortocoronary bypass grafts: a pooled analysis of five randomized clinical trials. *Circulation* **106**:3063–3067.

11 Reffelmann T, Kloner RA (2002). The 'no-reflow' phenomenon: basic science and clinical correlates. *Heart* **87**:162–168.

12 Reffelmann T, Kloner RA (2002). Microvascular reperfusion injury: rapid expansion of anatomic no reflow during reperfusion in the rabbit. *Am. J. Physiol. Heart Circ. Physiol.* **283**:H1099–1107.

13 Topol EJ, Neumann FJ, Montalescot G (2003). A preferred reperfusion strategy for acute myocardial infarction. *J. Am. Coll. Cardiol.* **42**:1886–1889.

14 Beran G, Lang I, Schreiber W, *et al.* (2002). Intracoronary thrombectomy with the X-sizer catheter system improves epicardial flow and accelerates ST segment resolution in patients with acute coronary syndrome: a prospective, randomized, controlled study. *Circulation* **105**:2355–2360.

15 Napodano M, Pasquetto G, Sacca S, *et al.* (2003). Intracoronary thrombectomy improves myocardial reperfusion in patients undergoing direct angioplasty for acute myocardial infarction. *J. Am. Coll. Cardiol.* **42**:1395–1402.

16 Limbruno U, Micheli A, De Carlo M, *et al.* (2003). Mechanical prevention of distal embolization during primary angioplasty: safety, feasibility, and impact on myocardial reperfusion. *Circulation* **108**:171–176.

Age and acute myocardial infarction
References

1 Gillum RF (1993). Trends in acute myocardial infarction and coronary heart disease death in the United States. *J. Am. Coll. Cardiol.* **23**:1273–1277.

2 Tresch DD (1998). Management of the older patient with acute myocardial infarction: difference in clinical presentations between older and younger patients. *J. Am. Geriatr. Soc.* **46**:1157–1162.

3 Maggioni AP, Maseri A, Fresco C, *et al.* (1993). Age-related increase in mortality among patients with first myocardial infarctions treated with thrombolysis. *N. Engl. J. Med.* **329**:1442–1448.

4 Aronow WS (1998). Effects of aging on the heart. In: *Brocklehurst's Textbook of Geriatric Medicine and Gerontology*, 5th edn. RC Tallis, HM Fillit, JC Brocklehurst (eds). Churchill Livingstone, Edinburgh, pp. 255–262.

5 Lesnefsky EJ, Lundergan CF, Hodgson J, *et al.* (1996). Increased left ventricular dysfunction in elderly patients despite successful thrombolysis: the GUSTO I angiographic experience. *J. Am. Coll. Cardiol.* **28**:331–337.

6 Rathore SS, Berger AK, Weinfurt KP, *et al.* (2000). Acute myocardial infarction complicated by atrial fibrillation in the elderly: prevalence and outcomes. *Circulation* **101**:969–974.

7 Aronow WS, Starling L, Etienne F, *et al.* (1985). Unrecognized Q wave myocardial infarction in patients older than 64 years in a long-term health care facility. *Am. J. Cardiol.* **56**:483.

8 Aronow WS (1987). Prevalence of presenting symptoms of recognized acute myocardial infarction and of unrecognized healed myocardial infarction in elderly patients. *Am. J. Cardiol.* **60**:1182.

9 Nadelmann J, Frishman WH, Ooi WL, *et al.* (1990). Prevalence, incidence, and prognosis of recognized and unrecognized myocardial infarction in persons aged 75 years or older: The Bronx aging study. *Am. J. Cardiol.* **66**:533–537.

10 Sigurdsson E, Thorgeirsson G, Sigvaldason H, Sigfusson N (1995). Unrecognized myocardial infarction: epidemiology, clinical characteristics, and the prognostic role of angina pectoris. The Reykjavik Study. *Ann. Intern. Med.* **22**:96–102.

11 Sheifer SE, Gersh BJ, Yanez ND III, *et al.* (2000). Prevalence, predisposing factors, and prognosis of clinically unrecognized myocardial infarction in the elderly. *JACC* **35**:119–126.

12 Aronow WS (1989). New coronary events at four-year follow-up in elderly patients with recognized or unrecognized myocardial infarction. *Am. J. Cardiol.* **63**:621–622.

13 Pathy MS (1967). Clinical presenation of myocardial infarction in the elderly. *Br. Heart J.* **29**:190–199.

14 Wroblewski M, Mikulowski P, Steen B (1986). Symptoms of myocardial infarction in old age: clinical case, retrospective and prospective studies. *Age & Aging* **15**:99–104.

15 Tresch DD, Brady WJ, Aufderheide TP, *et al.* (1996). Comparison of elderly and younger patients with out-of-hospital chest pain. *Arch. Intern. Med.* **156**:1089–1093.

16 Sheifer SE, Rathore SS, Gersh BJ, *et al.* (2000). Time to presentation with acute myocardial infarction in the elderly. Associations with race, sex, and socioeconomic characteristics. *Circulation* **102**:1651–1656.

17 Woodworth S, Nayak D, Aronow WS, *et al.* (2002). Comparison of acute coronary syndromes in men versus women ≥70 years of age. *Am. J. Cardiol.* **90**:1145–1147.

18 Ryan TJ, Antman EM, Brooks NH, *et al.* (1999). 1999 update: ACC/AHA guidelines for the management of patients with acute myocardial infarction: executive summary and recommendations. A report of the American College of Cardiology/American Heart Association Task Force on Practice Guidelines (Committee on Management of Acute Myocardial Infarction). *Circulation* **100**:1016–1030.

19 AIMS Trial Study Group (1988). Effect of intravenous APSAC on mortality after acute myocardial infarction: preliminary report of a placebo-controlled clinical trial. *Lancet* **1**:545–549.

20 Gruppo Italiano Per Lo Studio Della Streptochinasi Nell'Infarto Miocardico (GISSI) (1987). Long-term effects of intravenous thrombolysis in acute myocardial infarction: final report of the GISSI study. *Lancet* **2**:871–874.

21 Wilcox RG, von der Lippe G, Olsson CG, *et al.* (1990). Effects of alteplase in acute myocardial infarction: 6-month results from the ASSET Study. *Lancet* **335**:1175–1178.

22 Fibrinolytic Therapy Trialists'(FTT) Collaborative Group (1994). Indications for fibrinolytic therapy in suspected acute myocardial infarction: collaborative overview of early mortality and major morbidity results from all randomized trials of more than 1,000 patients. *Lancet* **343**:311–322.

23 Berger AK, Schulman KA, Gersh BJ, *et al.* (1999). Primary coronary angioplasty versus thrombolysis for the management of acute myocardial infarction in elderly patients. *JAMA* **282**:341–348.

24 ISIS-2 (Second International Study of Infarct Survival) Collaborative Group (1988). Randomized trial of intravenous streptokinase, oral aspirin, both, or neither among 17187 cases of suspected acute myocardial infarction: ISIS-2. *Lancet* **2**:349–360.

25 Krumholz HM, Radford MJ, Ellerbeck EF, *et al.* (1995). Aspirin in the treatment of acute myocardial infarction in elderly Medicare beneficiaries. Patterns of use and outcomes. *Circulation* **92**:2841–2847.

26 Aronow WS, Ahn C (2002). Reduction of coronary events with aspirin in older patients with prior myocardial infarction treated with and without statins. *Heart Dis.* **4**:159–161.

27 Antman EM, McCabe CH, Gurfinkel EP, *et al.* (1999). Enoxaparin prevents death and cardiac ischemic events in unstable angina/non-Q wave myocardial infarction. Results of the Thrombolysis in Myocardial Infarction (TIMI) 11B Trial. *Circulation* **100**:1593–1601.

28 Antman EM, Cohen M, Radley D, *et al.* (1999). Assessment of the treatment effect of enoxaparin for unstable angina/non-Q wave myocardial infarction. TIMI 11B-ESSENCE Meta-Analysis. *Circulation* **100**:1602–1608.

29 Cohen M, Demers C, Gurfinkel EP, *et al.* (1997). A comparison of low-molecular-weight heparin with unfractionated heparin for unstable coronary artery disease. *N. Engl. J. Med.* **337**:447–452.

30 Hjalmarson A, Herbiz J, Malek J, *et al.* (1981). Effect on mortality of metoprolol in acute myocardial infarction. *Lancet* **2**:823–827.

31 MIAMI Trial Research Group (1985). Metoprolol in acute myocardial infarction (MIAMI): a randomised placebo-controlled international trial. *Eur. Heart J.* **6**:199–226.

32 ISIS-1 (First International Study of Infarct Survival) Collaborative Group (1986). Randomized trial of intravenous atenolol among 16,027 cases of suspected acute myocardial infarction. *Lancet* **2**:57–66.

33 Beta Blocker Heart Attack Trial Research Group (1982). A randomized trial of propranolol in patients with acute myocardial infarction. *JAMA* **247**:1707–1714.

34 Gundersen T, Abrahamsen AM, Kjekshus J, *et al.* (1982). Timolol-related reduction in mortality and reinfarction in patients aged 65–75 years surviving acute myocardial infarction. *Circulation* **66**:1179–1184.

35 Gruppo Italiano per lo Studio della Sopravvivenza nell'Infarto Miocardico (1996). Six-month effects of early treatment with lisinopril and transdermal glyceryl trinitrate singly and together withdrawn six weeks after acute myocardial infarction: the GISSI-3 Trial. *J. Am. Coll. Cardiol.* **27**:337–344.

36 ISIS-4 (Fourth International Study of Infarct Survival) Collaborative Group (1995). ISIS-4: a randomized factorial trial assessing early oral captopril, oral mononitrate, and intravenous magnesium sulphate in 58,050 patients with suspected acute myocardial infarction. *Lancet* **345**:669–685.

37 Ambrosioni E, Borghi C, Magnani B, for the Survival of Myocardial Infarction Long-Term Evaluation (SMILE) Study Investigators (1995). The effect of the angiotensin-converting-enzyme inhibitor zofenopril on mortality and morbidity after anterior myocardial infarction. *N. Engl. J. Med.* **332**:80–85.

38 Pfeffer MA, Braunwald E, Moye LA, *et al.* (1992). Effect of captopril on mortality and morbidity in patients with left ventricular dysfunction after myocardial infarction. Results of the Survival and Ventricular Enlargement Trial. *N. Engl. J. Med.* **327**:669–677.

39 The Acute Infarction Ramipril Efficacy (AIRE) Study Investigators (1993). Effect of ramipril on mortality and morbidity of survivors of acute myocardial infarction with clinical evidence of heart failure. *Lancet* **342**:821–828.

40 Kober L, Torp-Pedersen C, Carlsen JE, *et al.* (1995). A clinical trial of the angiotensin-converting-enzyme inhibitor trandolapril in patients with left ventricular dysfunction after myocardial infarction. *N. Engl. J. Med.* **333**:1670–1676.

41 Yusuf S, Sleight P, Pogue J, *et al.* on behalf of the Heart Outcomes Prevention Evaluation Study Investigators (2000). Effects of an angiotensin-converting-enzyme inhibitor, ramipril, on cardiovascular events in high-risk patients. *N. Engl. J. Med.* **342**:145–153.

42 Miettinen TA, Pyorala K, Olsson AG, *et al.* (1997). Cholesterol-lowering therapy in women and elderly patients with myocardial infarction or angina pectoris. Findings from the Scandinavian Simvastatin Survival Study (4S). *Circulation* **96**:4211–4218.

43 Lewis SJ, Moye LA, Sacks FM, *et al.* (1998). Effect of pravastatin on cardiovascular events in older patients with myocardial infarction and cholesterol levels in the average range. Results of the Cholesterol and Recurrent Events (CARE) Trial. *Ann. Intern. Med.* **129**:681–689.

44 The Long-Term Intervention With Pravastatin in Ischaemic Disease (LIPID) Study Group (1998). Prevention of cardiovascular events and death with pravastatin in patients with coronary heart disease and a broad range of initial cholesterol levels. *N. Engl. J. Med.* **339**:1349–1357.

45 Pedersen TR, Kjekshus J, Pyorala K, *et al.* (1998). Effect of simvastatin on ischemic signs and symptoms in the Scandinavian Simvastatin Survival Study (4S). *Am. J. Cardiol.* **81**:333–336.

46 Kjekshus J, Pedersen TR, Olsson AG, *et al.* (1997). The effects of simvastatin on the incidence of heart failure in patients with coronary heart disease. *J. Card. Fail.* **3**:249–254.

47 Aronow WS, Ahn C (2002). Incidence of new coronary events in older persons with prior myocardial infarction and serum low-density lipoprotein cholesterol ≥125 mg/dl treated with statins versus no lipid-lowering drug. *Am. J. Cardiol.* **89**:67–69.

48 Aronow WS, Ahn C, Gutstein H (2002). Incidence of new atherothrombotic brain infarction in older persons with prior myocardial infarction and serum low-density lipoprotein cholesterol ≥125 mg/dl treated with statins versus no lipid-lowering drug. *J. Gerontol. Med. Sci.* **57A**:M333–M335.

49 Aronow WS, Ahn C (2002). Frequency of congestive heart failure in older persons with prior myocardial infarction and serum low-density lipoprotein cholesterol ≥125 mg/dl treated with statins versus no lipid-lowering drug. *Am. J. Cardiol.* **90**:147–149.

50 Heart Protection Study Collaborative Group (2002). MRC/BHF Heart Protection Study of cholesterol lowering with simvastatin in 20,536 high-risk individuals: a randomized placebo-controlled trial. *Lancet* **360**:7–22.

Gender differences in acute myocardial infarction
Further reading
Heer T, Schiele R, Schneider S, *et al.* (2002). Gender differences in acute myocardial infarction in the era of reperfusion (the MITRA registry). *Am. J. Cardiol.* **89**:511–517.

Herlitz J, Bang A, Karlson BW, Hartford M (1999). Is there a gender difference in etiology of chest pain and symptoms associated with acute myocardial infarction? *Eur. J. Emerg. Med.* **6**:311–315.

Karlson BW, Herlitz J, Hartford M (1994). Prognosis in myocardial infarction in relation to gender. *Am. Heart J.* **128**:477–483.

Maynard C, Every NR, Martin JS, Kudenchuk PJ, Weaver WD (1997). Association of gender and survival in patients with acute myocardial infarction. *Arch. Intern. Med.* **157**:1379–1384.

Diabetes and acute myocardial infarction
Further reading
Abbott RD, Donahue RP, Kannel WB, Wilson PW (1988). The impact of diabetes on survival following myocardial infarction. *JAMA* **260**:3456–3460.

Bahl VK, Seth S (2001). Management of coronary artery disease in patients with diabetes mellitus. *Indian Heart J.* **53**:147–154.

Haffner SM, Lehto S, Ronnemaa T, Pyorala K, Laakso M (1998). Mortality from coronary heart disease in subjects with type 2 diabetes and in nondiabetes subjects with and without prior myocardial infarction. *N. Engl. J. Med.* **339**:229–234.

Malmberg K, for the DIGAMI (Diabetes Mellitus, Insulin Glucose Infusion in Acute Myocardial Infarction) Study Group (1997). Prospective randomized study of intensive insulin treatment on long-term survival after acute myocardial infarction in patients with diabetes mellitus. *BMJ* **314**:1512–1515.

UK Prospective Diabetes Study Group (1998). Intensive blood glucose control with sulphonylureas or insulin compared with conventional treatment and risk of complications in patients with type II diabetes mellitus. *Lancet* **352**:837–853.

Smoking
References
1 Bøttcher M, Falk E (1999). Pathology of the coronary arteries in smokers and nonsmokers. *J. Cardiovasc. Risk* **6**:299–302.

2 Kannel WB, Higgins M (1990). Smoking and hypertension as predictors of cardiovascular risk in population studies. *J. Hypertens. Suppl.* **8**:S3–8.

3 Barbash GI, Reiner J, White HD, *et al.* (1995). Evaluation of paradoxic beneficial effects of smoking in patients receiving thrombolytic therapy for acute myocardial infarction: mechanism of the 'smoker's paradox' from the GUSTO-I trial, with angiographic insights. Global Utilization of Streptokinase and Tissue-Plasminogen Activator for Occluded Coronary Arteries. *J. Am. Coll. Cardiol.* **26**:1222–1229.

4 Czernin J, Sun K, Brunken R, Bottcher M, Phelps M, Schelbert H (1995). Effect of acute and long-term smoking on myocardial blood flow and flow reserve. *Circulation* **91**:2891–2897.

5 McGill HC Jr, McMahan CA, Malcom GT, Oalmann MC, Strong JP (1997). Effects of serum lipoproteins and smoking on atherosclerosis in young men and women. The PDAY Research Group. Pathobiological Determinants of Atherosclerosis in Youth. *Arterioscler. Thromb. Vasc. Biol.* **17**:95–106.

Acute myocardial infarction in normal coronary arteries
Further reading
Alpert JS, (1994). Myocardial infarction with angiographically normal coronary arteries. *Arch. Intern. Med.* **154**:265–269.

Da Costa A, Isaaz K, Faure E, Mourot S, Cerisier A, Lamaud M. (2001). Clinical characteristics, etiological factors, and long-term prognosis of myocardial infarction with an absolutely normal coronary angiogram: a 3-year follow-up study of 91 patients. *Eur. Heart J.* **22**:1459–1465.

Glagov S, Weisenberg E, Zarins CK, Stankunavicius R, Kolettis GJ (1987). Compensatory enlargement of human atherosclerotic coronary arteries. *N. Engl. J. Med.* **316**:1371–1373.

Prizel KR, Hutchins GM, Bulkley BH (1978). Coronary artery embolization and myocardial infarction. *Ann. Intern. Med.* **88**:155–161.

Zimmerman FH, Cameron A, Fisher LD, Ng G (1995). Myocardial infarction in young adults: angiographic characterization, risk factors, and prognosis (Coronary Artery Surgery Study Registry). *J. Am. Coll. Cardiol.* **26**:654–661.

CHAPTER 13 Heart Attack: Management Strategy
Prehospital
Further reading

Julian DG, Norris RM (2002). Myocardial infarction: is evidence-based medicine the best? *Lancet* **359**:1515–1516.

Pell JP, Sirel J, Marsden AK, Ford I, Walker NL, Cobbe S (2002). Potential impact of public access defibrillators on survival after out of hospital cardiopulmonary arrest: retrospective cohort study. *BMJ* **325**:515–517.

Terkelsen CJ, Lassen JF, Norgaard BL, Nielsen TT, Andersen HR (2003). Are we underestimating the full potential of early initiation of thrombolytic therapy, and is the golden hour in fact a golden two hours? *Heart* **89**:483–484.

Emergency Department
References

1 Erhardt L, Herlitz J, Bossaert L, *et al.* (2002). Task Force on the management of chest pain. *Eur. Heart J.* **23**:1153–1176.

2 Alpert JS, Thygesen K and the Joint ESC/ACC Committee (2000). A consensus document of the The Joint European Society of Cardiology/American College of Cardiology Committee for the redefinition of myocardial infarction. *Eur. Heart J.* **21**:1502–1513.

3 Van de Werf F, Ardissimo D, Betriu A, *et al.* (2003). Management of acute myocardial infarction in patients presenting with ST segment elevation. Recommendations of the Task Force on the management of acute myocardial infaction of the European Society of Cardiology. *Eur. Heart J.* **24**:28–66.

4 Bertrand ME, Simoons ML and the Task Force of the European Society of Cardiology (2000). Management of acute coronary syndromes: acute coronary syndromes without persistent ST segment elevation. *Eur. Heart J.* **21**:1406–1432.

5 Braunwald E, Antman EM, Beasley JW, *et al.* (2000). ACC/AHA guidelines for the management of patients with unstable angina and non-ST segment elevation myocardial infarction: a report of the American College of Cardiology/American Heart Association Task Force on practice guidelines. *J. Am. Coll. Cardiol.* **36**:970–1062.

Coronary Care Unit
References

1 Alpert JS, Thygesen K and the Joint ESC/ACC Committee (2000). A consensus document of the the Joint European Society of Cardiology/American College of Cardiology Committee for the redefinition of myocardial infarction. *Eur. Heart J.* **21**:1502–1513.

2 Van de Werf F, Ardissimo D, Betriu A, *et al.* (2003). Management of acute myocardial infarction in patients presenting with ST segment elevation. Recommendations of the Task Force on the management of acute myocardial infaction of the European Society of Cardiology. *Eur. Heart J.* **24**:28–66.

3 Bertrand ME, Simoons ML and the Task Force of the European Society of Cardiology (2000). Management of acute coronary syndromes: acute coronary syndromes without persistent ST segment elevation. *Eur. Heart J.* **21**:1406–1432.

4 Braunwald E, Antman EM, Beasley JW, *et al.* (2000). ACC/AHA guidelines for the management of patients with unstable angina and non-ST segment elevation myocardial infarction: a report of the American College of Cardiology/American Heart Association Task Force on practice guidelines. *J. Am. Coll. Cardiol.* **36**:970–1062.

Posthospital
Further reading

AHA/ACC guidelines for preventing heart attack and death in patients with atherosclerotic cardiovascular disease: 2001 Update (2001). *Circulation* **104**:1577–1579.

Core components of cardiac rehabilitation/secondary prevention programs. A statement for healthcare professionals from the American Heart Association and American Association of Cardiovascular and Pulmonary Rehabilitation (2000). *Circulation* **102**:1069–1073.

Goble AJ, Worchester MUC (1999). *Best Practice Guidelines for Cardiac Rehabilitation and Secondary Prevention.* Department of Human Services, Victoria, Australia.

Joliffe JA, Rees K, Taylor RS, Thompson D, Oldridge N, Ebrahim S (2002). Exercise-based rehabilitation for coronary heart disease (Cochrane Review). In: *The Cochrane Library*, Issue 2. Update Software, Oxford.

Prevention of coronary heart disease in clinical practice. Recommendations of the Second Joint Task Force of European and other Societies on Coronary Prevention (1998). *Eur. Heart J.* **19**:1434–1503.

CHAPTER 14 Silent Myocardial Ischemia
Silent Myocardial Ischemia
References

1 Mickley H, Nielsen JR, Berning J, *et al.* (1998). Serial Holter ST segment monitoring after first acute myocardial infarction. Prevalence, variability, and long-term prognostic importance of transient myocardial ischemia. *Cardiology* **9**:160–167.

2 Ditchburn CJ, Hall JA, de Belder M, *et al.* (2001). Silent myocardial ischemia in patients with proved coronary artery disease: a comparison of diabetic and nondiabetic patients. *Postgrad. Med. J.* **77**:395–398.

3 Forslund L, Hjemdahl P, Held C, *et al.* (1998). Ischemia during exercise and ambulatory monitoring in patients with stable angina pectoris and healthy controls. Gender differences and relationships to catecholamines. *Eur. Heart J.* **19**:578–587.

4 Sigwart U, Grbic M, Payot M, Essinger A, Fisher A (1984). Ischemic events during coronary artery balloon obstruction. In: *Silent Myocardial Ischemia.* W Rutishauser, H Roskam (eds). Springer-Verlag, Berlin, p. 29.

5 Knatterud GL, Bourassa MG, Pepine CJ, *et al.* (1994). Effects of treatment strategies to suppress ischemia in patients with coronary artery disease: 12-week results of the asymptomatic cardiac ischemia pilot (ACIP) study. *J. Am. Coll. Cardiol.* **24**:11–20.

6 Kathiresan S, Jordan MK, Gimelli G, *et al.* (1999). Frequency of silent myocardial ischemia following coronary stenting. *Am. J. Cardiol.* **84**:930–932.

7 Rocco MB, Nabel EG, Campbell S, *et al.* (1988). Prognostic importance of myocardial ischemia detected by ambulatory monitoring in patients with stable coronary artery disease. *Circulation* **78**: 877–884.

8 Mulcahy D, Knight C, Patel D, *et al.* (1995). Detection of ambulatory ischemia is not of practical clinical value in the routine management of patients with stable angina. A long term follow-up study. *Eur. Heart J.* **16**:317–324.

9 Mulcahy D (2005). The return of silent ischemia? Not really. *Heart* **91**:1249–1250.

10 Mulcahy D, Gunning M, Knight C, *et al.* (1998). Long-term (5 year) effects of transient (silent) ischemia on left ventricular systolic function in stable angina. Clinical and radionuclide study. *Eur. Heart J.* **19**:1342–1347.

11 Cohn PF, Fox KM, Daly C (2003). Silent myocardial ischemia. *Circulation* **108**:1263–1277.

CHAPTER 15 Chronic Arrhythmias and Conduction Disorders
Chronic Arrhythmias and Conduction Disorders
Further reading
ACC/AHA/NASPE (2002). 2002 guideline update for implantation of cardiac pacemakers and antiarrhythmia devices: summary article: a report of the American College of Cardiology/American Heart Association Task Force on practice guidelines (ACC/AHA/NASPE Committee to update the 1998 pacemaker guidelines). *Circulation* **106**:2145–2161.

Camm AJ, Yap YG (2001). Clinical trials of antiarrhythmic drugs in postmyocardial infarction and congestive heart failure patients. *J. Cardiovasc. Pharmacol. Ther.* **6**:99–106.

Fuster V, Ryden LE, Asinger RW, *et al.* (2001). ACC/AHA/ESC guidelines for the management of patients with atrial fibrillation: executive summary. A report of the American College of Cardiology/ American Heart Association Task Force on practice guidelines and the European Society of Cardiology Committee for practice guidelines and policy conferences (Committee to develop guidelines for the management of patients with atrial fibrillation): developed in collaboration with the North American Society of Pacing and Electrophysiology. *J. Am. Coll. Cardiol.* **38**:1231–1266; *Eur. Heart J.* **22**:1852–1923.

Hohnloser SH, Gersh BJ (2003). Changing late prognosis of acute myocardial infarction: impact on management of ventricular arrhythmias in the era of reperfusion and the implantable cardioverter-defibrillator. *Circulation* **107**:941–946.

International ECC and CPR Guidelines (2000). *Circulation* **102**:Supplement I.

Priori SG, Aliot E, Blomstrom-Lundqvist C, *et al.* (2003). Update of the guidelines on sudden cardiac death of the European Society of Cardiology. *Eur. Heart J.* **24**:13–15.

Tracy CM, Akhtar M, DiMarco JP, *et al.* (2000). American College of Cardiology/American Heart Association clinical competence statement on invasive electrophysiology studies, catheter ablation, and cardioversion: a report of the American College of Cardiology/American Heart Association/American College of Physicians/American Society of Internal Medicine Task Force on clinical competence. *Circulation* **102**:2309–2320.

Wellens HJ (2001). Electrophysiology: ventricular tachycardia: diagnosis of broad QRS complex tachycardia. *Heart* **86**:579–585.

CHAPTER 16 Left Ventricular Dysfunction
Heart failure
Further reading
Cleland JGF (2002). For debate: Preventing atherosclerotic events with aspirin. *BMJ* **324**(7329):103–105.

Cleland JGF (2002). Is aspirin 'The Weakest Link' in cardiovascular prophylaxis? The surprising lack of evidence supporting the use of aspirin for cardiovascular disease. *Prog. Cardiovasc. Dis.* **44**:275–292.

Cleland JGF, Alamgir F, Nikitin N, Clark A, Norell M (2001). What is the optimal medical management of ischemic heart failure? *Prog. Cardiovasc. Dis.* **43**:433–455.

Cleland JGF, Gemmel I, Khand A, Boddy A (1999). Is the prognosis of heart failure improving? *Eur. J. Heart Fail.* **1**:229–241.

Cleland JGF, Khand A, Clark AL (2001). The heart failure epidemic: exactly how big is it? *Eur. Heart J.* **22**(8):623–626.

Cleland JGF, Thackray S, Goodge L, Kaye GC, Cooklin M (2002). Outcome studies with device therapy in patients with heart failure. *J. Cardiovasc. Electrophysiol.* **13**:(Suppl):S73–91.

Cowburn PJ, Cleland JGF, Coats AJS, Komajda M (1998). Risk stratification in chronic heart failure. *Eur. Heart J.* **19**:696–710.

European Society of Cardiology Task Force for the diagnosis and treatment of chronic heart failure, Remme WJ, Swedberg K (2001). Guidelines for the diagnosis and treatment of chronic heart failure. *Eur. Heart J.* **22**:1527–1560.

Ischemic cardiomyopathy, hibernation, and viability
References

1 Gheorghiade M, Bonow RO (1998). Chronic heart failure in the United States: a manifestation of coronary artery disease. *Circulation* **97**:282–289.

2 Bourassa MG, Gurne O, Bangdiwala SI, *et al.* (1993). Natural history and patterns of current practice in heart failure. The Studies of LV Dysfunction (SOLVD) Investigators. *J. Am. Coll. Cardiol.* **22**:14A–19A.

3 Levy D, Kenchaiah S, Larson MG, *et al.* (2002). Long-term trends in the incidence of and survival with heart failure. *N. Engl. J. Med.* **347**:1397–1402.

4 Diamond GA, Forrester JS, deLuz PL, Wyatt HL, Swan HJC (1978). Post-extrasystolic potentiation of ischemic myocardium by atrial stimulation. *Am. Heart J.* **95**:204–209.

5 Rahimtoola SH (1985). A perspective on the three large multi-center randomized clinical trials of coronary bypass surgery for chronic stable angina. *Circulation* **72**:V123–135.

6 Rahimtoola SH (1989). The hibernating myocardium. *Am. Heart J.* **117**:211–221.

7 Canty JM Jr, Fallavollita JA (1999). Resting myocardial flow in hibernating myocardium: validating animal models of human pathophysiology. *Am. J. Physiol.* **277**:417H–422H.

8 Bax JJ, Poldermans D, Elhendy A, Boersma E, Rahimtoola SH (2001). Sensitivity, specificity, and predictive accuracies of various noninvasive techniques for detecting hibernating myocardium. *Curr. Probl. Cardiol.* **26**:141–186.

9 Bax JJ, Visser FC, Poldermans D, *et al.* (2001). Time course of functional recovery of stunned and hibernating segments after surgical revascularization. *Circulation* **104**:I314–318.

10 Pagano D, Bonser RS, Townend JN, Parums D, Camici PG (1996). Histopathological correlates of dobutamine echocardiography in hibernating myocardium. *Circulation* **94**(Suppl I):I543.

11 Wijns W, Vatner SF, Camici PG (1998). Hibernating myocardium. *N. Engl. J. Med.* **339**:173–181.

12 Cowie MR, Wood DA, Coats AJ, *et al.* (1999). Incidence and etiology of heart failure; a population-based study. *Eur. Heart J.* **20**:421–428.

13 Bax JJ, Poldermans D, Elhendy A, *et al.* (1999). Improvement of LV ejection fraction, heart failure symptoms, and prognosis after revascularization in patients with chronic coronary artery disease and viable myocardium detected by dobutamine stress echocardiography. *J. Am. Coll. Cardiol.* **34**:163–169.

14 Milano CA, White WD, Smith LR, *et al.* (1993). Coronary artery bypass in patients with severely depressed ventricular function. *Ann. Thorac. Surg.* **56**:487–493.

15 Pagley PR, Beller GA, Watson DD, Gimple LW, Ragosta M (1997). Improved outcome after coronary bypass surgery in patients with ischemic cardiomyopathy and residual myocardial viability. *Circulation* **96**:793–800.

16 Schinkel AFL, Bax JJ, Boersma E, Elhendy A, Roelandt JR, Poldermans D (2001). How many patients with ischemic cardiomyopathy exhibit viable myocardium? *Am. J. Cardiol.* **88**:561–564.

17 Bax JJ, Wijns W, Cornel JH, Visser FC, Boersma E, Fioretti PM (1997). Accuracy of currently available techniques for prediction of functional recovery after revascularization in patients with LV dysfunction due to chronic coronary artery disease: comparison of pooled data. *J. Am. Coll. Cardiol.* **30**:1451–1460.

18 Udelson JE, Coleman PS, Metherall J, *et al.* (1994). Predicting recovery of severe regional ventricular dysfunction: comparison of resting scintigraphy with 201Tl and 99m Tc-sestamibi. *Circulation* **89**:2552–2561.

19 La Canna G, Alfieri O, Giubbini R, Gargano M, Ferrari R, Visioli O (1994). Echocardiography during infusion of dobutamine for identification of reversible dysfunction in patients with chronic coronary artery disease. *J. Am. Coll. Cardiol.* **23**:617–626.

20 Kim RJ, Wu E, Rafael A, *et al.* (2000). The use of contrast-enhanced magnetic resonance imaging to identify reversible myocardial dysfunction. *N. Engl. J. Med.* **343**:1445–1453.

21 Keck A, Hertting K, Schwartz Y, *et al.* (2002). Electromechanical mapping for determination of myocardial contractility and viability. A comparison with echocardiography, myocardial single-photon emission computed tomography, and positron emission tomography. *J. Am. Coll. Cardiol.* **40**:1067–1074.

CHAPTER 17 Percutaneous Coronary Intervention
Indications, procedure, and technique
Further reading

Sidney C, Smith JR, Dove JT, *et al.* (2001). ACC/AHA guidelines for percutaneous coronary intervention (revision of the 1993 PCI guidelines). *J. Am. Coll. Cardiol.* **37**:2215–2238.

Results and complications
References

1 Serruys P, de Jaegere P, Kiemeneij F, *et al.* (1994). A comparison of balloon-expandable-stent implantation with balloon angioplasty in patients with coronary artery disease. *N. Engl. J. Med.* **331**:489–495.

2 Fischman D, Leon M, Baim D, *et al.* (1994). A randomized comparison of coronary-stent placement and balloon angioplasty in the treatment of coronary artery disease. Stent Restenosis Study Investigators. *N. Engl. J. Med.* **331**:496–501.

3 Hofma S, Whelan D, van Beusekom H, *et al.* (1998). Increasing arterial wall injury after long-term implantation of two types of stent in a porcine coronary model. *Eur. Heart J.* **19**:601–609.

4 van Beusekom H, Whelan D, Hofma S, *et al.* (1998). Long-term endothelial dysfunction is more pronounced after stenting than after balloon angioplasty in porcine coronary arteries. *J. Am. Coll. Cardiol.* **32**:1109–1117.

5 Serruys P, Unger F, Sousa J, *et al.* (2001). Comparison of coronary artery bypass surgery and stenting for the treatment of multi-vessel disease. *N. Engl. J. Med.* **344**:1117–1124.

6 Zijlstra F, de Boer JM, Hoorntje JC, *et al.* (1993). A comparison of immediate coronary angioplasty with intravenous streptokinase in acute myocardial infarction. *N. Engl. J. Med.* **328**:680–684.

7 Grines CL, Browne KF, Marco J, *et al.* (1993). A comparison of immediate angioplasty with thrombolytic therapy for acute myocardial infarction. *N. Engl. J. Med.* **328**:673–679.

8 Weaver W, Simes R, Betriu A, *et al.* (1997). Comparison of primary coronary angioplasty and intravenous thrombolytic therapy for acute myocardial infarction: a quantitative review. *JAMA* **278**:2093–2098.

9 Stone GW, Grines CL, Cox DA, *et al.* (2002). Comparison of angioplasty with stenting, with or without abciximab, in acute myocardial infarction. *N. Engl. J. Med.* **346**:957–966.

10 Zijlstra F, Hoorntje JC, de Boer MJ, *et al.* (1999). Long-term benefit of primary angioplasty as compared with thrombolytic therapy for acute myocardial infarction. *N. Engl. J. Med.* **341**:1413–1419.

11 Montalescot G, Barragan P, Wittenberg O, *et al.* (2001). Platelet glycoprotein IIb/IIIa inhibition with coronary stenting for acute myocardial infarction. *N. Engl. J. Med.* **344**:1895–1903.

12 Morice M, Serruys P, Sousa J, *et al.* (2002). A randomized comparison of a sirolimus-eluting stent with a standard stent for coronary revascularization. *N. Engl. J. Med.* **346**:1773–1780.

13 Topol EJ, Mark DB, Lincoff AM, *et al.* (1999). Outcomes at 1 year and economic implications of platelet glycoprotein IIb/IIIa blockade in patients undergoing coronary stenting: results from a multi-centre randomized trial. EPISTENT Investigators. Evaluation of platelet IIb/IIIa inhibitor for stenting. *Lancet* **354**:2019–2024.

14 Serruys PW, van Hout B, Bonnier H, *et al.* (1998). Randomized comparison of implantation of heparin-coated stents with balloon angioplasty in selected patients with coronary artery disease (Benestent II). *Lancet* **352**:673–681.

15 Seshadri N, Whitlow PL, Acharya N, *et al.* (2002). Emergency coronary artery bypass surgery in the contemporary percutaneous coronary intervention era. *Circulation* **106**:2346–2350.

16 Schindler J, Williams DO, Holmes DR, *et al.* (2002). Emergent and urgent coronary surgery after attempted percutaneous coronary intervention (PCI): an analysis of the NHLBI database in the era of stents. *J. Am. Coll. Cardiol.* (Suppl.): 418A.

17 Wiley JM, White CJ, Uretsky BF (1999). Noncoronary complications of coronary intervention. *Cathet. Cardiovasc. Intervent.* **47**:143–148.

Late restenosis

References

1 Serruys PW, Luijten HE, Beat KJ, *et al.* (1988). Incidence of restenosis after successful coronary angioplasty: a time related phenomenon. A quantitative angiographic study in 342 consecutive patients at 1, 2, 3, and 4 months. *Circulation* **77**:361–377.

2 Nobuyoshi M, Kimura T, Nosaka H, *et al.* (1988). Restenosis after successful percutaneous transluminal coronary angioplasty: serial angiographic follow-up of 299 patients. *J. Am. Coll. Cardiol.* **12**:616–623.

3 Serruys PW, de Jaegere P, Kiemeneij F, *et al.* (1994). A comparison of balloon-expandable implantation stent with balloon angioplasty in patients with coronary artery disease. Benestent Study Group. *N. Engl. J. Med.* **331**:489–495.

4 Mintz GS, Popma JJ, Pichard AD, *et al.* (1996). Arterial remodeling after coronary angioplasty: a serial intravascular ultrasound study. *Circulation* **94**:35–43.

5 Kimura T, Kaburagi S, Tamura T, *et al.* (1997). Remodeling of human coronary arteries undergoing coronary angioplasty or atherectomy. *Circulation* **96**:475–483.

6 Hoffmann R, Mintz GS, Dussaillant GR, *et al.* (1996). Patterns and mechanism of in-stent restenosis. A serial intravascular ultrasound study. *Circulation* **94**:1247–1254.

7 de Feyter PJ, Kay P, Disco C, Serruys PW (1999). Reference chart derived from poststent implantation intravascular ultrasound predictors of 6-month expected restenosis on quantitative coronary angiography. *Circulation* **100**:1777–1783.

8 Serruys PW, Kay IP, Disco C, Deshpande NV, de Feyter PJ (1999). Periprocedural quantitative coronary angiography after Palmaz-Schatz stent implantation predicts the restenosis rate at six months. *J. Am. Coll. Cardiol.* **34**:1067–1074.

9 Mehran R, Dangas G, Abizaid AS, *et al.* (1999). Angiographic patterns of restenosis. Classification and implications for long-term outcome. *Circulation* **100**:1872–1878.

10 Morice MC, Serruys PW, Sousa JE, *et al.* (2002). A randomized comparison of a sirolimus-eluting stent with a standard stent for coronary revascularization. *N. Engl. J. Med.* **346**:1778–1780.

11 Moses JW, Leon MB, Popma JJ, *et al.* (2003). Sirolimus-eluting stents in patients with stenosis in a native coronary artery. *N. Engl. J. Med.* **349**:1315–1323.

12 Stone G, Ellis SG, Cox DA, *et al.* (2004). A polymer-based, paclitaxel-eluting stent in patients with coronary artery disease. *N. Engl. J. Med.* **350**:221–231.

CHAPTER 18 Coronary Artery Bypass Graft Surgery
Procedures and indications
Further reading
See Complications and Outcomes.

Complications and outcomes
Further reading
Abu-Omar Y, Taggart DP (2002). Off-pump coronary artery bypass grafting. *Lancet* **360**:327–330.

Eagle KA, Guyton RA, Davidoff R, *et al.* (1999). ACC/AHA guidelines for coronary artery bypass graft surgery: executive summary and recommendations: a report of the American College of Cardiology/American Heart Association Task Force on practice guidelines (Committee to revise the 1991 guidelines for coronary artery bypass graft surgery). *Circulation* **100**:1464–1480.

Maisel WH, Rawn JD, Stevenson WG (2001). Atrial fibrillation after cardiac surgery. *Ann. Intern. Med.* **135**:1061–1073.

Pepper J (2000). Severe morbidity after coronary artery surgery. *Curr. Opin. Cardiol.* **15**:400–405.

Taggart DP, Westaby S (2001). Neurological and cognitive disorders after coronary artery bypass grafting. *Curr. Opin. Cardiol.* **16**:271–276.

CHAPTER 19 Ischemic Heart Disease: Special Problems
Women and hormones
Further reading
Douglas PS (2001). Coronary artery disease in women. In: *Heart Disease: A Textbook of Cardiovascular Medicine*, 6th edn. E Braunwald, DP Zipes, P Libby (eds). WB Saunders, Philadelphia, ch. 58, p. 2038.

Grady D, Herrington D, Bittner V, *et al.* (2002). Cardiovascular disease outcomes during 6.8 years of hormone therapy: Heart and estrogen/progestin replacement study follow-up (HERS II). *JAMA* **288**:49–57.

Hulley S, Grady D, Bush T, *et al.* (1998). Randomized trial of estrogen plus progestin for secondary prevention of coronary heart disease in postmenopausal women. Heart and Estrogen/progestin Replacement Study (HERS) Research Group. *JAMA* **280**:605–613.

Rossouw JE, Anderson GL, Prentice RL, *et al.* (2002). Risks and benefits of estrogen plus progestin in healthy postmenopausal women: principal results from the Women's Health Initiative randomized controlled trial. *JAMA* **288**:321–333.

Diabetic atherogenic dyslipidemias
Further reading
Colhoun HM, Betteridge DJ, Durrington PN, *et al.* for the CARDS Investigators (2004). Primary prevention of cardiovascular disease with atorvastatin in type 2 diabetes in the Collaborative Atorvastatin Diabetes Study (CARDS): multicenter randomized placebo-controlled trial. *Lancet* **364**(9435):685–696.

Sniderman AD, Furberg CD, Keech A, Roeters van Lennep JE, Frolich J, Jungner I (2003). Apoproteins versus lipids as indices of coronary risk and as targets for statin therapy: analysis of the evidence. *Lancet* **361**:777–780.

Sniderman AD, Scantlebury T, Cianflone K (2001). Hypertriglyceridemic hyper-apoB: the unappreciated atherogenic dyslipoproteinemia in type 2 diabetes mellitus. *Ann. Intern. Med.* **135**:447–459.

Revascularization: percutaneous coronary intervention versus coronary artery bypass grafting
References
1 Hamm C, Reimers J, Ischinger T, Rupprecht H, Berger J, Bleifeld W (1994). A randomized study of coronary angioplasty compared with bypass surgery in patients with symptomatic multivessel coronary disease. *N. Engl. J. Med.* **331**:1037–1043.

2 Hannan E, Racz M, McCallister B, *et al.* (1999). A comparison of 3-year survival after coronary artery bypass graft surgery and percutaneous transluminal coronary angioplasty. *J. Am. Coll. Cardiol.* **33**:63–72.

3 Henderson R, Pocock S, Sharp S, *et al.* (1998). Long-term results of RITA-1 trial: clinical and cost comparisons of coronary angioplasty and coronary artery bypass grafting. *Lancet* **352**:1419–1425.

4 Hueb W, Bellotti G, de Oliveira S (1995). The Medicine, Angioplasty, or Surgery Study (MASS): a prospective, randomized trial of medical therapy, balloon angioplasty, or bypass surgery for single proximal left anterior descending artery stenosis. *J. Am. Coll. Cardiol.* **26**:1600–1605.

5 The BARI Investigators (1996). Comparison of coronary bypass surgery with angioplasty in patients with multi-vessel disease. *N. Engl. J. Med.* **335**:217–225.

6 King S, Lembo N, Weintraub W, *et al.* (1994). A randomized trial comparing coronary angioplasty with coronary bypass surgery. *N. Engl. J. Med.* **331**:1044–1050.

7 Serruys P, Unger F, Sousa E, *et al.* (2001). Comparison of coronary artery bypass surgery and stenting for the treatment of multi-vessel disease. *N. Engl. J. Med.* **344**:1117–1124.

8 Pocock S, Henderson R, Rickards A, *et al.* (1995). Meta-analysis of randomized trials comparing coronary angioplasty with bypass surgery. *Lancet* **346**:1184–1189.

9 Hlatky M, Rogers W, Johnstone I, *et al.* (1997). Medical care costs and quality of life after randomization to coronary angioplasty or coronary bypass surgery. *N. Engl. J. Med.* **336**:92–99.

10 Eagle K, Guyton R, Davidoff R, *et al.* (1999). ACC/AHA guidelines for coronary artery bypass graft surgery: a report of the American College of Cardiology/American Heart Association Task Force on practice guidelines. *J. Am. Coll. Cardiol.* **34**:1262–1346.

11 Goy J, Eechhout E, Moret C, *et al.* (1999). Five-year outcome in patients with isolated proximal left anterior descending coronary artery stenosis treated by angioplasty or left internal mammary artery grafting. *Circulation* **99**:3255–3259.

12 Goy J, Kaufmann U, Goy-Eggenberger D, *et al.* (2000). A prospective randomized trial comparing stenting to internal mammary artery grafting for proximal isolated *de novo* left anterior coronary stenosis: The SIMA Trial. *Mayo Clin. Proc.* **75**:1116–1123.

13 Anderson H, Cannon C, Stone P, *et al.* (1995). One-year result of the Thrombolysis in Myocardial Infarction (TIMI) IIIB clinical trial. A randomized comparison of tissue-type plasminogen activator versus placebo and early invasive versus early conservative strategies in unstable angina and non-Q wave myocardial infarction. *J. Am. Coll. Cardiol.* **26**:1643–1650.

14 Morrison D, Sethi G, Sacks J, *et al.* (2001). Percutaneous coronary intervention versus coronary artery bypass graft surgery for patients with medically refractory myocardial ischemia and risk factors for adverse outcomes with bypass: a multicenter randomized trial. *J. Am. Coll. Cardiol.* **38**:143–149.

Allograft coronary artery disease
Further reading
Eisen HJ, Tuzen EM, Dorent R, *et al.* (2003). Everolismus for the prevention of allograft rejection and vasculopathy in cardial transplant recipients. *N. Engl. J. Med.* **349**:847–858.

Segovia J (2002). Update on cardiac allograft vasculopathy. *Curr. Opin. Organ Transplant* **7**:240–251.

Valentine H (2004). Cardiac allograft vasculopathy after heart transplantation: factors and management. *J. Heart Lung Transplant* **23**:S187–193.

Chronic refractory angina
Further reading
Kim MC, Kini A, Sharma SK (2002). Refractory angina pectoris: mechanism and therapeutic options. *J. Am. Coll. Cardiol.* **39**:923–934.

Mannheimer C, Camici P, Chester MR, *et al.* (2002). The problem of chronic refractory angina: report from the ESC Joint Study Group on the treatment of refractory angina. *Eur. Heart J.* **23**:355–370.

Ethnicity and cardiovascular disease
Further reading
Anand SS, Yusuf S, Vuksan V, *et al.* (2000). Differences in risk factors, atherosclerosis, and cardiovascular disease between ethnic groups in Canada: the study of health assessment and risk in ethnic groups. *Lancet* **356**:279–284.

Barker DJP (1994). *Mothers, Babies, and Disease in Later Life.* BMJ Publishing Group, London.

Bhatnagar D, Anand IS, Durrington PN, *et al.* (1995). Coronary risk factors in people from the Indian subcontinent living in West London and their siblings in India. *Lancet* **345**:405–409.

Hales CN, Barker DJ (1992). Thrifty genotype type 2 (noninsulin-dependent) diabetes mellitus: the thrifty phenotype hypothesis. *Diabetologia* **35**:595–601.

Kagan A, Harris BR, Winkelstein W Jr, *et al.* (1974). Epidemiologic studies of coronary heart disease and stroke in Japanese men living in Japan, Hawaii, and California: demographic, physical, dietary, and biochemical characteristics. *J. Chronic Dis.* **27**:345–364.

Menotti A, Keys A, Kromhout D, *et al.* (1993). Inter-cohort differences in coronary heart disease mortality in the 25-year follow-up of the Seven Countries Study. *Eur. J. Epidemiol.* **9**:527–536.

Omran AR (1971). The epidemiologic transition: a key of the epidemiology of population change. *Millbank Mem. Fund Quart.* **49**:509–538.

Vaz M, Kurpad A, Pais P, *et al.* (2002). Contrasting coronary heart disease risk profiles between urban and rural Indians: the PURE pilot study. World Congress of Cardiology. Sydney, Australia (Poster).

World Health Report (1999). *Making a Difference.* World Health Organization, Geneva.

1997–1999 World Health Statistics Annual (2000). World Health Organization, Geneva.

http://wwwnt.who.int/whosis/statistics/menu.cfm?path=statistics,whsa&language=english

Cardiovascular disease in chronic kidney disease
References
1 National Kidney Foundation (2002). K/DOQI Clinical practice guidelines on hypertension and antihypertensive agents in chronic kidney disease. *Am. J. Kidney Dis.* **39**(Suppl. 1):S1–S266.

2 Sarnak MJ, Levey AS, Schoolwerth AC, *et al.* (2003). Kidney disease as a risk factor for development of cardiovascular disease: a statement from the American Heart Association Councils on kidney in cardiovascular disease, high blood pressure research, clinical cardiology, and epidemiology and prevention. *Circulation* **108**:2154–2169.

3 Mann JFE, Gerstein HC, Pogue J, *et al.* (2001). Renal insufficiency as a predictor of cardiovascular outcomes and the impact of ramipril: the HOPE randomized trial. *Ann. Intern. Med.* **134**:629–636.

4 Gerstein HC, Mann JF, Yi Q, *et al.* (2001). Albuminuria and risk of cardiovascular events, death, and heart failure in diabetic and nondiabetic individuals. *JAMA* **286**(4): 421–426.

5 Levin A, Singer J, Thompson CR, *et al.* (1996). Prevalent left ventricular hypertrophy in the predialysis population: identifying opportunities for intervention. *Am. J. Kidney Dis.* **27**:347–354.

6 Foley RN, Parfrey PS, Sarnak MJ (1998). Epidemiology of cardiovascular disease in chronic renal disease. *Am. J. Kidney Dis.* **32**(Suppl. 3):S112–S119.

7 Herzog CA, Ma JZ, Collins AJ (1998). Poor long-term survival after myocardial infarction among patients on long-term hemodialysis. *N. Engl. J. Med.* **339**:799–805.

8 Levey AS, Beto JA, Coronado BE, *et al.* (1998). Controlling the epidemic of cardiovascular disease in chronic renal disease: what do we know, what do we need to learn, where do we go from here? National Kidney Foundation Task Force on Cardiovascular Disease. *Am. J. Kidney Dis.* **32**:853–906.

9 Boaz M, Smetana S, Weinstein T, *et al.* (2000). Secondary prevention with antioxidants of cardiovascular disease in endstage renal disease (SPACE): randomized placebo-controlled trial. *Lancet* **356**:1213–1218.

10 Tepel M, van der Griet M, Statz M, *et al.* (2003). The antioxidant acetylcysteine reduces cardiovascular events in patients with end-stage renal failure: a randomized controlled trial. *Circulation* **107**:992–995.

CHAPTER 20 Primary Prevention
Further reading

Grundy S, Becker D, Van Horn L, *et al.* (2002). Third report of the National Cholesterol Education Program (NCEP) Expert Panel on detection, evaluation, and treatment of high blood cholesterol in adults (Adult Treatment Panel III): Final Report. NIH Publication No. 02-5215; reprinted in *Circulation* **106**:3143–3421.

Pearson TA, Blair SN, Daniels SR, *et al.* (2002). AHA guidelines for primary prevention of cardiovascular disease and stroke: 2002 Update: Consensus Panel guide to comprehensive risk reduction for adult patients without coronary or other atherosclerotic vascular diseases. American Heart Association Science Advisory and Coordinating Committee. *Circulation* **106**:388–391.

Rossouw JE, Anderson GL, Prentice RL, *et al.* (2002). Risks and benefits of estrogen plus progestin in healthy postmenopausal women: principal results from the Women's Health Initiative randomized controlled trial. *JAMA* **288**:321–333.

Smith SC Jr, Greenland P, Grundy SM (2000). AHA Conference Proceedings. Prevention conference V: Beyond secondary prevention: Identifying the high-risk patient for primary prevention: executive summary. American Heart Association. *Circulation* **101**:111–116.

The DASH (Dietary Approaches to Stop Hypertension) Study (2001). NIH Publication No. 01-4082.

CHAPTER 21 Genetics of Ischemic Heart Disease
References

1 Carleton RA, Dwyer J, Finberg L, *et al.* (1991). Report of the expert panel on population strategies for blood cholesterol reduction: a statement from the National Cholesterol Education Program, National Heart, Lung, and Blood Institute, National Institutes of Health. *Circulation* **83**:2154–2232.

2 Pyörälä K, De Backer G, Graham I, Poole-Wilson P, Wood D (1994). Prevention of coronary heart disease in clinical practice: recommendations of the Task Force of the European Society of Cardiology, European Atherosclerosis Society, and European Society of Hypertension. *Eur. Heart J.* **15**:1300–1331.

3 Scandinavian Simvastatin Survival Study Group (1994). Randomized trial of cholesterol lowering in 4444 patients with coronary heart disease: the Scandinavian Simvastatin Survival Study (4S). *Lancet* **344**:1383–1389.

4 Shepherd J, Cobbe SM, Ford I, *et al.* (1995). Prevention of coronary heart disease with pravastatin in men with hypercholesterolemia. *N. Engl. J. Med.* **333**:1301–1307.

5 Sacks FM, Pfeffer MA, Moye LA, *et al.* (1996). The effect of pravastatin on coronary events after myocardial infarction in patients with average cholesterol levels. *N. Engl. J. Med.* **335**:1001–1009.

6 Goldstein JL, Hobbs HH, Brown MS (2001). Familial hypercholesterolemia. In: *The Metabolic and Molecular Basis of Inherited Disease*, 8th edn. CR Scriver, AL Beaudet, WS Sly, D Valle (eds). McGraw-Hill, New York, Vol. 2, pp. 2863–2913.

7 Soria LF, Ludwig EH, Clarke HRG, Vega GL, Grundy SM, McCarthy BJ (1989). Association between a specific apolipoprotein B mutation and familial defective apolipoprotein B-100. *Proc. Natl. Acad. Sci. USA* **86**:587–591.

8 Pullinger CR, Hennessy LK, Chatterton JE, *et al.* (1995). Familial ligand-defective apolipoprotein B: identification of a new mutation that decreases LDL receptor binding affinity. *J. Clin. Invest.* **95**:1225–1234.

9 Gaffney D, Reid JM, Cameron IM, *et al.* (1995). Independent mutations at codon 3500 of the apolipoprotein B gene are associated with hyperlipidemia. *Arterioscler. Thromb. Vasc. Biol.* **15**:1025–1029.

10 Borén J, Ekström U, Ågren B, Nilsson-Ehle P, Innerarity TL (2001). The molecular mechanism for the genetic disorder familial defective apolipoprotein B100. *J. Biol. Chem.* **276**:9214–9218.

11 Tybjærg-Hansen A, Gallagher J, Vincent J, *et al.* (1990). Familial defective apolipoprotein B-100: detection in the United Kingdom and Scandinavia and clinical characteristics of ten cases. *Atherosclerosis* **80**:235–242.

12 Tybjærg-Hansen A, Humphries SE (1992). Familial defective apolipoprotein B-100: a single mutation that causes hypercholesterolemia and premature coronary artery disease. *Atherosclerosis* **96**:91–107.

13 Tybjærg-Hansen A, Steffensen R, Meinertz H, Schnohr P, Nordestgaard BG (1998). Association of mutations in the apolipoprotein B gene with hypercholesterolemia and the risk of ischemic heart disease. *N. Engl. J. Med.* **338**:1577–1584.

14 Ludwig EH, McCarthy BJ (1990). Haplotype analysis of the human apolipoprotein B mutation associated with familial defective apolipoprotein B100. *Am. J. Hum. Genet.* **47**:712–720.

15 Tybjærg-Hansen A (1999). Familial defective apolipoprotein B-100. In: *Lipoproteins in Health and Disease*, 1st edn. DJ Betteridge, DR Illingworth, J Shepherd (eds). Arnold, London, pp. 701–718.

16 Lees RS, Cashin-Hemphill L, Lees AM (1999). Nonpharmacological lowering of low-density lipoprotein by apheresis and surgical techniques. *Curr. Opin. Lipidol.* **10**:575–579.

CHAPTER 22   Stem Cell Therapy in Acute Myocardial Infarction
References

1 Jiang Y, Jahagirdar BN, Reinhardt RL, *et al.* (2002). Pluripotency of mesenchymal stem cells derived from adult marrow. *Nature* **418**:41–49.

2 Orlic D, Kajstura J, Chimenti S, *et al.* (2001). Mobilized bone marrow cells repair the infarcted heart, improving function and survival. *Proc. Natl. Acad. Sci.* USA **98**:10344–10349.

3 Wang Y, Jørgensen E, Johnsen HE, Kastrup J (2003). The clinical impact of vascular growth factors and endothelial progenitor cells in the acute coronary syndrome. *Scand. Cardiovasc. J.* **37**:18–22.

4 Strauer BE, Brehm M, Zeus T, *et al.* (2002). Repair of infarcted myocardium by autologous intracoronary mononuclear bone marrow cell transplantation in humans. *Circulation* **106**:1913–1918.

5 Assmus B, Schächinger V, Teupe C, *et al.* (2002). Transplantation of progenitor cells and regeneration

enhancement in acute myocardial infarction (TOPCARE-AMI). *Circulation* **106**:3009–3017.

6 Britten MB, Abolmaali ND, Assmus B, *et al.* (2003). Infarct remodeling after intracoronary progenitor cell treatment in patients with acute myocardial infarction (TOPCARE-AMI). Mechanistic insights from serial contrast-enhanced magnetic resonance imaging. *Circulation* **108**:2212–2218.

7 Dobert N, Britten M, Assmus B, *et al.* (2004). Transplantation of progenitor cell after reperfused acute myocardial infarction: evaluation of perfusion and myocardial viability with FDG-PET and thallium SPECT. *Eur. J. Nucl. Mol. Imaging* **31**(8):1146–1151.

8 Fuchs S, Satler LF, Kornowski R, *et al.* (2003). Catheter-based autologous bone marrow myocardial injection in no-option patients with advanced coronary artery disease. A feasibility study. *J. Am. Coll. Cardiol.* **41**:1721–1724.

9 Stamm C, Westphal B, Kleine H-D, *et al.* (2003). Autologous bone-marrow stem-cell transplantation for myocardial regeneration. *Lancet* **361**:45–47.

10 Kastrup J, Joergensen E, Rück A, *et al.* (2005). Direct intramyocardial plasmid vascular endothelial growth factor-A165 gene therapy in patients with stable angina pectoris: a randomized, double-blind, placebo-controlled study. The Euroinject One Trial. *J. Am. Coll. Cardiol.* **45**:982–988.

CHAPTER 23   Guidelines and Recommendations
References

1 Giugliano RP, Lloyd-Jones DM, Camargo CA Jr, Makary MA, O'Donnell CJ (2000). Association of unstable angina guideline care with improved survival. *Arch. Intern. Med.* **160**:1775–1780.

2 Abookire SA, Karson AS, Fiskio J, Bates DW (2001). Use and monitoring of 'statin' lipid-lowering drugs compared with guidelines. *Arch. Intern. Med.* **161**:53–58.

3 Schwartz PJ, Breithardt G, Howard AJ, Julian DG, Rehnqvist AN (1999). Task Force Report: The legal implications of medical guidelines. Task Force of the European Society of Cardiology. *Eur. Heart J.* **20**:1152–1157.

4 Guidelines from the European Society of Cardiology can be found at www.escardio.org

5 Guidelines from the American Heart Association can be found at www.americanheart.org

6 Guidelines from the American College of Cardiology can be found at www.acc.org